SALEM HEALTH

COMPLEMENTARY
& ALTERNATIVE
MEDICINE

SALEM HEALTH

COMPLEMENTARY
& Alternative Medicine

Volume 1

Editors

Richard P. Capriccioso, M.D.
University of Phoenix

Paul Moglia, Ph.D.
South Nassau Communities Hospital

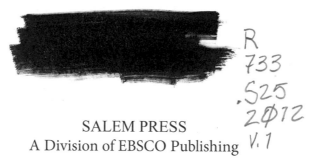

SALEM PRESS
A Division of EBSCO Publishing
Ipswich, Massachusetts   Hackensack, New Jersey

Note to Readers

The material presented in *Salem Health: Complementary and Alternative Medicine* is intended for broad informational and educational purposes. Readers who suspect that they or someone they know has any disorder, disease, or condition described in this set should contact a physician without delay. This set should not be used as a substitute for professional medical diagnosis. Readers who are undergoing or about to undergo any treatment or procedure described in this set should refer to their physicians and other health care providers for guidance concerning preparation and possible effects. This set is not to be considered definitive on the covered topics, and readers should remember that the field of health care is characterized by a diversity of medical opinions and constant expansion in knowledge and understanding.

Library of Congress Cataloging-in-Publication Data

Complementary & alternative medicine / editors, Richard P. Capriccioso, Paul Moglia.
    p. ; cm. — (Salem health)
Complementary and alternative medicine
Includes bibliographical references and indexes.
    ISBN 978-1-58765-870-9 (set : alk. paper) — ISBN 978-1-58765-871-6 (vol. 1) — ISBN 978-1-58765-872-3 (vol. 2) — ISBN 978-1-58765-873-0 (vol. 3) — ISBN 978-1-58765-874-7 (vol. 4)
    I. Capriccioso, Richard P. II. Moglia, Paul. III. Title: Complementary and alternative medicine. IV. Series: Salem health (Ipswich, Mass.)
    [DNLM: 1. Complementary Therapies–Encyclopedias–English. WB 13]
    LCclassification not assigned
    615.503–dc23
                              2011051023

Contents

Contents

Publisher's Note

Complementary and alternative medicine (CAM) has emerged as an important course of treatment in minor and major health care. Alternative medicine is broadly defined as medical practices outside traditional medicine, while complimentary medicine designates a more recent development in the intersection of traditional and nontraditional medical practices. Together, these practices influence preventative medicine, lifestyle choice, and innovative treatments of illness and disease. *Salem Health: Complimentary and Alternative Medicine* is a new addition to the Salem Health family of titles, which also includes both print and electronic versions of *Salem Health: Cancer* (2009), *Salem Health: Psychology and Mental Health* (2009), *Salem Health: Genetics and Inherited Conditions* (2010), *Salem Health: Infectious Diseases and Conditions* (2011), and the core set *Magill's Medical Guide* (revised every three years). All of them come with free online access with the purchase of the print set.

SCOPE AND COVERAGE

This A-Z encyclopedia includes 782 essays on all aspects of complimentary and alternative medicine—homeopathic techniques and methodologies, body-based practices, disease, nutrition, and non-Western practices. Written by professors and professional medical writers for nonspecialists, this comprehensive reference publication will interest students of Eastern medicine and philosophy, life sciences, and alternative medical practices; in addition, public library patrons and librarians building scientific collections will find this collection to be an important resource.

Salem Health: Complimentary and Alternative Medicine surveys this continually evolving discipline from a variety of perspectives, offering historical and technical background along with a balanced discussion of recent discoveries and developments. Basics of CAM—from the integrative treatment of disease to preventive lifestyle practices, from the use of natural products to movement therapies—constitute the core coverage. Medical topics are covered in a significant number of essays, as the relationship between traditional and nontraditional approaches to illness continues to grow in importance for many patients. In addition, the use of non-Western practices, evidenced in the popularity of homeopathy, veganism, and acupuncture, reveals the significance of alternative philosophies in determining approaches to health and lifestyle.

ORGANIZATION AND FORMAT

Essays vary in length from one to five pages. Each essay follows a standard format, including ready-reference top matter and the following standard features:

CATEGORY lists the aspect of CAM under which the topic falls:

- Conditions
- Drug Interactions
- Functional Foods
- Herbs and Supplements
- Homeopathy
- Issues and Overviews
- Organizations and Legislation
- Biographies
- Therapies and Techniques

Therapies & Techniques essays then provide standard information in these subsections:

- RELATED TERMS lists a broad range of relevant terms.
- DEFINITION introduces, defines, and describes the therapy or technique.
- PRINCIPLE USES lists the major illnesses and diseases that the therapy or technique is used to treat.
- OTHER PROPOSED USES lists secondary illnesses and diseases that the therapy or technique is used to treat.
- OVERVIEW provides an expanded definition and introduces background material on the therapy or technique.
- MECHANISM OF ACTION explains how the therapy or technique is believed to function in or on the body.
- USES AND APPLICATIONS lists the primary benefits and illnesses treated.
- SCIENTIFIC EVIDENCE summarizes the results of scientific studies of the efficacy of the therapy or technique.
- CHOOSING A PRACTITIONER provides guidance on selecting a practitioner of the therapy or technique.

- SAFETY ISSUES discusses the side effects and problems that may result from the therapy or technique.

Other types of essays are divided into these sections:
- INTRODUCTION provides a definition, summarizes the topic's importance, and offers background information.
- Topical subheads, chosen by the author, divide the main text and guide readers through the essay.

All essays conclude with the following material:
- The contributor's byline lists the area expert who wrote the essay, including his or her advanced degrees and other credentials.
- The SEE ALSO section lists cross-references to other essays of interest within the set.
- FURTHER READING lists sources for further study, often with annotations.

Some essays in the encyclopedia include sidebars, which appear in shaded boxes, that offer coverage of significant subtopics within overview essays.

SPECIAL FEATURES

The articles in the *Salem Health: Complimentary and Alternative Medicine* are arranged alphabetically by title. All four volumes offer a Complete List of Contents for easy identification of desired topics. In addition, appendixes appear at the end of the fourth volume. A Glossary provides hundreds of definitions of commonly used scientific, medical, and alternative medicine terms and concepts. The Bibliography offers citations for both classic and recently published sources for additional research. The Resources appendix provides a list of organizations and support groups. The importance of the Internet to general education in complementary and alternative medicine is reflected in the annotated Web Site Directory. The Timeline of Major Developments offers a chronological overview of CAM from ancient times to the present. The Biographical Dictionary features practitioners and critics of CAM. Category, personages, and comprehensive subject indexes can be found at the end of Volume 4.

ACKNOWLEDGMENTS

The editors wish to thank the many practitioners and other scholars who contributed to this set; their names and academic affiliations appear in the list of Contributors that follows.

ABOUT THE EDITORS

Dr. Paul Moglia holds a Ph.D. in counseling psychology from Boston College. He is currently the Director of Behavioral and Faculty Education at South Nassau Community Hospital. Dr. Moglia completed fellowships sponsored by the Harvard Medical School's Department of Psychiatry and the Albert Einstein College of Medicine. In addition to his role as director, he has published numerous articles and presented at dozens of national forums. He also maintains a full-time private practice.

Dr. Richard P. Capriccioso teaches science, health, psychology, and general studies courses at the University of Phoenix, where he has served as a Science Area Chairman. Dr. Capriccioso provided medical support for the Peace Sun and Peace Hawk programs (Department of Defense programs that provide technical support for fighter jets supplied to the Kingdom of Saudi Arabia). He is a member of the American Heart Association Council on Nutrition, Physical Activity & Metabolism and the American Medical Writer's Association. Dr. Capriccioso holds bachelor of science and doctor of medicine degrees from the University of Michigan. He has published several recent science and alternative medicine articles and gave a presentation on complementary and alternative medicine at a national conference for the American College of Emergency Physicians.

Contributors

Richard Adler, Ph.D.
University of Michigan—
    Dearborn

Rick Alan
Medical writer and editor

Deborah A. Appello, M.S.
Brick, NJ

Mihaela Appello, M.D., Ph.D.
Verlan Medical Communications

Michelle Badash, M.S.
Wakefield, MA

Dana K. Bagwell
Memory Health and Fitness
    Institute

Paul F. Bell, Ph.D.
Heritage Valley Health System

Alvin K. Benson, Ph.D.
Utah Valley University

Janet Ober Berman, M.S., C.G.C.
Temple University School of
    Medicine

Jigna Bhalla Pharm.D.
American Medical Writers
    Association

Zuzana Bic, M.D., D.P.H.
University of California, Irvine

Dawn M. Bielawski, Ph.D.
Wayne State University

Andrea Bozja
Medical writer

Steven Bratman, M.D.
Fort Collins, CO

James F. Breckenridge, Th.D.
Oral Roberts University

Kecia Brown, M.P.H.
Washington, DC

Michael A. Buratovich, Ph.D.
Spring Arbor University

Richard P. Capriccioso, M.D.
University of Phoenix

Christine M. Carroll, R.N.,
    M.B.A., B.S.N.
American Medical Writers
    Association

Jack Carter, Ph.D.
University of New Orleans

Rose Ciulla-Bohling, Ph.D.
Lansdale, PA

Barbara Williams Cosentino,
    R.N., CSW
New York, NY

Stephanie Eckenrode, L.L.B., B.A.
New York, NY

Lain Chroust Ehmann
Lexington, MA

Renée Euchner, R.N., B.S.N.
American Medical Writers
    Association

Merrill Evans, M.A.
Tucson, AZ

Fernando J. Ferrer, Ph.D.
Carlsbad, CA

Robert Flatley, M.L.S.
Kutztown University

Rebecca J. Frey, Ph.D.
Yale University

Roxanne Friedenfels, Ph.D.
Drew University

Cathy Frisinger, M.P.H.
Arlington, TX

Jeffrey S. Geller, M.D.
EBSCO CAM Review Board

Richard Glickman-Simon, M.D.
EBSCO CAM Review Board

Jackie Hart, M.D., FACPE
Boston, MA

Katherine Hauswirth, M.S.N., R.N.
Hauswirth Writing Solutions,
    LLC

Sandra C. Hayes, Ph.D.
Tougaloo College

David Hutto, Ph.D.
Tetrascribe

Christopher Iliades, M.D.
Centerville, MA

Gerald W. Keister, M.S.
American Medical Writers
    Association

Ing-Wei Khor, Ph.D.
Oceanside, CA

M. Barbara Klyde, Ph.D.P.H.,
    PA-C
House Call Physicians

Marylane Wade Koch, M.S.N.,
    R.N.
University of Memphis

Anita P. Kuan, Ph.D.
Lyme, CT

David J. Ladouceur, Ph.D.
University of Notre Dame

Dawn Laney, M.S., CGC, CCRC
Emory University

Scott O. Lilienfeld, Ph.D.
Emory University

Martha O. Loustaunau, Ph.D.
New Mexico State University

Marianne M. Madsen, M.S.
University of Utah

Mary E. Markland, M.A.
Argosy University

Mary Mihaly
Cleveland, OH

Deborah Mitchell
Tuscon, AZ

Deanna M. Neff, M.P.H.
Stow, MA

David A. Olle, M.S.
Eastshire Communications

Lisa Paddock, Ph.D.
Cape May Court House, NJ

Robert J. Paradowski, Ph.D.
Rochester Institute of Technology

Crystal L. Park, Ph.D.
University of Connecticut

Marie President, M.D.
Sequoia Medical Associates

Ganson Purcell, Jr., M.D., FACOG
Hartford, CT

Cynthia F. Racer, M.A., M.P.H.
New York Academy of Sciences

Brian Randall, M.D.
EBSCO Publishing

Jack B. Robinson Jr., Ph.D.
Duncanville, TX

Ana Maria Rodriguez-Rojas, M.S.
GXP Medical Writing, LLC

Elizabeth D. Schafer, Ph.D.
Loachapoka, AL

Amy Scholten, M.P.H.
Inner Medicine Publishing

Roger Smith, Ph.D.
Portland, OR

Bethany Thivierge, M.P.H.
Technicality Resources

Linda H. Underhill
Medical writer

Eugenia M. Valentine, Ph.D.
Xavier University of Louisiana

Vibu Varghese, M.S.
South Nassau Communities
    Hospital

Brandy Weidow, M.S.
Nashville, TN

Debra Wood, R.N.
Orlando, FL

Robin L. Wulffson, M.D., FACOG
FACOG (Faculty, American
    College of Obstetrics and
    Gynecology)

George D. Zgourides, M.D.,
    Psy.D.
John Peter Smith Hospital

Complete List of Contents

Volume 1

Volume 2

Volume 3

Volume 4

SALEM HEALTH

COMPLEMENTARY
& Alternative Medicine

A

Acerola

CATEGORY: Functional foods
RELATED TERM: *Malpighia glabra*
DEFINITION: Natural plant product promoted as a dietary supplement for specific health benefits.
PRINCIPAL PROPOSED USE: Source of vitamin C
OTHER PROPOSED USE: Antioxidant

OVERVIEW

Acerola is a small tree (*Malpighia glabra*) that grows in dry areas of the Caribbean and Central America and South America. Traditionally, its fruit has been used to treat diarrhea, arthritis, and fevers, and kidney, heart, and liver problems. Acerola contains ten to fifty times more vitamin C by weight than oranges. Other important substances found in acerola include bioflavonoids, magnesium, pantothenic acid, and vitamin A.

USES AND APPLICATIONS

Acerola is primarily marketed as a source of vitamin C and bioflavonoids. Because of these constituents, it has substantial antioxidant properties. One study found that acerola significantly increased the antioxidant activity of soy and alfalfa. It is not clear, however, that this rather theoretical finding indicates anything of significance to human health. Other powerful antioxidants such as vitamin E and beta-carotene have proved disappointing when they were subjected to studies that could discern whether their actions as antioxidants translated into actual health benefits.

Like many plants, acerola has antibacterial and antifungal properties, at least in the test tube. However, no studies in humans have been reported.

DOSAGE

A typical supplemental dosage of acerola is 40 to 100 milligrams daily.

SAFETY ISSUES

As a widely used food, acerola is believed to have a relatively high safety factor. However, it has been discovered that people who are allergic to latex may be allergic to acerola too. Maximum safe doses in young children, pregnant or nursing women, and people with severe liver or kidney disease have not been established.

EBSCO CAM Review Board

FURTHER READING

Cáceres, A. et al. "Plants Used in Guatemala for the Treatment of Dermatophytic Infections: Evaluation of Antifungal Activity of Seven American Plants." *Journal of Ethnopharmacology* 40 (1993): 207-213.

Hassimotto, N. M., et al. "Antioxidant Activity of Dietary Fruits, Vegetables, and Commercial Frozen Fruit Pulps." *Journal of Agricultural and Food Chemistry* 53 (2005): 2928-2235.

Hwang, J., H. N. Hodis, and A. Sevanian. "Soy and Alfalfa Phytoestrogen Extracts Become Potent Low-Density Lipoprotein Antioxidants in the Presence of Acerola Cherry Extract." *Journal of Agricultural and Food Chemistry* 49 (2001): 308-314.

Motohashi, N., et al. "Biological Activity of Barbados Cherry (Acerola Fruits, Fruit of *Malpighia emarginata* DC) Extracts and Fractions." *Phytotherapy Research* 18 (2004): 212-223.

Raulf-Heimsoth, M., et al. "Anaphylactic Reaction to Apple Juice Containing Acerola: Cross-Reactivity to Latex Due to Prohevein." *Journal of Allergy and Clinical Immunology* 109 (2002): 715-716.

See also: Antioxidants; Vitamin C.

Acetaminophen

CATEGORY: Drug interactions
DEFINITION: A common drug used to reduce pain and fever.
INTERACTIONS: Chaparral, citrate, coenzyme Q_{10}, coltsfoot, comfrey, methionine, milk thistle, vitamin C
TRADE NAMES: Apacet, Arthritis Foundation Aspirin Free, Arthritis Foundation Nighttime, Acephen,

Aceta, Amaphen, Anoquan, Aspirin Free Anacin, Aspirin Free Excedrin, Bayer Select, Dapacin, Dynafed, Endolor, Esgic, Excedrin P.M., Fem-Etts, Femcet, Feverall, Fioricet, Fiorpap, Genapap, Genebs, Halenol, Isocet, Liquiprin, Mapap, Maranox, Meda, Medigesic, Midol, Multi-Symptom Pamprin, Neopap, Nighttime Pamprin, Oraphen-PD, Panadol, Phrenilin, Repan, Ridenol, Sedapap, Silapap, Sominex Pain Relief, Tapanol, Tempra, Tylenol, Uni-Ace, Unisom with Pain Relief

MILK THISTLE, COENZYME Q_{10} (CoQ$_{10}$), METHIONINE

Effect: Possible Helpful Interactions

The herb milk thistle and the supplements CoQ$_{10}$ and methionine might help protect the liver against damage caused by excessive use of acetaminophen. However, it is extremely dangerous to take excessive amounts of acetaminophen.

VITAMIN C

Effect: Possible Increased Risk of Toxicity

One study from the 1970s suggests that very high doses of vitamin C (3 grams daily) might increase the levels of acetaminophen in the body. This could potentially put a person at higher risk for acetaminophen toxicity. Problems might occur if one takes higher-than-recommended doses or takes high doses of acetaminophen on a regular basis, such as for osteoarthritis. The risk increases if one has liver or kidney impairment or drinks alcoholic beverages regularly, which further harms the liver.

CHAPARRAL, COMFREY, AND COLTSFOOT

Effect: Possible Harmful Interaction

The herbs chaparral (*Larrea tridentata* or *L. mexicana*), comfrey (*Symphytum officinale*), and coltsfoot (*Tussilago farfara*) contain liver-toxic substances. Combined use with acetaminophen could accentuate the liver toxicity of the medication.

CITRATE

Effect: Possible Harmful Interaction

Potassium citrate, sodium citrate, and potassium-magnesium citrate are sometimes used to prevent kidney stones. These supplements reduce urinary acidity and can therefore lead to decreased blood levels and decreased effectiveness of acetaminophen.

EBSCO CAM Review Board

FURTHER READING

Muriel, P., et al. "Silymarin Protects Against Paracetamol-Induced Lipid Peroxidation and Liver Damage." *Journal of Applied Toxicology* 12 (1992): 439-442.

Neuvonen, P. J., et al. "Methionine in Paracetamol Tablets: A Tool to Reduce Paracetamol Toxicity." *International Journal of Clinical Pharmacology, Therapy, and Toxicology* 23 (1985): 497-500.

2011 PDR for Nonprescription Drugs, Dietary Supplements, and Herbs. Toronto, Ont.: Thomson Health Care, 2010.

See also: Food and Drug Administration; Herbal medicine; Pain management; Supplements: Introduction; Vitamin C.

Acne

CATEGORY: Condition

RELATED TERMS: Acne vulgaris, blackheads, pimples, whiteheads

DEFINITION: Treatment of a skin condition caused by clogged, inflamed, or infected pores.

PRINCIPAL PROPOSED NATURAL TREATMENTS: Niacinamide gel, tea tree oil, zinc

OTHER PROPOSED NATURAL TREATMENTS: Ayurvedic medicine, burdock, chromium, gugulipid, low-glycemic-load diet, red clover, selenium, vitamin E

INTRODUCTION

The blackheads and sometimes painful pimples known as acne occur most commonly during adolescence, but they also may persist into adulthood. Much remains to be learned about what causes acne. During adolescence and other times of hormonal imbalance, such as menopause, glands in the skin increase their levels of oil secretions. A combination of naturally occurring yeast and bacteria then breaks down these secretions, causing the skin to become inflamed and the pimples to eventually rupture. In severe cases, acne can cause permanent scarring.

Conventional treatment of acne, which usually is quite successful, consists primarily of oral or topical antibiotics, cleansing agents, and chemically modified versions of vitamin A. One should not use the natural treatments discussed here to treat severe acne in which scarring is a possibility.

Development of Acne

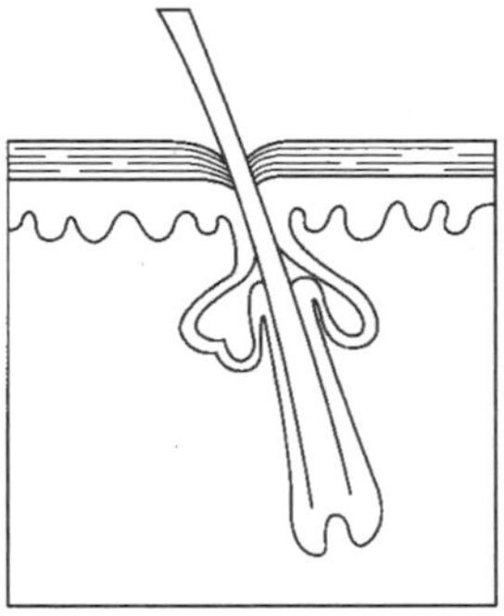

(1) Normal skin

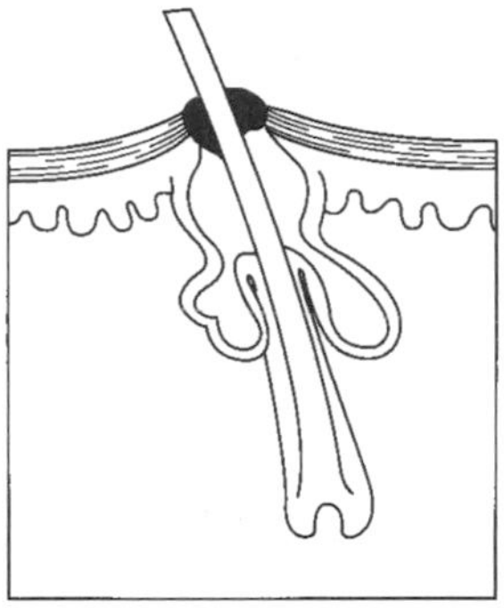

(2) Clogged sebaceous gland

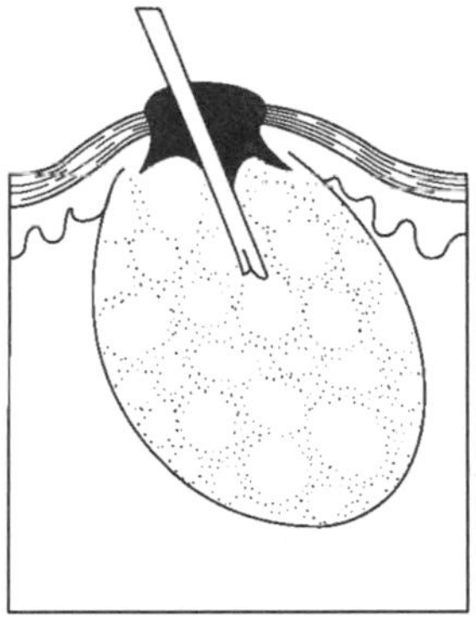

(3) Acne vulgaris

PRINCIPAL PROPOSED NATURAL TREATMENTS

Zinc. Studies suggest that people with acne have lower-than-normal levels of zinc in their bodies. This fact alone does not indicate that taking zinc supplements will help acne. Several double-blind, placebo-controlled studies have found zinc more effective than placebo but less effective than antibiotic therapy. In one of these studies, fifty-four people were given either placebo or 135 milligrams (mg) of zinc as zinc sulfate daily. Zinc produced slight but measurable benefits. Similar results have been seen in other studies using 90 to 135 mg of zinc daily, although other studies failed to find that zinc helped. Relatively weak evidence suggests that a lower and safer dose, 30 mg daily, may also be helpful.

A large double-blind trial (332 participants) compared 30 mg daily of zinc with a tetracycline-family medication often used for acne (minocycline at 100 mg daily). The results showed minocycline is more effective than zinc. Tetracycline taken at a dose of 250 mg daily appears to be no more effective than zinc, but when taken at 500 mg daily, it seems to be considerably more effective.

Dosages of zinc used in most of these studies are much higher than daily requirements and have the potential for causing toxicity. Case reports indicate that people have become extremely ill after taking zinc in hopes of treating their acne symptoms.

Tea tree oil. Tea tree oil has antiseptic properties and has been suggested as an alternative to benzoyl peroxide for direct application to the skin. The best evidence for benefits with tea tree oil comes from a randomized double-blind clinical trial of sixty people with mild to moderate acne. In this study, participants were divided into two groups and treated with placebo or 5 percent tea tree oil gel. During the forty-five-day study period, researchers evaluated acne severity in two ways: by counting the number of acne lesions and by rating acne severity on a standardized index. The results showed that tea tree oil gel was significantly more effective than placebo at reducing both the number of acne lesions and their severity.

Niacinamide. In a double-blind trial, seventy-six persons with moderately severe acne were treated with either 4 percent niacinamide gel or 1 percent clindamycin gel (a standard antibiotic treatment). Niacinamide proved to be just as effective as the antibiotic in an eight-week trial. However, because this study lacked a placebo group, its results are unreliable.

OTHER PROPOSED NATURAL TREATMENTS

Ayurvedic medicine has shown some promise for acne. One study evaluated the potential benefits of an herbal combination containing the following constituents: *Aloe barbadensis, Azardirachta indica, Curcuma longa, Hemidesmus indicus, Terminalia chebula, T. arjuna,* and *Withania somnifera.* In this four-week, double-blind, placebo-controlled study of fifty-three people with acne, combined topical and oral use of the herbal preparation significantly improved acne symptoms. Oral treatment alone was not effective.

Another controlled trial compared an extract of the Ayurvedic herb guggul with tetracycline for the treatment of acne and found them equally effective. The study report does not state whether this trial was double-blind, and for this reason the results are not reliable. Other commonly mentioned natural treatments for acne include chromium, vitamin E, selenium, burdock, and red clover. There have been no well-designed studies examining these treatments, however.

The effect of diet on acne is unclear. One far from definitive study compared a low-glycemic-load diet with a high-carbohydrate diet and found that the low-glycemic-load diet reduced acne symptoms.

HERBS AND SUPPLEMENTS TO USE ONLY WITH CAUTION

Various herbs and diet supplements may interact adversely with conventional (including prescription) drugs used to treat acne, so people should be cautious when considering the use of herbs and supplements.

EBSCO CAM Review Board

FURTHER READING

Bassett, I. B., D. L. Pannowitz, and R. S. Barnetson. "A Comparative Study of Tea-Tree Oil Versus Benzoylperoxide in the Treatment of Acne." *Medical Journal of Australia* 153 (1990): 455-458.

Dreno, B., et al. "Multicenter Randomized Comparative Double-Blind Controlled Clinical Trial of the Safety and Efficacy of Zinc Gluconate Versus Minocycline Hydrochloride in the Treatment of Inflammatory Acne Vulgaris." *Dermatology* 203 (2001): 135-140.

Enshaieh, S., et al. "The Efficacy of 5 Percent Topical Tea Tree Oil Gel in Mild to Moderate Acne Vulgaris." *Indian Journal of Dermatology, Venereology, and Leprology* 73 (2007): 22-25.

Igic, P. G., et al. "Toxic Effects Associated with Consumption of Zinc." *Mayo Clinic Proceedings* 77 (2002): 713-716.

Lalla, J. K., et al. "Clinical Trials of Ayurvedic Formulations in the Treatment of Acne Vulgaris." *Journal of Ethnopharmacology* 78 (2001): 99-102.

Meynadier, J. "Efficacy and Safety Study of Two Zinc Gluconate Regimens in the Treatment of Inflammatory Acne." *European Journal of Dermatology* 10 (2000): 269-273.

Porea, T. J., J. W. Belmont, and D. H. Mahoney, Jr. "Zinc-Induced Anemia and Neutropenia in an Adolescent." *Journal of Pediatrics* 136 (2000): 688-690.

Smith, R. N., et al. "A Low-Glycemic-Load Diet Improves Symptoms in Acne Vulgaris Patients." *American Journal of Clinical Nutrition* 86 (2007): 107-115.

Thappa, D. M., and J. Dogra. "Nodulocystic Acne: Oral Gugulipid Versus Tetracycline." *Journal of Dermatology* 21 (1994): 729-731.

See also: Tea Tree; Tetracycline; Zinc.

Active hexose correlated compound

CATEGORY: Herbs and supplements
RELATED TERMS: Basidiomycota, basidiomycetes
DEFINITION: Natural substance promoted as a dietary supplement for specific health benefits.
PRINCIPAL PROPOSED USE: Cancer treatment
OTHER PROPOSED USES: Cancer prevention, immune support, inflammatory bowel disease, reducing side effects of cancer chemotherapy

OVERVIEW

In Japan, various mushrooms and tree fungi have a long history of medicinal use. Active hexose correlated compound (AHCC) is a proprietary compound made from the mycelia (vegetative portion) of various mushrooms in the general family of basidiomycete (or basidiomycota). The exact composition of the mushrooms, and the method used to prepare them, is considered a trade secret. AHCC has been developed in Japan for use in the treatment of cancer.

USES AND APPLICATIONS

AHCC is primarily advocated as an aid to cancer treatment and is said to improve survival in people undergoing treatment for liver cancer and other forms of cancer. However, evidence that it works is far too preliminary to be taken as meaningful, consisting as it does only of animal studies and a few entirely inadequate human trials. Only double-blind studies can actually prove a treatment effective, and none have been performed on AHCC.

Other proposed uses of AHCC have even weaker supporting evidence. These proposed uses include decreasing chemotherapy side effects, reducing cancer risk, treating inflammatory bowel disease, and generally enhancing immune function.

DOSAGE

A typical dose of AHCC is 3 grams daily, often divided into three doses.

SAFETY ISSUES

While the use of AHCC has not been associated with any severe adverse effects, this substance has not undergone thorough safety testing. Safety in young children, pregnant or nursing women, or people with severe liver or kidney disease has not been established.

EBSCO CAM Review Board

FURTHER READING

Cowawintaweewat, S., et al. "Prognostic Improvement of Patients with Advanced Liver Cancer After Active Hexose Correlated Compound (AHCC) Treatment." *Asian Pacific Journal of Allergy and Immunology* 24 (2006): 33-45.

Gao, Y., et al. "Active Hexose Correlated Compound Enhances Tumor Surveillance Through Regulating Both Innate and Adaptive Immune Responses." *Cancer Immunology and Immunotherapy* 55 (2006): 1258-1266.

Matsui, Y., et al. "Improved Prognosis of Postoperative Hepatocellular Carcinoma Patients When Treated with Functional Foods." *Journal of Hepatology* 37 (2002): 78-86.

See also: Maitake; Reishi; Shiitaki.

Acupressure

CATEGORY: Therapies and techniques
RELATED TERMS: Acupoint, acupuncture, massage therapy, pressure points, qi, qigong, reflexology, shiatsu, Tai Chi Chuan, touch therapy, traditional Chinese medicine, *tui na*
DEFINITION: The noninvasive application of focused touch to specific points of the body.
PRINCIPAL PROPOSED USES: Arthritis, bursitis, headaches, injuries, postsurgical pain
OTHER PROPOSED USES: Addiction, anxiety, chronic fatigue, circulation, depression, eating disorders, enhance self-esteem, general well-being, hypertension, immune system, insomnia, irritable bowel syndrome, premenstrual and menopausal symptoms, relaxation, sexual dysfunctions, smoking, stress

OVERVIEW

Acupressure is sometimes thought of as acupuncture without needles. Because acupressure and acupuncture support the body's natural healing powers, many conditions can be improved, corrected, or even eliminated. Like other touch therapies, acupressure conveys the care and empathy that are necessary ingredients in healing. As such, holistic therapies like acupressure are especially appropriate for problems best suited to a biopsychosocial approach.

Acupressure is part of the healing system of traditional Chinese medicine (TCM), a unique and comprehensive system for diagnosing and treating disease, preventing illness, and promoting wellness. TCM encompasses many diverse health-enhancing and energy-balancing therapies, including acupuncture, herbal medicine, Tai Chi Chuan, qigong, *Gua Sha*, cupping, moxibustion, and *tui na* acupressure. All of these techniques, and many others, manipulate qi, the essential energy of life. Originating in China thousands of years ago, TCM continues to be practiced throughout the world.

To understand acupressure, one should study some basic principles of TCM, and one theory in particular necessitates elaboration: the notion that human beings are governed by opposing but complementing forces, yin and yang, a notion at the heart of Daoism, which forms the basis of TCM. According to Daoism, this balance of forces infiltrates and influences the entire universe, including those within. One of the basic aims of TCM is to correct imbalances of yin and yang to prevent sickness and restore health. Fully comprehending the principles behind yin and yang (and many other concepts) permits Chinese medical practitioners to diagnose accurately and treat effectively.

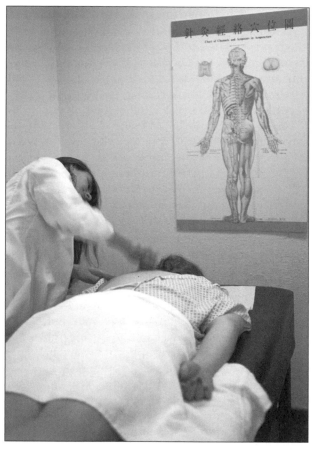

A patient receiving acupressure treatment. (PhotoDisc)

and allow the manipulation of qi are referred to as acupoints or acupressure points. During a typical acupressure session, these points are pressed, rubbed, tapped, or otherwise touched as a way of influencing qi to bring about desired results. The effects of acupressure are reinforced through a healthy diet, herbal formulas, exercise, fresh air, meditation, and spirituality.

USES AND APPLICATIONS

According to data published by the World Health Organization, TCM is helpful for ophthalmological, respiratory, gastrointestinal, neurological, and musculoskeletal disorders, and disorders of the ear, nose, and throat. In the United States, acupressure (and acupuncture) are used mostly to treat painful conditions such as headaches, arthritis, bursitis, injuries, and postsurgical pain.

The effectiveness of TCM in general extends beyond controlling pain. More recently, acupressure is being used to treat chronic fatigue, anxiety, stress, insomnia, depression, addictions, smoking, eating disorders, irritable bowel syndrome, hypertension, sexual dysfunctions, premenstrual and menopausal symptoms, and many other conditions. Also, acupressure appears to improve circulation, boost immune functioning, help eliminate metabolic waste products, promote relaxation, enhance self-esteem, and create a general sense of well-being.

In its most crucial role, however, TCM presents a theoretical and practical framework for engaging in a holistic understanding of health and illness.

SCIENTIFIC EVIDENCE

Controlled double-blind studies into the efficacy of acupressure per se have not been conducted. However, many smaller studies exist that affirm the positive role of acupressure in such conditions as pain, stroke, heart disease, cancer, smoking, obesity, insomnia, allergies, and menstrual disorders. Furthermore, scientific evidence supporting the efficacy of TCM in general–and acupuncture in particular–continues to grow. This is in addition to millennia of observational information gathered throughout China, Japan, Korea, and other Asian countries.

CHOOSING A PRACTITIONER

TCM is certainly more complex than the beginner or casual observer might think. This ancient discipline specifically emphasizes concepts of wellness, illness,

In short, TCM offers alternative explanations for how health problems develop in the first place, and it provides many approaches for treating these problems. Depending on a person's specific clinical presentation, acupressure and other modalities, used alone or with allopathic methods, can prove quite beneficial for many health conditions.

MECHANISM OF ACTION

Acupressure relies on touch rather than needles to manipulate the flow of qi in the body. Specifically, qi is thought to move through the body by means of a complex system of meridians, or energy channels. These meridians are known by the names of body organs (the bladder channel or liver channel) and refer to energetic patterns with particular characteristics based on TCM principles and practice.

Specific areas on the skin where the meridians pass

and recovery. It further emphasizes the best of medical ideas and methodologies from the past and the present--from the wisdom of everyday people to the advanced knowledge of the best-trained TCM physicians and other healing arts practitioners. For these reasons and more, actual treatment with TCM, including acupressure, requires the expertise of a trained and licensed clinician. Simple, everyday ailments, however, respond well to acupressure performed as self-therapy.

In the United States, licensed physicians, acupuncturists, and massage therapists practice acupressure. Practitioners can be found by contacting state licensing boards and such national groups as the American Academy of Medical Acupuncture, the American Association of Acupuncture and Oriental Medicine, and the American Massage Therapy Association.

SAFETY ISSUES

Acupressure is an exceptionally safe modality because of its noninvasive nature. Contraindications (that is, conditions for which acupressure is not recommended) typically include acute illness (such as hypertensive urgency and tachycardia), serious illness (such as cancer), pregnancy, bleeding (such as with open wounds), and skin diseases and lesions (such as infections and ulcers).

George D. Zgourides, M.D., Psy.D.

FURTHER READING

Deadman, P., M. al-Khafaji, and K. Baker. *A Manual of Acupuncture.* 2d ed. Vista, Calif.: Eastland Press, 2007. A standard acupuncture text. An encyclopedic reference for professionals. Contains excellent diagrams and clinical information. Also available in CD format that includes an invaluable search feature.

Gach, M. R. *Acupressure's Potent Points: A Guide to Self-Care for Common Ailments.* New York: Bantam Books, 1990. An excellent book for general readers about treating everyday ailments with acupressure.

_____, and B. A. Henning. *Acupressure for Emotional Healing: A Self-Care Guide for Trauma, Stress, and Common Emotional Imbalances.* New York: Bantam Dell, 2004. A thoughtful exploration of the applications of acupressure for emotional healing.

Mann, F. *Acupuncture: The Ancient Chinese Art of Healing and How It Works Scientifically.* Rev. 2d ed. New York: Vintage Books, 1973. An easy-to-read introduction to the art and science of acupuncture.

See also: Acupuncture; Biodynamic massage; Craniosacral therapy; Energy medicine; Manipulative and body-based practices; Massage therapy; Meridians; Metamorphic technique; Osteopathic manipulation; Pain management; Progressive muscle relaxation; Qigong; Reflexology; Relaxation therapies; Rolfing; Shiatsu; Soft tissue pain; Therapeutic touch.

Acupuncture

CATEGORY: Therapies and techniques

RELATED TERMS: Acupressure, electroacupuncture, shiatsu

DEFINITION: A treatment method in which fine needles are inserted into the skin at designated points.

EVIDENCE-BASED USES: Nausea, tendonitis

OTHER STUDIED USES: Alcoholism, allergic rhinitis (hay fever), anxiety, asthma, back pain, Bell's palsy, bladder infections, breast-feeding support, cancer chemotherapy support, childbirth, chronic fatigue syndrome, cigarette addiction, colic in infants, Crohn's disease, dental procedures, depression, dysmenorrhea, epilepsy, female infertility, fibromyalgia, headache, high blood pressure, insomnia, irritable bowel syndrome, menopause, menstrual pain, migraine headache, narcotic addiction, neck pain, osteoarthritis, pain during medical procedures, Parkinson's disease, peripheral neuropathy, post-traumatic stress disorder, pregnancy support, premenstrual syndrome, prostatitis, psoriasis, Raynaud's phenomenon, rheumatoid arthritis, shingles (postherpetic neuralgia), sleep apnea, sports performance enhancement, stroke, surgery support, tension headache, tinnitus, temporomandibular joint pain, ulcerative colitis, weight loss

OVERVIEW

Acupuncture has been part of the medical mainstream in countries such as China and Japan for centuries. It is also one of the most widely utilized forms of alternative therapy in the United States. More than ten million acupuncture treatments are administered annually in the United States alone. In addition, third-party insurance reimbursement and managed care coverage for acupuncture are increasing.

Because of acupuncture's popularity, scientific investigation of the method has grown dramatically, with many new studies reported every week. However, the results have been mixed at best.

WHAT IS ACUPUNCTURE?

Simply defined, acupuncture is a treatment method aimed at eliciting a response (such as pain relief) through the insertion of very fine needles in the body surface at sites called acupuncture points. A related technique called acupressure (or shiatsu) uses pressure on these points, and a related therapy known as electroacupuncture applies electricity to the points.

A variety of treatment methods, approaches, techniques, styles, and theoretical frameworks exist within the broad scope of acupuncture. Differences in forms of acupuncture are often cultural. The system of acupuncture practiced in Japan, for example, is quite different from that found in China. Many acupuncturists practice a more or less traditional style called traditional Chinese medicine (TCM). Others have adopted modern styles that have little or no reliance on traditional principles.

Acupuncture needles are most often inserted at specific locations on the skin called acupuncture points. These points are located on specific lines outlined by tradition, referred to as meridians or channels. According to Chinese medical theory, fourteen major meridians form an invisible network connecting the body surface with the internal organs. Meridians are to conduct qi, the energy or vital force of the body. Pain or illness is said to result from imbalances or blockages in the flow of qi through the meridians. Acupuncture is traditionally thought to remove such blockages, restore the normal circulation of qi, and improve overall health by promoting the balance of energy in the system. However, there is no scientific evidence for the existence of the meridians or qi itself. (Meridians are not visible under a microscope and, contrary to popular belief, they do not match major nerve pathways.)

In addition to meridians and qi, the concept of yin and yang is central to acupuncture theory, as it is to all of traditional Chinese philosophy. The terms "yin" and "yang" do not represent forces or substances; rather, they are, as one, a way to look at the world in terms of the interaction of polar opposites. According to this viewpoint, all movement, growth, and change in the world is a manifestation of the push and pull of these forces. Although seemingly in opposition, these forces are thought to complement and support each

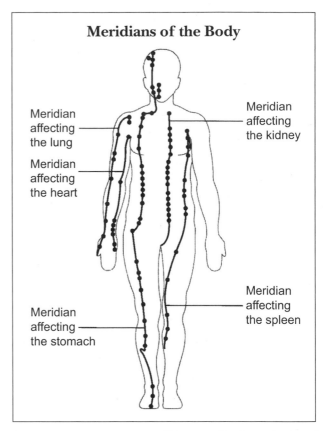

Meridians of the Body

Meridian affecting the lung

Meridian affecting the heart

Meridian affecting the stomach

Meridian affecting the kidney

Meridian affecting the spleen

Acupuncture is an ancient Chinese medical practice based on the concept of meridians, channels in the body through which flows the life force called qi; acupuncture involves the insertion and manipulation of tiny needles along these meridians.

other. For example, without rest one cannot exert energy; without becoming tired by exerting energy, it is difficult to sleep. This is just one illustration of the harmony and interaction of yin and yang.

Yang is traditionally associated with heat, power, daylight, summer, and many other active or energetic aspects of life; yin is cold, quiet, and dark. Many illnesses are characterized in terms of an excess or deficiency of either yin or yang, or of both at the same time. For example, when the body is feverish, it is too yang as a whole. There is also a yin and yang balance in each individual organ and part of the body; these can become excessive or deficient too.

Thus, in TCM, illnesses are described as complex patterns of imbalances and blockages. Treatment is based not on medical diagnosis, but on identifying these problems in the body's energy and seeking to correct them. Does this traditional analysis contain truths about human health or is it just archaic thinking? The answer remains unknown.

HISTORY OF ACUPUNCTURE

Primitive acupuncture needles dating to circa 1000 B.C.E. have been discovered in archeological finds of the Shan Dynasty in China. The theoretical framework underlying the practice of acupuncture was first set forth in the *Inner Classic of Medicine,* or *Nei Jing*, first published in 206 B.C.E. during the Han Dynasty.

As an active and growing tradition, the theory and practice of TCM evolved over the centuries, at times undergoing rapid changes. Acupuncture reached perhaps its golden age under the Ming Dynasty in the late sixteenth and early seventeenth centuries. Subsequently, it took second place to an ascending practice of herbal medicine. By the time acupuncture came back in vogue in twentieth-century China, it had undergone a major transformation, sometimes called the herbalization of acupuncture. Today's acupuncture methods given the name traditional Chinese medicine are derived to a great extent from this relatively modern revision of the theory. Present-day Japanese acupuncture, however, dates to earlier versions of acupuncture.

Another major change occurred after the Communist Revolution in China in 1949. The new leadership, while wanting to carry through a process of modernization, decided to support and preserve traditional medicine. During the Cultural Revolution, the famous "barefoot doctors" were trained in both modern and traditional medicine and sent out to the rural areas to provide medical care for the people. Today, in the largest and most modern Chinese hospitals, Western medicine and TCM, including acupuncture and herbal treatments, are practiced side by side.

Acupuncture entered France through its colonial rule of Vietnam. It was there that, in 1957, the French physician Paul Nogier conceived the notion of auricular (ear) acupuncture. According to his theory, the entire body is "mapped" onto the ear in the form of an inverted fetus. Using this system of correspondence, one can, according to Nogier, treat any part of the body by treating the corresponding part of the ear. This approach was subsequently taken up in China, even though it had been invented in the West and had no real foundation in traditional practice.

(Classic acupuncture includes only a few points on the ear and does not refer to any representation of the entire body.) Nogier claimed to have scientifically tested his theory, but the methods he used to accomplish this fall far short of anything recognizable as modern science. There are no properly designed studies to support the "little man on the ear" hypothesis, and the one well-designed study on the subject failed to find any correlation between pain in the body and tenderness in corresponding parts of the ear as predicted by Nogier's theory.

Acupuncture was virtually unheard of and unavailable in the United States until 1972, the year U.S. president Richard Nixon made his historic visit to China. Among the accompanying press was the well-known journalist James Reston, who was hospitalized while in China and received acupuncture anesthesia. Upon returning to the United States, Reston published an article about his experience, stimulating new interest in acupuncture among the public and within the medical community. Although it was later discovered that the drugs used with acupuncture anesthesia probably played a major role, the perception of acupuncture as a powerful treatment caused it to gain respect in the United States. Acupuncture schools began to open in the late 1970s and 1980s. With training available in the United States, the number of acupuncturists began to grow rapidly; there are now many thousands of certified and licensed acupuncturists.

MECHANISM OF ACTION

The exact mechanisms by which acupuncture might produce effects on the body remain unknown. Weak preliminary evidence from the 1970s hints that acupuncture encourages the release of endorphins (morphine-like compounds that function as the body's internal pain-regulating substances). Support for this theory comes from a study in which the use of the drug naloxone, which opposes the effects of endorphins, was found to block pain relief from acupuncture. However, the body releases endorphins in response to any sort of pain, and it may be that needle insertion per se, and not acupuncture, is responsible for the rise in endorphins. Furthermore, there is some evidence that the placebo effect itself works by means of endorphins; in one study, naloxone blocked the ability of a placebo treatment to reduce pain.

It has also been proposed that acupuncture may

influence other chemicals in the body that control various physiologic activities. Preliminary studies have shown possible effects of acupuncture on norepinephrine, acetylcholine, and cyclic AMP, all of which are "chemical messengers" that regulate key systems in the body. However, none of this evidence is strong.

SCIENTIFIC EVIDENCE

Although there have been numerous controlled studies of acupuncture, there is no condition for which acupuncture's supporting evidence is strong. There are several reasons for this, but one is fundamental: Even with the best of intentions, it is difficult to properly ascertain the effectiveness of a hands-on therapy such as acupuncture.

Only one form of study can truly prove that a treatment is effective: the double-blind, placebo-controlled trial. However, it is not easy to fit acupuncture into a study design of this type. One problem is designing a form of placebo acupuncture, and an even more challenging problem is to ensure that participants and practitioners do not know who is receiving real acupuncture and who is receiving fake. Without such blinding, the results of the study can be skewed by numerous factors.

In an attempt to approximate double-blind studies of acupuncture, researchers have resorted to a number of clever techniques. Perhaps the most common involves sham acupuncture. In such studies, a fake version of acupuncture is used. However, because the acupuncturist knows that this is a fake treatment, he or she may subtly convey a lack of confidence in the outcome. Such studies are called single-blind and are not fully trustworthy. (The only exceptions are studies in which the patient is anesthetized before the acupuncture and is, presumably, incapable of interpreting the possibly biased actions of the acupuncturist.)

To get around this problem and produce a truly double-blind study, some studies may employ trained technicians, and not real acupuncturists, to insert needles. Such technicians might be given a list of real acupuncture points or phony acupuncture points, without being told which is which. However, it is not reasonable to suppose that an essentially untrained technician can give an acupuncture treatment as effective as that of a real acupuncturist. Furthermore, using a fixed set of points to treat a problem is not true to traditional acupuncture, which always individualizes treatment to the person seeking care.

Another approach is to use real acupuncturists to deliver treatment, but to have a separate person evaluate the effects of that treatment. Such studies may be described as partially double-blind (or observer blind); they prevent researchers from biasing their own observations, but they still do not eliminate the problem that the acupuncturist might communicate confidence (or lack of it) to the participants. The placebo effect in acupuncture is very sensitive to expectation; in one study, persons who believed they were getting real acupuncture experienced benefits and those who believed they were getting fake acupuncture failed to experience benefits. Whether or not they were actually receiving real or fake acupuncture proved to be irrelevant; it was the belief that mattered. One doubts whether acupuncturists are sufficiently adept at hiding their true feelings from their patients. Osteopathic physician Kerry Kamer suggested a whimsical approach to testing acupuncture: For the placebo group, use actors trained to convey confidence while performing fake acupuncture. However, such studies have not been reported.

Despite their limitations, most of the best studies available are single-blind or partially double-blind designs. Although imperfect, they can give some idea whether true acupuncture might be effective.

There is another problem to consider. Acupuncture causes a very strong placebo effect, whether it is real or fake. This phenomenon tends to diminish the difference in results between the treatment group and the placebo group and can potentially hide a true benefit by making it too small to reach statistical significance. As an example, consider a study in which sixty-seven people with hip arthritis received either random needle placement or actual acupuncture. The results showed improvement in both groups, but to the same extent. Does this mean that traditional acupuncture is actually no better than random acupuncture? Not necessarily. The study could simply have been too small to identify benefits that did occur. In studies that show a strong placebo effect, it may be necessary to enroll hundreds of participants to show benefit above statistical "background noise." A small study can fail to find benefit, but it cannot actually prove lack of benefit.

Some studies have compared acupuncture to other therapies, such as physical therapy or massage. Trials of this kind are good for determining relative cost effectiveness, but they cannot be taken as proof of efficacy for one simple reason: These other therapies have never been proven effective themselves.

There is one additional problem in evaluating the evidence for acupuncture: Many of the studies were performed in China, and there is evidence of systematic bias in the Chinese medical literature. In 1998, researchers evaluating the acupuncture studies from China discovered that each study found acupuncture effective. This led researchers to look further into other Chinese medical research. Review of controlled trials involving other therapies, including standard drugs, showed that Chinese trials reported positive results 99 percent of the time. Although some bias exists in all medical publications, this finding suggests a particularly high rate of bias in the Chinese research record. A subsequent analysis in 2007 continued to find grossly inadequate standards of rigor in Chinese studies of Chinese medicine.

Given these caveats, the following sections address the science regarding acupuncture. They begin with conditions in which acupuncture research has been mostly positive, continue with those for which the record is mixed, and conclude with those in which the tested form of acupuncture has not proved effective. Studies of acupressure and electroacupuncture also are discussed.

EVIDENCE-BASED USES

Nausea and vomiting. Numerous studies have evaluated treatment on a single acupuncture point (P6), which is traditionally thought to be effective for relief of various forms of nausea and vomiting. This point is located on the inside of the forearm, about two inches above the wrist crease. Most studies have investigated the effects of pressure on this point (acupressure) rather than needling. The most common methods involve a wristband with a pearl-sized bead in it situated over P6. The band exerts pressure on the bead while it is worn, and the user can press on the bead for extra stimulation.

Although the research record is mixed, on balance it appears that P6 stimulation offers at least modest benefits for nausea. This approach has been studied in anesthesia-induced nausea, the nausea and vomiting of pregnancy, and other forms of nausea.

Anesthesia-induced nausea. General anesthetics and other medications used for surgery frequently cause nausea. A minimum of ten controlled studies enrolling about one thousand women undergoing gynecologic surgery found that P6 stimulation of various types reduced such postsurgical nausea compared with placebo.

On the negative side, a double-blind, placebo-controlled study of 410 women undergoing gynecologic surgery failed to find P6 acupressure more effective than fake acupressure (both were more effective than no treatment). A small trial of acupuncture in gynecologic surgery also failed to find benefit, as did three studies of acupressure for women undergoing cesarean section. Studies of acupuncture or acupressure in other forms of surgery have produced about as many negative results as positive ones.

A 2004 review of the entire literature regarding P6 stimulation for postoperative nausea found twenty-six studies. All of these studies suffered from significant flaws; however, on balance, the reviewers found that stimulation of P6 does reduce postoperative nausea compared with placebo. Similarly, a 2008 review of six placebo-controlled trials investigating the effectiveness of P6 stimulation on nausea and vomiting both during and after cesarean section found some benefit, though the authors concluded that the results were largely inconsistent.

One aspect of studies of acupressure for postsurgical nausea is that here a single-blind study is probably as good as a double-blind study. If the acupressure wrist band is not put on until after anesthesia has begun, no amount of confidence or lack of it by the practitioner is likely to alter the placebo effect experienced by the unconscious patient. Thus, studies of acupressure/acupuncture for this condition have a higher potential validity than studies for any of the other conditions listed here. The fact that benefits have been seen strongly suggests that stimulation of P6 does affect nausea. That there is no clear physiological reason why this should be so makes this an intriguing finding, even if the benefit is too slight to make much real difference in postoperative care.

Nausea and vomiting during pregnancy. Several controlled studies have evaluated the benefits of acupressure or acupuncture in the nausea and vomiting of pregnancy, commonly called morning sickness. The results for acupressure, though not for acupuncture, have generally been positive.

For example, a double-blind, placebo-controlled study of ninety-seven women found evidence that wristband acupressure may work. Participants wore either a real wristband or a phony one that appeared identical. Both real and fake acupressure caused noticeable improvement in more than one-half of the participants. However, women using the real wristband showed better results in terms of the duration of nausea. Intensity of the nausea symptoms was not significantly different between groups.

These results are consistent with other studies of acupressure for morning sickness, though two studies failed to find benefit for severe morning sickness. However, one large trial of acupuncture instead of acupressure failed to find benefit. This single-blind, placebo-controlled study of 593 pregnant women with morning sickness compared the effects of traditional acupuncture, acupuncture at P6 only, acupuncture at "wrong" points (sham acupuncture), and no treatment. As noted, the placebo effect of acupuncture is very strong. Women in all three treatment groups (including the fake acupuncture group) showed significant improvements in nausea and dry retching compared with the no-treatment group. However, neither form of real acupuncture proved markedly more effective than fake acupuncture.

Other forms of nausea. A single-blind, placebo-controlled study found acupressure helpful for motion sickness, though another, similar study did not. A single-blind, placebo-controlled trial of 104 people undergoing high-dose chemotherapy for breast cancer found that electrical stimulation on P6 significantly reduced episodes of vomiting. A small study in children receiving chemotherapy for a variety of cancers suggested that acupuncture may reduce the need for antinausea medication. Similar improvements were seen in four other studies of acupuncture or acupressure in persons undergoing chemotherapy or radiation. In a small sham-controlled study, acupressure wristbands showed promise, although the benefit seen just missed the conventional cutoff for statistical significance. However, equivocal or absent effectiveness was seen in three other studies of wristbands, and one study failed to find more benefit with real acupuncture than with fake acupuncture.

Tendonitis. Several small controlled studies have found acupuncture helpful for tendonitis. For example, a single-blind, placebo-controlled trial of fifty-two people with rotator cuff (shoulder) tendonitis found evidence that acupuncture is more effective than placebo. Benefits were also seen in four other studies of people with shoulder or elbow tendonitis. However, another study failed to find benefit.

In a sizable randomized trial, 425 persons receiving physical therapy for their persistent shoulder pain were divided into two groups: One group received single-point acupuncture while the other group received a sham treatment (mock transcutaneous electrical nerve stimulation) for three weeks. The acupuncture group showed significant improvement over the control group one week after treatment.

In a study of eighty-two people with elbow tendonitis, deep acupuncture was more effective than shallow acupuncture placebo in the short term, but by three months there was no difference between the groups. A comparative trial of twenty people found weak evidence that electroacupuncture may be more effective than ordinary acupuncture for elbow tendonitis. Two other trials failed to find laser acupuncture effective compared with either sham or other, similar treatments. Eight sessions of true acupuncture were no better than sham acupuncture in 123 persons treated for persistent arm pain caused by repetitive use.

A 2004 systematic review found five positive controlled studies on acupuncture for tennis elbow and concluded that "strong evidence" supports the use of acupuncture for this condition. However, this characterization of the evidence as "strong" would seem to be premature. For the reasons described in the beginning of this section, virtually all studies of acupuncture are single-blind, and such studies (except when performed on anesthetized patients) cannot exclude the possible effect of confidence conveyed by practitioners performing valid treatment, compared with lack of confidence conveyed by those delivering sham treatment.

Pregnancy support. As noted, acupuncture has shown some promise for reducing symptoms of morning sickness. This treatment has additionally been studied for aiding other aspects of pregnancy. However, the record is marred by poorly designed studies.

A well-controlled study of 210 women giving birth found that real acupuncture was more effective than sham acupuncture at reducing labor pain. Benefits were also seen in another well-controlled study. Two other studies of poorer quality also reported benefit. In one study, however, sterile water injections were found to be more effective than acupuncture for lower back pain and relaxation during labor. It is unclear whether or not the persons in the study knew what treatment they were receiving at the time. In one placebo-controlled trial and one review of ten mostly low quality trials, real acupuncture was no better than sham acupuncture in relieving pelvic pain during pregnancy before labor.

A study of forty-five pregnant women found that the use of acupuncture on the expected birth due date significantly sped up the actual date of delivery. However, this trial used a no-treatment control group instead of sham acupuncture. Another study that failed to use sham treatment found minimal evidence that the use of acupuncture may help stimulate normal term labor. A study of 106 women evaluated whether acupuncture can speed up delivery after prelabor rupture of membranes ("water breaking" too early) and failed to find benefit. However, again, no adequate control group was used; this is equally a problem for negative and for positive studies. Finally, in a placebo-controlled trial, real acupuncture administered for two days before a planned induction of labor (artificial stimulation of labor) was no better than sham acupuncture at preventing the need for induction or shortening the time of labor.

Acupuncture has also been studied for converting breech presentation of the unborn infant to normal positioning. In a study of 240 women at thirty-three to thirty-five weeks gestation, acupuncture combined with moxibustion caused the breech presentation to convert in 54 percent of women, while only 37 percent of women in the no-treatment control converted. Again, placebo acupuncture would have been better than no treatment. A much smaller study also found benefits with acupressure. In 2008, researchers published a review of six randomized-controlled trials that investigated acupuncture-like therapies (moxibustion, acupuncture, or electroacupuncture) applied to a specific point (BL67). They concluded that these therapies were effective at decreasing the incidence of breech presentations at the time of delivery. Again, however, not all of these studies employed a sham acupuncture group for comparison.

Osteoarthritis. Acupuncture has shown inconsistent benefit as a treatment for osteoarthritis. While the results of numerous smaller studies suggest that acupuncture is an effective treatment for osteoarthritis (of the knee, in particular), larger studies have generally found it be no more effective than sham acupuncture.

A 2006 meta-analysis (systematic statistical review) of studies on acupuncture for osteoarthritis found eight trials that were similar enough to be considered

together. A total of 2,362 people were enrolled in these studies. The authors of the meta-analysis concluded that acupuncture should be regarded as an effective treatment for osteoarthritis.

However, one study comprised almost one-half of all the people considered in this meta-analysis, and it failed to find real acupuncture more effective than sham acupuncture. In this study, published in 2006, 1,007 people with knee osteoarthritis were given either real acupuncture, fake acupuncture, or standard therapy for six weeks. Though both real acupuncture and fake acupuncture were more effective than no acupuncture, there was no significant difference in benefits between the two acupuncture groups. In general, larger studies are more reliable than small ones. For this reason, it is always somewhat questionable when meta-analysis combines one very large negative study and a number of smaller positive ones to come up with a positive outcome.

Another review, published in 2007, concluded differently. It concluded that real acupuncture produces distinct benefits in osteoarthritis compared with no treatment, but that fake acupuncture is very effective for osteoarthritis too. When real acupuncture is compared with fake acupuncture, the difference in outcome, while it might possibly be statistically significant, is so trivial as to make no difference in real life. In other words, virtually all of the benefit of acupuncture for osteoarthritis is a placebo effect.

The apparent slight statistical difference between real and fake acupuncture could easily have been caused by problems of single-blind studies. Acupuncturists who know they are performing real acupuncture may subconsciously convey more confidence to their patients than those who know they are performing fake acupuncture. The history of medical studies makes it clear that such unconscious communications can greatly affect results; because the evidence shows only a minute difference between the results of real and fake acupuncture, it is quite possible that this transmission of confidence (or lack of it) is the entire cause of the difference, and that the specific techniques and theories of acupuncture themselves play no role.

Headache. Acupuncture has shown some promise for various types of headaches, including migraines and tension headaches; however, the research record remains mixed, and the best-designed studies have generally failed to find benefit. In a 2008 analysis of five randomized-controlled trials that were considered highest in quality, researchers determined that real acupuncture has limited benefit over sham acupuncture for tension headache. Subsequently, in a large randomized trial involving 3,182 headache patients, the group that received fifteen acupuncture sessions in three months experienced significantly fewer headache days and less pain compared with the group receiving usual care. However, there was no placebo group. While it is clear that many headache patients benefit from acupuncture, it remains unclear whether or not this presents more than a placebo effect.

Neck pain. A 2006 review of the literature found ten controlled studies of acupuncture for chronic neck pain. The pooled results suggest that acupuncture may be more effective than fake acupuncture, in the short term. However, overall the study quality was fairly low.

In a study of 177 people with chronic neck pain, fake acupuncture proved more effective than massage. In a pilot study, ten weeks of acupuncture combined with physical therapy appeared to be more effective than either acupuncture or physical therapy alone for chronic neck pain, in the short term. There has been some study of acupuncture for acute neck pain; however, in one of the best of these studies, the use of laser acupuncture failed to provide benefit for whiplash injuries.

Dental procedures. The evidence regarding acupuncture treatment of dental pain is mixed. A literature review published in 1998 identified four meaningful studies on acupuncture for reducing pain during dental procedures. Three of the studies found positive results, but the largest (with 110 participants) found no benefit. It was largely on the basis of this review that acupuncture was discussed in the media as a "proven" treatment for dental pain. However, these mixed results do not constitute proof. More recent studies have also shown mixed results. At present, therefore, the available evidence does not provide a reliable basis for concluding that acupuncture is effective for dental pain.

Chemical dependency. Although some animal studies suggest that ear acupuncture or electroacupuncture may have some benefits for chemical dependency, study results in humans have been mixed at best, with the largest studies reporting no benefits. For example, while benefits were seen in a much smaller single-blind trial, a single-blind, placebo-controlled trial that evaluated 620 cocaine-dependent adults found acupuncture no more effective than sham acupuncture or relaxation training. Similarly, a single-blind, placebo-controlled study enrolling 236 residential clients found no benefit for cocaine addiction from ear acupuncture. Finally, in a placebo-controlled trial involving 83 people addicted to drugs attending a methadone detoxification clinic, the addition of ear acupuncture did not improve withdrawal symptoms or cravings. Methadone, a relatively weak narcotic, is commonly used to treat narcotic addition over the long-term.

The situation is much the same for alcohol addiction. A single-blind, placebo-controlled study of 503 alcoholics failed to find evidence of benefit with three weeks of ear acupuncture. In addition, a ten-week, single-blind, placebo-controlled study of 72 alcoholics found no difference in drinking patterns or cravings between sham acupuncture and real acupuncture groups. There are two other small trials that also failed to find significant benefits. However, one single-blind trial of 54 people did find some evidence of improvement.

A single-blind, controlled trial of one hundred people with heroin addiction evaluated the potential benefits of ear acupuncture. However, a high dropout rate makes the results difficult to interpret.

In a meta-analysis of 12 placebo-controlled trials, acupuncture was not found more effective than sham acupuncture for smoking cessation. A more recent observer-blind, sham-controlled study of 330 adolescent smokers also found no benefit. While most addiction studies involve ear acupuncture, a randomized trial compared real versus sham acupuncture on body points. The study found no difference in quit rates, depression, or anxiety. One study found that acupuncture may not be effective on its own but may (in some unknown manner) increase the effectiveness of stop-smoking education. In this sham-controlled study of 141 adults, acupuncture plus education was twice as effective as sham acupuncture plus education and four times as effective as acupuncture alone. However, these benefits were seen only in the short term; at long-term follow-ups, the relative advantage of acupuncture disappeared.

Back pain. Research has not produced convincing evidence that acupuncture is effective for back pain. Many studies widely cited as providing such evidence were actually invalid because of a lack of a proper control group. People with back pain given acupuncture report benefits, but the problem is that people given fake acupuncture also experience benefits, often to a similar degree. In a review of twenty-three randomized trials involving more than six thousand persons with chronic low back pain, researchers concluded that acupuncture is more effective than no treatment for short-term pain relief, but there was no significant difference between the effects of true and sham acupuncture. Researchers also found that acupuncture can be a useful addition to conventional therapies.

A six-month patient-blind and observer-blind trial of 1,162 people with back pain compared real acupuncture, fake acupuncture, and conventional therapy. Both real and fake acupuncture proved to be twice as effective as conventional therapy according to the measures used. However, there was only a minimal difference between real and fake acupuncture. These results do not indicate that acupuncture is effective per se; rather, they show the significant power of acupuncture as placebo.

Similarly, in a single-blind, controlled study (using sham acupuncture and no treatment) of 298 people with chronic back pain, the use of real acupuncture failed to prove significantly more effective than sham acupuncture. Also, in a fairly large randomized trial involving 638 adults with chronic back pain, there was no difference in pain at one year in persons receiving real acupuncture compared with fake acupuncture (with neither group improving significantly over standard care). Both real and sham acupuncture were, however, associated with improved function at one year. Other studies enrolling more than three hundred people also failed to find benefit.

A trial compared the effects of acupuncture, massage, and education (such as videotapes on back care) in 262 people with chronic back pain in a ten-week period. The exact type of acupuncture and massage was left to practitioners, but only ten visits were permitted. At the ten-week point, evaluations showed benefit with massage but not with acupuncture. One year later, massage and education were nearly equivalent, and both were superior to acupuncture.

One small study found chiropractic spinal manipulation more effective than anti-inflammatory medication or acupuncture for low back pain. In another trial, acupressure-style massage was found to be more effective for back pain than Swedish massage. However, Swedish massage has not been proven effective

for back pain, so this does not prove that acupressure-style massage is effective. Two single-blind, placebo-controlled trials, one with thirty participants and another with sixty, also failed to find evidence of benefit.

Two studies did find possible slight benefits with electrical acupuncture for chronic low back pain. An additional study found acupressure more effective than physical therapy for low back pain, and another found some potential benefit with electric acupuncture.

Low level laser therapy (LLLT) is a technique similar to electroacupuncture that uses precision laser energy instead of electricity conducted through a needle. In a detailed review of seven randomized trials, researchers were unable to draw any conclusions regarding the effectiveness of LLLT for nonspecific low back pain.

Several other studies have compared acupuncture with other treatments for back pain. Treatments such as transcutaneous electrical nerve stimulation (TENS), physical therapy, and chiropractic care were found equally effective. However, because TENS, physical therapy, and chiropractic care have not themselves been proven effective for back pain, studies of this type cannot be taken as evidence that acupuncture is effective. One study did find acupressure massage more effective than standard physical therapy; however, it was performed in a Chinese population that may have had more faith in this traditional approach than in physical therapy.

Stroke. Acupuncture is widely used in China for treatment of acute stroke. A few controlled studies have been published, but the best-designed and largest studies failed to find benefit.

For example, a single-blind, placebo-controlled trial of 104 people who had just experienced a stroke failed to find any benefit with ten weeks of twice-weekly acupuncture. Similarly, a single-blind, controlled study of 150 people recovering from stroke compared acupuncture (including electroacupuncture), high-intensity muscle stimulation, and sham treatment. All participants received twenty treatments for ten weeks. Neither acupuncture nor muscle stimulation produced any benefits. A ten-week study of 106 people that provided thirty-five traditional acupuncture sessions also failed to find benefit. Also, 92 persons who received either twelve acupuncture treatments or a comparable sham treatment demonstrated the same level of improvement up to one year later.

A few studies did find benefit, but they were very small, and some did not use a placebo group. One trial of sixty-two persons found that a three-week program of TENS of acupuncture points (beginning about nine days after stroke) improved muscle tone and strength in the affected leg. A large review including fifty-six mostly poor quality trials reported that acupuncture may benefit post-stroke rehabilitation (based on an analysis of thirty-eight trials), and another review of nine trials found limited evidence in support of moxibustion for stroke rehabilitation.

Surgery support. Acupuncture has been explored as a means of reducing pain after surgery with encouraging but not unequivocal results. A double-blind, placebo-controlled study of forty-two people undergoing arthroscopic knee surgery found that the use of acupuncture during surgery did not reduce pain levels during the subsequent twenty-four hours. Another double-blind, placebo-controlled trial of fifty women undergoing hysterectomy found no benefit with electroacupuncture, and a double-blind study of seventy-one people undergoing abdominal surgery failed to find acupressure helpful.

However, some benefits of acupressure were reported in a single-blind trial of forty persons undergoing arthroscopic knee surgery. In addition, a special form of needle insertion called intradermal acupuncture reduced postsurgical pain in 107 people undergoing abdominal surgery. Ear acupuncture has also shown promise. In a 2008 review of fifteen randomized-controlled trials, researchers determined that acupuncture is capable of reducing pain and the need for opioid medications (morphine and related agents) immediately following surgery compared with sham acupuncture.

Other studied uses. Bee venom acupuncture (BVA), which involves the injection of diluted bee venom directly into acupoints, has been used for the treatment of pain. An analysis of four well-designed, randomized trials, comparing bee venom plus classic acupuncture with saline injection plus classic acupuncture, found that the BVA-classic acupuncture combination was significantly more effective for musculoskeletal pain.

Acupressure and acupuncture have been tried for insomnia with mixed results. A single-blind, placebo-controlled study involving eighty-four residents of a nursing home found that real acupressure was superior to sham acupressure for improving sleep quality.

Treated participants fell asleep faster and slept more soundly. In a similar study, researchers found that performing acupressure on a single point on both wrists for five weeks improved sleep quality among residents of long-term care facilities compared with lightly touching the same point. Another single-blind, controlled study reported benefits with acupuncture but failed to include a proper statistical analysis of the results. For this reason, no conclusions can be drawn from the report. In another trial, ninety-eight people with severe kidney disease were divided into three groups: no extra treatment, twelve sessions of fake acupressure (not using actual acupuncture points), and twelve sessions of real acupressure. Participants receiving real acupressure experienced significantly improved sleep compared with those receiving no extra treatment. However, fake acupressure was just as effective as real acupressure.

In a fourth randomized trial involving twenty-eight women, six weeks of auricular (outer ear) acupuncture was more effective than sham acupuncture. In one study, magnetic pearls used to stimulate acupuncture points in the ear seemed to show some benefit compared with nonmagnetic stimulation of ear points. A small, single-blind, placebo-controlled study of sixty adults with primary insomnia found that three weeks of electroacupuncture improved sleep efficiency and decreased wake time after sleep onset.

One small, double-blind, placebo-controlled study found real acupuncture more effective than sham acupuncture for menstrual pain. (This study used nonacupuncturists who were given real or fake acupuncture protocols to apply, but they did not know which they were applying.) In addition, a controlled study of sixty-one women evaluated the effects of a special garment designed to stimulate acupuncture points related to menstrual pain. In this latter study, researchers chose to compare treatment to no treatment, rather than to sham treatment. For this reason, the results (which were positive) mean little. In another trial, a seed-pressure method of auricular acupressure appeared to improve menstrual pain compared with sham auricular acupressure in seventy-four women. The potentially inadequate blinding of participants in this study, however, may have limited these results. Indeed, in a review of thirty controlled trials on menstrual pain, researchers were unable to draw conclusions about the effectiveness of acupuncture and similar treatments for menstrual pain because of widespread study design problems. Also, a review of twenty-seven trials with 2,960 persons concluded that acupuncture might be more effective than medications or herbs for relieving menstrual pain, but the studies were of limited quality.

Although anesthesia apparently performed entirely with acupuncture first raised Western interest in acupuncture, the original demonstrations of acupuncture anesthesia have been discredited. It now appears that if acupuncture has any anesthetic effect, that effect is extremely modest. At most, acupuncture may be capable of slightly decreasing the required dose of general anesthetic necessary to induce anesthesia (but even this has not been consistently seen in studies).

A six-month, single-blind, controlled study of sixty-seven women with frequent bladder infections found that acupuncture therapy reduced the frequency of infection. Another study found that acupuncture may be helpful for hyperactive bladder (the frequent need to urinate but without the presence of an infection to cause the need).

A study of fifty-two people with allergic rhinitis (hay fever) found that acupuncture plus traditional Chinese herbal treatment was slightly more effective than fake acupuncture plus fake Chinese herbal treatment. However, another study failed to find acupuncture alone beneficial for allergic rhinitis. Moreover, a carefully conducted review of seven placebo-controlled trials failed to find convincing evidence for acupuncture's effectiveness against allergic rhinitis.

A Chinese study found that acupuncture plus moxibustion was more effective for Bell's palsy than was drug treatment. In a review of six studies involving 537 persons with Bell's palsy, researchers could draw no conclusions about the beneficial effects of acupuncture because of poor study quality.

Five small, controlled studies reported that acupuncture can improve menopausal symptoms, but most of these studies had significant problems in design or statistical analysis. Two additional trials failed to find acupuncture beneficial for hot flashes. One trial of 175 perimenopausal and postmenopausal women concluded that adding acupuncture to usual care reduced hot flash frequency compared with usual care alone in the first four weeks after treatment. However, another fairly large randomized trial involving 267 postmenopausal women found that while the addition of acupuncture to self-care advice significantly reduced the frequency and intensity of hot flashes in the first twelve weeks, the benefits were lost six months later. A 2009 review of six trials found that true acupuncture was no more effective than sham acupuncture for this indication. Finally, one small study found no benefit for the psychological distress associated with menopause.

Another small, placebo-controlled study in women with breast cancer who also had hot flashes caused by their treatments suggested some benefit for acupuncture, though the results were inconclusive for similar reasons. However, another study did not find acupuncture effective in these women, and a 2008 review of all existing studies on the subject concluded that the evidence does not support a beneficial effect for acupuncture in women with breast cancer who have hot flashes.

Acupuncture has been studied for use in cancer treatment support. In a small randomized trial of forty-three women with breast cancer, six weeks of acupuncture twice-weekly reduced joint pain attributed to aromatase-inhibitor therapy. Another small randomized trial of seventy persons found that acupuncture may decrease xerostomia and pain after neck dissection for cancer treatment.

A 2006 review of acupuncture for treatment of fibromyalgia found five controlled studies, none of which were of high quality. The authors of another review of seven trials could not determine the effectiveness of acupuncture for fibromyalgia because of the unreliability of the studies. Overall, the results do not provide reliable evidence that acupuncture is helpful.

Evidence for acupuncture's effectiveness for depression has been mixed. In a study of 151 depressed persons, twelve sessions of acupuncture failed to prove more effective than fake acupuncture. However, another sham-acupuncture controlled trial evaluated 43 people with depression and 13 people with generalized anxiety disorder. The results suggest that ten (but not five) acupuncture sessions can significantly improve symptoms.

One study of eight persons with major depressive disorder found that adding acupuncture to a lower dose of antidepressant (fluoxetine) improved anxiety and had an overall therapeutic effect similar to sham acupuncture with a higher dose of antidepressant. In a mathematical review of the results of eight randomized trials, the impact of acupuncture on depression was unconvincing. However, in another review of twenty trials involving two thousand persons with major depression, real acupuncture's effectiveness was comparable to that of antidepressants but no greater than that of sham acupuncture for this population.

Another trial compared real and sham ear acupuncture in healthy people and found some evidence that real acupuncture can relieve normal daily stress. A 2010 review of nine mostly poor quality trials determined that there is insufficient evidence to conclude that acupuncture is effective for premenstrual syndrome.

Although open trials appeared to show benefit, a minimum of three controlled studies failed to find acupuncture helpful for improving the success rate of in vitro fertilization (IVF). A 2008 analysis of seven randomized trials found that, on balance, acupuncture may significantly improve the odds of pregnancy in women undergoing IVF. However, because not all of these studies used sham acupuncture as a control, the reliability of this conclusion is questionable. Moreover, a second analysis in the same year of thirteen randomized-controlled trials investigating the effectiveness of acupuncture in 2,500 women undergoing a specialized IVF procedure, in which sperm is injected directly into the egg, found no evidence of any benefit. However, the story does not end here. In a subsequent review of thirteen trials, a different group of researchers concluded that acupuncture may improve the success rate of IVF, but only if it is used on the day of embryo transfer (when the fertilized egg is placed into the womb). According to this study, acupuncture is not effective when used up to three days after embryo transfer or when eggs are being retrieved from the ovaries.

Acupuncture may be more effective than sham acupuncture and as effective as standard treatments for temporomandibular joint (TMJ) pain. One study of 110 people with pain found acupuncture at least as effective as standard occlusal splint therapy. Another small study involving forty persons with TMJ pain, however, found no difference between placebo and low-level laser therapy (LLLT) directed at painful points; both groups benefitted equally. However, in a double-blind, randomized trial comparing real LLLT with sham LLLT, the real therapy was more effective for TMJ pain after eight sessions. Instead of needles, LLLT involves the use of laser energy directed on or off acupuncture points.

A single-blind trial tested acupuncture on a group of thirty-six healthy young men and found some evidence of improvement in sports performance. However, a single-blind, controlled study of forty-eight people found that the use of acupuncture did not reduce muscle soreness caused by exercise.

One study purportedly found that acupressure reduced fatigue in people with severe kidney disease. In fact, it found that both sham acupuncture and real acupuncture reduced fatigue compared with no treatment, but that real acupuncture was not more effective than fake acupuncture.

One study found minimal benefits for Parkinson's disease. Another study failed to find any benefits. In two comprehensive reviews of multiple clinical trials, independent sets of researchers concluded that there was no well-established evidence for acupuncture's effectiveness in this condition.

People with cancer often experience fatigue. Acupuncture has shown a bit of promise for improving this symptom. A Chinese study reported that acupuncture is helpful for vocal cord dysfunction.

A study that reported acupuncture's benefits for chronic prostatitis failed to use a control group and is, therefore, meaningless. However, another study found that real acupuncture was more effective than sham acupuncture at reducing the symptoms of chronic prostatitis both during treatment and for six months after treatment. Another study suggested that electroacupuncture may improve symptoms in men with chronic prostatitis (or a related condition called chronic pelvic pain syndrome), but this study was very small.

After an acute attack of shingles, pain may linger for months or years, causing what is known as postherpetic neuralgia. A single-blind, placebo-controlled study of sixty-two people with pain of this type failed to find any benefit with acupuncture. Two separate groups of researchers conducting detailed reviews of eight randomized controlled trials found some beneficial effects of acupuncture for rheumatoid arthritis, but they were unconvinced that it was more beneficial than sham acupuncture or other standard treatments. There have been numerous reports about acupuncture treatment for asthma, but most published studies are of low quality, with results being contradictory at best. One study failed to find acupuncture helpful for shortness of breath associated with advanced cancer.

Peripheral neuropathy (nerve pain in the extremities) is a common complaint for those with human immunodeficiency virus (HIV) infection. A placebo-controlled trial of 239 people with HIV found acupuncture no more effective than placebo in peripheral neuropathy. The study also tested drug therapy for peripheral neuropathy and also found it ineffective.

A substantial study (192 participants) failed to find acupuncture more helpful than fake acupuncture for high blood pressure. However, another study, this one enrolling 160 people, did report benefit. A much smaller study also reported benefits, but there were problems in its statistical analysis. In a review of eleven randomized-controlled trials on the subject, researchers determined that acupuncture's ability to lower blood pressure remains inconclusive.

Acupuncture is probably not effective for epilepsy. A single-blind, controlled trial of individualized acupuncture for thirty-four people with severe epilepsy found no benefit, and subsequently, a comprehensive review of eleven studies found no reliable evidence of its effectiveness.

One controlled study failed to find electroacupuncture effective for reducing discomfort during colonoscopy. A controlled study purportedly found acupuncture helpful for speeding recovery in people with spinal cord injuries, but it failed to use a sham-acupuncture control group. Several controlled and open trials of acupuncture for tinnitus (ringing in the ear) found no benefit.

A well-designed, single-blind, placebo-controlled study of sixty people with irritable bowel syndrome (IBS) compared traditional acupuncture to sham acupuncture. In the thirteen-week study period, both groups improved to the same extent. A larger trial of 230 adults with IBS found that acupuncture (six treatments in three weeks) was not associated with improved symptoms or severity compared with sham acupuncture. Two smaller studies have also failed to find acupuncture more effective than placebo acupuncture.

In a placebo-controlled trial, sixty nursing women received needle acupuncture, fifty-six women received laser acupuncture, and sixty women received placebo acupuncture. The results showed no differences in milk production. In one small study, light needling at one acupuncture point on both hands was more effective than no needling among forty infants with colic.

WHAT TO EXPECT DURING TREATMENT

Acupuncture therapy has its own style and atmosphere, both like and unlike an ordinary medical encounter. The first session will begin with a thorough analysis of the condition and the patient's health history. If the acupuncturist practices according to the principles of TCM, the patient will be asked a number of questions about his or her specific complaint and general health, including how well he or she sleeps, digests food, eliminates, and breathes, and about the level of his or her energy. All of these factors are considered relevant. The acupuncturist may ask questions that seem to have little bearing on the patient's condition, questions such as whether or not the patient feels cold or hot most of the time. TCM looks for overall patterns in both physical and emotional well-being, which guide the acupuncturist in developing a treatment plan that is specific not only for the patient's symptoms but also for the patient's overall health pattern.

Depending on the specific complaint and on the patient's individual symptom pattern, the acupuncturist may use only a few needles or as many as twenty or more. Acupuncture needle sizes are typically 32- to 36-gauge, which means they are about one-quarter millimeter in diameter, much smaller than a hypodermic needle. Unlike hollow hypodermic needles, acupuncture needles are solid, which allows them to penetrate the skin easily and relatively painlessly. Acupuncture needles may produce a mild pricking sensation when inserted, but sometimes nothing is felt at insertion. The needles are generally inserted to a depth ranging from a few millimeters to one-half inch. Insertion depth is greater at the more fleshy areas of the body, such as the thighs and buttocks.

Acupuncture needles are typically inserted through a plastic tube that guides the needle into the skin. This is a fairly modern needle insertion technique. Traditional freehand insertion is also used; most acupuncturists are trained in this method. Virtually all acupuncturists in the United States now use sterilized, one-time-use disposable needles, which eliminate any risk of cross-infection.

The acupuncturist may twirl the inserted needles and ask the patient to indicate when he or she feels a mild, achy, heavy sensation or when the area may feel slightly numb or tingly. These sensations, described in TCM as the arrival of qi, are regarded as a

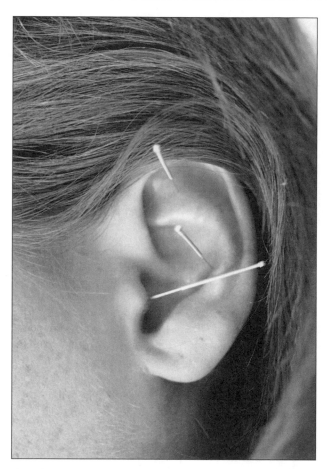

A patient receives an acupuncture treatment. (PhotoDisc)

positive response that will enhance the effectiveness of the treatment.

Whatever the sensation, it should be mild, should not be overly unpleasant, and should subside within a few minutes. If any needles are genuinely painful, one should inform the practitioner so he or she can adjust the depth or remove the needle altogether. The needles are generally left in place for twenty to thirty minutes. During this time, the patient should feel comfortable and relaxed and may fall asleep.

Acupuncturists may also employ a technique known as electroacupuncture, in which electrodes are attached to the needles and a mild current is applied. This is intended to increase the stimulation of the needle and is generally used for more painful conditions. Electroacupuncture produces a tingly, pulsating sensation. The acupuncturist can control the intensity and adjust it to a level that is comfortable.

Traditionally trained acupuncturists often use needles and heat to stimulate acupuncture points with a procedure called moxibustion, which involves a mixture of herbs rolled into a cigar-like shape. The roll is lit, and the burning end is held over the skin, allowing the heat to penetrate the area around the acupressure point. The moxa roll never touches the skin, so the patient will not be burned. The acupuncturist will ask the patient to inform him or her know before the moxa gets too hot. Moxibustion is generally quite pleasant. It is regarded as a "tonifying" treatment, which means it is intended to strengthen function.

CHOOSING A PRACTITIONER

Acupuncture is a licensed health profession in the United States in thirty-nine states and the District of Columbia. Most states require at least three years of training at an accredited school of acupuncture and passage of a national board certification examination administered by the National Certification Commission for Acupuncture and Oriental Medicine. Most states grant the title licensed acupuncturist, certified acupuncturist, registered acupuncturist, or simply acupuncturist upon certification. A few states allow acupuncturists who have a doctorate from an approved or accredited college to use the title doctor of Oriental medicine (D.O.M.) or Oriental medical doctor (O.M.D.).

In most states, medical doctors can practice acupuncture with no training; in many states, chiropractors may practice acupuncture with one hundred or fewer hours of training. Approximately one-third of the states that license acupuncturists require their clients to have a referral from a Western medical practitioner (a medical doctor, osteopath, chiropractor, or dentist) before or in conjunction with acupuncture treatment. In the remaining states, acupuncturists may accept persons for treatment without prior referral.

Training programs have become fairly standardized, so an acupuncturist with qualifications in one state has essentially the same training as those certified in other states. If a prospective patient is in a state that does not license acupuncturists, he or she should ask to see evidence that the acupuncturist has completed a minimum of three years of training at an accredited institution. One can check with the state's medical board for the exact licensure title and requirements.

SAFETY ISSUES

Serious adverse effects associated with the use of acupuncture are rare. The most commonly reported problems include short-term pain from needle insertion, tiredness, and minor bleeding. There is one report of infection caused by acupuncture given to a person with diabetes.

Some acupuncture points lie over the lungs, so insertion to an excessive depth could conceivably cause a pneumothorax (punctured lung). Because acupuncturists are trained to avoid this complication, it is a rare occurrence.

A report from China contained an example of another complication caused by excessively deep needling. A forty-four-year-old man was needled on the back of the neck at a commonly used acupuncture point just below the bony protuberance at the base of the skull. However, the acupuncturist inserted the needle too deeply and punctured a blood vessel in the skull. The client developed a severe headache with nausea and vomiting; a scan showed bleeding in the brain, and a spinal tap found a small amount of blood in the cerebrospinal fluid. The severe headache, along with neck stiffness, continued for twenty-eight days. The man was treated with standard pain medication, and the condition resolved itself without any permanent effects. Also, infection caused by the use of unclean needles has been reported, but the modern practice of using disposable sterile needles appears to have eliminated this risk.

EBSCO CAM Review Board

FURTHER READING

Alecrim-Andrade, J., et al. "Acupuncture in Migraine Prevention." *Clinical Journal of Pain* 24 (2008): 98-105.

Borud, E. K., et al. "The Acupuncture on Hot Flashes Among Menopausal Women Study." *Menopause* 17 (2010): 262-268.

Carrasco, T. G., et al. "Low Intensity Laser Therapy in Temporomandibular Disorder." *Cranio* 26 (2008): 274-281.

Cherkin, D. C., et al. "A Randomized Trial Comparing Acupuncture, Simulated Acupuncture, and Usual Care for Chronic Low Back Pain." *Archives of Internal Medicine* 169 (2009): 858-866.

Cho, S. H., and E. W. Hwang. "Acupuncture for Primary Dysmenorrhoea." *BJOG: An International Journal of Obstetrics and Gynaecology* 117 (2010): 509-521.

Cho, S. H., and J. Kim. "Efficacy of Acupuncture in Management of Premenstrual Syndrome." *Complementary Therapies in Medicine* 18 (2010): 104-111.

Davis, M. A., et al. "Acupuncture for Tension-Type Headache." *Journal of Pain* 9 (2008): 667-677.

Frey, U. H., et al. "P6 Acustimulation Effectively Decreases Postoperative Nausea and Vomiting in High-Risk Patients." *British Journal of Anaesthesiology* 102 (2009): 620-625.

Goldman, R. H., et al. "Acupuncture for Treatment of Persistent Arm Pain Due to Repetitive Use." *Clinical Journal of Pain* 24 (2008): 211-218.

Hollifield, M., et al. "Acupuncture for Post-traumatic Stress Disorder." *Journal of Nervous and Mental Disease* 195 (2007): 504-513.

Hsieh, L. L., et al. "Effect of Acupressure and Trigger Points in Treating Headache." *American Journal of Chinese Medicine* 38 (2010): 1-14.

La Touche, R., et al. "Effectiveness of Acupuncture in the Treatment of Temporomandibular Disorders of Muscular Origin." *Journal of Alternative and Complementary Medicine* 16 (2010): 107-112.

Langhorst, J., et al. "Efficacy of Acupuncture in Fibromyalgia Syndrome." *Rheumatology* 49 (2010): 778-788.

Lee, H., et al. "Acupuncture for Lowering Blood Pressure." *American Journal of Hypertension* 22 (2009): 122-128.

Sun, J. L., et al. "Effectiveness of Acupressure for Residents of Long-Term Care Facilities with Insomnia." *International Journal of Nursing Studies* 47 (2010): 798-805.

Zhang, Z. J., et al. "The Effectiveness and Safety of Acupuncture Therapy in Depressive Disorders." *Journal of Affective Disorders* 124 (2010): 9-21.

See also: Acupressure; Chinese medicine; Manipulative and body-based practices; Pain management; Traditional healing.

Adenosine monophosphate

CATEGORY: Herbs and supplements
DEFINITION: Natural substance promoted as a dietary supplement for specific health benefits.
PRINCIPAL PROPOSED USES: None
OTHER PROPOSED USES: Cold sores, photosensitivity, postherpetic neuralgia, shingles

OVERVIEW

Adenosine monophosphate (AMP) is a substance the body creates in the process of making adenosine triphosphate (ATP), a source of energy used throughout the body. ATP is so ubiquitous in the body that it is sometimes called the body's energy currency. Based on preliminary evidence, AMP has been recommended as a treatment for cold sores, shingles, and photosensitivity.

SOURCES

There is no nutritional requirement for AMP because it is already manufactured by the body.

THERAPEUTIC DOSAGES

A typical recommended dose of AMP is 100 to 200 milligrams daily. However, it is not clear that AMP can be absorbed orally, and most studies have involved an injected form of the substance.

THERAPEUTIC USES

In adults, infection by the virus herpes zoster (which causes chickenpox) can cause a condition known as shingles. The initial shingles attack generally abates in a couple of weeks, but symptoms can go on to become chronic. This condition is called postherpetic neuralgia (PHN). Some evidence hints that people with herpes zoster infection may have lower than normal levels of AMP. On this slim basis, AMP has been studied as a possible treatment for initial shingles symptoms and for preventing PHN.

In a double-blind, placebo-controlled study of thirty-two people with shingles, AMP was injected three times a week for four weeks. At the end of the treatment period, 88 percent of those treated with AMP were pain free versus only 43 percent in the placebo group; all participants still in pain were then given AMP, and no recurrence of pain was reported in three to eighteen months of follow-up.

However, this was a preliminary study, and more evidence is needed before AMP can be considered a proven treatment for shingles or PHN. Furthermore, oral AMP has not been tried for this condition. It is questionable whether AMP taken orally actually survives intact in the body.

Another study found weak evidence that injected AMP might be helpful for cold sores. However, this study was not a double-blind trial; it was an open study, in which the placebo effect and other confounding factors could have played a major role. For that reason, its results cannot be relied upon. Another open study hints that AMP, this time in an oral form, might be helpful for people with excessive sensitivity to the sun (photosensitivity) associated with a condition called porphyria cutanea tarda.

SAFETY ISSUES

In the human studies performed, the use of oral AMP has not been associated with any side effects. However, it has been suggested that the use of supplemental AMP could potentially decrease immunity. Safety in young children, pregnant or nursing women, or people with severe liver or kidney disease has not been established.

EBSCO CAM Review Board

FURTHER READING

Sherlock, C. H., and L. Corey. "Adenosine Monophosphate for the Treatment of Varicella Zoster Infections: A Large Dose of Caution." *Journal of the American Medical Association* 253 (1985): 1444-1445.

Sklar, S. H., et al. "Herpes Zoster: The Treatment and Prevention of Neuralgia with Adenosine Monophosphate." *Journal of the American Medical Association* 253 (1985): 1427-1430.

Sklar, S. H., and E. Buimovici-Klein. "Adenosine in the Treatment of Recurrent Herpes Labialis." *Oral Surgery, Oral Medicine, and Oral Pathology* 48 (1979): 416-417.

See also: Colds and flu; Photosensitivity; Shingles.

Adolescent and teenage health

CATEGORY: Issues and overviews
DEFINITION: Complementary and alternative medicines and therapies that are focused on adolescent health.

OVERVIEW

Adolescents and teenagers, those children and young adults between eleven and twenty years old, are faced with a number of physical and psychosocial challenges. Chronic medical conditions and other conditions related to poor lifestyle habits may manifest during this period, which lasts about nine or ten years.

Adolescents also face emotional issues concerning body image, identity, and relationships.

The National Health Interview Survey of 2007 found that nearly 17 percent of teenagers (age twelve to seventeen years) reported using a minimum of one form of complementary or alternative medicine (CAM). The survey also found that the most commonly used natural therapies among children (including teenagers) in the United States are, in descending order, herbal products, chiropractic/osteopathic care, deep breathing, yoga, homeopathic treatment, traditional healing, massage, meditation, diet-based therapies, and progressive relaxation. The majority of teenagers using CAM already have a chronic or incurable condition (or both) such as asthma, allergies, and cancer. Girls tend to use CAM more often than do boys.

While additional research needs to be done, evidence regarding CAM has increased for certain therapies. It is important to note, however, that many of these studies are based on the testing of adults, not children or adolescents. One should be cautious when embarking on any new therapy or treatment.

The National Center for Complementary and Alternative Medicine, part of the National Institutes of Health, divides CAM into four major categories: biologically based (supplementing one's diet with nutrients, herbs, particular foods, or extracts), manipulative and body-based (using touch and manipulation such as chiropractic or massage therapy), mind/body (connecting the mind to the body and spirit in practices such as yoga and meditation), and energy therapies (aiming to restore balance to the body's energy with therapies such as qigong). Other whole, ancient, medical systems include traditional Chinese medicine, Ayurveda, homeopathic medicine, and naturopathic medicine.

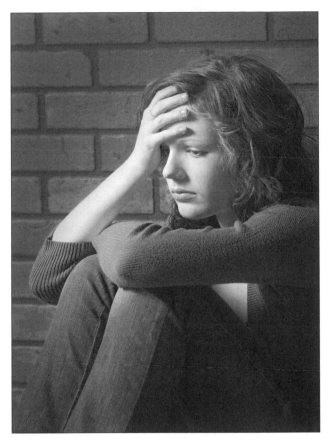

Mood disorders, depression, and anxiety are commonly seen in adolescence. (©Eric Simard/Dreamstime.com)

Common Health Issues

There are a number of issues that tend to arise during the teenage years, including eating disorders and concerns about sports performance; many of these issues continue into adulthood. CAM is one place to begin to address these issues. Other good starting points for optimum health during these years are proper nutrition, adequate rest, and good coping strategies.

Alternative therapies for eating disorders. Teenage girls and young women in middle and upper socioeconomic classes especially are affected by eating disorders. Cultural influences, such as the preoccupation with slimness and body image promoted in advertising, contribute to the preoccupation of girls and women with their looks and body size. Although there are no well-established natural treatments for eating disorders, some evidence exists that zinc supplements, when used in conjunction with conventional medical treatments, may help people with the eating disorder anorexia to gain weight. Improvements in the symptoms of bulimia, another eating disorder, have been shown in those girls and women who increase serotonin levels. In addition, the dietary supplement dehydroepiandrosterone (DHEA) provides help in protecting bone mass.

Alternative therapies for sports performance. There is some evidence that suggests creatine, one of the best-selling and best-documented supplements for enhancing athletic performance, has benefits for sports

Common Conditions Affecting Teenagers

Girls and Young Women

Acne
Asthma
Athlete's foot
Bladder infections
Canker sores
Cervical dysplasia
Cigarette addiction
Colds and flu
Depression
Dysmennorhea
Eating disorders
Endometriosis
Fatigue
Herpes

Immune function
Insomnia
Irritable bowel syndrome (IBS)
Migraine headaches
Minor injuries
Premenstrual syndrome (PMS)
Rosacea
Sports performance
Strep throat
Sunburn
Vaginal infections
Weight control

Boys and Young Men

Acne
Attention deficit disorder (ADD)
Athlete's foot
Canker sores
Cigarette addiction
Colds and flu
Fatigue
Herpes

Immune function
Insomnia
Minor injuries
Sports performance
Strep throat
Stress
Sunburn

performance. Overall, however, the benefits are slight and are limited to brief, intermittent, intense forms of exercise rather than including exercise that increases endurance. Creatine is a naturally occurring substance that plays an important role in the production of energy in the body. The body converts creatine to stored energy for muscles (phosphocreatine). It is thought that ingesting extra creatine will enhance the reserve of energy in the muscle tissue and help athletes to perform better. Supplemental creatine may also help the body make new phosphocreatine faster following intense physical activity. Caffeine, often included in creatine supplements, offsets the uptake and activity of creatine.

HERBAL AND NUTRITION THERAPIES

Surveys have indicated that 30 to 41 percent of adolescents report having used herbs and supplements. Teenagers commonly use herbal therapies for weight loss, depression, anxiety, respiratory illness, and athletic performance issues.

It is recommended that teenagers use caution when taking herbs or supplements, most of which have not been tested on adolescents. Herbalists may suggest taking one-half the adult dose. Many common herbs, such as ephedra, kava kava, lavender, monkshood, wormwood, deadly nightshade, foxglove, desert herb, star anise, lobelia, mistletoe, and Ayurvedic herbal remedies have been shown to be toxic to the cardiac and central nervous systems.

Teenagers should discuss with their doctors any alternative treatments being used or considered, because these alternatives may alter the effectiveness of traditional medication or pose other health threats. A national survey showed that 10 percent of adolescents reported using supplements at the same time as prescribed medication.

Adolescents commonly use home remedies such as

warm honey and lemon or special teas. Echinacea is also commonly used among adolescents for colds and flu. Double-blind, placebo-controlled studies enrolling more than one thousand people have found that various forms and species of echinacea can reduce the symptoms and duration of a common cold, in adults. It is thought that echinacea works by temporarily stimulating, strengthening, and nourishing the immune system. There is limited evidence, however, that this is the case, and other studies have not supported the claims. Although echinacea may stimulate the immune system temporarily, no evidence shows any benefit from long-term use.

As with all herbal medicine, the precise species and part or parts of the plant in question are key. There are three main species of echinacea: *E. purpurea*, *E. angustifolia*, and *E. pallida*. The flowers, leaves, and stems of *E. purpurea*, when used together, provide the best supporting evidence for benefits in treating colds and influenza. The root of *E. purpurea* has not been shown to be effective, while the root of *E. pallida* may be the active, and effective, part of that species.

Echinacea may be beneficial in reducing symptoms or halting a cold once those symptoms have started. However, echinacea does not appear to prevent colds. It may not be effective in children and adolescents and has not been studied in these populations. As with all herbal supplements, the actual dosing, potency, and quality of the over-the-counter product are not regulated or guaranteed.

Mood disorders, depression, and anxiety are commonly seen in adolescence. A national survey found that many teenagers report using St. John's wort, the most common CAM herbal treatment used for depression. Its effectiveness is unproven, and there are possible adverse effects in persons also using commonly prescribed medications (such as contraceptives and prescription antidepressants). A National Institutes of Health study showed that St. John's wort was not more effective than a placebo in treating major depression. A systematic review of research has shown, however, that the supplement may be beneficial in treating minor depression, as are synthetic antidepressants.

Taking a multivitamin regularly is a good place to start a healthy lifestyle and may enhance mood and vitality. B vitamins (including folate) help to metabolize tryptophan to serotonin, a mood stabilizer. Research has shown that many teenagers are vitamin D-deficient because of indoor lifestyles and inadequate consumption of food rich in vitamin D, such as fortified milk, eggs, and sardines.

Calcium, magnesium, chromium, zinc, and iron are also important minerals for mind and body health. Low levels of calcium and vitamin D are associated with depressive symptoms and premenstrual symptoms. Many youth do not meet their recommended intake for calcium (1,200 to 1,500 milligrams per day). Magnesium is also important for the metabolism of serotonin and may alleviate premenstrual mood changes.

Chromium is a dietary trace mineral that aids in sugar and fat metabolism and has been shown to alleviate depression in some persons. Chromium can be found in breads, cereals, fresh vegetables, meat, fish, and brewer's yeast. Zinc is found in nearly every cell in the body. Low zinc levels are associated with major depression. It is recommended that teenagers have 11 milligrams per day of zinc. Alcohol decreases the absorption of zinc.

Iron is key to energy metabolism and can affect mood and learning. Young women, particularly, should take in adequate amounts of iron to replace iron lost through menstruation.

A number of fatty acids (linoleic, eicosapentaenoic, and docosahexaenoic) found in fish oil have been associated with a protective effect from depression and suicide. Amino acids (L-tryptophan and S-adenosyl-L-methionine, or SAMe) have also been studied extensively and have been shown to fight depression.

MIND/BODY THERAPIES

The power of the mind to heal and bring about well-being has been demonstrated in self-reported quality-of-life measures. Strong evidence in the form of randomized controlled trials is lacking, however, in part because of the difficulty in devising placebo therapies and because of funding obstacles. Many practices, such as yoga, meditation, and Tai Chi, may help adolescents experience a sense of relaxation and help them cope with their individual stressors.

Stress changes the body's chemistry and releases cortisone into the bloodstream. It alters the balance of hormones that lower resistance to disease. As a result, teenagers can become more susceptible to colds, influenza, and other types of illness. Too much stress can bring on outbreaks of cold sores or genital herpes for adolescents who carry these viruses in their systems. Other chronic conditions, such as irritable bowel syndrome (IBS), asthma, inflammatory bowel disease (IBD), and rheumatoid arthritis may also flare up during times of stress.

Yoga emphasizes a healthy spine for a healthy body. Different poses and movements involving twist and balance are said to stimulate the nerves along the spine and promote circulation and the flow of energy. Many professional athletes practice some form of yoga for increased flexibility, and it is often incorporated into cross-training exercise routines.

Meditation is beneficial because it can be done anywhere and does not require equipment or much time. There are many books and Web sites that provide guidance on meditation for teenagers. To meditate, one needs only a quiet location, a comfortable position, and mental focus, or mantra. A 2007 government survey found that 1 percent of children, including adolescents (750,000 nationally), had used meditation as a form of therapy in the year before the survey. Another study showed that adolescents between the ages of twelve and nineteen with IBS were likely to engage in or consider meditation or prayer (or both) for symptom management. (Peppermint oil, probiotics, and acupuncture have been associated with symptom relief in persons with IBD or IBS as well.)

As with all physical and mental therapies, one should have proper expert guidance to avoid injury and should discuss plans to use CAM with a primary care doctor.

Deanna M. Neff, M.P.H.

FURTHER READING

American Academy of Pediatrics: Provisional Section for Complementary, Holistic, and Integrative Medicine. http://www.aap.org/sections/chim.

Cotton, S., et al. "Mind-Body Complementary Alternative Medicine Use and Quality of Life in Adolescents with Inflammatory Bowel Disease." *Inflammatory Bowel Disease* 16, no. 3 (2010): 501-506. Discussion of CAM therapies focused on adolescents affected by inflammatory bowel disease.

EBSCO Publishing. *Health Library: Adolescent Health.* Available through http://www.ebscohost.com. A comprehensive review of adolescent health topics.

Freeman, Lyn. *Mosby's Complementary and Alternative Medicine: A Research-Based Approach.* 3d ed. St. Louis, Mo.: Mosby/Elsevier, 2009. A comprehensive resource on CAM, from a research perspective.

Kemper, K., and P. Gardiner. "Herbal Medicines." In *Nelson Textbook of Pediatrics,* edited by Richard E. Behrman, Robert M. Kliegman, and Hal B. Jenson. 18th ed. Philadelphia: Saunders/Elsevier, 2007. A thorough chapter examining the use of herbal medicines for children and adolescents.

Kemper, K., and S. Shannon. "Complementary and Alternative Medicine Therapies to Promote Healthy Moods: Primary Care from Infancy to Adolescence." *Pediatric Clinics of North America* 54, no. 6 (2007). A look at CAM therapies for child and adolescent mental health.

Natural Medicines Comprehensive Database. http://www.naturaldatabase.com.

See also: Acne; Children's health; Compulsive overeating; Creatine; Dehydroepiandrosterone (DHEA); Depression, mild to moderate; Eating disorders; Herbal medicine; Mental health; Premenstrual syndrome (PMS); Sports and fitness support: Enhancing performance; Sports-related injuries: Homeopathic remedies.

Adrenal extract

CATEGORY: Herbs and supplements

RELATED TERM: Glandular extract (adrenal)

DEFINITION: Natural substance promoted as a dietary supplement for specific health benefits.

PRINCIPAL PROPOSED USES: Adrenal exhaustion, stress

OTHER PROPOSED USES: Allergies, asthma, fatigue, rheumatoid arthritis

OVERVIEW

The adrenal gland, an endocrine gland situated near the kidneys, is divided into two parts: the inner and outer. The inner portion (medulla) of the adrenal gland secretes epinephrine (adrenaline) and norepinephrine (adrenaline). The outer portion (the cortex) manufactures the hormones cortisone and aldosterone. All these hormones are necessary for life.

Adrenal extracts are made from the adrenal glands of cows, pigs, or other animals. According to a theory prevalent in alternative medicine, the consumption of adrenal extracts can strengthen the function of an underperforming or exhausted adrenal gland. How-

COMPLEMENTARY AND ALTERNATIVE MEDICINE

ever, there is no scientific evidence to support this belief and no rational justification to indicate that it might be true.

Early in the twentieth century, physicians used glandular extracts as an actual source of hormones. For example, extracts of ovaries were used to supply female hormones such as progesterone. Similarly, animal adrenal glands may contain significant levels of adrenal hormones. This is the basis for some of the recommended uses of adrenal extracts, such as allergies, asthma, and rheumatoid arthritis (conditions that respond to cortisone). However, modern adrenal extracts are manufactured in such a way that they do not contain significant levels of adrenal hormones. Therefore, it is difficult to find any justification for their use along these lines.

USES AND APPLICATIONS

Some manufacturers of glandular products claim that the animal version of an organ provides nutrients that support the corresponding organ in humans. However, there is no evidence that the human adrenal gland requires any nutrients that are uniquely available in animal adrenals.

SCIENTIFIC EVIDENCE

It has been suggested by one manufacturer of glandular products that consuming extracts of an organ might offer immune-related benefits. According to this theory, some people may possess antibodies to some of their own glands; the consumption of an animal version of the gland will divert these antibodies from their target. However, this explanation does not make much sense. Antibodies are primarily produced against proteins, and even if cow adrenal glands had the same proteins as human adrenal glands, which is unlikely, proteins are not absorbed whole into the bloodstream.

It may be that, on an unconscious level, those who recommend glandular extracts are being influenced by the ancient notion of "sympathetic magic," the idea that eating a lion's heart, for example, will create courage. However, this is a prescientific form of thinking that is difficult to take seriously in the modern era.

Not only is the proposed action of adrenal glandular extracts questionable, their primary proposed purpose for use is questionable too. Adrenal glandular extracts are most often recommended for the treatment of a purported condition called adrenal exhaustion. In adrenal exhaustion, the adrenal glands are supposedly weakened by the chronic stresses of modern life and incapable of performing at full capacity. However, there is no scientific basis for believing this to be true. The notion of adrenal exhaustion developed as a result of studies done in the mid-twentieth century that involved extreme, life-threatening stress; the studies do not support the existence of a milder, common adrenal fatigue. (Even if adrenal fatigue did exist, there is no scientific reason to think that adrenal extracts would help.)

Finally, there are no meaningful scientific studies that have found benefit with adrenal gland extracts in their modern, nonhormonal form. Only double-blind, placebo-controlled studies can show a treatment effective, and none have been reported for adrenal extracts.

EBSCO CAM Review Board

FURTHER READING

Sneader, Walter. "Adrenal Cortex Hormones." In *Drug Discovery: A History*. Hoboken, N.J.: Wiley, 2005.
WebMD. "Adrenal Extract." Available at http://www.webmd.com/vitamins-supplements/default.aspx.

See also: Allergies; Asthma; Chronic fatigue syndrome; Fatigue; Rheumatoid arthritis; Spleen extract; Stress; Thymus extract; Thyroid hormone.

Aging

CATEGORY: Issues and overviews
RELATED TERMS: Life extension, seniors' health
DEFINITION: Complementary and alternative treatments that focus on the aging process and on the health of the elderly.

OVERVIEW

Marginal nutritional deficiencies occur more often in older people. For this reason, many elderly persons could benefit from enhancing nutrition.

Some proponents of alternative medicine advocate products and treatments for the purpose of life extension. Despite some promising results in test tube and other preliminary studies, however, no meaningful evidence shows that alternative treatment can prolong life. Numerous natural supplements have been

Aging and the Brain

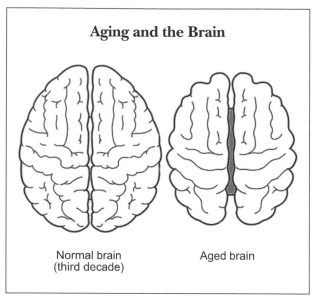

Normal brain
(third decade)   Aged brain

The human brain shrinks with age as nerve cells are lost and brain tissue atrophies.

promoted as fountains of youth for the elderly and are said to enhance life in multiple ways and to restore youthful levels of energy, well-being, and mental function. No evidence indicates that any of these supplements are effective. One widely advocated hormone, dehydroepiandrosterone (DHEA), has been shown ineffective for this purpose.

TREATMENTS

A study published in 1990 created hopes that the human growth hormone (somatotropin, or HGH) could increase strength and reverse many symptoms of aging in men. However, subsequent evidence suggests that HGH is not useful for this purpose. In any case, despite widespread marketing, HGH cannot be successfully used as an oral supplement because it is destroyed by stomach acid. (In the positive trial, HGH was administered intravenously.) Various amino acids and other supplements are marketed as HGH-releasers on the premise that they cause the body to increase HGH production. However, there is no reliable

Natural Treatments for Specific Conditions

Even though natural treatments have not proven helpful for fighting the effects of aging in general, they have shown considerable promise for treating specific health conditions of relevance to older persons. Some of these possible applications are listed here.

In Women
Aging skin
Alzheimer's disease and related conditions
Back pain
Cancer prevention
Cancer treatment
Cataracts
Diverticular disease
Fatigue
General well-being
Heart attack
Heart disease prevention
Immune support
Insomnia
Macular degeneration
Memory and mental function
Menopausal symptoms
Osteoarthritis
Osteoporosis
Sciatica
Sexual dysfunction
Varicose veins

In Men
Aging skin
Alzheimer's disease and related conditions
Back pain
Cancer prevention
Cancer treatment
Cataracts
Diverticular disease
Fatigue
General well-being
Heart attack
Heart disease prevention
Immune support
Insomnia
Macular degeneration
Memory and mental function
Osteoarthritis
Prostate cancer
Prostate enlargement
Sciatica
Sexual dysfunction

evidence that they actually do so to any meaningful extent; because HGH itself is no fountain of youth, this potential effect is of little significance.

Anabolic hormones have also failed to prove useful for enhancing strength in older people. The supplements creatine and hydroxymethyl butyrate have shown some promise for this purpose, but the evidence for benefit remains weak.

One natural approach is guaranteed to enhance strength in seniors: exercise. Increasing exercise is one of the most health-positive steps available for people of any age.

Some evidence suggests that vitamin D supplements may improve balance (technically, reduce body sway) in frail seniors and, thereby, help prevent falls. However, not all studies have found benefits.

SAFETY CONCERNS

Many people implicitly believe that "natural" means "safe." However, there is no scientific reason to believe that this should be the case. Many conventional drugs are safe, while some herbs and supplements present real safety risks. Perhaps the biggest issue of concern here is the interaction between natural supplements and conventional medications.

EBSCO CAM Review Board

FURTHER READING

Chrusch, M. J., et al. "Creatine Supplementation Combined with Resistance Training in Older Men." *Medicine and Science in Sports and Exercise* 33 (2001): 2111-2117.

Gotshalk, L. A., et al. "Creatine Supplementation Improves Muscular Performance in Older Men." *Medicine and Science in Sports and Exercise* 34 (2002): 537-543.

Janssen, H. C., M. M. Samson, and H. J. Verhaar. "Vitamin D Deficiency, Muscle Function, and Falls in Elderly People." *American Journal of Clinical Nutrition* 75 (2002): 611-615.

Latham, N. K., et al. "A Randomized, Controlled Trial of Quadriceps Resistance Exercise and Vitamin D in Frail Older People: The Frailty Interventions Trial in Elderly Subjects (FITNESS)." *Journal of the American Geriatrics Society* 51 (2003): 291-299.

Percheron, G., et al. "Effect of One-Year Oral Administration of Dehydroepiandrosterone to Sixty- to Eighty-Year-Old Individuals on Muscle Function
and Cross-sectional Area." *Archives of Internal Medicine* 163 (2003): 720-727.

Pfeifer, M., et al. "Effects of a Short-Term Vitamin D and Calcium Supplementation on Body Sway and Secondary Hyperparathyroidism in Elderly Women." *Journal of Bone and Mineral Research* 15 (2000): 1113-1118.

Van Niekerk, J. K., F. A. Huppert, and J. Herbert. "Salivary Cortisol and DHEA: Association with Measures of Cognition and Well-Being in Normal Older Men and Effects of Three Months of DHEA Supplementation." *Psychoneuroendocrinology* 26 (2001): 591-612.

Vance, M. L. "Can Growth Hormone Prevent Aging?" *New England Journal of Medicine* 348 (2003): 779-780.

Wiroth, J. B., et al. "Effects of Oral Creatine Supplementation on Maximal Pedalling Performance in Older Adults." *European Journal of Applied Physiology* 84 (2001): 533-539.

See also: Elder health; Vitamins and minerals.

Alcoholism

CATEGORY: Condition

RELATED TERMS: Alcohol addiction, alcohol dependency

DEFINITION: Treatment of addiction to alcoholic beverages.

PRINCIPAL PROPOSED NATURAL TREATMENTS: General nutritional support, milk thistle, S-adenosylmethionine

OTHER PROPOSED NATURAL TREATMENTS: Acupuncture, honey, kudzu, passionflower, phosphatidylcholine, prickly pear cactus (*Opuntia ficus indica*), trimethylglycine

HERBS AND SUPPLEMENTS TO AVOID: Arginine; beta-carotene (excessive doses); kava; kombucha; prepackaged Chinese herbal combinations; vitamin A (excessive doses); white willow

INTRODUCTION

Alcoholic beverages present a perfect example of the ancient virtue of moderation. While small amounts of alcohol (the equivalent of one to two drinks daily) may actually enhance health, excessive consumption of alcohol wreaks gradual havoc throughout the entire body. The liver is often the first organ to show injury, followed by (in no set order) the brain, circulatory system, pancreas, stomach, and throat.

Conventional treatment of alcoholism involves nutritional support and various means to induce and maintain abstinence. The program Alcoholics Anonymous is the most effective known abstinence-promoting method, but other programs and techniques are also in use. The drugs acamprosate (Campral) and naltrexone (ReVia) have shown considerable promise. It is not clear whether disulfiram (Antabuse) actually offers any benefit.

PRINCIPAL PROPOSED NATURAL TREATMENTS

The herb milk thistle and the supplement S-adenosylmethionine (SAMe) have been recommended for protecting the liver from alcohol-induced damage. However, none of these treatments have been conclusively proven effective; abstinence have proven more effective than any treatment.

In addition to damaging the liver, alcoholism causes a general depletion of nutrients. People who drink to excess (either because they have not quit drinking or because they are in the process of quitting) may benefit from supplementation.

Milk thistle. Numerous double-blind, placebo-controlled studies enrolling several hundred people have evaluated whether milk thistle can successfully counter alcohol-induced liver damage. Most of the studies, however, were flawed in design and reporting, and their results were less than consistent. A 2007 review of published and unpublished studies on milk thistle as a treatment for liver disease concluded that benefits were seen only in low-quality trials, and even in these trials, milk thistle did not show more than a slight benefit. A subsequent 2008 review of nineteen randomized trials drew a similar conclusion for alcoholic liver disease generally, although it did find a modest reduction in mortality for persons with severe liver cirrhosis. It is not possible to draw firm conclusions about milk thistle's usefulness for people who consume too much alcohol.

SAMe. The supplement SAMe has been proposed for the treatment of alcoholic liver disease, but there is no meaningful evidence that it is effective. A two-year, double-blind, placebo-controlled study of 117 people with alcoholic liver cirrhosis found that treatment with SAMe reduced mortality or the need for a liver transplant (or both) in those with less advanced disease but not in the group as a whole.

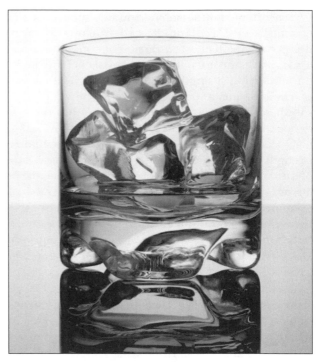

Alcohol has been linked to several cancers, although a direct causal relationship has not been established. (PhotoDisc)

Nutritional support. Chronic overconsumption of alcohol may lead to improper metabolism or outright deficiencies of numerous vitamins and minerals. For this reason, the use of a general nutritional supplement may be advisable.

OTHER PROPOSED NATURAL TREATMENTS

In a double-blind study of sixty-four people, the use of an extract made from the skin of the fruit of the prickly pear cactus *Opuntia ficus indica* significantly reduced hangover symptoms compared with placebo. The greatest improvements were seen in symptoms of nausea, loss of appetite, and dry mouth. Overall, the rate of severe hangover symptoms was 50 percent lower in the treatment group compared with the placebo group. The researchers involved in this study hypothesized that hangovers are caused by inflammation and that the herb reduced inflammation.

Artichoke leaf is much better known than prickly pear cactus as a means of preventing hangover symptoms. However, the one double-blind study on the subject failed to find artichoke any more effective than placebo.

The supplement trimethylglycine stimulates the formation of SAMe and might be helpful for alcoholic liver disease. However, no meaningful double-blind, placebo-controlled clinical trials have been reported.

The supplement phosphatidylcholine has been advocated as a treatment for early alcohol-related liver damage (especially fatty liver), but the results of preliminary studies have been inconsistent. One study in baboons even found evidence of increased liver toxicity.

Other herbs and supplements that have been proposed for protecting the liver, but only on the basis of extremely weak evidence, include andrographis, barberry, beet leaf, boldo, dandelion, inositol, licorice, lipoic acid, liver extracts, N-acetylcysteine, *Picrorhiza kurroa*, schisandra, taurine, thymus extract, and turmeric.

The herb kudzu has been widely advocated as an aid for quitting alcohol, based on studies using hamsters or rats. However, small double-blind studies in humans have yielded inconsistent results.

Acupuncture has also been proposed as an aid to alcohol withdrawal. However, study results have been contradictory, and the largest trial failed to find any benefit. This three-week, single-blind trial study of 503 alcoholics failed to find any difference between actual ear acupuncture and placebo ear acupuncture. In addition, a ten-week, single-blind, placebo-controlled study of 72 alcoholics found no difference in drinking patterns or cravings between sham acupuncture and real acupuncture groups. Negative results were also seen in a similar trial of 56 participants, and in 1 of 48 people. A study of 109 people compared acupuncture with aromatherapy (intended by these researchers as a placebo) and failed to find that acupuncture was more effective. However, a single-blind trial of 54 people did find acupuncture more effective than placebo, as did a single-blind trial of 80 people.

The herb passionflower has been proposed as an aid to alcohol withdrawal, primarily on the basis of the study of people addicted to opiates. Another study suggests that honey consumption might increase the body's ability to metabolize alcohol, thereby limiting intoxication and more rapidly reducing blood alcohol levels to a safer (or legal) zone.

Herbs and Supplements to Avoid

High doses of the supplements beta-carotene and vitamin A might cause alcoholic liver disease to develop more rapidly in people who abuse alcohol. Nutritional supplementation at the standard daily requirement level should not cause a problem.

All forms of vitamin B_3, including niacin, niacinamide (nicotinamide), and inositol hexaniacinate, may damage the liver when taken in high doses. Again, nutritional supplementation at the standard daily requirement level should not cause a problem.

One animal study suggests that the herb kava may have value as an aid to alcohol withdrawal. However, people who abuse alcohol should probably not take kava; even in healthy people, the herb has caused severe liver damage.

Numerous herbs and supplements have known or suspected liver-toxic properties, including barberry, borage, chaparral, coltsfoot, comfrey, germander, germanium (a mineral), greater celandine, kombucha, mistletoe, noni, pennyroyal, pokeroot, sassafras, and various herbs and minerals used in traditional Chinese herbal medicine. In addition, herbs that are not liver-toxic in themselves are sometimes adulterated with other herbs of similar appearance accidentally harvested in a misapprehension of their identity (for example, germander found in skullcap products). Other forms of contamination also are possible. Blue-green algae species, such as spirulina, may at times be contaminated with liver-toxic substances called microcystins (for which no highest safe level is known).

Some articles claim that the herb echinacea is potentially liver-toxic, but this concern appears to have been based on a misunderstanding of its constituents. (Echinacea contains substances in the pyrrolizidine alkaloid family. However, while many pyrrolizidine alkaloids are liver toxic, those found in echinacea are not believed to have that property.)

Whole valerian contains liver-toxic substances called valepotriates. However, valepotriates are thought to be absent from most commercial valerian products, and case reports suggest that even very high doses of valerian do not harm the liver. Herbs and supplements with the potential to irritate the stomach, such as white willow and arginine, should be used only with caution by people who consume excessive alcohol.

EBSCO CAM Review Board

Further Reading

Akhondzadeh, S., et al. "Passionflower in the Treatment of Opiates Withdrawal." *Journal of Clinical Pharmacy and Therapeutics* 26 (2001): 369-373.

Bullock, M. L., et al. "A Large, Randomized, Placebo-Controlled Study of Auricular Acupuncture for Alcohol Dependence." *Journal of Substance Abuse Treatment* 22 (2002): 71-77.

Keung, W. M., and B. L. Vallee. "Kudzu Root: An Ancient Chinese Source of Modern Antidipsotropic Agents." *Phytochemistry* 47 (1998): 499-506.

Kunz, S., et al. "Ear Acupuncture for Alcohol Withdrawal in Comparison with Aromatherapy." *Alcoholism: Clinical and Experimental Research* 31 (2007): 436-442.

Lukas, S. E., et al. "An Extract of the Chinese Herbal Root Kudzu Reduces Alcohol Drinking by Heavy Drinkers in a Naturalistic Setting." *Alcoholism: Clinical and Experimental Research* 29 (2005): 756-762.

O'Keefe, J. H., K. A. Bybee, and C. J. Lavie. "Alcohol and Cardiovascular Health: The Razor-Sharp Double-Edged Sword." *Journal of the American College of Cardiology* 50 (2007): 1009-1014.

Onyesom, I. "Honey-Induced Stimulation of Blood Ethanol Elimination and Its Influence on Serum Triacylglycerol and Blood Pressure in Man." *Annals of Nutrition and Metabolism* 49 (2005): 319-324.

Pittler, M. H., et al. "Effectiveness of Artichoke Extract in Preventing Alcohol-Induced Hangovers." *Canadian Medical Association Journal* 169 (2003): 1269-1273.

Rambaldi, A., and C. Gluud. "S-adenosyl-L-methionine for Alcoholic Liver Diseases." *Cochrane Database of Systematic Reviews* (2001): CD002235. Available through *EBSCO DynaMed Systematic Literature Surveillance* at http://www.ebscohost.com/dynamed.

Rambaldi, A., B. Jacobs, and C. Gluud. "Milk Thistle for Alcoholic and/or Hepatitis B or C Virus Liver Diseases." *Cochrane Database of Systematic Reviews* (2007): CD003620. Available through *EBSCO DynaMed Systematic Literature Surveillance* at http://www.ebscohost.com/dynamed.

Saller, R., et al. "An Updated Systematic Review with Meta-analysis for the Clinical Evidence of Silymarin." *Forschende Komplementärmedizin* 15 (2008): 9-20.

Shebek, J., and J. P. Rindone. "A Pilot Study Exploring the Effect of Kudzu Root on the Drinking Habits of Patients with Chronic Alcoholism." *Journal of Alternative and Complementary Medicine* 6 (2000): 45-48.

Trumpler, F., et al. "Acupuncture for Alcohol Withdrawal." *Alcohol and Alcoholism* 38 (2003): 369-375.

Wiese, J., et al. "Effect of *Opuntia ficus indica* on Symptoms of the Alcohol Hangover." *Archives of Internal Medicine* 164 (2004): 1334-1340.

See also: Alcoholism; Beta-carotene; Cirrhosis; Milk thistle; SAMe; Vitamin A.

Alexander technique

CATEGORY: Therapies and techniques
DEFINITION: An alternative therapy that is focused on improving a person's posture and movement.
PRINCIPAL PROPOSED USES: Improved posture, pain relief, stress elimination

OVERVIEW

The Alexander technique (AT) is a system of body alignment, movement, and thought that was developed in the early twentieth century. The technique focuses on posture, poise, breathing, body awareness, efficiency of movement, and elegance of stride. AT is used extensively by singers, musicians, and actors.

The technique was developed Frederick Matthias Alexander, a Shakespearean actor and orator whose chronic hoarseness had threatened to derail his career. Doctors could do nothing to help him, but, determined not to give up, he tried to discover the cause of his chronic voice problems by observing himself in a mirror as he spoke in his stage voice. What he saw was poor body alignment: His head was pulled back, his neck muscles were tensed, and his breathing was awkward and gasping. In effect, his larynx had been compressed by the extreme tension in his neck muscles.

Alexander knew that changing his posture would not be easy. Just thinking that he was about to speak would cause his neck muscles to tense. He ended up using a sort of reverse psychology to retrain his body. "Don't speak," he would tell himself, noticing a release of tension in his neck. His retraining would become the Alexander technique. AT, as it is still taught, is not only about posture and movement but also about mind and thought.

MECHANISM OF ACTION

Students of AT will typically meet individually with a teacher for 20 to 30 minutes, once each week. Lessons are hands-on, with the instructor gently guiding the student to lengthen and widen the body through gentle pressure. Particular attention is paid to the neck and head. The neck should be loose, with the head forward and raised. The shoulders should be lowered ("untensed") and raised. Each session typically includes time to sit, to stand, and then to lie on a treatment table with one's head resting lightly on a book; the knees are bent. A lesson will also include specific training for the particular body movement that brought the student to the class (breathing and vocalizing, for instance, for a student who is a singer). Lessons are usually repeated weekly for several months or several years.

USES AND APPLICATIONS

Those seeking the technique may range from violinists experiencing intermittent shoulder pain, to office workers who have upper back and neck problems from extended computer use, to overweight persons who feel pain in their hips after walking as little as one block. AT instructors are careful to refer to their clients as "students," not as "patients," even though the majority of people who seek out lessons are suffering either from specific aches or pains or from generalized physical symptoms associated with stress and could, thus, be considered medical "patients."

AT is widely accepted in Europe, especially in England, where Alexander lived and taught. In all countries, the technique is especially popular among performers. Many music schools, including that at the prestigious Juilliard School in New York City, have certified AT instructors as faculty. It is not surprising that actors, such as Alexander himself, frequently practice AT. Famous actors who are said to have studied the Alexander technique include Paul Newman, Kevin Kline, Mary Steenburgen, Ralph Fiennes, John Cleese, and William Hurt. Another person who studied and practiced AT long-term was American philosopher-educator John Dewey.

SCIENTIFIC EVIDENCE

No scientific studies of the Alexander technique have been conducted.

SAFETY ISSUES

No known safety concerns are associated with the Alexander technique.

Cathy Frisinger, M.P.H.

FURTHER READING

American Society for the Alexander Technique. http://www.amsatonline.org.

Bloch, Michael. *F. M: The Life of Frederick Matthias Alexander, Founder of the Alexander Technique.* Boston: Little, Brown, 2004.

Vineyard, Missy. *How You Stand, How You Move, How You Live: Learning the Alexander Technique to Explore Your Mind-Body Connection and Achieve Self-Mastery.* New York: Marlowe, 2007.

See also: Acupressure; Acupuncture; Applied kinesiology; Aston-Patterning; Back pain; Dance movement therapy; Feldenkrais method; Manipulative and body-based practices; Meridians; Metamorphic technique; Mind/body medicine; Neck pain; Pain management; Progressive muscle relaxation; Qigong; Reflexology; Relaxation therapies; Rolfing; Shiatsu; Soft tissue pain; Tai Chi; Therapeutic touch.

Alfalfa

CATEGORY: Functional foods
RELATED TERMS: Alfalfa seeds, alfalfa sprouts, *Medicago sativa*
DEFINITION: Natural plant product consumed as a nutritional and dietary supplement for specific health benefits.
PRINCIPAL PROPOSED USE: Nutritional support
OTHER PROPOSED USES: Allergies, diabetes, lowering cholesterol, menopausal symptoms

OVERVIEW

Alfalfa is one of the earliest cultivated plants, used for centuries for feeding livestock. The plant is easy to grow, thrives in many varied climates throughout the world, and provides an excellent protein-rich food source for cattle, horses, sheep, and other animals. The name "alfalfa" comes from the Arabic *al-fac-facah*, meaning "father of all foods." Its high protein content and abundant stores of vitamins make it a good nutritional source for humans too. Historical (but undocumented) medicinal uses of alfalfa include treatment of stomach upset, arthritis, bladder and kidney problems, boils, and irregular menstruation.

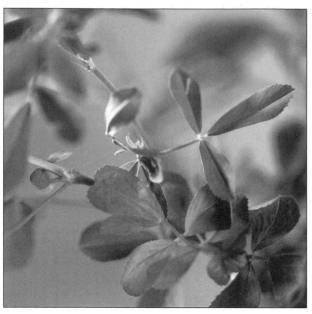

Pills containing alfalfa leaves or seeds are sold in pharmacies and health-food stores. (Cristina Pedrazzini/Photo Researchers, Inc.)

REQUIREMENTS AND SOURCES

Alfalfa sprouts appear in many salad bars and in the produce section of grocery stores. Bulk powdered herb or capsules and tablets containing alfalfa leaves or seeds are available in pharmacies and health-food stores.

THERAPEUTIC DOSAGES

A typical dose of alfalfa for tea is one to two teaspoons per cup, steeped in boiling water for ten to twenty minutes. Tablets and capsules of whole alfalfa or alfalfa extracts should be taken according to the manufacturer's recommendations. Certain products are said to be free of canavanine and other potentially harmful constituents; these products may be preferable.

THERAPEUTIC USES

Alfalfa is high in vitamin content. It provides beta-carotene, various B vitamins, and vitamins C, E, and K, and it can be used as a nutritional supplement. However, high doses of alfalfa may present some health risks.

Numerous animal studies and preliminary human trials indicate that extracts from alfalfa seeds, leaves, and roots might be helpful for lowering cholesterol levels. However, there exist no well-designed, double-blind, placebo-controlled trials demonstrating alfalfa is useful for this (or any other) purpose.

Studies using mice to investigate alfalfa's traditional use for diabetes found that it improved some symptoms. Alfalfa also has been investigated in the laboratory (but not evaluated in people) as a source of plant estrogens, which might make it helpful for menopause. Alfalfa may also have some use in fighting fungi. Rats fed a disease-causing fungus were able to eliminate more of the fungus from their systems when fed a diet high in alfalfa. It has been suggested that one of the saponins from alfalfa causes damage to the cell membranes of fungi. Finally, alfalfa has been proposed as a treatment for hay fever, but there is no scientific evidence that it is helpful for this purpose.

SAFETY ISSUES

Alfalfa, in its various forms, may present some health risks. Powdered alfalfa herb, alfalfa sprouts, and alfalfa seeds all contain L-cavanine, a substance that may cause abnormal blood-cell counts, spleen enlargement, or recurrence of lupus in persons with controlled disease. However, heating alfalfa may correct this problem.

Researchers investigating alfalfa seeds' ability to lower cholesterol levels discovered that it had another effect on the lab animals used for testing. In some of the monkeys, alfalfa seeds caused a disease very similar to lupus. Further research on this effect revealed that monkeys that had abnormal blood-cell counts when eating either alfalfa seeds or sprouts, and then recovered when alfalfa was no longer part of their diet, developed the symptoms again when given an isolated component of alfalfa called L-canavanine. Alfalfa seeds and sprouts have a higher concentration of L-canavanine than the leaves or roots.

In a clinical trial of alfalfa seeds for lowering cholesterol involving only three human volunteers, one man who participated developed pancytopenia (an abnormally low number of all of the various types of blood cells) and enlargement of the spleen. Additionally, there are two published case reports of persons, who had lupus that was controlled with drug therapy, suffering relapses after consuming alfalfa tablets. Again, L-canavanine is thought to be responsible for these effects.

When alfalfa seeds were autoclaved (heated to extremely high temperatures) and fed to monkeys for one year, no ill effects were seen, and the monkeys' cholesterol levels decreased. It may be that the L-canavanine can be destroyed by extreme heat, while the saponins that seem to be responsible for the beneficial effects of alfalfa remain intact. If so, a heat-treated product might prove safe.

It seems prudent that people who have been diagnosed with lupus, or those who suspect a predisposition to it based on family history, should probably avoid alfalfa. This includes the tablets used for supplements and the sprouts on the salad bar.

Because of the estrogenic effects of some of alfalfa's components, alfalfa is not recommended for pregnant or nursing women or young children. In addition, the high vitamin K content in alfalfa could, in theory, make the drug warfarin (Coumadin) less effective.

Finally, a number of cases of food poisoning have been documented from fresh sprouts infected with bacteria that was present on the seeds before germination. Sprouts can appear fresh and yet host enough bacteria to cause illness in people who eat them. Some health care workers recommend that those at higher risk for such infections, such as young children, those with chronic diseases, and the elderly, should avoid eating sprouts altogether.

IMPORTANT INTERACTIONS

Persons taking warfarin should note that the high vitamin K content of alfalfa might make warfarin less effective.

EBSCO CAM Review Board

FURTHER READING

Akaogi, J., et al. "Role of Non-protein Amino Acid L-canavanine in Autoimmunity." *Autoimmunity Reviews* 5 (2006): 429-435.

Colodny, L. R., A. Montgomery, and M. Houston. "The Role of Esterin Processed Alfalfa Saponins in Reducing Cholesterol." *Journal of the American Nutraceutical Association* 3 (2001): 6-15.

Inami, G. B., and S. E. Moler. "Detection and Isolation of *Salmonella* from Naturally Contaminated Alfalfa Seeds Following an Outbreak Investigation." *Journal of Food Protection* 62 (1999): 662-664.

Loui, C., et al. "Bacterial Communities Associated with Retail Alfalfa Sprouts." *Journal of Food Protection* 71 (2008): 200-204.

Van Beneden, C. A., et al. "Multinational Outbreak of *Salmonella enterica* Serotype Newport Infections Due to Contaminated Alfalfa Sprouts." *Journal of the American Medical Association* 13 (1999): 158-162.

See also: Allergies; Cholesterol, high; Diabetes; Menopause.

Allergies

CATEGORY: Condition

RELATED TERMS: Respiratory allergies, allergic conjunctivitis, allergic pharyngitis, allergic rhinitis, allergic sinusitis, hay fever, perennial rhinitis, pollen allergy, seasonal allergy

DEFINITION: Treatment for an allergic reaction best known as hay fever.

PRINCIPAL PROPOSED NATURAL TREATMENTS: Butterbur, sublingual immunotherapy

OTHER PROPOSED NATURAL TREATMENTS: Acupuncture, adrenal extract, antioxidants, Ayurvedic medicine, *Bacopa monniera* (brahmi), barberry, bee pollen, betaine hydrochloride, cat's claw, *Coleus forskohlii*, conjugated linoleic acid, enzyme potentiated desensitization, fish oil, gamma-linolenic acid, hops, hypnosis, methyl sulfonyl methane, nettle leaf, oligomeric proanthocyanidins, other flavonoids, including citrus bioflavonoids, probiotics, quercetin, rosmarinic acid/*Perilla frutescens*, royal jelly, soy sauce extract, spirulina, *Tinospora cordifolia*, topical capsaicin, traditional Chinese medicine, vitamin B_6, vitamin B_{12}, vitamin C, vitamin E

INTRODUCTION

About 7 percent of all Americans have hay fever, an allergic condition that can cause runny nose, sneezing, and teary eyes. It is known officially as allergic rhinitis, allergic sinusitis, or allergic conjunctivitis, depending on whether symptoms manifest mainly in the nose, sinuses, or eyes, respectively. Hay fever usually peaks when particular plants are pollinating or when molds are flourishing. People who have year-round hay fever (perennial rhinitis) may be allergic to persistent allergens in the environment coming from such sources as dust mites, mice, and cockroaches.

In response to the foregoing triggers, a person prone to allergies develops an exaggerated immune

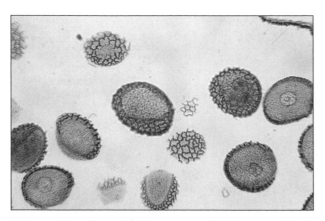

Microscopic pollens, which are responsible for many allergic reactions. (PhotoDisc)

response. Substances known as IgEs flood the nasal passages; white blood cells called eosinophils arrive by the millions and billions; and inflammatory substances such as histamine, prostaglandins, and leukotrienes are released in massive amounts. The overall effect is the familiar one of swelling, dripping, itching, and aching.

The mechanism of allergic response is fairly well understood. Why allergic people react so excessively to innocent bits of pollen, however, remains a complete mystery.

Conventional treatment for hay fever primarily involves nonsedating antihistamines and nasal steroids and is usually quite effective.

PRINCIPAL PROPOSED NATURAL TREATMENTS

The herb butterbur is best known as a promising new treatment for migraine headaches. However, butterbur may also be helpful for allergic rhinitis.

In a two-week, double-blind, placebo-controlled study of 186 people with intermittent allergic rhinitis, the use of butterbur at a dose of three standardized tablets daily, or one tablet daily, reduced allergy symptoms compared with placebo. Significantly greater benefits were seen in the higher dose group. Such "dose dependency" is taken as a confirming sign that a treatment really works.

In another double-blind study, 330 people were given either butterbur extract (one tablet three times daily), the antihistamine fexofenadine (Allegra), or placebo. The results showed that butterbur and fexofenadine were equally effective, and both were more effective than placebo.

A two-week double-blind (and earlier) study of 125 persons with hay fever (technically, seasonal allergic rhinitis) compared a standardized butterbur extract with the antihistamine drug cetirizine. According to ratings by both doctors and patients, the two treatments proved about equally effective. This study did not use a placebo group. Two much smaller studies produced inconsistent results.

An alternative to allergy shots known as sublingual immunotherapy (SLIT) involves using allergenic substances placed under the tongue. Numerous double-blind, placebo-controlled studies indicate that SLIT can improve all major symptoms of allergic rhinitis when the offending allergens are known. However, in a 2008 comprehensive review of SLIT for grass pollen and house dust mite allergies, researchers raised questions regarding the quality and consistency of these and other studies.

If SLIT is effective, it may require two to three years for significant benefit to develop. One placebo-controlled study found that three years of treatment was more effective than two years. In addition, to provide benefits for grass allergy season, SLIT must be started at least eight weeks before the onset of the grass allergy season; even longer lead times lead to even better results. Putting all this evidence together, it appears that SLIT may work best if used year round, and year after year.

One study suggests that SLIT is not only effective for treating allergy but also effective in preventing the development of new allergies or mild persistent asthma in children with allergic rhinitis or intermittent asthma.

While SLIT is fairly well accepted in conventional medicine, another form of alternative allergy shots remains firmly in the alternative medicine field: enzyme potentiated desensitisation (EPD). This method involves injections of allergens combined with certain enzymes. In one double-blind, placebo-controlled study, EPD failed to prove more helpful than placebo for seasonal allergic rhinitis.

OTHER PROPOSED NATURAL TREATMENTS

Several natural products have shown potential benefit for allergic rhinitis in one or more preliminary controlled trials. These include a water-extract of hops, a freeze-dried extract of stinging nettle, various probiotics, an extract of soy sauce (Shoyu polysaccharides), the herbs *Tinospora cordifolia* and *Astragalus*

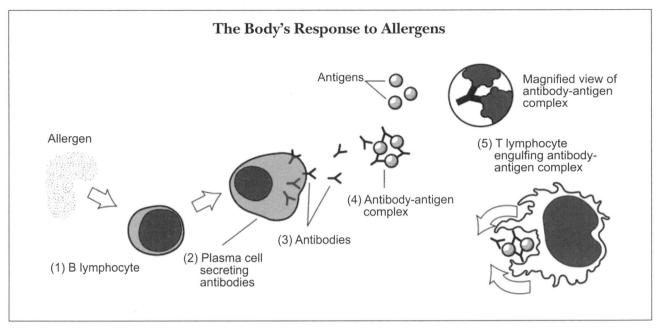

The Body's Response to Allergens

An allergic reaction is caused when foreign materials, or antigens, enter the immune system, which produces B lymphocytes (1) that cause blood plasma cells to secrete antibodies (2). The antibodies (3) link with antigens to form antigen-antibody complexes (4), which then are engulfed and destroyed by a T lymphocyte (5).

membranaceus, rosmarinic acid (a substance found in rosemary and other herbs, including *Perilla frutescens*), and an Ayurvedic herbal formula containing *Commiphora mukul, T. cordifolia, Rubia cordifolia, Emblica officinalis, Moringa pterygosperma,* and *Glycyrrhiza glabra.*

Traditional Chinese herbal medicine also has shown some promise for allergies. Another traditional Chinese treatment, acupuncture, is commonly recommended for allergies, but a controlled trial of forty people failed to find significantly more benefit with real acupuncture than with fake acupuncture. However, another study found benefit with real acupuncture plus real traditional Chinese herbs as opposed to placebo acupuncture and nonspecific Chinese herbs. A carefully conducted review of seven placebo-controlled trials failed to find convincing evidence for acupuncture's effectiveness against allergic rhinitis.

One rather unusual study tested a nasal spray containing capsaicin, the "hot" in cayenne and other hot peppers. It is not clear how practical this spray would be (researchers had to use local anesthetic in the nose before administering the spray).

Preliminary evidence suggests that spirulina may counter allergic reactions of the type involved in hay fever. A sizable (112-participant) double-blind study of vitamin E at a dose of 800 milligrams daily for hay fever found modest benefits at best. A smaller study failed to find any benefits.

A twelve-week, double-blind, placebo-controlled study of forty people tested the supplement conjugated linoleic acid as a treatment for people with allergies to birch pollen and found some evidence of benefit. Vitamin C is often suggested as a treatment for allergies, but the research results are preliminary and somewhat contradictory.

Test tube studies suggest that flavonoids (biologically active compounds found in many plants) may help reduce allergy symptoms. A particular flavonoid, quercetin, seems to be one of the most active. Many texts on natural medicine claim that quercetin works like the drug cromolyn (Intal) by stopping the release of allergenic substances in the body. However, while there is direct evidence that cromolyn is effective, there have not been any published studies in which people were given quercetin and their allergic symptoms decreased.

Tomato extract has been advocated for the treatment of allergic rhinitis, but the one double-blind study said to demonstrate benefit actually proves almost nothing because of major flaws in its statistical analysis.

Oligomeric proanthocyanidins (OPCs) from grape seed or pine bark are also often said to be effective. However, an eight-week double-blind trial of forty-nine persons found no benefit from grape seed extract (the dose was not stated).

The last several substances discussed (vitamins E and C, flavonoids, and OPCs) are antioxidants. One study failed to find evidence of benefit with a mixture of antioxidants: beta-carotene (9 mg per day), vitamin C (1,500 mg per day), vitamin E (130 mg per day), zinc (45 mg per day), selenium (76 mg per day), and garlic (150 mg per day).

Adrenal extracts, bee pollen, *Bacopa monniera* (brahmi), barberry, vitamin B_6, vitamin B_{12}, cat's claw, *Coleus forskohlii*, methyl sulfonyl methane, and betaine hydrochloride are sometimes recommended for hay fever, but there is no significant evidence that they are effective. A 2009 review of six high-quality trials with more than one thousand children found that neither omega-3 nor omega-6 oil consumption prevented allergic diseases in high-risk children. Allergic diseases included eczema, asthma, allergic rhinitis, and food allergy, and omega-3 and omega-6 sources included gamma-linolenic acid, fish oil, canola oil, and borage oil.

It has often been suggested that consumption of honey can reduce symptoms of hay fever. However, the one published study designed to test this suggestion failed to find benefit. Another study failed to find the bee product royal jelly effective.

EBSCO CAM Review Board

FURTHER READING

Anandan, C., U. Nurmatov, and A. Sheikh. "Omega 3 and 6 Oils for Primary Prevention of Allergic Disease." *Allergy* 64 (2009): 840-848.

Badar, V. A., et al. "Efficacy of *Tinospora cordifolia* in Allergic Rhinitis." *Journal of Ethnopharmacology* 96 (2004): 445-449.

Brinkhaus, B., et al. "Acupuncture and Chinese Herbal Medicine in the Treatment of Patients with Seasonal Allergic Rhinitis." *Allergy* 59 (2004): 953-969.

Cox, L. S., et al. "Sublingual Immunotherapy." *Journal of Allergy and Clinical Immunology* 117 (2006): 1021-1035.

Dahl, R., et al. "Sublingual Grass Allergen Tablet Immunotherapy Provides Sustained Clinical Benefit with Progressive Immunologic Changes over Two Years." *Journal of Allergy and Clinical Immunology* 121 (2008): 512-518.

Giovannini, M., et al. "A Randomized Prospective Double-Blind Controlled Trial on Effects of Long-Term Consumption of Fermented Milk Containing *Lactobacillus casei* in Pre-school Children with Allergic Asthma and/or Rhinitis." *Pediatric Research* 62 (2007): 215.

Kobayashi, M., et al. "Shoyu Polysaccharides from Soy Sauce Improve Quality of Life for Patients with Seasonal Allergic Rhinitis." *International Journal of Molecular Medicine* 15 (2005): 463-467.

Langewitz, W., et al. "Effect of Self-Hypnosis on Hay Fever Symptoms." *Psychotherapy and Psychosomatics* 74 (2005): 165-172.

Magnusson, A. L., et al. "The Effect of Acupuncture on Allergic Rhinitis." *American Journal of Chinese Medicine* 32 (2004): 105-115.

Marogna, M., et al. "Preventive Effects of Sublingual Immunotherapy in Childhood." *Annals of Allergy, Asthma, and Immunology* 101 (2008): 206-211.

Matkovic, Z., V. Zivkovic, and M. Korica. "Efficacy and Safety of *Astragalus membranaceus* in the Treatment of Patients with Seasonal Allergic Rhinitis." *Phytotherapy Research* 24 (2010): 175-181.

Pfaar, O., and L. Klimek. "Efficacy and Safety of Specific Immunotherapy with a High-Dose Sublingual Grass Pollen Preparation." *Annals of Allergy, Asthma, and Immunology* 100 (2008): 256-263.

Rajan, T. V., et al. "Effect of Ingestion of Honey on Symptoms of Rhinoconjunctivitis." *Annals of Allergy, Asthma, and Immunology* 88 (2002): 198-203.

Roberts, J., et al. "A Systematic Review of the Clinical Effectiveness of Acupuncture for Allergic Rhinitis." *BMC Complementary and Alternative Medicine* 8 (2008).

Shahar, E., G. Hassoun, and S. Pollack. "Effect of Vitamin E Supplementation on the Regular Treatment of Seasonal Allergic Rhinitis." *Annals of Allergy, Asthma, and Immunology* 92 (2004): 654-658.

Yoshimura, M., et al. "An Evaluation of the Clinical Efficacy of Tomato Extract for Perennial Allergic Rhinitis." *Allergology International* 3 (2007): 225-230.

See also: Butterbur.

Aloe

CATEGORY: Herbs and supplements
RELATED TERMS: Aloe vera, drug aloe
DEFINITION: Natural plant product used as a dietary supplement for specific health benefits.
PRINCIPAL PROPOSED USES: Burns, diabetes, genital herpes, psoriasis, seborrhea
OTHER PROPOSED USES: Asthma, cancer treatment support, human immunodeficiency virus infection support, immune support, lichen planus, radiation therapy side-effect prevention, ulcers, wound healing

OVERVIEW

The succulent aloe plant has been valued since prehistoric times for the treatment of burns, wound infections, and other skin problems. Medicinal aloe is pictured in an ancient cave painting in South Africa, and Alexander the Great is said to have captured an island off Somalia for the sole purpose of possessing the luxurious crop of aloe found there.

Most uses of aloe involve the gel inside its cactus-like leaves. However, the skin of the leaves themselves can be condensed to form a sticky substance known as drug aloe or aloes. It is a powerful laxative too, but it is seldom used for this purpose because its effects are unpleasant. The uses described here are intended to refer only to aloe gel, not to drug aloe. However, to make matters trickier, some aloe gel products contain small amounts of drug aloe, and it is possible that this contaminant is the actual source of benefits seen in some studies.

USES AND APPLICATIONS

Millions of people might swear by their own experience that applying aloe to the skin can drastically reduce the time it takes for burns (including sunburn) to heal. However, scientific evidence fails to support this belief. Studies suggest that aloe is not effective for treating sunburn and may actually impair the healing of second-degree burns.

Aloe also appears to be ineffective for treating the burn-like skin damage caused by radiation therapy for cancer. In a double-blind, placebo-controlled study of 194 women undergoing radiation therapy for breast cancer, the use of aloe gel failed to protect the skin from radiation-induced damage. Lack of benefit was also seen in an open trial of 225 women. One study

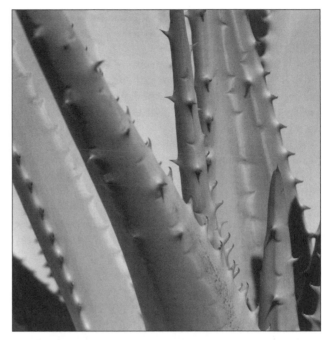

Aloe vera leaves. (Lawrence Lawry/Photo Researchers, Inc.)

evaluated aloe soap in 73 men and women undergoing radiation therapy for various forms of cancer and, overall, failed to find benefit except possibly at the highest doses. Another study failed to find aloe gel helpful for mouth inflammation caused by radiation therapy for head and neck cancer.

Aloe also has been widely recommended for aiding wound healing. However, while the results of test tube and animal studies of aloe for wounds have been positive, one clinical report in people suggests that aloe can actually impair the healing of severe wounds. Does topical aloe provide any benefit? There is some evidence (although quite incomplete) that it might help genital herpes, lichen planus, psoriasis, and seborrhea.

Aloe gel has also been tried as a treatment to be taken internally by mouth. Two studies suggest that aloe gel taken in this way might be helpful for type 2 diabetes. One study found possible benefits for ulcerative colitis. Weak evidence hints that regular intake of aloe might decrease risk of kidney stones.

Oral aloe is also sometimes recommended as an aid in the treatment of asthma and stomach ulcers and for general immune support, but there is no meaningful evidence that it is effective for any of these purposes. One of the constituents of aloe gel, acemannan, has shown some promise in test tube and animal studies for stimulating immunity and inhibiting the growth of viruses. These findings have led to the suggestion that acemannan can help human immunodeficiency virus (HIV) infection. However, the one reported double-blind, placebo-controlled trial failed to show benefits.

SCIENTIFIC EVIDENCE

Genital herpes. A two-week, double-blind, placebo-controlled trial enrolled sixty men with active genital herpes. Participants applied aloe cream (0.5 percent aloe) or placebo cream three times daily for five days. Use of aloe cream reduced the time necessary for lesions to heal (4.9 days versus 12 days) and also increased the percentage of those persons who were fully healed by the end of two weeks (66.7 percent versus 6.7 percent). A previous double-blind, placebo-controlled study by the same author, enrolling 120 men with genital herpes, found that cream made from aloe was more effective than pure aloe gel or placebo.

Seborrhea. Seborrhea is a fairly common skin condition leading to oily, red, and scaly eruptions in such areas as the eyebrows, eyelids, nose, ear, upper lip, chest, groin, and chin. A double-blind, placebo-controlled study of forty-four persons found that four to six weeks of treatment with aloe ointment could significantly reduce symptoms of seborrhea.

Psoriasis. According to a double-blind study that enrolled sixty men and women with mild to moderate symptoms of psoriasis, aloe cream may be helpful for this chronic skin condition. Participants were treated with either topical aloe extract (0.5 percent) or a placebo cream, applied three times daily for four weeks. Aloe treatment produced significantly better results than placebo, and these results were said to endure for almost one year after treatment was stopped. The study authors also reported a high level of complete "cure," but what exactly they meant by this was not reported clearly.

However, another study failed to replicate these results. During four weeks of treatment, marked improvement was seen in 72.5 percent of skin patches treated with aloe, but in 82 percent of those treated with placebo. This was a statistically significant difference in favor of placebo. Further studies are needed to sort out these contradictory results.

Lichen planus. Lichen planus is a chronic skin condition characterized by itchy, flat, scaly patches. It can occur in various parts of the body, including the wrists, legs, trunk, mouth, and vagina.

One study evaluated the potential value of aloe vera as a topical treatment for oral lichen planus. In this double-blind, placebo-controlled study of fifty-four people with oral lichen planus, the use of aloe vera gel was significantly more effective than placebo in alleviating symptoms. In another study involving thirty-four women with lichen planus of the vulva (just outside the vagina), aloe vera led to significantly more improvement than placebo.

Diabetes. Evidence from two human trials suggests that aloe gel can improve blood sugar control in persons with type 2 diabetes. A single-blind, placebo-controlled trial evaluated the potential benefits of aloe in either seventy-two or forty persons with diabetes (the study report appears to contradict itself). The results showed significantly greater improvements in blood sugar levels among those given aloe over the two-week treatment period.

Another single-blind, placebo-controlled trial evaluated the benefits of aloe in persons who had failed to respond to the oral diabetes drug glibenclamide. Of the thirty-six persons who completed the study, those taking glibenclamide and aloe showed definite improvements in blood sugar levels over forty-two days compared with those taking glibenclamide and placebo. Although these are promising results, large studies that are double- rather than single-blind are needed to establish aloe as an effective treatment for hypoglycemia.

Ulcerative colitis. In a double-blind, placebo-controlled study of forty-four people with active ulcerative colitis, use of oral aloe gel at a dose of 100 milliliters twice daily for four weeks appeared to improve both subjective symptoms and objective measurements of disease severity. About one-half of the people given aloe showed response to treatment; about 30 percent experienced full remission. Benefits occurred only rarely in the placebo group. However, this was a small study, and its results cannot be taken as conclusive.

THERAPEUTIC DOSAGES

Topical aloe vera cream typically contains 0.5 percent aloe and is applied three times daily. For the treatment of diabetes, a dosage of 1 tablespoon of aloe juice twice daily has been used in studies.

Safety Issues

Other than occasional allergic reactions, no serious problems have been reported with aloe gel, whether used internally or externally. However, comprehensive safety studies are lacking. Safety in young children, pregnant or nursing women, or those with severe liver or kidney disease has not been established.

If aloe is used as a treatment for diabetes, and it proves effective, blood sugar levels could fall too low, necessitating a reduction in medication dosage. Close monitoring of blood sugar levels is, therefore, advised.

In addition, there is one report of an herb-drug interaction between aloe and the anesthesia drug sevoflurane, in which it appeared that aloe may have increased sevoflurane's blood-thinning effect. Another isolated report appears to connect aloe to liver inflammation in one person. (Because aloe does not appear to possess any liver toxicity in general, this report would seem to suggest an idiosyncratic, in other words, a highly personal, reaction to the herb.)

Important Interactions

In persons using medications for diabetes, the oral use of aloe vera might cause blood sugar levels to fall too low. Aloe gel might increase the effectiveness of hydrocortisone cream.

EBSCO CAM Review Board

Further Reading

Bottenberg, M. M., et al. "Oral Aloe Vera-Induced Hepatitis." *Annals of Pharmacotherapy* 41 (2007): 1740-1743.

Heggie, S., et al. "A Phase III Study on the Efficacy of Topical Aloe Vera Gel on Irradiated Breast Tissue." *Cancer Nursing* 25 (2002): 442-451.

Kirdpon, S., et al. "Changes in Urinary Compositions Among Children After Consuming Prepared Oral Doses of Aloe (*Aloe vera* Linn.)." *Journal of the Medical Association of Thailand* 89 (2006): 1199-1205.

_____. "Effect of Aloe (*Aloe vera* Linn.) on Healthy Adult Volunteers: Changes in Urinary Composition." *Journal of the Medical Association of Thailand* 89, suppl. 2 (2006): S9-S14.

Langmead, L., et al. "Randomized, Double-Blind, Placebo-Controlled Trial of Oral Aloe Vera Gel for Active Ulcerative Colitis." *Alimentary Pharmacology and Therapeutics* 19 (2004): 739-748.

See also: Asthma; Burns, minor; Cancer treatment support; Diabetes; Herpes; HIV support: Homeopathic remedies; Immune support; Psoriasis; Radiation therapy support: Homeopathic remedies; Seborrheic dermatitis; Ulcers; Wounds, minor.

Alopecia

Category: Condition
Related terms: Alopecia areata, alopecia universalis, androgenetic alopecia, baldness, hair loss, hair thinning
Definition: Treatment of the loss or thinning of hair.
Principal proposed natural treatments: Essential oils (combination of thyme, lavender, rosemary, and cedarwood)
Other proposed natural treatments: Biotin, khellin, melatonin, nickel sulfate, *Primula obconica*, zinc

Introduction

Alopecia, or hair loss, can occur in several forms. One of the most common forms is male pattern hair loss, or androgenetic alopecia. As one might expect from the name, this type of hair loss occurs most commonly in men, where it appears as the well-known receding hairline. It can also occur in women, however, generally in the form of overall hair thinning (diffuse hair loss). Conventional treatment includes the drugs minoxidil and finasteride and medical diagnostic techniques to rule out potential underlying problems (especially in women).

Hair loss that occurs in patchy areas is referred to as alopecia areata. It can occur in both men and women at any age but usually starts during childhood. Alopecia areata typically starts with one or more small, round, smooth patches in the scalp or beard area. Rarely, it causes total body hair loss, a condition called alopecia universalis. Alopecia areata has no medical cure. However, in many cases, hair grows back on its own without treatment. Widespread hair loss is less likely to reverse itself. Corticosteroids injected under the skin may promote some hair growth, but the results usually do not last. One approach to the treatment of alopecia areata involves inducing mild allergic reactions using either nickel sulfate or the leaves of the plant *Primula obconica*. It appears that

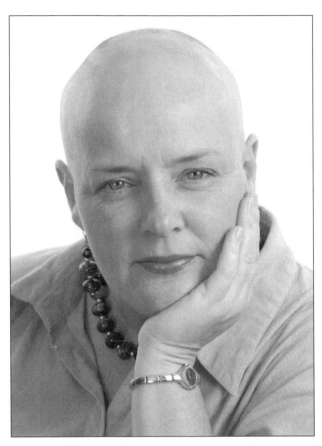

Chemotherapy has caused this woman to lose her hair. (©Lisa F. Young/Dreamstime.com)

when these substances irritate the skin they trigger new hair growth, but larger studies are needed to confirm the findings.

Other forms of hair loss include anagen effluvium and telogen effluvium. Anagen effluvium is typically caused by chemotherapy but may occur as a result of various medical conditions. Telogen effluvium is generally caused by severe physiological stress, such as major illness.

PRINCIPAL PROPOSED NATURAL TREATMENTS

One study suggests that a combination of essential oils applied topically may stimulate hair growth in people with alopecia areata. In this double-blind, placebo-controlled trial, eighty-four people massaged either essential oils or a nontreatment oil into their scalps each night for seven months. The results showed that 44 percent of those in the treatment group had

new hair growth; only 15 percent of the control group had new hair growth. The treatment oil contained essential oils of thyme, rosemary, lavender, and cedarwood, in a base of grape seed and jojoba oils.

Although there are no reported side effects associated with using thyme, rosemary, lavender, and cedarwood oils topically, essential oils can be toxic if taken internally. They can also cause allergic reactions, which may be severe, when applied topically.

OTHER PROPOSED NATURAL TREATMENTS

Preliminary evidence suggests that topical khellin, an extract of the fruit of the Mediterranean plant khella (*Ammi visnaga*), may promote new hair growth when combined with ultraviolet light (UVA) therapy in people with alopecia areata. Khellin selectively sensitizes the skin to UVA and is related to drugs used to treat psoriasis.

The supplements zinc aspartate and biotin, taken together in high (and possibly dangerous) doses, have been tried for alopecia areata in children. For women, one double-blind study found that the hormone melatonin, applied topically to the scalp as a 0.1 percent solution, may be helpful for those with diffuse hair loss. A proprietary form of silicon (choline-stabilized orthosilicic acid) has shown some promise. Hypnotherapy has been proposed as a treatment for alopecia areata, but a small study found it had no effect.

EBSCO CAM Review Board

FURTHER READING

Barel, A., et al. "Effect of Oral Intake of Choline-Stabilized Orthosilicic Acid on Skin, Nails, and Hair in Women with Photodamaged Skin." *Archives of Dermatological Research* 297 (2005): 147-153.

Camacho, F. M., and M. J. Garcia-Hernandez. "Zinc Aspartate, Biotin, and Clobetasol Propionate in the Treatment of Alopecia Areata in Childhood." *Pediatric Dermatology* 16 (1999): 336-338.

Fischer, T. W., et al. "Melatonin Increases Anagen Hair Rate in Women with Androgenetic Alopecia or Diffuse Alopecia." *British Journal of Dermatology* 150 (2004): 341-345.

Hay, I. C., M. Jamieson, and A. D. Ormerod. "Randomized Trial of Aromatherapy: Successful Treatment for Alopecia Areata." *Archives of Dermatology* 134 (1998): 1349-1352.

Wickett, R. R., et al. "Effect of Oral Intake of Choline-Stabilized Orthosilicic Acid on Hair Tensile Strength and Morphology in Women with Fine Hair." *Archives of Dermatological Research* 299 (2007): 499-505.

See also: Aging; Cancer chemotherapy support: Homeopathic remedies; Essential oil monoterpenes.

Alternative versus traditional medicine

Category: Issues and overviews
Definition: Comparing and contrasting nontraditional medicine with conventional, or Western, medicine.

Overview

Alternative and traditional medicine have a great deal to learn from each other, and health practitioners and consumers have much to gain in bringing the two fields closer together. Alternative medicine is defined in many ways: as medicine that is "complementary," "alternative," "nontraditional," "nonconventional," and "unorthodox," and as those "practices that are not in conformity with the beliefs or standards of the dominant group of medical practitioners in a society."

Traditional medicine is defined as "allopathic," "conventional," "orthodox," and "Western." The term "traditional," although used quite commonly, is somewhat inaccurate, given that many alternative medical disciplines have been practiced for thousands of years, while many conventional types of medicine have been practiced for one century or less. Also, most of these terms are relevant only in the context of Western culture. In some cultures, the so-called traditional approach is considered alternative and a particular alternative approach is considered traditional.

The U.S. National Institutes of Health (NIH) and other organizations use the term "complementary and alternative medicine" (CAM) to refer to these therapies and techniques collectively.

Alternative Medicine's Appeal

Although the approach and focus of different types of alternative therapies may differ, they all share the following characteristics, which make them appealing to health consumers and practitioners willing to try alternative approaches: empowerment of the individual to participate in and take responsibility for his or her own health; recognition and emphasis on lifestyle issues, such as proper nutrition, exercise, adequate rest, and emotional and spiritual balance; treatment of the individual as a whole person; and an emphasis on preventing disease and maintaining health.

Criticisms of Traditional Medicine

Traditional medicine is commonly criticized for treating symptoms, such as pain or fever, instead of causes and for prescribing medications to try to mask these symptoms. However, this criticism is not entirely fair. Although it is true that doctors of traditional medicine often prescribe drugs or use other approaches to control symptoms, they also search for causes of symptoms, such as infection or inflammation, to be able to treat them allopathically.

Criticisms of Alternative Medicine

Alternative medical practices are commonly criticized for sensationalizing the merits of a particular nontraditional medical approach. For example, books about certain dietary approaches claim to cure a whole host of ailments, and similar claims are sometimes made about particular dietary supplements.

Alternative practitioners also are criticized for the way they report the outcomes of patient cases: often through anecdote. However, this practice is not limited to alternative practitioners: Any medical doctor, traditional or nontraditional, can relate a story about a patient who did either quite well or quite poorly with one or another method of treatment.

To counter some of these criticisms, both CAM and allopathic medicine are moving to an evidence-based approach to treatment. Evidence-based medicine is the application of a scientific process to distinguish chance outcomes from outcomes that are reproducible and, therefore, presumably more reliable.

Joining the Disciplines: Integrative Medicine

Integrative medicine was created to bring alternative and traditional medicines together. Victoria Maizes, a family doctor with the University of Arizona and one of the key persons responsible for the success of integrative medicine, has stated that "integrative medicine honors the innate ability of the body to heal, values the relationship between patient and physician, and integrates complementary and alternative medicine when appropriate to facilitate healing."

Integrative medicine refocuses medicine on health and healing. It insists on patients being treated as whole persons—as minds and spirits, and as physical bodies—who participate actively in their own health care.

Many medical schools in the United States now teach the principles and practices of integrative medicine. Clinics and private practices are embracing its philosophy. Also, integrative medicine research studies have been published in peer-reviewed medical journals.

Skeptics in both CAM and traditional medical communities blame integrative medicine for being either too scientific or not scientific enough. For health consumers who would like "the best of both worlds," integrative medicine may be a good choice. Health consumers should share with their practitioners any other treatments they are receiving.

CONCLUSION

In 1847, the American Medical Association was established to regulate medical care. This governing body controls state medical boards and determines whether doctors can receive or maintain hospital privileges and whether they can keep their medical license. A medical license can be revoked for a reason secondary to incompetence, which is essentially defined as "deviating from what is known as the standard of care." As long as Western medical practice is considered the definitive standard of care, alternative medical practices will continue to face the challenges of recognition, acceptance, and respect.

Jackie Hart, M.D.; reviewed by Brian Randall, M.D.

FURTHER READING

American Academy of Family Physicians. http://www. aafp.org.

Bell, I., et al. "Integrative Medicine and Systematic Outcomes Research: Issues in the Emergence of a New Model for Primary Health Care." *Archives of Internal Medicine* 162 (2002): 133-140.

Kliger, B., et al. "Core Competencies in Integrative Medicine for Medical School Curricula: A Proposal." *Academic Medicine* 79, no. 6 (2004).

Maizes, V., and O. Caspi. "The Principles and Challenges of Integrative Medicine: More Than a Combination of Conventional and Alternative Medicine." *Western Journal of Medicine* 171 (1999): 148-149.

National Center for Complementary and Alternative Medicine. http://nccam.nih.gov.

See also: Education and training of CAM practitioners; Folk medicine; Herbal medicine; Health freedom movement; History of alternative medicine; History of complementary medicine; Integrative medicine; Licensing and certification of CAM practitioners; National Center for Complementary and Alternative Medicine; Popular practitioners; Regulation of CAM; Scientific method; Traditional healing; Whole medicine.

Altitude sickness

CATEGORY: Condition

RELATED TERMS: Acute mountain sickness, high-altitude sickness, mountain sickness

DEFINITION: Treatment of symptoms caused by the lower pressure and reduced amount of oxygen at high altitudes.

PRINCIPAL PROPOSED NATURAL TREATMENTS: None

OTHER PROPOSED NATURAL TREATMENTS: Antioxidants (vitamin C, vitamin E, lipoic acid), arginine, *Ginkgo biloba*, glutamine, high-carbohydrate diet, magnesium, milk thistle, *Rhodiola rosea*

INTRODUCTION

Altitude sickness, which is caused by reduced oxygen at high altitudes, includes symptoms such as headache, dizziness, shortness of breath, fatigue, and nausea, and, in serious cases, extreme fatigue, impaired motor control, and fluid accumulation in the brain and lungs. In general, the greater the altitude and the more rapid the ascent, the greater the likelihood of severe symptoms.

Many deaths on Mount Everest in the Himalaya and on other high mountains can be attributed to the effects of altitude sickness on climbers. In most cases, however, altitude sickness is a benign condition that afflicts people who live at relatively low elevations but who travel to higher elevations (to ski or hike, for example).

The best treatment for altitude sickness is prevention. Persons planning an ascent of high mountains should take as much time as possible to acclimate to the starting elevation. Full adjustment to the reduced oxygen content of the air may take several weeks. In general, ascents should be gradual. One recommendation suggests taking two days to adjust to an 8,000-foot elevation gain, plus one day for each 1,000 to 2,000 feet beyond 8,000.

Such recommendations, however, are not practical for people who fly to a vacation destination, such as a ski resort, and must deal with the effects of reduced oxygen all at once. To prevent or treat mild cases of altitude sickness, one should drink plenty of water and avoid alcohol, caffeine, and salty foods. If severe symptoms develop, the best response is to descend as rapidly as possible.

Conventional treatments for altitude sickness include acetazolamide or dexamethasone for prevention or treatment of mild cases and nifedipine for people prone to pulmonary edema. Ibuprofen and related drugs may help with headache.

PROPOSED NATURAL TREATMENTS

A double-blind trial of eighteen mountaineers climbing to one of two Mount Everest base camps (both are at about 18,000 feet) found that the use of an antioxidant vitamin supplement (providing 1,000 milligrams [mg] of vitamin C, 400 IU (international units) of vitamin E, and 600 mg of lipoic acid daily) significantly improved symptoms of altitude sickness compared with placebo. Treatment was begun three weeks before ascent and continued during the ten days of climbing. This was a small study, however, and its results cannot be taken as reliable. Another small study using similar antioxidants in a similar manner found that the use of antioxidants might offer benefits in the first couple of days of high altitude ascent but that these benefits decline with acclimatization.

Three small double-blind trials that enrolled about one hundred people (in total) found preliminary evidence that the use of the herb *Ginkgo biloba* can help prevent altitude sickness. A large scale double-blind study that enrolled 614 people however, failed to find benefit. The same study found that the drug acetazolamide did provide significant benefits compared with placebo. A similarly designed smaller study that enrolled fifty-seven people also failed to find ginkgo effective. Overall, the balance of evidence suggests that ginkgo is not effective for this purpose.

High-carbohydrate meals are sometimes recommended for preventing altitude sickness. The reasoning is that carbohydrate ingestion increases carbon dioxide production, which in turn stimulates an increased rate of breathing. However, studies on this treatment have resulted in contradictory results.

Magnesium, glutamine, and milk thistle, alone or in combination, have been suggested for altitude sickness, but there is no meaningful evidence that they work. The herb *Rhodiola rosea* has also been proposed as an altitude sickness treatment, but evidence is more negative than positive. One study of the supplement arginine found that it increased elevation-related headaches.

EBSCO CAM Review Board

FURTHER READING

Bailey, D. M., and B. Davies. "Acute Mountain Sickness: Prophylactic Benefits of Antioxidant Vitamin Supplementation at High Altitude." *High Altitude Medicine and Biology* 2 (2001): 21-29.

Chow, T., et al. "*Ginkgo biloba* and Acetazolamide Prophylaxis for Acute Mountain Sickness." *Archives of Internal Medicine* 165 (2005): 296-301.

Gertsch, J. H., et al. "*Ginkgo biloba* for the Prevention of Severe Acute Mountain Sickness (AMS) Starting One Day Before Rapid Ascent." *High Altitude Medicine and Biology* 3 (2002): 29-37.

_____. "Randomised, Double Blind, Placebo Controlled Comparison of *Ginkgo biloba* and Acetazolamide for Prevention of Acute Mountain Sickness Among Himalayan Trekkers: The Prevention of High Altitude Illness Trial." *British Medical Journal* 328 (March 11, 2004).

Moraga, F. A., et al. "*Ginkgo biloba* Decreases Acute Mountain Sickness in People Ascending to High Altitude at Ollague (3696 m) in Northern Chile." *Wilderness and Environmental Medicine* 18 (2007): 251-257.

Subudhi, A. W., et al. "Changes in Ventilatory Threshold at High Altitude: Effect of Antioxidants." *Medicine and Science in Sports and Exercise* 38 (2006): 1425-1431.

Wing, S. L., et al. "Lack of Effect of *Rhodiola* or Oxygenated Water Supplementation on Hypoxemia and Oxidative Stress." *Wilderness and Environmental Medicine* 14 (2003): 9-16.

See also: Antioxidants; Fatigue; Headache, cluster; Morning sickness; Nausea; *Rhodiola rosea*; Sports and fitness support: Enhancing recovery; Sports-related injuries: Homeopathic remedies; Strokes; Vitamins and minerals.

Alzheimer's disease and non-Alzheimer's dementia

CATEGORY: Condition

DEFINITION: Treatment of mental and cognitive decline in the elderly.

PRINCIPAL PROPOSED NATURAL TREATMENTS: Acetyl-L-carnitine, *Ginkgo biloba*, huperzine A, phosphatidylserine, vinpocetine

OTHER PROPOSED NATURAL TREATMENTS: Aromatherapy, carnosine, citrulline, choline or phosphatidylcholine, fish oil, treating high homocysteine, dehydroepiandrosterone, lemon balm, N-acetylcysteine, sage, vitamin E

INTRODUCTION

Alzheimer's disease is the most common cause of severe mental deterioration (dementia) in the elderly. It has been estimated that 30 to 50 percent of people older than age eighty-five years have this condition. Its cause is not known. However, microscopic examination of the brains of people who have died of Alzheimer's shows loss of cells in the thinking part of the brain, particularly cells that release a chemical called acetylcholine.

Alzheimer's begins with subtle symptoms, such as loss of memory for names and recent events. It progresses from difficulty learning new information to a few eccentric behaviors to depression, loss of spontaneity, and anxiety. Over the course of the disease, the person gradually loses the ability to carry out the activities of everyday life. Disorientation, asking questions repeatedly, and an inability to recognize friends are characteristics of moderately severe Alzheimer's. Eventually, virtually all mental functions fail.

Similar symptoms may be caused by conditions other than Alzheimer's disease, such as multiple small strokes (called multi-infarct or vascular dementia), severe alcoholism, and certain rarer causes. It is critical to begin with an examination to discover what is causing the symptoms of mental decline. Various treatable conditions, such as depression, can mimic the symptoms of dementia.

Four drugs have shown at least modest benefit for Alzheimer's disease or non-Alzheimer's dementia: Reminyl, Exelon, Aricept, and Cognex. These medications usually produce a modest improvement in mild to moderate Alzheimer's disease by increasing the

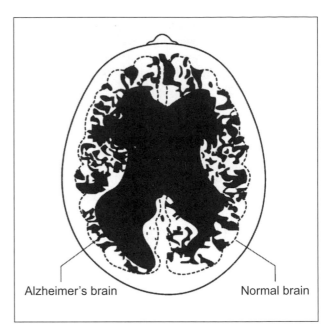

Alzheimer's disease causes the volume of the brain to shrink substantially.

duration of action of acetylcholine. However, they can sometimes cause severe side effects because of the exaggeration of acetylcholine's action in other parts of the body.

PRINCIPAL PROPOSED NATURAL TREATMENTS

There are two natural treatments for Alzheimer's disease with significant scientific evidence behind them: *Ginkgo biloba* and phosphatidylserine. Huperzine A and vinpocetine, while more like drugs than natural remedies, may also improve mental function in people with dementia. Acetyl-L-carnitine was once considered a promising option for this condition too, but evidence suggests that it does not work.

Ginkgo biloba. The best-established herbal treatment for Alzheimer's disease is the herb *Ginkgo biloba.* Numerous high quality double-blind, placebo-controlled studies indicate that ginkgo is effective for treating various forms of dementia. One of the largest studies was a 1997 trial in the United States that enrolled more than three hundred people with Alzheimer's disease or non-Alzheimer's dementia. Participants were given 40 milligrams (mg) of either ginkgo extract or a placebo three times daily for fifty-two weeks. The results showed significant but not entirely consistent improvements in the treated group.

Another study published in 2007 followed four hundred people for twenty-two weeks and used twice the dose of ginkgo employed in the foregoing study. The results of this trial indicated that ginkgo was significantly superior to placebo. The areas in which ginkgo showed the most marked superiority compared with placebo included "apathy/indifference, anxiety, irritability/lability, depression/dysphoria and sleep/nighttime behavior."

One fairly large study of ginkgo extract drew headlines for concluding that ginkgo is ineffective. This twenty-four-week, double-blind, placebo-controlled study of 214 participants with either mild to moderate dementia or ordinary age-associated memory loss found no effect with ginkgo extract at a dose of 240 or 160 mg daily. However, this study has been sharply criticized for a number of serious flaws in its design. In another community-based study among 176 elderly persons with early-stage dementia, researchers found no beneficial effect for 120 mg of ginkgo extract given daily for six months.

The ability of ginkgo to prevent or delay a decline in cognitive function is less clear. In a placebo-controlled trial of 118 cognitively intact adults age eighty-five years or older, ginkgo extract seemed to effectively slow the decline in memory function during a forty-two-month period. The researchers also reported a higher incidence of stroke in the group that took ginkgo, a finding that requires more investigation.

In a 2009 review of thirty-six randomized trials involving 4,423 persons with declining mental function (including dementia), researchers concluded that ginkgo appears safe but added that there is inconsistent evidence of its effectiveness.

Phosphatidylserine. Phosphatidylserine is one of the many substances involved in the structure and maintenance of cell membranes. Double-blind studies involving more than one thousand people suggest that phosphatidylserine is an effective treatment for Alzheimer's disease and other forms of dementia.

The largest of these studies followed 494 elderly persons in northeastern Italy for six months. All had moderate to severe mental decline, as measured by standard tests. Treatment consisted of 300 mg daily of either phosphatidylserine or placebo. The group that took phosphatidylserine did significantly better in both behavior and mental function than the placebo group. Symptoms of depression also improved.

These results agree with those of numerous smaller double-blind studies involving more than five hundred people with Alzheimer's and other types of age-related dementia. However, the form of phosphatidylserine available as a supplement has altered since the studies described above were performed, and the available form may not be equivalent.

Huperzine A. Huperzine A is a chemical derived from a particular type of club moss (*Huperzia serrata*). Like caffeine and cocaine, huperzine A is a medicinally active, plant-derived chemical that belongs to the class known as alkaloids. This substance is really more a drug than an herb, but it is sold over-the-counter as a dietary supplement for memory loss and mental impairment.

According to three Chinese double-blind trials enrolling more than 450 people, the use of huperzine A can significantly improve symptoms of Alzheimer's disease and other forms of dementia. However, one double-blind trial failed to find evidence of benefit, but it was a relatively small study. In a review of six randomized, controlled trials, researchers concluded that, on balance, huperzine A is probably of some benefit in Alzheimer's disease, but the variable quality of these studies weakens this conclusion.

Vinpocetine. Vinpocetine is a chemical derived from vincamine, a constituent found in the leaves of common periwinkle (*Vinca minor*) and in the seeds of various African plants. It is used as a treatment for memory loss and mental impairment.

Developed in Hungary, vinpocetine is sold in Europe as a drug called Cavinton. In the United States, it is available as a dietary supplement, although the substance probably does not fit that category. Vinpocetine does not exist to any significant extent in nature. Producing it requires significant chemical work performed in the laboratory.

Several double-blind studies have evaluated vinpocetine for the treatment of Alzheimer's disease and related conditions. Most of these studies had significant flaws in design and reporting. A review of the literature found three studies of acceptable quality, enrolling 583 people. Perhaps the best of these was a sixteen-week, double-blind, placebo-controlled trial of 203 people with mild to moderate dementia that found significant benefit in the treated group. However, even this trial had several technical limitations, and the authors of the review concluded that vinpocetine cannot be regarded as a proven treatment.

Acetyl-L-carnitine. Carnitine is a vitamin-like substance

that is often used for angina, congestive heart failure, and other heart conditions. A special form of carnitine, acetyl-L-carnitine, has been extensively tested for the treatment of dementia; double-blind or single-blind studies involving more than fourteen hundred people have been reported.

While early studies found evidence of modest benefit, two large and well-designed studies failed to find acetyl-L-carnitine effective. The first of these was a double-blind, placebo-controlled trial that enrolled 431 people for one year. Overall, acetyl-L-carnitine proved no better than placebo. However, because a close look at the data indicated that the supplement might help people who develop Alzheimer's disease at an unusually young age, researchers performed a follow-up trial. This one-year, double-blind, placebo-controlled trial evaluated acetyl-L-carnitine in 229 persons with early-onset Alzheimer's. No benefits were seen here either.

One review of literature interpreted the cumulative results to mean that acetyl-L-carnitine may be mildly helpful for mild Alzheimer's disease. However, another review concluded that if acetyl-L-carnitine does offer benefits for any form of Alzheimer's disease, they are too minor to make much of a practical difference.

OTHER PROPOSED NATURAL TREATMENTS

Two small double-blind studies performed by a single research group found evidence that the herbs sage and lemon balm can improve cognitive function in people with mild to moderate Alzheimer's disease.

One study found that vitamin E (dl-alpha-tocopherol) may slow the progression of Alzheimer's disease, but another study did not. Another, large study failed to find that the use of vitamin E reduced the risk of general mental decline (whether caused by Alzheimer's or not) in women older than age sixty-five years. Preliminary evidence suggests that N-acetylcysteine (NAC) might also be helpful for slowing the progression of Alzheimer's disease.

Lavender oil used purely as aromatherapy (treatment involving inhaling essential oils) has been advocated for reducing agitation in people with dementia; however, people with dementia tend to lose their sense of smell, making this approach seem somewhat unlikely to work. Topical use of essential oil of the herb lemon balm has also shown promise for reducing agitation in people with Alzheimer's disease;

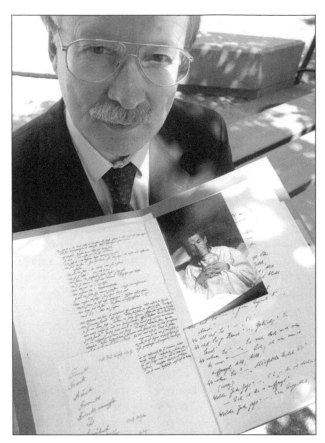

Physician Konrad Maurer displays Alois Alzheimer's handwritten file describing the first documented case of the disease named for him. (AP Photo)

the researchers who tested it considered their method aromatherapy because the fragrance wafts up from the skin, but essential oils are also absorbed through the skin; this mechanism of action seems more plausible. Oral use of lemon balm extract has also shown promise.

Drugs used for Alzheimer's disease affect levels of acetylcholine in the body. The body makes acetylcholine out of the nutrient choline. On this basis, supplements containing choline or the related substance phosphatidylcholine have been proposed for the treatment of Alzheimer's disease, but the results of studies have not been positive. One special form of choline, however, has shown more promise. In a six-month double-blind study of 261 people with Alzheimer's disease, the use of choline alfoscerate at a dose of 400 mg three times daily significantly improved cognitive function compared with placebo. Colistrinin, a substance derived from colostrum, has shown some promise for the treatment of Alzheimer's.

Bee pollen, carnosine, citrulline, 2-dimethylamino-ethanol, inositol, magnesium, pregnenolone, vitamin B_1, and zinc have also been suggested as treatments for Alzheimer's disease. However, there is no reliable scientific evidence to support their use. Elevated blood levels of the substance homocysteine have been suggested as a contributor to Alzheimer's disease and multi-infarct dementia. However, a double-blind, placebo-controlled study failed to find that homocysteine-lowering treatment using B vitamins was helpful for multi-infarct dementia. Similarly, two studies failed to find benefits in people with Alzheimer's disease. In another study, a mixture of B vitamins did not improve the quality of life in people with mild cognitive impairment of various causes. Early reports suggested that declining levels of the hormone dehydroepiandrosterone (DHEA) cause impaired mental function in the elderly. On this basis, DHEA has been promoted as a cognition-enhancing supplement. However, the one double-blind study that tested DHEA for Alzheimer's disease found little to no benefit. Studies of fish oil have failed to find it helpful for Alzheimer's disease, whether for delaying its onset, slowing its progression, or improving its symptoms.

In a sizable Danish trial, researchers investigated the effects of melatonin and light therapy (bright light exposure during daylight hours) on mood, sleep, and cognitive decline in elderly persons, most of whom had dementia. They found that melatonin 2.5 mg, given nightly for an average of fifteen months, slightly improved quality of sleep, but it worsened mood. Melatonin apparently had no significant effect on cognition. Light therapy alone slightly decreased cognitive and functional decline and improved mood. Combining melatonin with light therapy improved mood and quality of sleep.

EBSCO CAM Review Board

FURTHER READING

Aisen, P. S., et al. "High-Dose B Vitamin Supplementation and Cognitive Decline in Alzheimer Disease." *Journal of the American Medical Association* 300 (2008): 1774-1783.

Ballard, C. G., et al. "Aromatherapy as a Safe and Effective Treatment for the Management of Agitation in Severe Dementia." *Journal of Clinical Psychiatry* 63 (2002): 553-558.

Bilikiewicz, A., and W. Gaus. "Colostrinin (A Naturally Occurring, Proline-Rich, Polypeptide Mixture) in the Treatment of Alzheimer's Disease." *Journal of Alzheimer's Disease* 6 (2004): 17-26.

Birks, J., and J. G. Evans. "*Ginkgo biloba* for Cognitive Impairment and Dementia." *Cochrane Database of Systematic Reviews* (2009): CD003120. Available through *EBSCO DynaMed Systematic Literature Surveillance* at http://www.ebscohost.com/dynamed.

Dodge, H. H., et al. "A Randomized Placebo-Controlled Trial of *Ginkgo biloba* for the Prevention of Cognitive Decline." *Neurology* 70 (2008): 1809-1817.

Freund-Levi, Y., et al. "Omega-3 Supplementation in Mild to Moderate Alzheimer's Disease: Effects on Neuropsychiatric Symptoms." *International Journal of Geriatric Psychiatry* 23 (2008): 161-169.

Holmes, C., et al. "Lavender Oil as a Treatment for Agitated Behaviour in Severe Dementia." *International Journal of Geriatric Psychiatry* 17 (2002): 305-308.

Jia, X., G. McNeill, and A. Avenell. "Does Taking Vitamin, Mineral, and Fatty Acid Supplements Prevent Cognitive Decline?" *Journal of Human Nutrition and Dietetics* 21 (2008): 317-336.

Kang, J. H., et al. "A Randomized Trial of Vitamin E Supplementation and Cognitive Function in Women." *Archives of Internal Medicine* 166 (2006): 2462-2468.

Li, J., et al. "Huperzine A for Alzheimer's Disease." *Cochrane Database of Systematic Reviews* (2008): CD005592. Available through *EBSCO DynaMed Systematic Literature Surveillance* at http://www.ebscohost.com/dynamed.

Riemersma-Van der Lek, R. F., et al. "Effect of Bright Light and Melatonin on Cognitive and Noncognitive Function in Elderly Residents of Group Care Facilities." *Journal of the American Medical Association* 299 (2008): 2642-2655.

Snow, L. A., L. Hovanec, and J. Brandt. "A Controlled Trial of Aromatherapy for Agitation in Nursing Home Patients with Dementia." *Journal of Alternative and Complementary Medicine* 10 (2004): 431-437.

Sun, Y., et al. "Efficacy of Multivitamin Supplementation Containing Vitamins B(6) and B(12) and Folic Acid as Adjunctive Treatment with a Cholinesterase Inhibitor in Alzheimer's Disease." *Clinical Therapeutics* 29 (2007): 2204-2214.

See also: Carnitine; Ginkgo; Huperzine A; Phosphatidylserine; Vinpocetine.

Amenorrhea

CATEGORY: Condition

RELATED TERM: Absence of menstruation

DEFINITION: Treatment of the absence of menstrual bleeding that is not associated with menopause.

PRINCIPAL PROPOSED NATURAL TREATMENTS: None

OTHER PROPOSED NATURAL TREATMENTS: Alfalfa seed, angelica, asafetida, blue cohosh, bugleweed, chasteberry, motherwort, parsley, progesterone, rue, vitamin B_6, zinc

HERBS AND SUPPLEMENTS TO AVOID: Flaxseed, lignans

INTRODUCTION

The term "amenorrhea" literally means an "absence of menstrual bleeding." In medicine, amenorrhea indicates one of two conditions: the cessation of the menstrual cycle in a woman of menstrual age (secondary amenorrhea) or the lack of a menstrual cycle in a girl who has reached the age of sixteen years.

There are many causes of amenorrhea. Severe weight loss, such as may occur in a woman with anorexia nervosa, and extreme exercise, such as marathon running, bodybuilding, or professional-caliber ballet dancing, can cause the menstrual period to stop. Young college women may develop amenorrhea, possibly from stress or perhaps as a reflex reaction to what the body considers a "migration." Pregnancy and nursing stop the menstrual cycle by design, and women who have used oral contraceptives may find that it takes a while for a normal menstrual cycle to return after discontinuing them.

More rarely, amenorrhea may indicate a serious medical condition, such as a disorder of the pituitary gland, the hypothalamus, or the ovaries. For this reason, a woman should check with her doctor if she misses more than one menstrual period. Medical treatment for amenorrhea depends on the cause. If an examination reveals no underlying cause, physicians may recommend oral contraceptives to restart the menstrual cycle.

PROPOSED NATURAL TREATMENTS

The hormone progesterone, available (probably inappropriately) as an ingredient in some "natural" creams, may help restore the menstrual cycle. In one double-blind, placebo-controlled trial, oral use of a micronized form of progesterone restored a normal menstrual cycle in women with secondary amenor-

rhea. Although progesterone is marketed as a "natural hormone," it is as much a drug as estrogen and should never be used without medical supervision.

In some women, the pituitary gland produces excess levels of prolactin. Prolactin is a hormone that naturally rises during pregnancy to stimulate milk production; prolactin can also cause amenorrhea. Excessive pituitary prolactin release is a condition that must be investigated medically because it may indicate the presence of a tumor. It is possible, however, that slight abnormalities in prolactin level without a dangerous medical cause may trigger amenorrhea in some women. The herb chasteberry is thought to reduce prolactin levels, and for this reason it has been tried for amenorrhea. No double-blind, placebo-controlled trials on this potential use of chasteberry have been reported. The herb bugleweed is also thought to reduce prolactin levels, but it too has not been tested for amenorrhea.

Other commonly proposed natural treatments for amenorrhea include the supplements vitamin B_6 and zinc and the herbs blue cohosh, angelica, asafetida, alfalfa seed, motherwort, parsley, and rue. However, there is no meaningful scientific evidence to indicate whether they are effective.

For reasons that are not entirely clear, women who have developed amenorrhea because of heavy exercise tend to experience an accelerated rate of bone loss, which may lead to osteoporosis. Calcium and vitamin D supplements are not sufficient to protect bone mass under these circumstances. Stronger measures, such as reducing exercise or using medications, may be necessary.

HERBS AND SUPPLEMENTS TO AVOID

Substances called lignans, which are found in many foods but most especially in flax seeds, may increase levels of prolactin. Certain herbs and supplements may interact with oral contraceptive drugs used to treat amenorrhea.

EBSCO CAM Review Board

FURTHER READING

Baer, J. T., et al. "Diet, Hormonal, and Metabolic Factors Affecting Bone Mineral Density in Adolescent Amenorrheic and Eumenorrheic Female Runners." *Journal of Sports Medicine and Physical Fitness* 32 (1992): 51-58.

Hutchins, A. M., et al. "Flaxseed Consumption Influences Endogenous Hormone Concentrations in Postmenopausal Women." *Nutrition and Cancer* 39 (2001): 58-65.

Shangold, M. M., et al. "Factors Associated with Withdrawal Bleeding After Administration of Oral Micronized Progesterone in Women with Secondary Amenorrhea." *Fertility and Sterility* 56 (1991): 1040-1047.

Sulik, Sandra M., and Cathryn B. Heath. *Primary Care Procedures in Women's Health.* New York: Springer, 2010.

Zoorob, J. R. "CAM and Women's Health: Selected Topics." *Primary Care* 37, no. 2 (2010): 367-387.

See also: Adolescent and teenage health; Alfalfa; Blue cohosh; Bugleweed; Chasteberry; Dysmenorrhea; Eating disorders; Flaxseed; Lignans; Motherwort; Parsley; Premenstrual syndrome (PMS); Progesterone; Vitamin B_6; Women's health; Zinc.

American Academy of Anti-Aging Medicine

CATEGORY: Organizations and legislation
DEFINITION: Promotes the field of antiaging medicine and its recognition as a medical speciality.
DATE: Founded in 1993

PURPOSE

The American Academy of Anti-Aging Medicine (A4M) was founded by osteopaths Ronald Klatz and Robert Goldman in 1993 to advocate for the practice of antiaging medicine and its recognition as a legitimate medical specialization. In addition to recommending healthy diet and exercise, A4M endorses the use of antioxidants and other dietary supplements and recommends human growth hormone (HGH) treatments to slow, or even reverse, biological aging. A4M claims this new science can dramatically extend human longevity to 150 years and that it will eventually create "ageless societies" by applying currently available methods and promoting research to produce technological advances in antiaging medicine.

A4M promotes antiaging medicine in a number of ways, including through its certification program, publications, and conferences. Although the mainstream medical establishment does not recognize antiaging medicine as a medical specialty, A4M has certified more than twenty thousand practitioners, including medical doctors, dentists, nurses, dieticians, fitness trainers, and those with doctorates. The organization publishes the periodicals *Anti-aging Therapeutics* and *Anti-aging Medical News*. In addition to its annual A4M Conference, the organization sponsors the Annual World Conference on Anti-Aging Medicine and the World Anti-Aging Congress and Exposition. The latter two events are cosponsored by the World Anti-Aging Academy of Medicine, which is made up of a number of antiaging organizations from countries around the world; this academy is headed by A4M cofounder Goldman. A4M reportedly has tens of thousands of members worldwide.

CONTROVERSIES

The American Medical Association and the American Board of Medical Specialities refuse to recognize antiaging medicine as legitimate. The two organizations and numerous medical researchers claim that the reputed benefits of dietary supplements and HGH therapy are exaggerated, unproven, and potentially dangerous. The author of a 1990 study cited by A4M as support for its assertions has stated that he did not conclude that HGH could or should be used to slow aging, and he warned of the side effects of its indiscriminate use.

Many articles in established, refereed scientific journals also argue that research has shown that the risks of HGH therapy far outweigh the possible benefits. A 2002 position paper, endorsed by fifty-one scientists, posited that there is no research evidence to support the claims of antiaging doctors and entrepreneurs.

Also, critics assert that A4M's current and former affiliations with marketing organizations have generated large profits for A4M, and that the organization's non-peer-reviewed publications have allowed paid advertisers of antiaging products to assert scientific support for their advertised claims. Indeed, the U.S. Food and Drug Administration warns that it is a felony to provide HGH for antiaging therapy.

In response, A4M contends that its critics, including the media and medical and political establishments, are motived by conflicting professional and financial interests in trying to undermine the practice of antiaging medicine.

Jack Carter, Ph.D.

FURTHER READING
American Academy of Anti-Aging Medicine. http://www.worldhealth.net.
Giampapa, Vincent C., Frederic F. Buechel, and Ohan Kratoprak. *The Gene Makeover: The Twenty-First Century Anti-aging Breakthrough.* Laguna Beach, Calif.: Basic Health, 2007.
Klatz, Ronald, and Robert Goldman, eds. *The Science of Anti-aging Medicine.* Chicago: American Academy of Anti-Aging Medicine, 2003.
National Institute on Aging. http://www.nia.nih.gov.
Weil, Andrew. *Healthy Aging: A Lifelong Guide to Your Well-Being.* New York: Anchor Books, 2007.
Weintraub, Arlene. *Selling the Fountain of Youth: How the Anti-aging Industry Made a Disease Out of Getting Old.* New York: Basic Books, 2010.

See also: Aging; Antioxidants; Elder health; Pseudoscience.

Aminoglycosides

CATEGORY: Drug interactions
DEFINITION: Antibiotics given intravenously to treat certain infections.
INTERACTIONS: Calcium, ginkgo, magnesium, N-acetylcysteine, vitamin B$_{12}$
TRADE NAMES: Amikacin, Gentamycin, Tobramycin

GINKGO
Effect: Possible Harmful Interaction
The herb ginkgo is thought to increase circulation and protect nerve cells from damage. On this basis, it has been proposed as a possible treatment to help protect the auditory nerve from damage caused by aminoglycosides. However, the one animal study performed to evaluate this potential benefit found instead that the herb increased damage to the auditory nerve. Based on this finding, persons using aminoglycoside drugs should avoid ginkgo.

MINERALS: MAGNESIUM AND CALCIUM
Effect: Possible Harmful Interaction
Weak evidence from animal studies hints that the use of gentamicin may reduce levels of magnesium and calcium. Supplementation may therefore be helpful on general principles if gentamicin treat-ment is used for an extended time. One animal study suggests that calcium supplements in particular might help prevent gentamicin-induced kidney damage.

VITAMIN B$_{12}$
Effect: Supplementation Possibly Helpful
One animal study weakly hints that vitamin B$_{12}$ might help prevent hearing damage caused by gentamicin.

N-ACETYLCYSTEINE
Effect: May Decrease Effectiveness of the Drug
One exceedingly preliminary animal study suggests that N-acetylcysteine might help protect the kidneys from damage caused by gentamicin.

EBSCO CAM Review Board

FURTHER READING
Jin, X., and X. Sheng. "Methylcobalamin as Antagonist to Transient Ototoxic Action of Gentamicin." *Acta-Oto-Laryngologica* 121 (2001): 351-354.
Kes, P., and Z. Reiner. "Symptomatic Hypomagnesemia Associated with Gentamicin Therapy." *Magnesium and Trace Elements* 9 (1990): 54-60.
Miman, M. C., et al. "Amikacin Ototoxicity Enhanced by *Ginkgo biloba* Extract (EGb 761)." *Hearing Research* 169 (2002): 121-129.

See also: Antibiotics, general; Calcium; Food and Drug Administration; Ginkgo; Magnesium; Supplements: Introduction; Vitamin B$_{12}$; Vitamins and minerals.

Amiodarone

TRADE NAMES: Cordarone, Pacerone
CATEGORY: Drug interactions
DEFINITION: Drug used to restore normal heart rhythm.
INTERACTIONS: Chaparral, coltsfoot, comfrey, dong quai, St. John's wort, vitamin E

VITAMIN E
Effect: May Protect Against Side Effects
One of the problems with amiodarone is that it can cause injury to the lungs. One study suggests that vitamin E supplements might help prevent this side effect.

CHAPARRAL, COMFREY, AND COLTSFOOT

Effect: Possible Harmful Interaction

The herbs chaparral (*Larrea tridentata* or *L. mexicana*), comfrey (*Symphytum officinale*), and coltsfoot (*Tussilago farfara*) contain liver-toxic substances. Because amiodarone can also affect the liver, combining these herbs with the medication is not advisable.

DONG QUAI, ST. JOHN'S WORT

Effect: Possible Harmful Interaction

Amiodarone has been reported to cause increased sensitivity to the sun, amplifying the risk of sunburn or skin rash. Because St. John's wort and dong quai may also cause this problem, taking these herbal supplements during amiodarone therapy might add to this risk. It may be a good idea to use sunscreen or wear protective clothing during sun exposure if taking one of these herbs while using amiodarone.

EBSCO CAM Review Board

FURTHER READING

Kachel, D. L., et al. "Amiodarone-Induced Injury of Human Pulmonary Artery Endothelial Cells: Protection by Alpha-Tocopherol." *Journal of Pharmacology and Experimental Therapeutics* 254 (1990): 1107-1112.

See also: Chaparral; Coltsfoot; Comfrey; Dong quai; Food and Drug Administration; St. John's wort; Supplements: Introduction; Vitamin E.

Amoxicillin

CATEGORY: Drug interactions
DEFINITION: Relative of the antibiotic penicillin but modified to have a broader spectrum of effect.
INTERACTIONS: Bromelain, vitamin K
TRADE NAMES: Amoxil, Trimox, Wymox

BROMELAIN

Effect: Possible Helpful Interaction

According to two studies, the supplement bromelain (from pineapple stems) may increase the absorption of amoxicillin. This effect might help the antibiotic work better.

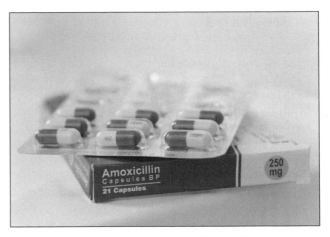

Amoxicillin is a moderate-spectrum antibiotic. (Gustoimages/ Photo Researchers, Inc.)

VITAMIN K

Effect: Possible Nutritional Depletion

There are concerns that antibiotic treatment might reduce levels of vitamin K in the body. However, this effect seems to be slight and only significant in persons who are already considerably deficient in vitamin K.

EBSCO CAM Review Board

FURTHER READING

Cohen, H., et al. "The Development of Hypoprothrombinaemia Following Antibiotic Therapy in Malnourished Patients with Low Serum Vitamin K1 Levels." *British Journal of Haematology* 68 (1988): 63-66.

Conly, J., and K. Stein. "Reduction of Vitamin K2 Concentrations in Human Liver Associated with the Use of Broad Spectrum Antimicrobials." *Clinical and Investigative Medicine* 17 (1994): 531-539.

Goss, T. F., et al. "Prospective Evaluation of Risk Factors for Antibiotic-Associated Bleeding in Critically Ill Patients." *Pharmacotherapy* 12 (1992): 283-291.

Shearer, M. J., et al. "Mechanism of Cephalosporin-Induced Hypoprothrombinemia: Relation to Cephalosporin Side Chain, Vitamin K Metabolism, and Vitamin K Status." *Journal of Clinical Pharmacology* 28 (1988): 88-95.

See also: Bromelain; Food and Drug Administration; Supplements: Introduction; Vitamin K.

Andrographis

CATEGORY: Herbs and supplements
RELATED TERMS: *Andrographis paniculata*, Indian echinacea
DEFINITION: Natural plant product used as a dietary supplement for specific health benefits.
PRINCIPAL PROPOSED USE: Common cold prevention and treatment
OTHER PROPOSED USES: Familial Mediterranean fever, heart disease prevention, immune support, liver protection, stimulating gallbladder contraction

OVERVIEW

Andrographis is a shrub found throughout India and other Asian countries that is sometimes called Indian echinacea. It has been used historically in epidemics, including the Indian flu epidemic in 1919, during which andrographis was credited with stopping the spread of the disease.

USES AND APPLICATIONS

A proprietary extract of andrographis (sold with *Eleutherococcus*) has become popular in Scandinavia as a treatment for colds. It is also available in other regions. Reasonably good evidence shows that either form of this extract can reduce the severity of cold symptoms. It may also help prevent colds.

Although it is not known how andrographis might work for colds, preliminary evidence suggests that it might stimulate immunity, potentially making it useful for general immune support.

Andrographis combined with *Eleutherococcus*, licorice, and schisandra has shown promise for a genetic disease called familial Mediterranean fever. Preliminary studies in animals weakly suggest that andrographis may offer benefits for preventing heart disease too. In addition, highly preliminary studies suggest that andrographis may help protect the liver from toxic injury, perhaps more successfully than the better known milk thistle, a liver-protective herb. Andrographis also appears to stimulate gallbladder contraction. Andrographis does not appear to have any antibacterial effects.

SCIENTIFIC EVIDENCE

Reducing cold symptoms. A meta-analysis (statistically rigorous review of studies) published in 2004 found seven double-blind, controlled trials of reasonable

---

Selected Vernacular Names for Andrographis

Akar cerita bidara, alui, *Andrographidis,* bidara, bhoonimba, bhuinimo, bhulimb, bhuninba, charita, cheranta, cherota, chiretta, chuan-hsin-lien, công công, fathalaai, fathalaichon, halviva, herba sambiloto, hinbinkohomba, I-chienhsi, kalafath, kalmegh, kanjang, kariyat, khee-pang-hee, king of bitters, kiriathu, kirta, kiryata, lanhelian, mahatikta, naynahudandi, nelavemu, quasab-uz-zarirah, rice bitters, sambilata, senshinren, sinta

---

quality, enrolling 896 persons and evaluating the use of a proprietary andrographis extract for the treatment of acute respiratory infections. The combined results indicate that this andrographis extract is more effective than placebo for reducing symptoms.

For example, a four-day, double-blind, placebo-controlled study of 158 adults with colds found that treatment with andrographis extract significantly reduced cold symptoms. Participants were given either placebo or 1,200 milligrams (mg) daily of an andrographis extract standardized to contain 5 percent andrographolide. The results showed that by day two of treatment, and even more by day four, participants who were given the actual treatment experienced significant improvements in symptoms, compared with participants in the placebo group. The greatest response was seen in reduced symptoms of earache, sleeplessness, nasal drainage, and sore throat, but other cold symptoms improved too.

Three other double-blind, placebo-controlled studies, enrolling about four hundred people, evaluated a related proprietary herbal combination treatment containing both andrographis and *Eleutherococcus senticosus*. (This proprietary combination is sold under the name Kan Jang. The manufacturer claims that this combination is more effective than andrographis alone.) Another study found this combination more effective than echinacea for colds in children.

A different formulation of andrographis has been compared with acetaminophen (Tylenol). In a double-blind study of 152 adults with a sore throat and fever, participants received andrographis (in doses of 3 or 6 grams [g] per day for seven days) or acetaminophen. The higher dose of andrographis (6 g) decreased symptoms of fever and throat pain to about the same extent as acetaminophen, but the lower dose of andrographis (3 g) was not as effective. There were no significant side effects in either group. A Russian study of questionable quality apparently found andrographis extract approximately as effective as the drug amanditine for influenza infections.

Preventing colds. According to one double-blind, placebo-controlled study, andrographis may increase resistance to colds. A total of 107 students, all eighteen years old, participated in this three-month trial, which used the same proprietary extract of andrographis as already noted. Fifty-four of the participants took two 100-mg tablets standardized to 5.6 percent andrographolide daily, which is considerably less than the 1,200 to 6,000 mg per day that has been used in studies on the treatment of colds. The other 53 students were given placebo tablets with a coating identical to the treatment. Then, once a week throughout the study, a clinician evaluated all the participants for cold symptoms.

By the end of the trial, only 16 people in the group using andrographis had experienced colds, compared with 33 of the placebo-group participants. This difference was statistically significant, indicating that andrographis reduces the risk of catching a cold by a factor of two compared with placebo.

DOSAGE

A typical dosage of andrographis is 400 mg three times a day. Doses as high as 1,000 to 2,000 mg three times daily have been used in some studies. Andrographis is usually standardized to its content of andrographolide, typically 4 to 6 percent. Note that virtually all published studies of andrographis have involved a single proprietary product. It is not clear that the results of these studies apply to products using different andrographis sources or different methods of extraction.

SAFETY ISSUES

Andrographis has not been associated with any side effects in human studies. In one study, participants were monitored for changes in liver function, blood counts, kidney function, and other laboratory measures of toxicity. No problems were found.

However, some animal studies have raised concerns that andrographis may impair fertility. One study found that male rats became infertile when fed

20 mg of andrographis powder daily. In this case, the rats stopped producing sperm and showed physical changes in some of the testicular cells involved in sperm production. Researchers also detected evidence of degeneration of other anatomical structures in the testicles. However, another study showed no evidence of testicular toxicity in male rats that were given up to 1 g per kilogram of body weight daily for sixty days, so this issue remains unclear. Furthermore, a human trial using the widely tested andrographis-*Eleutherococcus* combination found no adverse effect on male fertility measurements such as sperm quality and number.

One group of female mice also did not fare well on high dosages of andrographis. When fed 2 g per kilogram of body weight daily for six weeks (thousands of times higher than the usual human dose), all female mice failed to get pregnant when mated with males of proven fertility. Meanwhile, of the control females, 95 percent got pregnant when mated with a similar group of male mice. Another study found a potential explanation for this in evidence that andrographis relaxes the uterus. While andrographis is probably not a useful form of birth control, these results are worrisome regarding the use of andrographis by pregnant women.

Finally, if andrographis does indeed stimulate the immune system, this would lead to a whole host of potential risks. The immune system is carefully balanced. An immune system that is too relaxed fails to defend the body against infections, but an immune system that is too active attacks healthy tissues, causing autoimmune diseases. A universal immune booster might cause or exacerbate lupus, Crohn's disease, asthma, Graves' disease, Hashimoto's thyroiditis, multiple sclerosis, and rheumatoid arthritis, among other illnesses.

Safety in young children, nursing women, or those with severe liver or kidney disease has also not been established. Also, because andrographis may stimulate gallbladder contraction, it should not be used by persons with gallbladder disease except under physician supervision.

EBSCO CAM Review Board

FURTHER READING

Amaryan, G., et al. "Double-Blind, Placebo-Controlled, Randomized, Pilot Clinical Trial of Immunoguard, a Standardized Fixed Combination of *Andrographis paniculata Nees*, with *Eleutherococcus senticosus Maxim, Schizandra chinensis Bail*, and *Glycyrrhiza glabra* L. Extracts in Patients with Familial

Mediterranean Fever." *Phytomedicine* 10 (2003): 271-285.

Coon, J. T., and E. Ernst. "Andrographis Paniculata in the Treatment of Upper Respiratory Tract Infections: A Systematic Review of Safety and Efficacy." Planta Med. 70 (2004): 293-298.

Mkrtchyan, A., et al. "A Phase I Clinical Study of *Andrographis paniculata* Fixed Combination Kan Jang Versus Ginseng and Valerian on the Semen Quality of Healthy Male Subjects." *Phytomedicine* 12 (2005): 403-409.

Panossian, A., et al. "Plasma Nitric Oxide Level in Familial Mediterranean Fever and Its Modulations by Immuno-Guard." *Nitric Oxide* 9 (2003): 103-110.

Spasov, A. A., et al. "Comparative Controlled Study of *Andrographis paniculata* Fixed Combination, Kan Jang, and an Echinacea Preparation as Adjuvant, in the Treatment of Uncomplicated Respiratory Disease in Children." *Phytotherapy Research* 18 (2004): 47-53.

See also: Colds and flu; Echinacea; Immune support; Liver disease.

Androstenedione

CATEGORY: Herbs and supplements
DEFINITION: Natural substance used as a dietary supplement for specific health benefits.
PRINCIPAL PROPOSED USE: Sports performance enhancement

OVERVIEW

Androstenedione is a hormone produced naturally in the body by the adrenal glands, the ovaries (in women), and the testicles (in men). The body first manufactures dehydroepiandrosterone (DHEA), then turns DHEA into androstenedione, and finally transforms androstenedione into testosterone, the principal male sex hormone. Androstenedione is also transformed into estrogen.

Androstenedione is widely used by athletes who believe that it can build muscle and increase strength. However, there is no evidence that it works. Furthermore, androstenedione supplements may cause positive urine tests for illegal steroid use because it commonly contains a contaminant (19-norandrostenedione).

SOURCES

Androstenedione is not an essential nutrient, because the body manufactures it. It is found in meat and in some plants, but to get a therapeutic dosage, supplements are needed.

THERAPEUTIC DOSAGES

The typical recommended dose of androstenedione is 100 milligrams two times daily with food.

THERAPEUTIC USES

Androstenedione is said to enhance athletic performance and strength by increasing testosterone production, thereby building muscle. However, in double-blind studies, when androstenedione was given to men, it did not alter total testosterone levels or improve sports performance, strength, or lean body mass. It did, however, increase estrogen levels, an effect that would not be considered favorable. Some evidence suggests that androstenedione does raise testosterone levels in women; again, this is not likely to produce favorable results, and it could cause harm. The most consistent effect of androstenedione is to increase estrogen levels.

SAFETY ISSUES

There are concerns that androstenedione, like related hormones, might increase the risk of liver cancer and heart disease. In support of this last consideration, there is some evidence that androstenedione can adversely affect cholesterol levels. In addition, because androstenedione may raise testosterone levels in women, it could cause women to develop facial hair and other male-pattern appearance changes.

According to one case report, the use of androstenedione was associated with loss of libido and decreased sperm count in a twenty-nine-year-old bodybuilder. While a single case report does not prove cause and effect, androstenedione's apparent ability to raise estrogen levels in men would be consistent with these symptoms.

Another case report suggests an additional potential complication with the use of androstenedione. A man who was using androstenedione to improve his physique experienced priapism (painful continuous erection) for more than thirty hours, requiring emergency care. Previously, also while using androstenedione, he had experienced an episode lasting two to three hours that spontaneously resolved itself. It is not certain that androstenedione was the cause, but this appears to be the most likely possibility.

EBSCO CAM Review Board

FURTHER READING

Ballantyne, C. S., et al. "The Acute Effects of Androstenedione Supplementation in Healthy Young Males." *Canadian Journal of Applied Physiology* 25 (2000): 68-78.

Broeder, C. E., et al. "The Andro Project: Physiological and Hormonal Influences of Androstenedione Supplementation in Men 35 to 65 Years Old Participating in a High-Intensity Resistance Training Program." *Archives of Internal Medicine* 160 (2000): 3093-3104.

Catlin, D. H., et al. "Trace Contamination of Over-the-Counter Androstenedione and Positive Urine Test Results for a Nandrolone Metabolite." *JAMA* 284 (2000): 2618-2621.

Di Luigi, L. "Supplements and the Endocrine System in Athletes." *Clinics in Sports Medicine* 27 (2008): 131-151.

Kachhi, P. N., and S. O. Henderson. "Priapism After Androstenedione Intake for Athletic Performance Enhancement." *Annals of Emergency Medicine* 35 (2000): 391-393.

Kicman, A. T., et al. "Effect of Androstenedione Ingestion on Plasma Testosterone in Young Women: A Dietary Supplement with Potential Health Risks." *Clinical Chemistry* 49 (2003): 167-169.

Leder, B. Z., et al. "Effects of Oral Androstenedione Administration on Serum Testosterone and Estradiol Levels in Postmenopausal Women." *Journal of Clinical Endocrinology and Metabolism* 87 (2002): 5449-5454.

Ritter, R. H., A. K. Cryar, and M. R. Hermans. "Oral Androstenedione-Induced Impotence and Severe Oligospermia." *Fertility and Sterility* 84 (2005): 217.

See also: Sports and fitness support: Enhancing performance.

Angina

CATEGORY: Condition
RELATED TERMS: Angina pectoris, atherosclerosis, coronary artery disease

DEFINITION: Treatment of muscle cramping of the heart.
PRINCIPAL PROPOSED NATURAL TREATMENTS: L-carnitine and L-propionyl-carnitine, magnesium
OTHER PROPOSED NATURAL TREATMENTS: Arginine, chelation therapy, coenzyme Q_{10}, *Coleus forskohlii*, fish oil, glutamine, hawthorn, khella, *Terminalia arjuna*, traditional Chinese herbal medicine, vitamin E

INTRODUCTION

Essentially, angina is a muscle cramp in the heart, the one muscle that cannot take a rest. Angina develops when the heart muscle does not receive enough oxygen for its needs from the coronary arteries. Angina is, therefore, a symptom of coronary artery disease. Atherosclerosis (hardening of the arteries) is the most common cause of coronary artery disease; it causes thickened arterial walls and impaired blood flow.

People usually experience angina as a squeezing chest pain, as if a heavy weight rested on the chest or a tight band wrapped around it. This is often accompanied by sweating, shortness of breath, and possibly pain radiating into the left arm or neck. Usually, angina is brought on by exercise; the more rapidly the heart pumps, the more oxygen it needs. Atherosclerosis is the most common cause of angina.

People with angina are at high risk for a heart attack, and treatment must take that into account. Drugs that expand (dilate) the heart's arteries, such as nitroglycerin, can give immediate relief. Other drugs help over the long-term by making the heart's work easier. It is also important to slow or reverse the progression of atherosclerosis by treating high blood pressure and high cholesterol and by reducing other risk factors. Surgical treatments (such as angioplasty and coronary artery bypass grafting) physically widen the blood vessels that feed the heart.

PRINCIPAL PROPOSED NATURAL TREATMENTS

Angina is a serious disease that absolutely requires conventional medical evaluation and supervision. No one should self-treat for angina. However, alternative treatments may provide a useful adjunct to standard medical care when monitored by an appropriate health-care professional. Dosages are not provided in this section because they should be individualized by a doctor.

L-carnitine. The vitamin-like substance L-carnitine

Foods Containing Carnitine

Animal products, such as meat, fish, poultry, and milk, are the best sources of carnitine, a substance believed by some to aid in angina therapy. In general, as the table here shows, the redder the meat, the higher its carnitine content. The carnitine content of several foods is listed here.

Food	Milligrams
Beef steak, cooked, 4 ounces	56-162
Ground beef, cooked, 4 ounces	87-99
Milk, whole, 1 cup	8
Codfish, cooked, 4 ounces	4-7
Chicken breast, cooked, 4 ounces	3-5
Ice cream, ½ cup	3
Cheese, cheddar, 2 ounces	2
Whole-wheat bread, 2 slices	0.2
Asparagus, cooked, ½ cup	0.1

might be a good addition to standard therapy for angina. Carnitine plays a role in the cellular production of energy. Although carnitine does not address the cause of angina, it appears to help the heart produce energy more efficiently, thereby enabling it to get by with less oxygen.

In one controlled study, two hundred persons with angina (the exercise-induced variety) either received a daily dose of L-carnitine or were left untreated. All the study participants continued to take their usual medication for angina. Those taking carnitine showed improvement in several measures of heart function, including a significantly greater ability to exercise without chest pain. They were also able to reduce the dosage of some of their heart medications (under medical supervision) as their symptoms decreased. The results of this study cannot be fully trusted because it did not use a double-blind, placebo-controlled design.

A smaller trial that did use a double-blind, placebo-controlled format evaluated fifty-two people with angina. The results showed that daily use of L-carnitine significantly improved symptoms compared with placebo. Other studies (both single-blind and double-blind) used a special form of L-carnitine called L-pro-

pionyl-carnitine, and researchers found evidence of benefit.

Magnesium. Magnesium has actions in the body that resemble those of drugs in the calcium channel blocker family, although much weaker. Because these drugs are useful for angina, magnesium has been tried too.

In a six-month, double-blind, placebo-controlled study, 187 persons with angina were given either daily oral magnesium or placebo. The results showed that the use of magnesium significantly improved exercise capacity, lessened exercise-induced chest pain, and improved general quality of life. Similarly, two double-blind, placebo-controlled studies, enrolling about one hundred people with coronary artery disease, found that supplementation with magnesium significantly improved exercise tolerance.

OTHER PROPOSED TREATMENTS

A one-week, double-blind, placebo-controlled crossover trial of fifty-eight people evaluated the effectiveness of the herb *Terminalia arjuna* for angina by comparing it with placebo and with the standard drug isosorbide mononitrate. The results indicated that the herb reduced anginal episodes and increased exercise capacity. It was more effective than placebo and approximately as effective as the medication. A subsequent three-month study compared the effectiveness of *T. arjuna* with placebo in forty people who had recently had a heart attack. All participants in this study had a particular complication of a heart attack, called ischaemic mitral regurgitation. The results showed that the use of the herb improved heart function and reduced angina symptoms. Another study found benefits with an Ayurvedic herbal combination containing *T. arjuna*.

Preliminary evidence suggests that the amino acids arginine and glutamine might improve exercise tolerance in angina. Coenzyme Q_{10} (CoQ_{10}) is best known as a treatment for congestive heart failure, but it may offer benefits in angina too. N-acetylcysteine may be helpful when taken with the drug nitroglycerin, but severe headaches may develop.

Results are conflicting on whether the omega-3 fatty acids found in fish oil are helpful for people with angina. The herbs hawthorn, khella, and *Coleus forskohlii* are often recommended for angina by herbalists, but there is no meaningful evidence that they work. Vitamin E has been found only slightly effective for angina, and beta-carotene may actually increase angina. Chelation therapy is widely promoted for the treatment of angina, but there is no meaningful evidence that it is effective, and there is some evidence that it is not.

In a randomized trial of sixty-six adults with angina, four weeks of daily Chinese herbal Shenshao tablets (containing ginsenosides and white peony) were found to reduce angina frequency and improve quality-of-life scores. One should be cautious of taking certain herbs and supplements, which may interact adversely with drugs used to treat angina.

EBSCO CAM Review Board

Further Reading

Anderson, T. J., et al. "Effect of Chelation Therapy on Endothelial Function in Patients with Coronary Artery Disease: PATCH Substudy." *Journal of the American College of Cardiology* 41 (2003): 420-425.

Bednarz, B., et al. "Effects of Oral L-Arginine Supplementation on Exercise-Induced QT Dispersion and Exercise Tolerance in Stable Angina Pectoris." *International Journal of Cardiology* 75 (2000): 205-210.

Bharani, A., et al. "Efficacy of *Terminalia arjuna* in Chronic Stable Angina: A Double-Blind, Placebo-Controlled, Crossover Study Comparing *Terminalia arjuna* with Isosorbide Mononitrate." *Indian Heart Journal* 54 (2002): 170-175.

Burr, M. L., et al. "Is Fish Oil Good or Bad for Heart Disease? Two Trials with Apparently Conflicting Results." *Journal of Membrane Biology* 206 (2006): 155-163.

Dwivedi, S., et al. "Role of *Terminalia arjuna* in Ischaemic Mitral Regurgitation." *International Journal of Cardiology* 100 (2005): 507-508.

Ernst, E. "Chelation Therapy for Coronary Heart Disease: An Overview of All Clinical Investigations." *American Heart Journal* 140 (2000): 4-5.

Khogali, S. E., et al. "Is Glutamine Beneficial in Ischemic Heart Disease?" *Nutrition* 18 (2002): 123-126.

Knudtson, M. L., et al. "Chelation Therapy for Ischemic Heart Disease." *Journal of the American Medical Association* 287 (2002): 481-486.

Maxwell, A. J., et al. "Randomized Trial of a Medical Food for the Dietary Management of Chronic, Stable Angina." *Journal of the American College of Cardiology* 39 (2002): 37-45.

Pokan, R., et al. "Oral Magnesium Therapy, Exercise Heart Rate, Exercise Tolerance, and Myocardial Function in Coronary Artery Disease Patients."

British Journal of Sports Medicine 40, no. 9 (2006): 773-778.

Shechter, M., et al. "Effects of Oral Magnesium Therapy on Exercise Tolerance, Exercise-Induced Chest Pain, and Quality of Life in Patients with Coronary Artery Disease." *American Journal of Cardiology* 91 (2003): 517-521.

Wang, J., Q. Y. He, and Y. L. Zhang. "Effect of Shenshao Tablet on the Quality of Life for Coronary Heart Disease Patients with Stable Angina Pectoris." *Chinese Journal of Integrative Medicine* 15 (2009): 328.

Yokoyama, M., et al. "Effects of Eicosapentaenoic Acid on Major Coronary Events in Hypercholesterolaemic Patients (JELIS)." *The Lancet* 369 (2007): 1090-1098.

See also: Aging; Atherosclerosis and heart disease prevention; Carnitine; Cholesterol, high; Congenital heart failure; Diet-based therapies; Elder health; Heart attack; Magnesium; Strokes.

Angiotensin-converting enzyme (ACE) inhibitors

Category: Drug interactions

Definition: Medications that block the conversion of a naturally occurring substance, angiotensin, to a more active form.

Interactions: Arginine, dong quai, iron, licorice, potassium, St. John's wort, zinc

Drugs in this family: Benazepril hydrochloride (Lotensin, Lotrel), captopril (Capoten), enalapril maleate (Lexxel, Teczem, Vaseretic, Vasotec), fosinopril (Monopril), lisinopril (Prinivil, Prinzide, Zestoretic, Zestril), moexipril hydrochloride (Uniretic, Univasc), quinapril hydrochloride (Accupril), ramipril (Altace), trandolapril (Mavik, Tarka)

Arginine

Effect: Possible Harmful Interaction

Arginine is an amino acid that has been used to improve immunity in hospitalized persons and used for many other conditions. Based on experience with intravenous arginine, it is possible that the use of high-dose oral arginine might alter potassium levels in the body, especially in people with severe liver disease.

This is a potential concern for persons who take ACE inhibitors.

LICORICE

Effect: Possible Harmful Interaction

Licorice root, a member of the pea family, has been used since ancient times as both food and medicine. Whole licorice (*Glycyrrhiza glabra* or *G. uralensis*) can cause sodium retention and increase blood pressure, thus counteracting the intended effects of ACE inhibitors. An often unrecognized source of licorice is chewing tobacco. A special form of licorice known as DGL (deglycyrrhizinated licorice) is a deliberately altered form of the herb that should not cause these problems.

POTASSIUM

Effect: Possible Harmful Interaction

ACE inhibitors cause the body to retain more potassium than usual. This could raise blood levels of potassium too high, a condition called hyperkalemia, which can be dangerous. Depending on how high a person's potassium levels, the symptoms could include irregular heart rhythm, muscle weakness, nausea, vomiting, irritability, and diarrhea. Persons taking any ACE inhibitors should not take potassium supplements except on medical advice.

Because ingesting more potassium makes the problem worse, it is important to be aware of the various sources of extra potassium. Besides potassium supplements, sources include high-potassium diets, salt substitutes containing potassium, and potassium-sparing diuretics (diuretics that cause the body to retain potassium).

DONG QUAI, ST. JOHN'S WORT

Effect: Possible Harmful Interaction

St. John's wort (*Hypericum perforatum*) is primarily used to treat mild to moderate depression. The herb dong quai (*Angelica sinensis*) is often recommended for menstrual disorders such as dysmenorrhea, PMS, and irregular menstruation.

ACE inhibitors have been reported to cause increased sensitivity to the sun, amplifying the risk of sunburn or skin rash. Because St. John's wort and dong quai may also cause this problem, taking these herbal supplements during treatment with ACE inhibitors might add to this risk. It may be a good idea to wear sunscreen or protective clothing during sun

exposure if also taking one of these herbs while using an ACE inhibitor.

IRON

Effect: Possible Benefits and Risks

Persons taking ACE inhibitors frequently develop a dry cough as a side effect. One study suggests that iron supplementation can alleviate this symptom. In this four-week, double-blind, placebo-controlled trial of nineteen persons, use of iron as ferrous sulfate significantly reduced cough symptoms compared with placebo.

One should keep in mind that it is not healthy to get too much iron. For this reason, it is recommended that one seek medical advice before starting iron supplements. However, iron supplements can interfere with the absorption of captopril and perhaps other ACE inhibitors. Iron appears to bind with captopril, resulting in a compound that the body cannot absorb. This also impairs iron absorption. To minimize any potential problems, one should take iron supplements and ACE inhibitors two to three hours apart.

ZINC

Effect: Supplementation Possibly Helpful

ACE inhibitors may cause zinc depletion. The ACE inhibitors captopril and enalapril attach to the trace mineral zinc. Because zinc in this bound form cannot replace the zinc that the body uses to meet its normal needs, a gradual loss of zinc from body tissues may result. Continued drug therapy could lead to zinc deficiency.

It has been suggested, though not proven, that zinc deficiency might account for some of the side effects seen with ACE inhibitors. These side effects include taste disturbances, poor appetite, and skin numbness or tingling.

Whether zinc supplementation will prevent ACE inhibitor-induced zinc deficiency has not been examined, so it seems that taking extra zinc could help. Generally, zinc supplements should also contain copper to prevent zinc-induced copper deficiency.

FURTHER READING

AHFS Drug Information. Bethesda, Md.: American Society of Health-System Pharmacists, 2000.

Golik, A., et al. "Effects of Captopril and Enalapril on Zinc Metabolism in Hypertensive Patients." *Journal of the American College of Nutrition* 17 (1998): 75-80.

Good, C. B., L. McDermott, and B. McCloskey. "Diet and Serum Potassium in Patients on ACE Inhibitors." *Journal of the American Medical Association* 274 (1995): 538.

Lee, S. C., et al. "Iron Supplementation Inhibits Cough Associated with ACE Inhibitors." *Hypertension* 38 (2001): 166-170.

EBSCO CAM Review Board

See also: Atherosclerosis and heart disease prevention; Congestive heart failure; Food and Drug Administration; Hypertension; Supplements: Introduction.

Antacids

CATEGORY: Drug interactions

DEFINITION: Compounds that directly neutralize stomach acid.

INTERACTIONS: Calcium citrate, folate, minerals

DRUGS IN THIS FAMILY: Aluminum carbonate (Basaljel), aluminum hydroxide (ALternaGEL, Alu-Cap, Alu-Tab, Amphojel, Dialume, Nephrox), aluminum hydroxide/magnesium carbonate (Duracid), aluminum hydroxide/magnesium hydroxide (Alamag, Almacone, Aludrox, Gaviscon Liquid, Gelusil, Kudrox, Maalox Advanced Regular Strength, Magalox, Mintox, Mylanta, Rulox), aluminum hydroxide/magnesium hydroxide/calcium carbonate (Tempo), aluminum hydroxide/magnesium trisilicate (Alenic Alka, Gaviscon, Genaton, Foamicon), calcium carbonate (Alkets, Amitone, Chooz, Equilet, Gas-Ban, Mallamint, Mylanta Lozenges, Titralac, Tums), calcium carbonate/magnesium carbonate (Marblen, Mi-Acid Gelcaps, Mylanta Gelcaps, Mylagen Gelcaps), magnesium hydroxide (Milk of Magnesia, Phillips' Chewable), magaldrate or aluminum magnesium hydroxide sulfate (Iosopan, Riopan), magnesium oxide (Mag-Ox, Maox, Uro-Mag), sodium bicarbonate (Bell/ans, Bromo Seltzer), sodium citrate (Citra pH)

FOLATE

Effect: Supplementation Possibly Helpful

Research suggests that antacids physically bind to folate and reduce its absorption by the body. However, the decrease in folate absorption is relatively small, and this interaction may be clinically significant only in persons who take antacids regularly and whose diets are low in folate content.

MINERALS

Effect: Supplementation Possibly Helpful

Different types of antacids can interfere with the absorption of various minerals. Supplements containing the U.S. Dietary Reference Intake (formerly known as the Recommended Dietary Allowance) of these minerals should be helpful, especially if one takes them at a different time of day than the antacid (a minimum of two hours before or after taking the antacid).

Any antacid can interfere with the absorption of iron, zinc, and possibly other minerals by neutralizing stomach acid. Aluminum-containing antacids can bind with phosphorus and interfere with its absorption, and this can further lead to calcium depletion.

Antacids that contain calcium may also compete for absorption with iron. Although calcium antacids

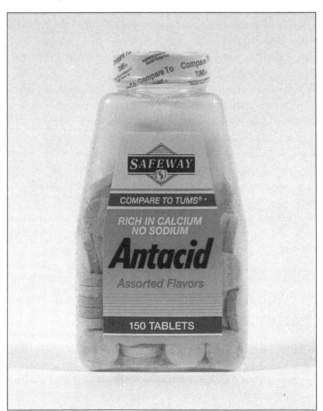

Research suggests that antacids physically bind to folate and reduce its absorption by the body. (Time & Life Pictures/ Getty Images)

may alter the absorption of magnesium, the clinical importance of this effect appears to be minimal. Calcium-containing antacids, when taken with zinc supplements, might substantially decrease zinc absorption. However, the presence of a meal appears to mitigate this effect. Finally, calcium antacids might also impair the absorption of manganese and chromium.

CITRATE

Effect: May Increase Aluminum Absorption

Concerns have been raised that the aluminum in some antacids may be harmful. Because there is some evidence that calcium citrate supplements might increase the absorption of aluminum, one should not take calcium citrate at the same time of day as aluminum-containing antacids. Another option is to use other forms of calcium, or to avoid antacids containing aluminum.

EBSCO CAM Review Board

FURTHER READING

Andon, M. B., et al. "Magnesium Balance in Adolescent Females Consuming a Low- or High-Calcium Diet." *American Journal of Clinical Nutrition* 63 (1996): 950-953.

U.S. Food and Drug Administration. "Maalox Total Relief and Maalox Liquid Products: Medication Use Errors." Available at http://www.fda.gov/safety/medwatch/safetyinformation.

Spencer, H., and L. Kramer. "Antacid-Induced Calcium Loss." *Archives of Internal Medicine* 143 (1983): 657-658.

See also: Calcium; Folate; Food and Drug Administration; H$_2$ blockers; Proton pump inhibitors; Supplements: Introduction; Vitamins and minerals.

Anthroposophic medicine

CATEGORY: Therapies and techniques

RELATED TERMS: Anthroposophical nursing, anthroposophy, art therapy, eurythmy, integrative oncology, mistletoe therapy, rhythmical massage

DEFINITION: A holistic, human-centered extension of conventional medical practice that promotes a spiritual understanding of the human being in health and illness.

PRINCIPAL PROPOSED USES: Cancer, immune and inflammatory disorders, pediatric disorders, psychiatric disorders

OTHER PROPOSED USE: Developmental disabilities

OVERVIEW

Rudolf Steiner built on his philosophical system, anthroposophy (from the Greek words *anthropos*, meaning "human," and *sophia*, meaning "wisdom"), to lay the foundations of a new medical system. Designed to be both art and science, this system reaches the spiritual side of existence and stimulates the body's natural healing forces. Steiner collaborated with medical doctors (such as Ita Wegman) and teachers to develop a "curative" educational system based on the idea that education is essential to maintaining health and preventing illness.

Several important principles guide the anthroposophical approach in medicine. Each person has a divinely guided destiny that includes individual freedom with the potential for error and illness. Illness can provide positive opportunities for development and change. Steiner recognized four manifestations of the human body that need to be considered as a whole if a person is to be treated efficiently. These manifestations are the etheric body (life force), the astral body (conscious awareness), the spiritual body (self-awareness or ego), and the physical body. The three main functional systems of the body are considered to be the sense-nervous system (conscious), the reproductive-metabolic (unconscious) system, and the rhythmic system (dreamlike). During life, the invisible bodies (three of the four manifestations) intimately connect with the organs and physiological processes of the physical body. The etheric body is especially active in growth and nutrition, the astral body functions in the nervous system, and the ego expresses itself in blood and muscular activity. Anthroposophic practitioners strive to understand a person's condition in terms of the way the four bodies interact.

MECHANISM OF ACTION

The conventional approach to medicine is limited by a materialistic view of the human body and an insufficient understanding of the ultimate causes of illness. In anthroposophic medicine (AM), illness is analyzed in terms of interrelationships between the physical and spiritual elements of the person. The therapeutic process seeks to influence and rebalance one or more of these elements. Every treatment aims to enhance the person's healing force, to improve health and deepen self-knowledge. From a pathological point of view, two main categories of disorders are distinguished in AM: metabolic pole disorders, in which physical and etheric forces predominate and build bodily substance (by generating inflammatory or feverish conditions such as childhood infectious illnesses), and head pole disorders, in which ego and astral activity predominate and destroy bodily substance (by generating disorders of late life such as degenerative illnesses and cancer).

Modern AM, an evolving discipline, retains its holistic character. The diagnostic process, however, now includes conventional methods (such as laboratory investigations and imaging), coupled with assessing a multitude of factors, such as the patient's constitution, lifestyle, diet, body rhythms (eating, sleeping, menstruation), behavioral patterns, and affinities (such as artistic inclinations). The physician's own spiritual state is important too, and she or he will often employ meditative techniques in the diagnostic process. Overall, the therapeutic process relies on the collaboration of professionally trained doctors, nurses, pharmacists, and therapists.

USES AND APPLICATIONS

AM is considered particularly suitable for inflammatory and immune conditions, childhood illnesses, developmental abnormalities, cancer, and psychiatric disorders. Therapeutic approaches include diet, special medications, and special artistic and physical therapies. Whenever possible, the treatments should support a person's own healing forces, with minimal resort to symptomatic medication.

Remedies are derived from minerals, plants, animals, and chemically defined substances. These remedies are prepared in concentrated form or in homeopathic potencies and are administered in various ways (oral, rectal, vaginal, nasal, percutaneous, or by injection). Medication can be standardized or individualized, and it may be administered alone or combined with conventional therapies. One of the most popular AM remedies remains the Iscador anticancer range of products, derived from mistletoe (*Viscum album*). The Weleda Group (in Arlesheim, Switzerland) is the biggest producer and exporter of anthroposophic medicines.

Artistic therapies (such as painting, clay modeling,

music, and speech exercises), biographic work, curative eurythmy (an artistic, deliberate method of movement), rhythmical massage, hydrotherapy, and anthroposophic nursing also belong to the AM therapeutic armamentarium.

SCIENTIFIC EVIDENCE

Hundreds of clinical trials of variable design, mostly observational and sometimes of low technical quality, have shown good clinical outcomes and safety for AM treatments. Study randomization is difficult, however, and the double-blind paradigm is rarely used. According to anthroposophic practitioners, this is due to the highly individualized nature of the treatment and the difficulty in conducting rigorous investigations on a relatively small scale.

One-half of all AM trials target cancer remedies, especially mistletoe preparations. In preclinical studies, mistletoe extracts have been shown to have immunostimulant and cytostatic effects. Many clinical trials of mistletoe anthroposophic preparations have been conducted, using various designs. The best evidence on the efficacy of mistletoe therapy exists for the improvement of quality of life and improved tolerability of conventional therapies (such as chemotherapy, radiotherapy, and surgery). In addition, tumor remission induced by injecting mistletoe extracts is well substantiated. However, the efficacy of the remedy is often called into question because of the absence of double-blinding in these studies.

Apart from studies looking at AM cancer therapy, two evaluations of AM naturalistic systems were conducted in Europe. In German outpatients with mental, musculoskeletal, respiratory, and other chronic conditions, anthroposophic treatment led to sustained improvements of symptoms and quality of life. In primary care patients from four European countries and the United States treated for acute respiratory and ear infections by anthroposophic or conventional physicians, AM was associated with a reduced use of antibiotics and antipyretics, faster recovery, and fewer adverse reactions.

Numerous studies show that persons receiving anthroposophic art therapy enjoy a long-term reduction of chronic disease symptoms and an improvement of life quality. In one Swedish study, the prevalence of atopy (predisposition to allergic reactions) in children from anthroposophic-practicing families was lower than in children from other types of families.

The study authors suggested that lifestyle factors associated with anthroposophy (such as probiotic foods, reduced exposure to antibiotics, and a lack of vaccination during infancy) may reduce the risk of atopy in children.

Choosing a Practitioner

All anthroposophic doctors must qualify first in conventional medicine and then undergo further specific training to gain a thorough understanding of the spiritual dimension of health and illness. The same pathway is followed by anthroposophic nurses.

A leading holistic health movement throughout Europe, AM is widely established and accepted in Germany, Switzerland, and the Netherlands, where many hospitals and general practitioners exist. German researchers found that anthroposophic doctors had more time for their patients and relied less on the use of technical tools.

The English-speaking world exhibits a growing interest in this practice. In the United Kingdom, both the national health system and the private sector include AM practitioners. In the United States, practitioners reside in many large cities, but the overall number of anthroposophic physicians is relatively small.

Interested persons and practitioners can contact anthroposophic professional associations or a residential clinic, such as the Rudolph Steiner Health Center in Ann Arbor, Michigan.

Safety Issues

AM is an adjunct to conventional medicine, rather than an alternative, and is largely considered safe. In recent years, German-government-funded studies of the safety of complementary medicine have reached positive conclusions regarding AM.

Anthroposophic treatment is generally well tolerated, with rare adverse reactions of mild to moderate severity. The most commonly described phenomena include local reactions from topical application, systemic hypersensitivity (with very rare cases of anaphylactic reactions), and aggravation of preexisting symptoms in sensitive persons.

Mistletoe therapy for cancer has generated some concern in the mainstream medical community, albeit mostly regarding persons who do not receive conventional treatment. Sixty percent of all persons with cancer in Germany and Switzerland, for example, are prescribed mistletoe as part of a comprehensive treatment regimen.

Mihaela Avramut, M.D., Ph.D.

Further Reading

Eurythmy Association in North America. http://www.eana.org.

Evans, Michael, and Iain Rodger. *Complete Healing: Regaining Your Health Through Anthroposophical Medicine.* Hudson, N.Y.: Anthroposophic Press, 2000. A well-written introduction to the scope of AM for general readers and health care practitioners.

Hamre, Harald J., et al. "Clinical Research in Anthroposophic Medicine." *Alternative Therapies in Health and Medicine* 15 (2009): 52-55. An authoritative review of AM for health practitioners.

Physicians' Association for Anthroposophic Medicine. http://www.paam.net.

Steiner, Rudolf. *Introducing Anthroposophic Medicine.* Hudson, N.Y.: Anthroposophic Press, 1999. A compilation of Steiner's lectures to doctors and students, describing his new art of healing.

See also: Art therapy; Dance movement therapy; Esoteric healing; Mind/body medicine; Spirituality.

Antibiotics, general

Category: Drug interactions

Definition: Substances produced naturally by microorganisms that inhibit the growth of other microorganisms, especially harmful bacteria.

Interactions: Acidophilus, *Bifidobacterium longum*, *Lactobacillus acidophilus*, probiotics, vitamin K

Drugs in this family: Amoxicillin (Amoxil, Trimox, Wymox), amoxicillin/potassium clavulanate (Augmentin), ampicillin (Omnipen, Principen, Totacillin, Marcillin), azithromycin (Zithromax), bacampicillin (Spectrobid), carbenicillin indanyl sodium (Geocillin), chloramphenicol (Chloromycetin Kapseals), cinoxacin (Cinobac), clarithromycin (Biaxin), clindamycin (Cleocin), clofazimine (Lamprene), cloxacillin sodium (Cloxapen), colistin sulfate (Coly-Mycin S), dapsone, dicloxacillin sodium (Dycill, Dynapen, Pathocil), dirithromycin (Dynabac), erythromycin (E-Base, Ilosone, EryPed, E. E. S., Ery-Tab, E-Mycin, Eryc, Erythrocin,

PCE), fosfomycin tromethamine (Monurol), kanamycin (Kantrex), lincomycin (Lincocin), metronidazole (Flagyl, Protostat), nafcillin sodium (Unipen), nalidixic acid (NegGram), neomycin (Neo-Tabs, Mycifradin, Neo-fradin), novobiocin (Albamycin), oxacillin sodium, paromomycin (Humatin), penicillin V (Pen Vee K Beepen-VK, Penicillin VK, Veetids), troleandomycin (Tao), vancomycin (Vancocin)

VITAMIN K
Effect: Possible Nutritional Depletion

Vitamin K plays a crucial role in blood clotting and also seems to be important for proper bone formation. There are concerns, however, that antibiotic treatment might reduce levels of vitamin K in the body. However, this effect seems to be slight, and only significant, if at all, in persons who are already considerably deficient in vitamin K.

ACIDOPHILUS AND OTHER PROBIOTICS
Effect: Probable Helpful Interactions

One common side effect of antibiotic therapy is diarrhea (about 25 to 30 percent of people taking antibiotics report this problem). The diarrhea is primarily caused by the antibiotic killing many of the "friendly" bacteria that normally live in the intestines. Changes in bacteria can also cause yeast infections. However, using helpful microorganisms (probiotics) such as *Saccharomyces boulardii*, *L. acidophilus*, or *Bifidobacterium*

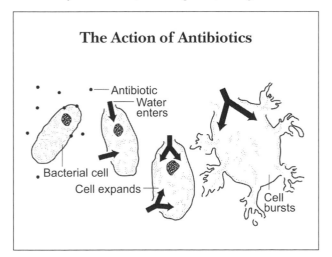

The Action of Antibiotics

Antibiotic
Water enters

Bacterial cell
Cell expands

Cell bursts

An antibiotic destroys a bacterium by causing its cell walls to deteriorate; water will then enter the bacterium unchecked until it bursts.

longum at the same time one starts antibiotics, and if continuing antibiotics for some time afterward, may reduce the risk of these complications.

EBSCO CAM Review Board

FURTHER READING
Beniwal, R. S., et al. "A Randomized Trial of Yogurt for Prevention of Antibiotic-Associated Diarrhea." *Digestive Diseases and Sciences* 48 (2003): 2077-2082.

Correa, N. B., et al. "A Randomized Formula Controlled Trial of *Bifidobacterium lactis* and *Streptococcus thermophilus* for Prevention of Antibiotic-Associated Diarrhea in Infants." *Journal of Clinical Gastroenterology* 39 (2005): 385-389.

Kotowska, M., et al. "*Saccharomyces boulardii* in the Prevention of Antibiotic-Associated Diarrhoea in Children." *Alimentary Pharmacology and Therapeutics* 21 (2005): 583-590.

Wullt, M., M. L. Hagslatt, and I. Odenholt. "*Lactobacillus plantarum* 299v for the Treatment of Recurrent *Clostridium difficile*-Associated Diarrhoea." *Scandinavian Journal of Infectious Diseases* 35 (2003): 365-367.

See also: Antacids; Children's health; Diarrhea; Food and Drug Administration; Probiotics; Supplements: Introduction; Vitamin K; Vitamins and minerals.

Anti-inflammatory diet

CATEGORY: Therapies and techniques
RELATED TERMS: Diet-based therapy, nutritional medicine
DEFINITION: Therapy that uses food with anti-inflammatory activities to treat and prevent chronic degenerative diseases.
PRINCIPAL PROPOSED USES: Arthritis, cancer, cardiovascular disease, diabetes, obesity
OTHER PROPOSED USES: Headaches, pain management

OVERVIEW
Numerous evidence-based research studies in the twenty-first century support the use of anti-inflammatory diets for the treatment and prevention of chronic degenerative diseases. These studies examined dietary properties that included raw versus processed,

organic versus commercially grown, and natural versus genetically modified. The studies also looked at the dietary effects of herbs and spices, fruits and vegetables, nuts and seeds, grains and legumes, minerals and vitamins, and phytochemicals and polyunsaturated fatty acids such as omega-3.

MECHANISM OF ACTION

There are few direct or indirect pathways (based on the specific inflammatory biomarkers) that explain how the anti-inflammatory diet works. The eicosanoid-related anti-inflammatory pathway is typical for foods with high omega-3 fatty acid content. This pathway decreases levels of arachidonic acid and inflammatory mediators such as cytokines, related prostaglandins, and related metabolites. This process also decreases the activities of inflammatory cells in the immune system.

Food with active phytochemicals (for example, resveratol and epigallocatechin galate) works through an inhibitory effect on nuclear transcription (for example, nuclear transcription factor) and through a signaling process.

THERAPEUTIC USES

Based on recent research studies, the anti-inflammatory diet could be used as a therapy for chronic degenerative diseases that have chronic inflammation as a common denominator. These diseases include diabetes, cardiovascular diseases, obesity, and certain cancers, as well as arthritis, osteoporosis, and other immune system disorders.

SCIENTIFIC EVIDENCE

Evidence-based research shows that an anti-inflammatory diet is beneficial in treating many chronic degenerative disease conditions. A 2003 double-blind, cross-over study included sixty-eight persons with a diagnosis of rheumatoid arthritis. Participants were divided into two groups for eight months of observation. One group was on a regular Western diet, and the other group was on an anti-inflammatory diet with specific regulations on arachidonic acid (low intake). Both groups received placebo or fish oil capsules for three months. Persons on the anti-inflammatory diet, but not those on the typical Western diet, showed improvements in tender and swollen joints and showed even higher improvements when fish oil was added. The basic anti-inflammatory diet can aug-

ment the beneficial effects of any single, added anti-inflammatory food component.

In a 2010 double-blind, placebo-controlled, cross-over study with a treatment period of five weeks, thirty-six healthy overweight persons received what was called an anti-inflammatory dietary mix (AIDM), which included green tea extract, resveratol (grape extract), vitamin C, vitamin E (alpha-tocopherol), tomato extract, and omega-3 fatty acid. All of these food components are described as anti-inflammatory by human and animal research studies. Serum and urine inflammatory biomarkers were measured. The AIDM brought about a decrease in inflammation and in oxidative stress (a marker for risk of inflammation) and changes in lipid metabolism (with a decrease of triglycerides and with improvement of endothelial function).

In a 2010 single-blind, randomized study, thirty-five persons diagnosed with obesity and metabolic syndrome were put on either an anti-inflammatory diet (consisting of green tea or green tea extract) or no diet for eight weeks. The group on green tea beverages or green tea extract showed lower interleukin (one of the biomarkers for inflammation) levels.

SAFETY ISSUES

No adverse side effects have been reported with the use of the anti-inflammatory diet. Beneficial changes in bowel habits can occur in the beginning, however.

Zuzana Bic, M.D., D.P.H.

FURTHER READING

Adam, O., et al. "Anti-inflammatory Effects of a Low Arachidonic Acid Diet and Fish Oil in Patients with Rheumatoid Arthritis." *Rheumatology International* 23, no. 1 (2003): 27-36.

Bakker, G. C. M., et al. "An Anti-inflammatory Dietary Mix Modulates Inflammation and Oxidative and Metabolic Stress in Overweight Men: A Nutrigenomic Approach." *American Journal of Clinical Nutrition* 91 (2010): 1044-1059.

Basu, A., et al. "Green Tea Minimally Affects Biomarkers of Inflammation in Obese Subjects with Metabolic Syndrome." *Nutrition,* June, 2010.

Calder, P. C., et al. "Polyunsaturated Fatty Acids, Inflammation, and Immunity." *European Journal of Clinical Nutrition* 56, suppl. 3 (2002): S14-S19.

Dandona, P., et al. "The Anti-inflammatory and Potential Anti-atherogenic Effect of Insulin: A New Paradigm." *Diabetologia* 45 (2002): 924-930.

Libby, P. "Inflammatory Mechanisms: The Molecular Basis of Inflammation and Disease." *Nutrition Reviews* 65, no. 12 (2007): 140-146.

Roberts, C. K., et al. "Effects of a Short-Term Diet and Exercise Intervention on Inflammatory/Anti-inflammatory Properties of HDL in Overweight/Obese Men with Cardiovascular Risk Factors." *Journal of Applied Physiology* 101 (2006): 1727-1732.

See also: Arthritis; Cancer risk reduction; Diabetes; Diet-based therapies; Green tea; Heart attack; Obesity and excess weight.

Antioxidants

CATEGORY: Functional foods

DEFINITION: Essential natural substances thought to help prevent illness and disease caused by free radicals, molecules that can damage cells.

OVERVIEW

Antioxidants are substances that inactivate free radicals, which are highly unstable molecules that can damage cell membranes and scramble the genetic information (DNA, or deoxyribonucleic acid) in cells. Free radicals are produced in the body during normal cell metabolism and at a higher rate following tissue injury or exposure to tobacco smoke, sunlight, X rays, and other environmental influences. To fight these dangerous chemicals, the body deploys a powerful antioxidant defense system, but it is hypothesized that in some cases the quantity of free radicals may overwhelm the body's natural defenses. This in turn could theoretically accelerate or cause various illnesses.

Beta-carotene, the mineral selenium, and vitamins A, C, and E function as antioxidants, agents with the ability to deactivate the naturally occurring toxic compounds called free radicals. Other substances in foods (such as lutein, astaxanthin, and lycopene) also have antioxidant activity; in addition, the body produces its own antioxidants.

The antioxidant hypothesis states that herbs and supplements with antioxidant properties may prevent illnesses and health problems associated with excess free-radical activity. For example, heart disease, cancer,

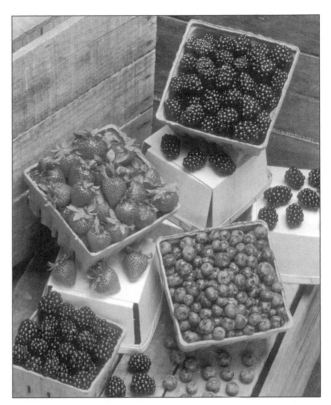

Berries contain flavonoids, a group of antioxidant compounds. (U.S. Department of Agriculture)

macular degeneration, and aging skin are just a few of the hundreds of illnesses in which free radicals are thought to play a role. Based on this hypothesis, some of the largest double-blind, placebo-controlled studies in history were set up and performed to evaluate the potential disease-preventive benefits of various antioxidant supplements. The results, however, have been quite disappointing. There is no firm evidence that antioxidants provide any meaningful health benefits.

In a 2008 detailed review of sixty-seven randomized trials involving 232,550 participants, researchers found no evidence that antioxidant supplements could reduce mortality in either healthy or diseased persons. On the contrary, there was some evidence that vitamin A, beta-carotene, and vitamin E supplementation may actually increase mortality.

What is the reason for this discrepancy? It is possible that studies have not involved the right combinations of antioxidants. It is also possible that the antioxidant hypothesis is wrong.

EBSCO CAM Review Board

FURTHER READING

Bardia, A., et al. "Efficacy of Antioxidant Supplementation in Reducing Primary Cancer Incidence and Mortality." *Mayo Clinic Proceedings* 83 (2008): 23-34.

Bjelakovic, G., A. Nagorni, et al. "Meta-analysis: Antioxidant Supplements for Primary and Secondary Prevention of Colorectal Adenoma." *Alimentary Pharmacology and Therapeutics* 24 (2006): 281-291.

Bjelakovic, G., D. Nikolova, L. L. Gluud, et al. "Mortality in Randomized Trials of Antioxidant Supplements for Primary and Secondary Prevention." *Journal of the American Medical Association* 297 (2007): 842-857.

Bjelakovic, G., D. Nikolova, L. L. Gluud, R. G. Simonetti, et al. "Antioxidant Supplements for Prevention of Mortality in Healthy Participants and Patients with Various Diseases." *Cochrane Database of Systematic Reviews* (2008): CD007176. Available through *EBSCO DynaMed Systematic Literature Surveillance* at http://www.ebscohost.com/dynamed.

Bleys, J., et al. "Vitamin-Mineral Supplementation and Then Progression of Atherosclerosis." *American Journal of Clinical Nutrition* 84 (2006): 880-887, 954-955.

Coulter, I. D., et al. "Antioxidants Vitamin C and Vitamin E for the Prevention and Treatment of Cancer." *Journal of General Internal Medicine* 21 (2006): 735-744.

Pham, D. Q., and R. Plakogiannis. "Vitamin E Supplementation in Cardiovascular Disease and Cancer Prevention: Part 1." *Annals of Pharmacotherapy* 39 (2005): 1870-1878.

See also: Astaxanthin; Beta-carotene; Lutein; Lycopene; Selenium; Vitamin A; Vitamin C; Vitamin E; Vitamins and minerals; Well-being: Homeopathic remedies; Wellness, general; Wellness therapies.

Anxiety and panic attacks

CATEGORY: Condition
RELATED TERM: Nervousness
DEFINITION: Treatment of anxiety and panic disorders.
PRINCIPAL PROPOSED NATURAL TREATMENTS: None
OTHER PROPOSED NATURAL TREATMENTS: Acupuncture; arginine plus lysine; aromatherapy; bach flower remedies; biofeedback; chamomile; Chinese skullcap; 5-hydroxytryptophan; flaxseed oil; *Galphimia glauca*; gamma oryzanol; gotu kola; hops; inositol; kava; lemon balm; linden; magnesium, hawthorn, and *Eschscholtzia californica* (California poppy) combination; massage; melatonin; multivitamin-multimineral supplements; passionflower; relaxation therapies (meditation and guided imagery); selenium; suma; valerian

INTRODUCTION

As the British-born American poet W. H. Auden pointed out in the early twentieth century, modern humans live in an age of anxiety. Most have a certain level of chronic anxiety because modern life is jagged, fast-paced, and divorced from the natural rhythms that tend to create a harmonious inner life. For some, this existential unease goes further and becomes a psychological disorder.

Typical symptoms of anxiety disorder include feelings of tension, irritability, worry, frustration, turmoil, and hopelessness, along with insomnia, restless sleep, grinding of teeth, jaw pain, an inability to sit still, and an incapacity to cope. Physical sensations frequently arise too and include a characteristic feeling of being unable to take a full, satisfying breath; dry mouth; rapid heartbeat; heart palpitations; a lump in the throat; tightness in the chest; and cramping in the bowels.

Anxiety can also give rise to panic attacks. These may be so severe that they are mistaken for heart attacks. The heart pounds and palpitates, the chest feels tight and painful, and the whole body tenses with unreasonable fear. Such attacks can be triggered by anxiety-provoking situations, but they may also arise suddenly and seemingly without cause, perhaps even awakening a person from his or her sleep. A person who tends to have panic attacks more so than generalized anxiety is said to have panic disorder.

The medical treatment of anxiety involves antianxiety drugs in the benzodiazepine family, the unique drug BuSpar (buspirone), and antidepressants. Panic attacks are generally more difficult to treat than other forms of anxiety.

PROPOSED NATURAL TREATMENTS

There are no natural treatments for anxiety that have been shown to be safe and effective. However, some treatments have shown promise for generalized anxiety disorder and related conditions. No

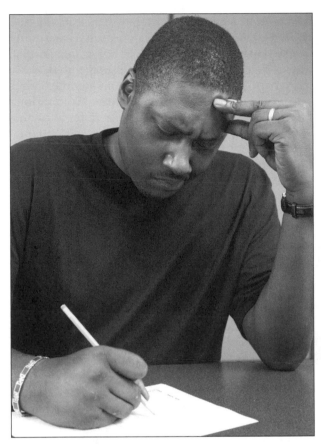

Taking exams can be a source of anxiety for some people.
(©Lisa F. Young/Dreamstime.com)

natural treatment is likely to be effective for panic disorder.

Valerian. The herb valerian is best known as a remedy for insomnia. However, because many drugs useful for insomnia also reduce anxiety, valerian has been proposed as an anxiety treatment.

In a double-blind, placebo-controlled study, thirty-six people with generalized anxiety disorder were given either valerian extract, valium, or placebo for four weeks. The study failed to find statistically significant differences among the groups, presumably because of its small size. However, a careful analysis of the results hints that valerian was helpful.

In addition, a preliminary double-blind study found that valerian may produce calming effects in stressful situations. Again, though, this study was too small to provide definitive results. Another study evaluated the anxiety-relieving effects of a combination containing valerian and lemon balm taken in various doses; some benefits were seen with doses of 600 milligrams (mg) or 1,200 mg three times daily, but the highest dose (1,800 mg three times daily) actually appeared to increase anxiety symptoms during stressful situations. Furthermore, people taking the herbal treatment at any dose showed slightly decreased cognitive function compared with those given placebo.

Kava. Until 2002, the herb kava was widely used in Europe as a medical treatment for anxiety, based on the evidence of a substantial body of double-blind, placebo-controlled studies. However, because of concerns involving its potential effects on the liver, it has been withdrawn from the market in many countries. Its use is not recommend.

Other herbs and supplements. A large (264-participant) three-month, double-blind, placebo-controlled study tested the possible antianxiety benefits of a combination therapy containing the mineral magnesium (150 mg twice daily), the herb hawthorn (150 mg twice daily of a standardized extract), and the seldom-studied herb *Eschscholtzia californica* (California poppy, 40 mg twice daily). Study participants all had generalized anxiety disorder of mild-to-moderate intensity. The results indicated that the combination treatment was more effective than placebo. No significant side effects were seen. This particular combination therapy is used in France.

A double-blind, placebo-controlled trial of eighty healthy male volunteers found that twenty-eight days of treatment with a multivitamin-multimineral supplement (containing calcium, magnesium, and zinc) significantly reduced anxiety and the sensation of stress.

The supplement 5-hydroxytryptophan (5-HTP) is best known as a proposed treatment for depression. An eight-week, double-blind, placebo-controlled study compared 5-HTP and the drug clomipramine in forty-five persons with anxiety disorder. The results indicated that 5-HTP was effective but clomipramine was more effective.

Based on its apparent ability to promote sleep, melatonin has been tried as a treatment for reducing anxiety. However, while four studies performed by Saudi researchers reported benefits, other researchers have been unable to confirm these results.

A four-week double-blind study of thirty-six persons with anxiety (specifically, generalized anxiety disorder) compared the herb passionflower to the standard drug oxazepam. Oxazepam worked more quickly, but by the end of the four-week trial, both treatments proved equally effective. Furthermore, passionflower showed a comparative advantage in terms of side effects: The use of oxazepam was associated with more impairment of job performance. Also, in a placebo-controlled trial involving sixty persons undergoing surgery, passionflower significantly reduced anxiety up to ninety minutes before surgery. The only other supporting evidence for passionflower comes from animal studies.

Several small double-blind studies by a single research group have found preliminary evidence that the oral use of lemon balm (*Melissa officinalis*) may reduce anxiety levels. Like other antianxiety agents, it may also impair mental function to some degree. A combination of lemon balm and valerian has also been tested, with generally positive results.

One study found that one week of oral treatment with lysine (2.64 grams per day) and arginine (2.64 grams per day) could reduce general levels of anxiety. A double-blind, placebo-controlled trial of forty persons found that gotu kola reduced the "startle" response to sudden loud noises. This suggests, but does not prove, that gotu kola may be helpful for anxiety.

A small, double-blind, placebo-controlled, crossover study found that the use of the herb European skullcap reduced general anxiety levels. The herb *Galphimia glauca* is traditionally used as a "nerve tonic" by Mexican herbalists. One substantial double-blind study purportedly found that a standardized galphimia extract is as effective as the standard medication lorazepam. However, because this study failed to use a placebo group, these results mean little.

Two preliminary studies that evaluated linden flower for potential sedative or antianxiety effects returned contradictory results. Another study found weak evidence that sage might reduce anxiety.

Other herbs or supplements that are frequently recommended for anxiety attacks include Chinese skullcap, flaxseed oil, chamomile, gamma oryzanol, hops, selenium, and suma, as well as inositol for panic disorder. However, there is no reliable supporting evidence to indicate that they work.

The substance gamma-aminobutyric acid (GABA) is a naturally occurring neurotransmitter that is used within the brain to reduce the activity of certain nerve systems, including those related to anxiety. For this reason, GABA supplements are sometimes recommended for treatment of anxiety-related conditions. However, there are no studies supporting the use of GABA supplements for anxiety. In fact, it appears that, when taken orally, GABA cannot pass the blood-brain barrier and, therefore, does not even enter the brain.

Alternative therapies. Various alternative therapies have shown some promise for the treatment of anxiety. These therapies include acupuncture (for generalized anxiety and for situational anxiety), aromatherapy (either alone or with massage), biofeedback, and music therapy (for terminally ill persons). However, the supporting evidence to indicate that these treatments work remains weak.

There is a fair amount of evidence in support of relaxation therapies and massage (either alone or with aromatherapy) to treat the symptoms of anxiety, at least in the short term. In a 2008 review of twenty-seven studies, for example, researchers concluded that relaxation therapies (including Jacobson's progressive relaxation, autogenic training, applied relaxation, and meditation) were effective against anxiety. (However, not all of the studies were randomized, controlled trials.) In a randomized trial involving sixty-eight persons with generalized anxiety disorder, ten sessions of therapeutic massage, thermotherapy (the application of heat), and relaxation were all found to be beneficial at reducing anxiety, though none was superior to the others. Finally, three studies failed to find that Bach flower remedies are helpful for situational anxiety.

HERBS AND SUPPLEMENTS TO USE ONLY WITH CAUTION

Various herbs and supplements may interact adversely with drugs used to treat anxiety, so persons should be cautious when considering the use of herbs and supplements.

HOMEOPATHIC REMEDIES

A double-blind, placebo-controlled study of forty-four people with generalized anxiety disorder found that the use of constitutional, or classical, homeopathy did not significantly improve symptoms.

EBSCO CAM Review Board

FURTHER READING

Andreatini, R., et al. "Effect of Valepotriates (Valerian Extract) in Generalized Anxiety Disorder." *Phytotherapy Research* 16 (2002): 650-654.

Bonne, O., et al. "A Randomized, Double-Blind, Placebo-Controlled Study of Classical Homeopathy in Generalized Anxiety Disorder." *Journal of Clinical Psychiatry* 64 (2003): 282-287.

Capuzzo, M., et al. "Melatonin Does Not Reduce Anxiety More Than Placebo in the Elderly Undergoing Surgery." *Anesthesia and Analgesia* 103 (2006): 121-123.

Coleta, M., et al. "Comparative Evaluation of *Melissa officinalis* L., *Tilia europaea* L., *Passiflora edulis* Sims., and *Hypericum perforatum* L. in the Elevated plus Maze Anxiety Test." *Pharmacopsychiatry* 34, suppl. 1 (2001): S20-S21.

Cooke, B., and E. Ernst. "Aromatherapy." *British Journal of General Practice* 50 (2000): 493-496.

Evans, S., et al. "Mindfulness-Based Cognitive Therapy for Generalized Anxiety Disorder." *Journal of Anxiety Disorders* 22 (2008): 716-721.

Hanus, M., J. Lafon, and M. Mathieu. "Double-Blind, Randomised, Placebo-Controlled Study to Evaluate the Efficacy and Safety of a Fixed Combination Containing Two Plant Extracts (*Crataegus oxyacantha* and *Eschscholtzia californica*) and Magnesium in Mild-to-Moderate Anxiety Disorders." *Current Medical Research and Opinion* 20 (2004): 63-71.

Horne-Thompson, A., and D. Grocke. "The Effect of Music Therapy on Anxiety in Patients Who Are Terminally Ill." *Journal of Palliative Medicine* 11 (2008): 582-590.

Karst, M., et al. "Auricular Acupuncture for Dental Anxiety." *Anesthesia and Analgesia* 104 (2007): 295-300.

Lahmann, C., et al. "Brief Relaxation Versus Music Distraction in the Treatment of Dental Anxiety." *Journal of the American Dental Association* 139 (2008): 317-324.

Manzoni, G. M., et al. "Relaxation Training for Anxiety." *BMC Psychiatry* 8 (2008): 41.

Movafegh, A., et al. "Preoperative Oral *Passiflora incarnata* Reduces Anxiety in Ambulatory Surgery Patients." *Anesthesia and Analgesia* 106 (2008): 1728-1732.

Nyklicek, I., and K. F. Kuijpers. "Effects of Mindfulness-Based Stress Reduction Intervention on Psychological Well-Being and Quality of Life: Is Increased Mindfulness Indeed the Mechanism?" *Annals of Behavioral Medicine* 35 (2008): 331-340.

Samarkandi, A., et al. "Melatonin vs. Midazolam Premedication in Children." *European Journal of Anaesthesiology* 22 (2005): 189-196

Sherman, K. J., et al. "Effectiveness of Therapeutic Massage for Generalized Anxiety Disorder." *Depression and Anxiety* 27 (2010): 441-450.

Sury, M. R. J., and K. Fairweather. "The Effect of Melatonin on Sedation of Children Undergoing Magnetic Resonance Imaging." *British Journal of Anaesthesiology* 97 (2006): 220-225.

Wachelka, D., and R. C. Katz. "Reducing Test Anxiety and Improving Academic Self-Esteem in High School and College Students with Learning Disabilities." *Journal of Behavior Therapy and Experimental Psychiatry* 30 (1999): 191-198.

See also: Biofeedback; Depression, mild to moderate; European skullcap; Guided imagery; Kava; Meditation; Seasonal affective disorder; Relaxation response; Relaxation therapies; Stress; Valerian.

Applied kinesiology

CATEGORY: Therapies and techniques
RELATED TERMS: Contact reflex analysis, functional neurologic assessment, kenesitherapy, kinesiology
DEFINITION: The use of techniques such as muscle testing to identify health problems.
PRINCIPAL PROPOSED USES: Allergies, disease diagnosis, neurologic evaluation, nutritional deficiencies, organ dysfunction
OTHER PROPOSED USES: Dyslexia, handwriting performance, mastalgia

OVERVIEW

The modern practice of applied kinesiology (AK) began in 1964 when chiropractor George J. Goodheart, Jr., observed that poor posture is often associated with weak muscles. Through his work, he linked specific diseases to the strength or weakness of muscles. Although many practitioners of AK refer to their work as kinesiology, AK should not be confused with standard kinesiology, which is the scientific study of the principles of mechanics and anatomy in relationship to human movement.

MECHANISM OF ACTION

The fundamental idea of AK is that every organ dysfunction in the body is accompanied by a specific muscle weakness. Particular disease states in the body can then be tied directly to the corresponding internal organs by determining what factor weakened a previously strong muscle.

USES AND APPLICATIONS

AK believes that muscle-testing procedures can be used to diagnose whatever illness might be afflicting a person. Treatment with appropriate nutrients, special diets, acupressure, various reflex procedures, and spinal or joint manipulation may be used in an effort to improve health.

SCIENTIFIC EVIDENCE

Although there is little doubt that muscle movements detected by AK are unconsciously triggered, no published scientific studies establish specific links between muscle responses and diseases that affect organs. Researchers who have conducted elaborate double-blind trials have concluded that connections between muscle weakness and particular diseases are random phenomena. Diagnoses of nutritional deficiencies by AK are not verified by the nutrient levels determined by blood serum analysis.

Other studies demonstrate that the power of suggestion, and distractions, variations in the amount of force or leverage applied to muscles, and muscle fatigue, all play a significant role in the outcome of muscle testing. Results from the scientific review of twenty research papers published by the International College of Applied Kinesiology concluded that none of the papers included statistical analyses rigorous enough to confer validity on their findings.

Although AK has been suggested for the treatment of many conditions, high-quality scientific research and findings are very limited. AK has not been shown to provide an effective diagnosis or treatment of any disease. No differences were found in controlled studies using nutrient substances versus placebos.

SAFETY ISSUES

AK techniques are generally safe but can produce temporary pain. Also, persons using AK could find that their illness has been left undetected and untreated. Sole AK use could delay the time it takes for a person to see a qualified health-care provider about a potentially life-threatening condition. One should not rely solely on AK for diagnosis; instead, AK should be used to enhance standard medical diagnosis and therapy.

Alvin K. Benson, Ph.D.

FURTHER READING

"Applied Kinesiology: Phony Muscle-Testing for 'Allergies' and 'Nutrient Deficiencies.'" Available at http://www.quackwatch.com/01quackeryrelatedtopics/tests/ak.html.

Frost, Robert. *Applied Kinesiology: A Training Manual and Reference Book of Basic Principles and Practices.* Berkeley, Calif.: North Atlantic Books, 2002.

International College of Applied Kinesiology. http://www.icak.com.

Neumann, Donald A. *Kinesiology of the Musculoskeletal System: Foundations for Rehabilitation.* 2d ed. St. Louis, Mo.: Mosby/Elsevier, 2010.

Walther, David S. *Applied Kinesiology: Synopsis.* 2d ed. Pueblo, Colo.: Systems DC, 2000.

See also: Alexander technique; Aston-Patterning; Feldenkrais method; Manipulative and body-based practices; Osteopathic manipulation; Progressive muscle relaxation; Reflexology; Rolfing; Shiatsu; Therapeutic touch.

Arginine

CATEGORY: Herbs and supplements
RELATED TERMS: Arginine hydrochloride, L-arginine
DEFINITION: Natural substance used as a dietary supplement for specific health benefits.
PRINCIPAL PROPOSED USES: Angina, congestive heart failure, intermittent claudication, sexual dysfunction in men, sexual dysfunction in women
OTHER PROPOSED USES: Common cold prevention, cystic fibrosis, diabetes, female infertility, heart attack (aiding recovery), interstitial cystitis, maintaining effectiveness of nitrate drugs, male infertility, osteoporosis, preeclampsia, Raynaud's phenomenon, sickle cell disease, surgery support
PROBABLY NOT EFFECTIVE USES: Altitude sickness, intermittent claudication

OVERVIEW

Arginine is an amino acid found in many foods, including dairy products, meats, poultry, fish, nuts, and chocolate. It plays a role in several important mechanisms in the body, including cell division, wound healing, removal of ammonia from the body, immunity to illness, and the secretion of important hormones.

The body also uses arginine to make nitric oxide (NO), a substance that relaxes blood vessels and also exerts numerous other effects in the body. Based on this, arginine has been proposed as a treatment for various cardiovascular diseases, including congestive heart failure and intermittent claudication, as well as impotence, female sexual dysfunction, interstitial cystitis, and many other conditions. Arginine's potential effects on immunity have also created an interest in using it as part of an immune "cocktail" given to severely ill hospitalized persons and also for preventing colds.

Requirements and Sources

Normally, the body either gets enough arginine from food or manufactures what it needs from other widely available nutrients. Certain stresses, such as severe burns, infections, and injuries, can deplete the body's supply of arginine. For this reason, arginine (combined with other nutrients) is used in a hospital setting to help enhance recovery from severe injury or illness.

Therapeutic Dosages

A typical supplemental dosage of arginine is 2 to 8 grams (g) per day. For congestive heart failure, higher dosages up to 15 g have been used in trials. However, one should not try to self-treat congestive heart failure.

Therapeutic Uses

Small double-blind, placebo-controlled studies suggest that arginine might be helpful for the treatment of several seemingly unrelated conditions that are all linked by arginine's effects on NO: congestive heart failure, intermittent claudication, angina, impotence, and sexual dysfunction in women. The first three conditions in this list are life-threatening. Persons with angina, congestive heart failure, or intermittent claudication should not attempt to self-treat with arginine except under a physician's supervision.

Arginine has been proposed for use after a heart attack to aid recovery. In one study, arginine did not cause harm and showed potential modest benefit. However, in another study, arginine failed to prove helpful for treatment of people who had just had a heart attack, and it possibly increased the post-heart-attack death rate.

A small, double-blind, placebo-controlled study suggests that use of arginine (700 milligrams [mg] four times daily) may support transdermal nitroglycerin therapy for angina. Ordinarily, the drug nitroglycerin becomes less effective over time, as the body develops a tolerance to it. However, arginine supplements appear to help prevent the development of tolerance.

The results of one controlled (but not blinded) study in women suggest that arginine might help standard fertility therapy for women (specifically, in vitro fertilization) work better. However, studies have not found any benefit in male infertility.

Weak evidence suggests that arginine might improve insulin action in people with type 2 diabetes. Nutritional mixtures containing arginine have shown promise for enhancing recovery from major surgery, injury, or illness, perhaps by enhancing immunity. Highly preliminary evidence suggests that arginine might be worth investigating as a treatment for pulmonary hypertension in people with sickle cell disease.

Conflicting results have been seen in preliminary double-blind studies of arginine for preeclampsia. Preliminary double-blind studies have failed to find arginine helpful for asthma, cystic fibrosis, interstitial cystitis, kidney failure, osteoporosis, or Raynaud's phenomenon. One study found that an arginine-rich food bar did not help relax arteries or thin the blood in people with high cholesterol.

A study of 133 people with intermittent claudication (pain in the legs caused by atherosclerosis) failed to find arginine helpful; in fact, arginine was less effective than placebo, suggesting that it actually increases symptoms to some extent. Two earlier studies had reported benefit, but they were small and poorly designed and reported.

One preliminary, double-blind study suggests that arginine supplementation might help prevent colds. Also, arginine has been proposed for preventing altitude sickness, but the one reported study found harmful effects (increase in headache) rather than beneficial ones.

Scientific Evidence

The first three conditions in this section are life-threatening. Persons with angina, congestive heart failure, or intermittent claudication should not self-treat with arginine except under a physician's supervision.

What Is Heart Failure?

Heart failure, thought by some to be treatable with arginine, is a condition in which the heart cannot pump enough blood to meet the body's needs. In some cases, the heart cannot fill with enough blood. In other cases, the heart cannot pump blood to the rest of the body with enough force. Some people have both problems. The term "heart failure" does not mean that the heart has stopped or is about to stop working. However, heart failure is a serious condition that requires medical care.

Heart failure develops over time as the heart's pumping action grows weaker. The condition can affect the right side of the heart only, or it can affect both sides of the heart. Most cases involve both sides of the heart. The leading causes of heart failure are diseases that damage the heart. These include coronary heart disease, also called coronary artery disease; high blood pressure; and diabetes.

Congestive heart failure. Three small double-blind, placebo-controlled studies enrolling a total of about seventy persons with congestive heart failure found that oral arginine at a dose of 5 to 15 g daily could significantly improve symptoms and objective measurements of heart function.

Intermittent claudication. People with advanced hardening of the arteries, or atherosclerosis, often have difficulty walking because of a lack of blood flow to the legs, a condition known as intermittent claudication. Pain may develop after walking less than half a block.

In a double-blind study of forty-one persons, two weeks of treatment with a high dose of arginine improved walking distance by 66 percent; no benefits were seen in the placebo group or in a low-dose arginine group. Good results also were seen in another study, although its convoluted design makes interpreting the results somewhat difficult.

Angina. A double-blind study of twenty-five persons with angina pectoris found that treatment with arginine at a dose of 6 g per day improved exercise tolerance, but not objective measurements of heart function. A double-blind, placebo-controlled crossover trial of thirty-six persons with heart disease found that the use of arginine (along with antioxidant vitamins and minerals) at a daily dose of 6.6 g reduced symptoms of angina.

Impotence. The substance NO plays a role in the development of an erection. Drugs such as Viagra increase the body's sensitivity to the natural rise in NO that occurs with sexual stimulation. A simpler approach might be to raise levels of this substance, and one way to accomplish this involves use of the amino acid L-arginine. Oral arginine supplements may increase NO levels in the penis and elsewhere. Based on this, L-arginine has been advertised as "natural Viagra." However, there is little evidence that it works. Drugs based on raising NO levels in the penis have not worked for pharmaceutical developers; the body seems simply to adjust to the higher levels and maintain the same level of response.

Nonetheless, some small studies have found possible evidence of benefit. In a double-blind trial, fifty men with erectile dysfunction received 5 g of either arginine or a placebo per day for six weeks. More men in the treated group experienced improvement in sexual performance than in the placebo group.

A double-blind crossover study of thirty-two men found no benefit with 1,500 mg of arginine daily for seventeen days. However, the lower dose of arginine and the shorter course of treatment may explain the discrepancy between these two studies.

Arginine also has been evaluated in combination with the drug yohimbine (as opposed to the herb yohimbe). A double-blind, placebo-controlled trial of forty-five men found that one-time use of this combination therapy one hour or two before intercourse improved erectile function, especially in those with only moderate erectile dysfunction scores. Arginine and yohimbine were both taken at a dose of 6 g. Note, however, that one should not use the drug yohimbine (or the herb yohimbe) except under physician supervision, because it presents a number of safety risks.

One study reportedly found that arginine plus oligomeric proanthocyanidins (OPCs) can improve male sexual function, but because the study lacked a placebo group, it did not find anything. A small, unpublished, double-blind study listed on a manufacturer's Web site reported benefits with a proprietary combination of arginine; the herbs ginseng, ginkgo, and damiana; and vitamins and minerals.

Sexual dysfunction in women. Some postmenopausal women have difficulty experiencing sexual arousal. One small double-blind study of yohimbine combined with arginine found an increase in measured physical arousal among twenty-three women with this condition. However, the women themselves did not report any noticeable subjective effects, suggesting that the effect was slight. In addition, only the combination of yohimbine and arginine produced results; neither substance was effective when taken on its own. Slight benefits were also seen in preliminary double-blind, placebo-controlled trials that evaluated a combination therapy containing arginine; the herbs ginseng, ginkgo, and damiana; and vitamins and minerals.

Interstitial cystitis. Interstitial cystitis is a condition in which a person feels like he or she has symptoms of a bladder infection, but no infection is present. Medical treatment for this condition is less than satisfactory.

A three-month, double-blind trial of fifty-three persons with interstitial cystitis found only weak indications that arginine might improve symptoms. Several participants dropped out of the study; when this was properly taken into account using a statistical method called ITT analysis, no benefit could be proven.

Colds. A two-month, double-blind study involving forty children with a history of frequent colds concluded that arginine seemed to provide some protection against respiratory infections. Of the children who were given arginine, fifteen stayed well during the sixty days of the study. By contrast, only five of the children who took placebo stayed well, a significant difference.

Nutritional support in hospitalized persons. Several nutritional products that contain arginine and other substances have been tried in hospital settings to enhance recovery following major surgery, illness, or injury. These mixtures are delivered enterally, through a tube into the stomach. A review of fifteen studies, about one-half of them double-blind and involving 1,557 persons, found that such products can reduce episodes of infection, time on ventilator machines, and length of stay in the hospital. However, because of the many nutrients contained in these so-called immunonutrient mixtures, it is not clear whether arginine deserves the credit.

SAFETY ISSUES

There is good evidence that arginine is safe and well tolerated at levels up to 20 g per day, although minor gastrointestinal upset can occur. However, there are some potential safety issues regarding high-dose arginine. These cautions are based on findings from animal studies and hospital experiences of intravenous administration.

For example, arginine may stimulate the body's production of gastrin, a hormone that increases stomach acid. For this reason, there are concerns that arginine could be harmful for people who have ulcers or take drugs that are hard on the stomach. In addition, a double-blind trial found that arginine (30 g/day) may increase the risk of esophageal reflux (heartburn) by relaxing the sphincter at the bottom of the esophagus.

Arginine might also alter potassium levels in the body, especially in people with severe liver disease. This is a potential concern for persons who take drugs that also alter potassium balance (such as potassium-sparing diuretics and angiotensin-converting enzyme, or ACE, inhibitors) and for those with severe kidney disease. Persons in any of these categories should not use high-dose arginine except under physician supervision.

Evidence that arginine can improve insulin sensitivity raises theoretical concerns that if a patient has diabetes and takes arginine, his or her blood sugar could fall too low. However, one study suggests that arginine is safe for use by people with stable type 2 diabetes.

The amino acid lysine has been advocated for use in oral or genital herpes. According to the theory behind this recommendation, it is important to simultaneously restrict arginine intake. If true, this would tend to suggest that arginine supplements would be harmful for people with a tendency to develop herpes. However, there is no meaningful evidence to support this hypothesis.

Maximum safe doses in pregnant or nursing women, young children, and those with severe liver or kidney disease have not been established.

IMPORTANT INTERACTIONS

Persons taking lysine to treat herpes should note that arginine use might counteract the potential benefit of the lysine. For persons using drugs that are hard on the stomach (such as nonsteroidal anti-inflammatory medications), taking high doses of arginine might stress the stomach additionally.

High doses of arginine should be used only under physician supervision in persons also taking medications that can alter the balance of potassium in the body (such as potassium-sparing diuretics or ACE inhibitors). For persons taking transdermal nitroglycerin, arginine may help prevent the development of tolerance.

EBSCO CAM Review Board

FURTHER READING

Baecker, N., et al. "L-Arginine, the Natural Precursor of NO, Is Not Effective for Preventing Bone Loss in Postmenopausal Women." *Journal of Bone and Mineral Research* 20 (2005): 471-479.

Bednarz, B., et al. "Efficacy and Safety of Oral L-Arginine in Acute Myocardial Infarction." *Kardiologia polska* 62 (2005): 421-427.

Grasemann, H., et al. "Oral L-Arginine Supplementation in Cystic Fibrosis Patients." *European Respiratory Journal* 25 (2005): 62-68.

Ito, T. Y., et al. "The Enhancement of Female Sexual Function with ArginMax, a Nutritional Supplement, Among Women Differing in Menopausal Status." *Journal of Sex and Marital Therapy* 32 (2006): 369-378.

Mansoor, J. K., et al. "L-Arginine Supplementation Enhances Exhaled NO, Breath Condensate VEGF, and Headache at 4342 m." *High Altitude Medicine and Biology* 6 (2005): 289-300.

Moriguti, J. C., et al. "Effects of Arginine Supplementation on the Humoral and Innate Immune Response of Older People." *European Journal of Clinical Nutrition* 59 (2005): 1362-1366.

Stanislavov, R., and V. Nikolova. "Treatment of Erectile Dysfunction with Pycnogenol and L-Arginine." *Journal of Sex and Marital Therapy* 29 (2003): 207-213.

See also: Angina; Congestive heart failure; Sexual dysfunction in men; Sexual dysfunction in women; Supplements: Introduction.

Arjun

CATEGORY: Herbs and supplements
RELATED TERMS: Arjun tree, *Terminalia arjuna*
DEFINITION: Natural plant product used as a dietary supplement for specific health benefits.
PRINCIPAL PROPOSED USE: Angina
OTHER PROPOSED USES: High cholesterol, intestinal parasites

OVERVIEW

Terminalia arjuna is a common herbal plant (known as the Arjun tree) in Central and South India. Its bark has a long history of use in Ayurvedic medicine (the traditional medicine of India) for the treatment of heart problems. Other uses of various parts of the Arjun tree include hemorrhage, diarrhea, irregular menstruation, skin ulcers, acne, wounds, and fractures.

USES AND APPLICATIONS

Evidence suggests that *Terminalia arjuna* (or arjun) may have properties for relaxing blood vessels. Arjun has shown promise in the treatment of angina, a condition in which blood vessels in the heart cannot carry adequate oxygen to the heart muscle. In addition, weak evidence suggests that arjun may have antimicrobial effects, providing benefits against amoebas and other microorganisms. One study has been used to indicate that arjun can improve cholesterol levels, but this study proves little because it was not double-blind.

SCIENTIFIC EVIDENCE

A one-week, double-blind, placebo-controlled, crossover trial of fifty-eight persons evaluated the effectiveness of arjun for angina by comparing it with placebo and also with the standard drug isosorbide mononitrate. The results indicated that the herb reduced anginal episodes and increased exercise capacity. It was more effective than placebo and approximately as effective as the medication.

A subsequent three-month study compared the effectiveness of arjun with placebo in forty people with a recent heart attack. All participants in this study had a particular complication of a heart attack called ischaemic mitral regurgitation. The results showed that the use of the herb improved heart function and reduced angina symptoms. Also, a combination Ayurvedic therapy containing arjun and approximately forty other herbs has also shown some promise for angina.

DOSAGE

A typical dosage of *Terminalia arjuna* is 500 milligrams two or three times daily.

SAFETY ISSUES

The use of arjun has not been associated with any severe adverse effects. However, comprehensive safety studies have not been performed. Safety in young children, pregnant or nursing women, or people with severe liver or kidney disease has not been established.

EBSCO CAM Review Board

FURTHER READING

Bharani, A., et al. "*Terminalia arjuna* Reverses Impaired Endothelial Function in Chronic Smokers." *Indian Heart Journal* 56 (2004): 123-128.

Hemalatha, T., et al. "Arjunolic Acid: A Novel Phytomedicine with Multifunctional Therapeutic Applications." *Indian Journal of Experimental Biology* 48 (2010): 238-247.

Khan, R., et al. "Antimicrobial Activity of Five Herbal Extracts Against Multi Drug Resistant (MDR) Strains of Bacteria and Fungus of Clinical Origin." *Molecules* 14 (2009): 586-597.

See also: Angina; Cholesterol, high; Herbal medicine; Parasites, intestinal.

Aromatherapy

CATEGORY: Therapies and techniques
RELATED TERM: Essential oils
DEFINITION: A form of herbal medicine in which an herb's essential oil is inhaled, applied to the skin, or taken orally.

PRINCIPAL PROPOSED USES:

- *Inhaled:* Reducing anxiety, decreasing agitation in Alzheimer's disease and other forms of dementia
- *Oral:* Acute bronchitis, acute sinusitis, chronic bronchitis, common cold

OTHER PROPOSED USES

- *Inhaled:* Chronic bronchitis, common cold, insomnia, memory and mental function enhancement, menstrual pain, nausea, pregnancy support, smoking cessation, stroke recovery
- *Topical:* Alopecia, athlete's foot, insect bites, photosensitivity, pregnancy support, tension headaches, vaginal infections
- *Oral:* Gingivitis, dyspepsia, irritable bowel syndrome

OVERVIEW

Aromatherapy is a form of herbal medicine. However, instead of using the entire herb, it employs the fragrant essential oil that is released when a fresh herb is compressed or subjected to chemical extraction. Essential oils also are often used as fragrances in cosmetics and bath products.

When employed medicinally, essential oils are often evaporated into the air through the use of a humidifier. The common Vicks VapoRub is a gel form of the essential oils of peppermint, eucalyptus, and camphor. Essential oils may also be applied directly to the skin or clothes so they will release their odor near the person using the oils. Essential oils may be inhaled, taken by mouth, or applied to the skin.

MECHANISM OF ACTION

It is not clear how inhaled aromatherapy works (assuming that it does). Possibly, enough is inhaled through the lungs to produce meaningful concentrations of herbal chemicals in the body. It is also possible that aromatherapy works through the olfactory centers of the brain. In other words, a pleasant fragrance may be soothing, refreshing, calming, and stimulating.

USES AND APPLICATIONS

Inhaled aromatherapy has become a popular, gentle treatment to reduce mild anxiety. It has also been tried for a variety of other conditions, including respiratory problems, postsurgical nausea, menstrual pain, and tension headaches. Topical treatment with essential oils has shown possible value for fungal infections and hair loss. Oral use of essential oils has shown promise for various digestive and respiratory problems.

SCIENTIFIC EVIDENCE

There is a major difficulty in studying aromatherapy by inhalation: how to conduct a double-blind, placebo-controlled trial. For the results of a study to be truly reliable, both participants and researchers must not known which participants received real treatment and which received placebo. This is a problem because it has been shown that when researchers create expectations about the effects of certain aromas, those effects may occur simply because of those expectations. Researchers have used various clever compromises in an effort to partially solve this problem. For example, some studies used a control group that received an aromatic substance believed to be ineffective, without informing the members of the control group that this alternate aromatic substance would work. It is just as difficult to prove that an aromatic substance is ineffective as to prove that it is effective. If the placebo in a study is just as effective as the tested treatment, the study will falsely indicate that the tested treatment is ineffective. Furthermore, many odors already have associations attached them, based on cultural patterns. Lavender oil, for example, conjures up for many people memories of their grandmother. It simply is not possible to remove such expectations.

In other studies, researchers tricked participants in the control group and told them that they might be receiving an active but odorless treatment, when in fact they were simply given an inactive treatment without much in it. Still other studies managed to find ethical ways of keeping their study participants in the dark regarding whether they were enrolled in a study at all, and then introduced the odors surreptitiously. Partially effective compromises such as these are necessary. Most published studies on aromatherapy fail even to achieve this level of rigor, falling far below minimal scientific standards of reliability.

Thus, everything discussed here on true aromatherapy—that is, inhalation of an aroma—must be understood cautiously. These problems do not arise to the same extent in studies of essential oils taken by mouth or applied directly to the skin.

Inhalation of essential oils: Calming effects. Preliminary controlled trials suggest that various forms of aromatherapy might be helpful for calming people with Alzheimer's disease and other forms of dementia. For example, in one small study, a hospital ward was suffused with either lavender oil or water for two hours. An investigator who was unaware of the study's design and who wore a device to block inhalation of odors entered the ward and evaluated the behavior of the fifteen residents, all of whom had dementia. The results indicated that the use of lavender oil aromatherapy modestly decreased agitated behavior. A less rigorous study also reported benefit with lavender. However, people with dementia tend to lose their sense of smell, making this approach seem somewhat limited in its usefulness.

Essential oil of lemon balm has also shown promise for this purpose; in a double-blind study of seventy-one people with severe dementia, the use of a lotion containing essential oil of lemon balm reduced agitation compared with placebo lotion. Here, absorption through the skin may have played a role.

Several relatively poorly designed studies hint that aromatherapy combined with massage may help to relieve anxiety in people without Alzheimer's disease. Another study suggests that aromatherapy with geranium oil might modestly reduce anxiety levels (again in people without Alzheimer's). However, in a trial of sixty-six women waiting to have abortions, ten minutes of inhaling the essential oils of vetivert, bergamot, and geranium failed to reduce anxiety significantly more than placebo treatment. In another study, rosemary oil failed to reduce tension during an anxiety-provoking task, and it may have actually increased anxiety.

One study evaluated the effects of massage therapy done with essential oils on people with anxiety or depression while undergoing treatment for cancer. The treatment did appear to provide some short-term benefits.

Cigarette addiction. A controlled study suggests that inhalation of black pepper vapor may reduce the craving for cigarettes. In this trial, forty-eight smokers used cigarette substitute devices that delivered black pepper vapor, menthol, or no fragrance. The results showed that the use of the black-pepper-based dummy cigarette reduced symptoms of craving for the first morning cigarette.

Tension headaches. Weak evidence hints that peppermint oil applied to the forehead might relieve tension headaches. A topical ointment known as Tiger Balm has also shown promise for headaches. Tiger Balm contains camphor, menthol, cajaput, and clove oil. A double-blind study enrolling fifty-seven people with acute tension headache compared the application of Tiger Balm to the forehead with placebo ointment and the drug acetaminophen (Tylenol). The placebo ointment contained mint essence to make it smell similar to Tiger Balm. Real Tiger Balm proved more effective than placebo and just as effective and more rapid-acting than acetaminophen.

Other conditions. Weak evidence suggests that inhaled peppermint oil might relieve postsurgical nausea. Inhaled peppermint oil may also be helpful for relieving mucus congestion of the lungs and sinuses; however, there is only weak supporting evidence for this use.

In one study, abdominal massage with lavender,

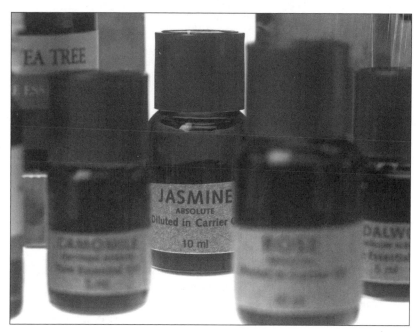

During aromatherapy, essential oils may be inhaled, taken by mouth, or applied to the skin. (Steve Horrell/Photo Researchers, Inc.)

rose, and clary sage reduced menstrual pain to a greater extent than an almond oil placebo. In another study, acupressure combined with lavender, rosemary, and peppermint aromatherapy was more effective than acupressure alone for treating the shoulder pain caused by a certain form of stroke.

Controlled studies have evaluated proprietary-inhaled aromatherapy preparations for treating the common cold and for preventing flare-ups of chronic bronchitis, but the results were marginal at best. A controlled study evaluated rosemary and also lavender aromatherapy for enhancing memory and mental function but found results that were mixed at best.

In a large controlled trial (more than six hundred participants), lavender oil in bath water failed to improve pain after childbirth. However, lavender oil has shown some promise for insomnia. Another large study failed to find aromatherapy more helpful than placebo for reducing psychological distress among people undergoing radiation therapy for cancer.

Oral use of essential oils: Respiratory problems. Eucalyptus is a standard ingredient in cough drops and cough syrups and in oils added to humidifiers. A standardized combination of eucalyptus oil plus two other essential oils has been studied for effectiveness in a variety of respiratory conditions. This combination therapy contains cineole from eucalyptus, d-limonene from citrus fruit, and alpha-pinene from pine. Because these oils are all in a chemical family called monoterpenes, the treatment is called essential oil monoterpenes.

Most double-blind studies, some of which were quite large, indicate that the oral use of essential oil monoterpenes can help colds, sinus infections, and acute bronchitis. For example, a three-month double-blind trial of 246 people with chronic bronchitis found that the consumption of essential oil monoterpenes helped prevent the typical worsening of chronic bronchitis that occurs during the winter. Another study evaluated 676 male and female outpatients with acute bronchitis and found that essential oil monoterpenes were more effective than placebo. Essential oil monoterpenes are thought to work by thinning mucus, though they may have other effects.

Eucalyptus oil alone also may be helpful for respiratory problems. In a double-blind trial, thirty-two people on steroids to control severe asthma (steroid-dependent asthma) were given either placebo or essential oil of eucalyptus for twelve weeks. The results showed that people using eucalyptus were able to gradually reduce their steroid dosage to a greater extent than those taking placebo. In another study, eucalyptus oil proved helpful for the treatment of "head cold" symptoms (technically, nonpurulent rhinosinusitis). In this double-blind, placebo-controlled study of 152 people, the use of cineole at a dose of 200 milligrams (mg) three times daily markedly improved cold symptoms compared with placebo.

Digestive problems. A double-blind, placebo-controlled study of thirty-nine people found that an enteric-coated peppermint-caraway oil combination taken three times daily by mouth for four weeks significantly reduced dyspepsia pain compared with placebo. Of the treatment group, 63.2 percent of participants were pain-free after four weeks, compared with 25 percent of the placebo group. Similarly, results from a double-blind comparative study of 118 people suggest that the combination of peppermint and caraway oil is comparable to the standard drug cisapride, which is no longer available. After four weeks, the herbal combination reduced dyspepsia pain by 69.7 percent, whereas the conventional treatment reduced pain by 70.2 percent.

A preparation of peppermint, caraway, fennel, and wormwood oil was compared with the drug metoclopramide in a double-blind study enrolling sixty people. After seven days, 43.3 percent of the treatment group was pain-free, compared with 13.3 percent of the metoclopramide group.

The oral use of peppermint oil has shown considerable promise for irritable bowel syndrome. However, most studies were relatively poorly designed.

Other oral uses for essential oils. One study found preliminary evidence that a complicated mixture of essential oils (taken by gargle or mouth spray) might be helpful for reducing snoring symptoms. A thorough review of eleven randomized, controlled trials found that the use of mouth rinses containing essential oils is effective against gingivitis and dental plaque formation when used with regular oral hygiene.

Topical use of essential oils. Tea tree oil, an essential oil from the plant *Melaleuca alternifolia*, possesses antibacterial and antifungal properties. It has been tried for various forms of vaginal infection, but the only supporting evidence for this use comes from an uncontrolled trial. There is slightly better evidence to support the use of tea tree oil for the treatment of fibromyalgia and athlete's foot and related fungal infections. One open study hints that oil of bitter orange, a flavoring agent from dried bitter orange peel, might have some effectiveness against athlete's foot when applied topically.

Topical essential oils might be helpful for alopecia areata, a form of hair loss that can occur in men and women. In a seven-month, double-blind, placebo-controlled trial, eighty-four people with alopecia areata massaged either essential oils or a nontreatment oil into their scalps each night for seven months. The treatment oil contained essential oils of thyme, rosemary, lavender, and cedarwood. The results showed that 44 percent of the treatment group experienced new hair growth, compared with only 15 percent of the control group.

Cineol (from eucalyptus) has shown some effectiveness for repelling mosquito bites. Also, in a preliminary double-blind study, coriander oil applied topically protected the skin from the harmful effects of ultraviolet radiation more than a placebo cream (photosensitivity).

People with fibromyalgia experience chronic muscle pain in many parts of, if not throughout, the body. A pilot double-blind study found that the topical application of a proprietary mixture containing camphor, rosemary, eucalyptus, peppermint, aloe vera, lemon, and orange oils could reduce fibromyalgia pain more effectively than placebo. Another study found that massage combined with the topical application of ginger and orange essential oils was no better than massage plus olive oil at relieving pain, reducing stiffness, or improving function in persons with osteoarthritis of the knee.

One study in rats indicates that under some circumstances essential oils instilled into the ear may be able to penetrate the eardrum. While this supports the idea of treating otitis media (the typical ear infection of childhood) with herbal ear drops, it also raises concerns about possible harm to the middle ear.

Finally, for literally hundreds of essential oils, test-tube studies show antimicrobial effects (activity against fungi, bacteria, and viruses). Presumably, essential oils are part of a plant's own defenses against such organisms. However, contrary to widespread claims, such studies do not indicate that these essential oils can work as antibiotics; innumerable substances (bleach is one good example) kill microorganisms in the test tube but not when taken orally by people.

CHOOSING A PRACTITIONER

Licensure in aromatherapy does not exist. The best way to find a qualified practitioner is to seek a referral from a health care professional.

SAFETY ISSUES

Essential oils can be toxic when taken internally, producing unpleasant and even fatal effects. Toxicity studies have not been performed for many essential oil products, and maximum safe dosages remain unknown. Infants, children, the elderly, and people with severe illnesses should not use essential oils internally except under the supervision of a physician; healthy adults should use only well-established products (such as peppermint oil) for which safe dosages have been determined.

Inhaled or topical use of essential oils is much safer than oral use. However, allergic reactions to inhaled or topical plant fragrances are not uncommon. Furthermore, when applied to the skin, some essential oils might also promote sunburning (photosensitization), raise the risk of skin cancer, or be absorbed sufficiently to cause toxic effects. In addition, one report suggests that a combination of lavender oil and tea tree oil applied topically caused gynecomastia (breast enlargement) in three young boys.

EBSCO CAM Review Board

FURTHER READING

Han, S. H., et al. "Effect of Aromatherapy on Symptoms of Dysmenorrhea in College Students." *Journal of Alternative and Complementary Medicine* 12 (2006): 535-541.

Howard, S., and B. M. Hughes. "Expectancies, Not Aroma, Explain Impact of Lavender Aromatherapy on Psychophysiological Indices of Relaxation in Young Healthy Women." *British Journal of Health Psychology* 13 (2008): 603-617.

Hur, M. H., et al. "Aromatherapy for Treatment of Hypertension." *Journal of Evaluation in Clinical Practice* (July 29, 2010).

Ko, G. D., et al. "Effects of Topical O24 Essential Oils on Patients with Fibromyalgia Syndrome." *Journal of Musculoskeletal Pain* 15 (2007): 11-19.

Moss, L., et al. "Differential Effects of the Aromas of *Salvia* Species on Memory and Mood." *Human Psychopharmacology* 25 (2010): 388-396.

Patel, R. M., and Z. Malaki. "The Effect of a Mouth Rinse Containing Essential Oils on Dental Plaque and Gingivitis." *Evidence-Based Dentistry* 9 (2008): 18-19.

Wilkinson, S. M., et al. "Effectiveness of Aromatherapy Massage in the Management of Anxiety and Depression in Patients with Cancer." *Journal of Clinical Oncology* 25 (2007): 532-539.

See also: Herbal medicine; History of alternative medicine.

Arrhythmia

CATEGORY: Condition

RELATED TERMS: Atrial fibrillation, cardiac arrhythmia, heart arrhythmia, heart palpitations, irregular heartbeat, palpitations, sinus arrhythmia

DEFINITION: Treatment of irregular heart rhythms.

PRINCIPAL PROPOSED NATURAL TREATMENTS: None

OTHER PROPOSED NATURAL TREATMENTS: Fish oil, hawthorn, magnesium, vitamin C

INTRODUCTION

Under the control of a complex internal electrical system, the heart beats out a continuous rhythm from a few weeks after conception until death. This rhythm is ordinarily even and regular, changing speed as necessary to adjust to the body's need for oxygen.

Sometimes, however, the heart's rhythm becomes disturbed (arrhythmic). The most common and benign form of arrhythmia is the common heart palpitation, known technically as sinus arrhythmia. Generally, these palpitations are felt as a short run of thumps or flutters in the chest. Sinus arrhythmia is often caused by stress and anxiety. It poses no danger, although it can be annoying.

More serious forms of heart arrhythmia may occur as well. In later life, many people develop atrial fibrillation, a condition in which part of the heart contracts at excessive speed and another part follows along irregularly. Although some people live for years in a state of atrial fibrillation, this is a potentially dangerous condition that requires medical attention.

Other forms of heart arrhythmia are more dangerous and include ventricular tachycardia and ventricular fibrillation. These frequently occur after a heart attack. They are often heralded by ventricular premature complexes.

Conventional treatment for arrhythmia depends on the type involved. Sinus arrhythmia is often left untreated. More serious rhythm disturbances are addressed through the use of medications, defibrillation, or a pacemaker.

Heart arrhythmias are far too dangerous for self-treatment. In all but the most obviously benign cases, one should immediately seek medical care.

PROPOSED NATURAL TREATMENTS

Although the evidence is conflicting on whether fish oil helps prevent dangerous heart arrhythmias, on balance fish oil probably does provide some benefit in certain persons. The mineral magnesium tends to stabilize the heart, and intravenous infusions of magnesium are sometimes given to people in cardiac intensive care. However, a six-month, double-blind, placebo-controlled study of 170 people did not find oral magnesium effective for maintaining normal heart rhythm in people with a tendency to develop atrial fibrillation.

Diuretic drugs in the thiazide family tend to deplete the body of the minerals potassium and magnesium. People using such drugs are usually advised to take potassium supplements because potassium deficiency can cause arrhythmias. One small double-blind study failed to find that additional supplementation with magnesium further stabilized the heart. Apparently, the extent of magnesium deficiency caused by thiazide diuretics is not severe enough to destabilize the heart's rhythm.

However, the drug digoxin appears to sensitize the heart to magnesium deficiency. People with congestive heart failure (CHF) are likely to use both digoxin and loop diuretics (another type of diuretic that depletes magnesium), and the net result can be cardiac arrhythmias. One small, double-blind, placebo-controlled study found that magnesium supplements reduced episodes of ventricular arrhythmia in people with CHF.

A controlled study found preliminary evidence that vitamin C may help prevent one of the types of arrhythmia (atrial fibrillation) that can follow coronary artery bypass grafting. However, because this trial failed to include a placebo group, its results are suspect.

The herb hawthorn is widely used to treat mild palpitations, but scientific evidence to show that it is effective consists only of partially relevant test-tube studies. N-acetylcysteine, a modified version of a dietary amino acid, was shown in a pilot placebo-controlled study (115 participants) to reduce the incidence of atrial fibrillation following open-heart surgery, a common complication of this kind of procedure.

When palpitations are caused by anxiety or stress, some herbs and supplements used for those conditions may be helpful. Other herbs and supplements sometimes recommended for palpitations, but which have little supporting evidence, include vitamin D, calcium, corydalis, valerian, skullcap, and lady's slipper.

Herbs and Supplements to Avoid

Caffeine stimulates the heart and may cause minor palpitations. Herbs containing caffeine, such as guarana and cola nut, would be expected to cause similar problems. The herb ephedra also stimulates the heart and should be avoided by people with palpitations. A few reports suggest that the supplement creatine could, at times, cause heart arrhythmias. Numerous herbs and supplements may interact adversely with drugs used to prevent or treat arrhythmias, so one should be cautious when considering the use of herbs and supplements.

EBSCO CAM Review Board

Further Reading

Calo, L., et al. "N-3 Fatty Acids for the Prevention of Atrial Fibrillation After Coronary Artery Bypass Surgery." *Journal of the American College of Cardiology* 45 (2005): 1723-1728.

Eslami, M., et al. "Oral Ascorbic Acid in Combination with Beta-blockers Is More Effective Than Beta-blockers Alone in the Prevention of Atrial Fibrillation After Coronary Artery Bypass Grafting." *Texas Heart Institute Journal* 34 (2007): 268-274.

Frick, M., et al. "The Effect of Oral Magnesium, Alone or as an Adjuvant to Sotalol, After Cardioversion in Patients with Persistent Atrial Fibrillation." *European Heart Journal* 21 (2000): 1177-1185.

Geelen, A., et al. "Effects of N-3 Fatty Acids from Fish on Premature Ventricular Complexes and Heart Rate in Humans." *American Journal of Clinical Nutrition* 81 (2005): 416-420.

Jenkins, D. J., et al. "Fish-Oil Supplementation in Patients with Implantable Cardioverter Defibrillators." *Canadian Medical Association Journal* 178 (2008): 157-164.

Kammer, R. T. "Lone Atrial Fibrillation Associated with Creatine Monohydrate Supplementation." *Pharmacotherapy* 25 (2005): 762-764.

Nodari, S., et al. "The Role of N-3 PUFAs in Preventing the Arrhythmic Risk in Patients with Idiopathic Dilated Cardiomyopathy." *Cardiovascular Drugs and Therapy* 23 (2008): 5-15.

Ozaydin, M., et al. "N-acetylcysteine for the Prevention of Postoperative Atrial Fibrillation." *European Heart Journal* 29 (2008): 625-631.

Raitt, M. H., et al. "Fish Oil Supplementation and Risk of Ventricular Tachycardia and Ventricular Fibrillation in Patients with Implantable Defibrillators." *Journal of the American Medical Association* 293 (2005): 2884-2891.

Saravanan, P., et al. "Omega-3 Fatty Acid Supplementation Does Not Reduce Risk of Atrial Fibrillation After Coronary Artery Bypass Surgery." *Circulation: Arrhythmia and Electrophysiology* 3 (2010): 46-53.

See also: Angina; Atherosclerosis and heart disease prevention; Cholesterol, high; Congestive heart failure; Heart attack; Hypertension; Strokes.

Artichoke

CATEGORY: Functional foods
RELATED TERMS: *Cynara scolymus*, cynarin, luteolin
DEFINITION: Natural plant product consumed as a dietary supplement for specific health benefits.
PRINCIPAL PROPOSED USES: Dyspepsia, high cholesterol
OTHER PROPOSED USE: Liver protection

OVERVIEW

The artichoke is one of the oldest cultivated plants. It was first grown in Ethiopia and then was brought to southern Europe via Egypt. Its image is found on ancient Egyptian tablets and sacrificial altars. The ancient Greeks and Romans considered it a valuable digestive aid and reserved what was then a rare plant for consumption in elite circles. In sixteenth century Europe, the artichoke was also considered a "noble" vegetable, meant for consumption by the royal and the rich.

In traditional European medicine, the leaves of the artichoke (not the flower buds, which are the parts commonly cooked and eaten as a vegetable) were used as a diuretic to stimulate the kidneys and as a "choleretic" to stimulate the flow of bile from the liver and gallbladder. (Bile is a yellowish-brown fluid manufactured in the liver and stored in the gallbladder; it consists of numerous substances, including several that play a significant role in digestion.)

In the first half of the twentieth century, French scientists began modern research into these traditional medicinal uses of the artichoke plant. Their work suggested that the plant does indeed stimulate the kidney and gallbladder. Midcentury, Italian scientists isolated a compound from artichoke leaf called cynarin, which appeared to duplicate many of the effects of whole artichoke. Synthetic cynarin preparations were used as a drug to stimulate the liver and gallbladder and to treat elevated cholesterol from the 1950s to the 1980s; competition from newer pharmaceuticals has since eclipsed the use of cynarin.

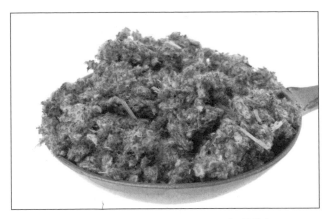

Artichoke leaf may help lower cholesterol. (Bildagentur-online/TH Foto-Werbung/Photo Researchers, Inc.)

USES AND APPLICATIONS

Artichoke leaf (as opposed to cynarin) continues to be used in many countries. Germany's Commission E has authorized its use for "dyspeptic problems." Dyspepsia is a rather vague term that corresponds to the common word "indigestion," indicating a variety of digestive problems including discomfort in the stomach, bloating, lack of appetite, nausea, and mild diarrhea or constipation. One substantial double-blind study indicates that artichoke leaf is indeed helpful for this condition. Another fairly substantial study indicates that artichoke leaf may help lower cholesterol.

Based on a general notion that artichoke leaf is good for the liver, it has become a popular treatment for alcohol-induced hangovers. However, a small, double-blind, placebo-controlled study failed to find it more effective than placebo.

A number of animal studies suggest that artichoke protects the liver from damage by chemical toxins. Artichoke's liver-protective effects, however, have not been proven in controlled clinical trials.

SCIENTIFIC EVIDENCE

High cholesterol. In a double-blind, placebo-controlled study of 143 people with high cholesterol, artichoke leaf extract significantly improved cholesterol readings. Total cholesterol fell by 18.5 percent compared with 8.6 percent in the placebo group, LDL (bad) cholesterol fell by 23 percent versus 6 percent, and LDL-to-HDL (good cholesterol) ratios fell by 20 percent versus 7 percent. In a subsequent study of seventy-five otherwise healthy people with high cholesterol, artichoke leaf extract significantly reduced total cholesterol compared with placebo, but it did not affect LDL, HDL, or triglycerides levels.

Another placebo-controlled study, this one involving forty-four healthy people, failed to find any improvement in cholesterol levels attributable to artichoke leaf. The researchers note, however, that study participants, on average, started the trial with lower-than-normal cholesterol levels (due to a statistical accident); improvement, therefore, could not be expected.

Artichoke leaf may work by interfering with cholesterol synthesis. In addition to cynarin, a compound in artichoke called luteolin may play a role in reducing cholesterol.

Dyspepsia. In Europe, vague digestive symptoms are commonly attributed to inadequate flow of bile from the gallbladder. Evidence shows that artichoke leaf does indeed stimulate the gallbladder. This by itself does not prove artichoke helpful for dyspepsia. In 2003, however, a large (247-participant) double-blind study evaluated artichoke leaf as a treatment for dyspepsia. In this carefully conducted study, artichoke leaf extract proved significantly more effective than placebo for alleviating digestive symptoms. A previous study of an herbal combination containing artichoke leaf also found benefits.

DOSAGE

Germany's Commission E recommends 6 grams of the dried herb or its equivalent per day, usually divided into three doses. Artichoke leaf extracts should be taken according to label instructions. People with gallbladder disease should use artichoke only under medical supervision.

SAFETY ISSUES

Artichoke leaf has not been associated with significant side effects in studies, but full safety testing has not been completed. For this reason, it should not be used by pregnant or nursing women. Safety in young children or in people with severe liver or kidney disease has also not been established.

In addition, because artichoke leaf is believed to stimulate gallbladder contraction, persons with gallstones or other forms of gallbladder disease could be put at risk by using this herb. Such persons should use artichoke leaf only under the supervision of a physician. It is possible that increased gallbladder

contraction could lead to obstruction of ducts or even rupture of the gallbladder. Finally, persons with known allergies to artichokes or related plants in the Asteraceae family, such as arnica or chrysanthemums, should avoid using artichoke or cynarin preparations.

EBSCO CAM Review Board

FURTHER READING

Bundy, R., et al. "Artichoke Leaf Extract (*Cynara scolymus*) Reduces Plasma Cholesterol in Otherwise Healthy Hypercholesterolemic Adults." *Phytomedicine* 15 (2008): 668-675.

Holtmann, G., et al. "Efficacy of Artichoke Leaf Extract in the Treatment of Patients with Functional Dyspepsia." *Alimentary Pharmacology and Therapeutics* 18 (2003): 1099-1105.

Pittler, M. H., et al. "Effectiveness of Artichoke Extract in Preventing Alcohol-Induced Hangovers." *CMAJ: Canadian Medical Association Journal* 169 (2003): 1269-1273.

See also: Cholesterol, high; Dyspepsia; Liver disease.

Art therapy

CATEGORY: Therapies and techniques
RELATED TERM: Art psychotherapy
DEFINITION: The combined use of psychotherapy and creative processes such as painting and drawing to enhance health and well-being.
PRINCIPAL PROPOSED USES: None
OTHER PROPOSED USES: Chronic pain, depression, eating disorders, post-traumatic stress disorder, schizophrenia, substance abuse

OVERVIEW

According to the American Art Therapy Association (AATA), art therapy is based on knowledge of human developmental and psychological theories and is an effective treatment for people with developmental, medical, educational, social, or psychological problems. The theory behind art therapy is based partially on the belief that creativity and healing may come from the same place. According to experts, art therapy is not merely arts and crafts, or purely recreational; it is multisensory and teaches people to use

Art Therapy in Practice

It can be difficult for a six-year-old, or for a sixty-year-old, to find the words to articulate painful memories. However, children and adults who have been exposed to unspeakable trauma, and those suffering from depression, anxiety, or other serious mental or physical illnesses, can reap enormous benefits from the healing process of art therapy, a therapy that uses paint and paper, glue and scissors, images and colors to symbolically express the depth and intensity of emotional pain.

Ava Charney-Danysh finds art therapy useful in her work with children and adults who have eating disorders. "Obsessions with food and weight are often attempts to cope with unresolved emotional issues such as depression, rage, powerlessness, and loss," she explains. "Art therapy is a special tool that can help provide access to those hidden feelings that contain the key to our struggles."

"Beginning with scribbles and lines, children express their feelings and needs through art even before verbal language is learned," says Noah Hass-Cohen. "Art therapy provides a nonthreatening place to release feelings and pent up emotions and may be especially useful for children and adolescents in times of family and individual crisis and/or change."

Janette, for example, is six years old, her brown eyes weary with the haunted wisdom of a child who has seen more than any six-year-old should ever see. She witnessed her father, in the frenzy of an alcoholic rage, kick her pregnant mother in the stomach and saw the police come and drag her father out of the room. Janette was home when her bruised and tearful mother returned from the hospital and told her that she was not going to have a baby sister after all.

New York art therapist Sandy Izhakoff works with neurologically impaired adults in nursing homes and in senior centers. She uses art therapy techniques such as free-drawing, mask-making, and finger-painting to help people (even persons who have problems verbalizing) perform life review, express regrets, resolve unresolved losses, and come to terms with issues such as aging, grief, and the fear of death.

Barbara Williams Cosentino, R.N., CSW

objects purposefully and to communicate their pain with the outside world.

Although human beings have used art as a mode of expression for thousands of years, art therapy was not recognized as a distinct profession until the late 1930s, when Margaret Naumberg, now considered the founder of art therapy, advocated using art as a gateway to the subconscious in conjunction with free association and psychoanalytic interpretation.

Artist Adrian Hill took credit for inventing the term "art therapy" in 1942. While recovering from tuberculosis in a sanitarium, he felt that his own foray into art led to his emotional recovery. Introducing painting to his fellow patients, he found that they used artistic expression not only for enjoyment but also for expressing fears and emotions.

Recognizing that artwork could be useful in helping patients express internal conflicts, the psychiatric staff at the Menninger Clinic in Kansas began to employ art as therapy. The first journal in the field, *Bulletin of Art Therapy*, began publishing in 1961, and the AATA, a national professional organization that regulates educational, professional, and ethical standards for art therapists, was established in 1969.

MECHANISM OF ACTION

There are two different poles of art therapy: art psychotherapy and art as therapy. Proponents of art as therapy suggest that the process of creating art itself is curative and that verbal reflection, discussions, or interpretations about the art itself are not necessary. Advocates believe that creative activity increases brain levels of serotonin, a hormone associated with feelings of well-being, and gives rise to the alpha brainwave patterns typically seen during periods of relaxed alertness.

USES AND APPLICATIONS

Art psychotherapy proponents believe that artwork is most effective when used as a tool to elicit feelings, fears, and fantasies, which can then be worked through in traditional talk therapy. Regardless of their orientation, most contemporary art therapists integrate a variety of approaches, individualizing the treatment to best meet the needs of a specific client.

Special techniques are often particularly useful in helping people express their feelings, develop social skills, solve problems, reduce anxiety, or resolve emotional conflicts. In the unstructured approach, patients might select from a variety of materials and media (such as paint, pastels, and clay) and use them however they choose, allowing unconscious material to rise to the surface. Then the therapist might ask the client to draw a family picture, which can help elicit complex family dynamics such as unhealthy patterns of relating or poor communication skills. Groups of people who share similar issues, such as having had cancer, might work together to create a collage or mural that can then be used to stimulate discussion of coping strategies.

Art therapists can practice alone or may be part of a treatment team that includes physicians, psychologists, nurses, social workers, counselors, and teachers. Art therapy, conducted in individual or group sessions, can be used with people of all ages, races, and ethnic backgrounds who have any one of a number of physical and emotional disorders.

CHOOSING A PRACTITIONER

Art therapists must possess a minimum of a master's degree and undergo a supervised practicum and a postgraduate internship before being certified for practice. Art therapists are registered (the credential ATR) or board certified (BC), or both, and practice in a variety of settings, including community mental health centers and psychiatric clinics; hospitals, rehabilitation facilities, and hospices; correctional facilities; nursing homes and senior centers; schools and early intervention programs; disaster relief centers; homeless shelters; and drug and alcohol rehabilitation programs.

SAFETY ISSUES

There are no known safety concerns with art therapy.

Barbara Williams Cosentino, R.N., CSW;
reviewed by Brian Randall, M.D.

FURTHER READING

American Art Therapy Association. http://www.arttherapy.org.
Art Therapy Credentials Board. http://www.atcb.org.
Art Therapy in Canada. http://www.artsintherapy.com/links.asp.
Canadian Art Therapy Association. http://www.catainfo.ca.
Craig, Claire. *Exploring the Self Through Photography Activities for Use in Group Work.* Philadelphia: Jessica Kingsley, 2009.
Edwards, David. *Art Therapy.* Thousand Oaks, Calif.: Sage, 2004.
Malchiodi, Cathy A. *The Art Therapy Sourcebook.* Rev. ed. New York: McGraw-Hill, 2007.
Rubin, Judith Aron. *The Art of Art Therapy: What Every Art Therapist Needs to Know.* New York: Brunner-Routledge, 2011.

See also: Aging; Aromatherapy; Children's health; Color therapy; Dance movement therapy; Hypnotherapy; Magnet therapy; Mind/body medicine; Music therapy; Relaxation therapies; Traditional healing.

Ashwagandha

CATEGORY: Herbs and supplements
RELATED TERMS: Indian ginseng, *Withania somniferum*
DEFINITION: Natural plant product used as a dietary supplement for specific health benefits.
PRINCIPAL PROPOSED USE: Adaptogen
OTHER PROPOSED USES: Anxiety, depression, immune support, infertility in men or women, insomnia, male sexual dysfunction, mental function enhancement, reducing cancer risk, sports performance enhancement

OVERVIEW

Ashwagandha is sometimes called Indian ginseng, not because it is related botanically (it is closer to potatoes and tomatoes) but because its traditional uses were similar. Like ginseng, ashwagandha was thought to be a tonic herb that could strengthen the body. On this basis it had been used in hopes of prolonging life, improving overall health, enhancing mental function, increasing fertility and libido, augmenting physical energy, and preventing infections.

In addition, as its species name *somniferum* suggests, ashwagandha had been used traditionally for inducing sleep.

USES AND APPLICATIONS

Modern herbalists classify ashwagandha as an adaptogen, a substance said to increase the body's ability to withstand stress of all types. However, the evidence for an adaptogenic effect is limited to test tube and animal studies.

Other proposed uses of ashwagandha, which are based on even weaker evidence, include preventing cancer, improving immunity, enhancing mental function, and combating anxiety and depression.

Some traditional uses of ashwagandha are also invoked today, such as enhancing sexual function in men, increasing fertility in men and women, aiding sleep, and enhancing sports performance. However, there is no supporting scientific evidence for these uses.

DOSAGE

A typical traditional dosage of ashwagandha is 1 to 2 grams of the root (boiled in milk or water for fifteen to twenty minutes) taken three times daily.

SAFETY ISSUES

Ashwagandha is believed to be safe; however, formal safety studies have not been reported. Therefore, it should not be used by pregnant or nursing women, young children, or those with severe kidney or liver disease.

According to one study in animals, ashwagandha may raise thyroid hormone levels. For this reason, it should not be used by people with hyperthyroidism. In addition, based on traditional beliefs that ashwagandha has sedative effects, interactions with sedative drugs are a potential concern.

IMPORTANT INTERACTIONS

Persons who are taking sedative drugs should not take ashwagandha at the same time except under a doctor's supervision.

EBSCO CAM Review Board

FURTHER READING

Bhattacharya, S. K., et al. "Anxiolytic-Antidepressant Activity of *Withania somnifera* Glycowithanolides." *Phytomedicine* 7 (2000): 463-469.

Davis, L., and G. Kuttan. "Effect of *Withania somnifera* on DMBA Induced Carcinogenesis." *Journal of Ethnopharmacology* 75 (2001): 165-168.

Singh, B., et al. "Adaptogenic Activity of a Novel, Withanolide-Free Aqueous Fraction from the Roots of *Withania somnifera* Dun. (Part I)." *Phytotherapy Research* 15 (2001): 311-318.

Singh, B., B. K. Chandan, and D. K. Gupta. "Adaptogenic Activity of a Novel, Withanolide-Free Aqueous Fraction from the Roots of *Withania somnifera* Dun. (Part II)." *Phytotherapy Research* 17 (2003): 531-536.

See also: Anxiety and panic attacks; Cancer risk reduction; Depression, mild to moderate; Ginseng; Immune support; Infertility, female; Infertility; male; Insomnia; Memory and mental function impairment; Sexual dysfunction in men; Sports and fitness support: Enhancing performance.

Astaxanthin

CATEGORY: Herbs and supplements
RELATED TERM: *Haematococcus pluvialis*
DEFINITION: Natural substance used as a dietary supplement for specific health benefits.
PRINCIPAL PROPOSED USES: None
OTHER PROPOSED USES: Cataracts prevention, dyspepsia, heart disease prevention, high blood pressure, high cholesterol, macular degeneration prevention, male infertility, sports and fitness support

OVERVIEW

Astaxanthin, a substance in the carotenoid family, provides the pink color of salmon and many other sea creatures. Like other carotenoids, astaxanthin is a strong antioxidant. It has been advocated for treating or preventing a number of health conditions, but none of these proposed uses is supported by meaningful scientific evidence.

REQUIREMENTS AND SOURCES

Astaxanthin is not an essential nutrient. However, it is possible that increased intake of astaxanthin could provide health benefits.

Salmon is an excellent source of astaxanthin. A typical serving of Atlantic salmon provides approximately 1 milligram (mg) of astaxanthin, while a similar serving of Pacific salmon might provide 4 to 5 mg. Krill oil is another good food source of astaxanthin.

When consistently exposed to high levels of ultraviolet light, the alga *Haematococcus pluvialis* produces very large quantities of astaxanthin, presumably to protect itself from injury. *Haematococcus* raised in this way is used as a commercial source of astaxanthin.

THERAPEUTIC DOSAGES

In studies, astaxanthin has been given in doses ranging from 4 to 16 mg daily. Some evidence suggests that astaxanthin is better absorbed when consumed in an oily base.

THERAPEUTIC USES

Many health claims for astaxanthin are based on its strength as an antioxidant. However, scientific confidence in the medical benefits of antioxidants has waned; study after study of antioxidants such as vitamin E and beta-carotene have failed to find the hoped-for benefits.

Other proposed uses of astaxanthin have some marginal supporting evidence from double-blind studies. In one such study, thirty men with infertility were given either placebo or 16 mg of astaxanthin daily for three months. The results showed possible small benefits on laboratory measures of fertility.

Another study tested astaxanthin combined with the carotenoid lutein as a possible supplement for enhancing recovery from exercise. In this small trial, twenty bodybuilders were given either placebo or the carotenoid combination for three weeks. Participants then engaged in intense exercise. The results failed to show that the use of the astaxanthin and lutein combination reduced muscle soreness or signs of muscle injury.

Weak evidence additionally hints that astaxanthin might reduce blood pressure, help prevent heart disease, lower cholesterol, protect the lens of the eye against cataracts, protect the stomach against ulcers, and reduce the risk of macular degeneration. However, for none of these uses (or any other) can astaxanthin be remotely called a proven treatment. Also, two studies failed to find astaxanthin significantly more effective than placebo for treating stomach irritation in people with dyspepsia (nonspecific stomach pain).

SAFETY ISSUES

As a widely consumed nutritional substance, astaxanthin is expected to have a low order of toxicity. In human studies, no serious adverse effects have been seen. Maximum safe doses in pregnant or nursing women, young children, or persons with severe liver or kidney disease have not been determined.

EBSCO CAM Review Board

FURTHER READING

Bloomer, R. J., et al. "Astaxanthin Supplementation Does Not Attenuate Muscle Injury Following Eccentric Exercise in Resistance-Trained Men." *International Journal of Sport Nutrition and Exercise Metabolism* 15 (2005): 401-412.

Comhaire, F. H., et al. "Combined Conventional/Antioxidant 'Astaxanthin' Treatment for Male Infertility." *Asian Journal of Andrology* 7 (2005): 257-262.

Higuera-Ciapara, I., L. Felix-Valenzuela, and F. M. Goycoolea. "Astaxanthin: A Review of Its Chemistry and Applications." *Critical Reviews in Food Science and Nutrition* 46 (2006): 185-196.

Kupcinskas, L., et al. "Efficacy of the Natural Antioxidant Astaxanthin in the Treatment of Functional Dyspepsia in Patients with or Without *Helicobacter pylori* Infection." *Phytomedicine* 15 (2008): 391-399.

Spiller, G. A., and A. Dewell. "Safety of an Astaxanthin-Rich *Haematococcus pluvialis* Algal Extract." *Journal of Medicinal Food* 6 (2003): 51-56.

Wu, T. H., et al. "Astaxanthin Protects Against Oxidative Stress and Calcium-Induced Porcine Lens Protein Degradation." *Journal of Agricultural and Food Chemistry* 54 (2006): 2418-2423.

See also: Cataracts; Cholesterol, high; Dyspepsia; Infertility, male; Macular degeneration; Sports and fitness support: Enhancing performance.

Asthma

RELATED TERM: Bronchial asthma

CATEGORY: Condition

DEFINITION: Treatment of severe breathing difficulties caused by bronchial inflammation and contraction.

PRINCIPAL PROPOSED NATURAL TREATMENTS: Boswellia, *Coleus forskohlii*, tylophora, ephedra (unsafe), vitamin C

OTHER PROPOSED NATURAL TREATMENTS: Acupuncture, adrenal extract, aloe, antioxidants, astha-15 (an Ayurvedic herbal combination), brahmi (*Bacopa monniera*), beta-carotene, betaine hydrochloride, butterbur, *Carum copticum* (ajwain), chamomile, coenzyme Q_{10}, damiana, elecampane, elimination diet, essential fatty acids (omega-3 and omega-6 fatty acids), essential oil of eucalyptus, fish oil, flaxseed oil, food allergen elimination diet, garlic, gamma-linolenic acid from evening primrose oil, green-lipped mussel, grindelia, horehound, hyssop, hypnosis, ivy leaf, licorice, *Lobelia inflata*, magnesium, marshmallow, massage, melatonin, mullein, onion, oligomeric proanthocyanidins, osteopathic manipulation, picrorhiza, quercetin, reishi, relaxation therapy, selenium, sublingual immunotherapy, vitamin B_6, vitamin B_{12}, vitamin E, yerba santa, yoga

INTRODUCTION

People who have an asthma attack have real trouble taking a breath. Many people with stuffy noses from hay fever or colds say "I can't breathe," but they retain the option of breathing through the mouth. For asthmatics, the bronchial tubes in their lungs become swollen and clogged. Breathing can become frighteningly difficult.

Asthma involves two conditions: contraction of the small muscles surrounding the bronchial tubes and inflammation of the lining of those tubes. Traditionally, treatment primarily addressed the first aspect of asthma; recently, however, it has become clear that tissue swelling is the underlying cause.

The conventional treatment of asthma is highly effective for most people. Treatments include both short- and long-acting bronchodilators, which relax the bronchial muscles, and anti-inflammatory medication, which helps relieve the swelling of tissue. Bronchodilators alone may be sufficient treatment for mild asthma or asthma that occurs only with exercise. Anti-inflammatory steroids in the cortisone family taken by inhalation are the mainstay of treatment for moderate to severe asthma. Although these are much safer than oral steroids, they may still increase risk of osteoporosis and other problems when they are taken in high doses or for a long time. Other drugs used to reduce inflammation include montelukast (Singulair), nedocromil (Tilade) and cromolyn (Intal). (Intal is derived from a Mediterranean herb named khella.) The newest drug treatment for asthma, omalizumab (Xolair), appears to be safe and effective, but it is extremely expensive, and for this reason, it is seldom used.

PRINCIPAL PROPOSED NATURAL TREATMENTS

None of these treatments has been shown to be effective for severe asthma. One should not stop

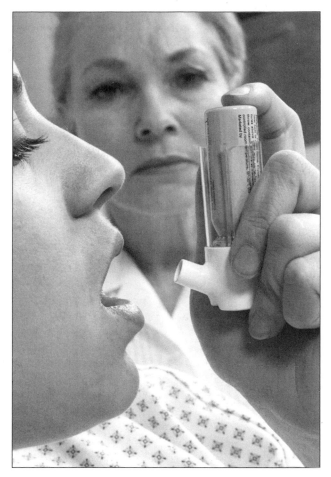

Many asthma medications are delivered using an inhaler. (PhotoDisc)

standard asthma medication except on the advice of a physician.

The herb *Tylophora indica* (also called *T. asthmatica*) appears to offer some promise as a treatment for asthma. It has a long history of use in the traditional Ayurvedic medicine of India. However, all of the studies on this herb were performed in India long ago and failed to reach modern standards of design and reporting.

In a double-blind, placebo-controlled study of 195 persons with asthma, the participants who were given 40 milligrams (mg) of a tylophora alcohol extract daily for six days showed significant improvement compared with placebo. Similar results were seen in two double-blind, placebo-controlled studies involving more than two hundred persons with asthma.

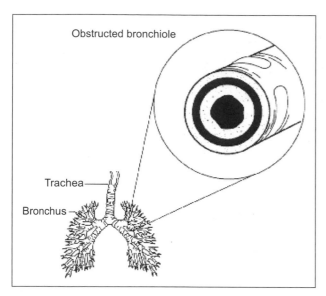

During an asthma attack, obstructed bronchioles limit or halt airflow, resulting in severely restricted breathing.

However, the design of these studies was a bit convoluted, and various pieces of information are missing from the reports, causing some difficulty in evaluating the validity of these trials.

Another double-blind study that enrolled 135 persons and followed a more straightforward design found no benefit from tylophora. Although tylophora is promising, larger and better studies are necessary to discover whether tylophora is truly effective.

Boswellia. The herb boswellia has shown promise as a treatment for rheumatoid arthritis. It is thought to work by inhibiting inflammation. Because asthma involves inflammation and can be treated by some of the same drugs that treat rheumatoid arthritis, boswellia has been tried for this purpose too.

One six-week, double-blind, placebo-controlled study of eighty persons with relatively mild asthma found that treatment with boswellia at a dose of 300 mg three times daily reduced the frequency of asthma attacks and improved objective measurements of breathing capacity. However, further research needs to be performed to follow up this pilot study before boswellia can be described as a proven treatment for asthma.

Coleus forskohlii. Another herb sometimes recommended for asthma also comes from India, *Coleus forskohlii.* While there is some preliminary evidence that

it might have value, this evidence is far too weak to be relied on. Furthermore, as sold, the herb is more like a drug than an herb. Natural *C. forskohlii* contains small amounts of a potent chemical called forskolin. Manufacturers deliberately modify the herb to dramatically increase its forskolin content; therefore, when using such products, one is essentially using an unlicensed drug. Forskolin appears to be safe, but more studies need to be undertaken before it can be recommended for self-treatment.

Ma huang. The Chinese herb ma huang, also called ephedra, is definitely effective for mild asthma because it contains the drug ephedrine. However, it is not recommended because of safety concerns. This Chinese herb is a member of a primitive family of plants that look like thin, branching, connected straws. A related species, *Ephedra nevadensis,* grows wild in the American Southwest and is widely called Mormon tea. However, only the Asian species of ephedra contains the active compounds ephedrine and pseudoephedrine.

Ma huang was traditionally used by Chinese herbalists in the early stages of respiratory infections and for the short-term treatment of certain kinds of asthma, eczema, hay fever, narcolepsy, and edema. Japanese chemists isolated ephedrine from ma huang around the beginning of the twentieth century, and it soon became a primary treatment for asthma in the United States and abroad. Ephedra's other major ingredient, pseudoephedrine, became the decongestant Sudafed.

Although ephedrine can still be found in a few over-the-counter asthma drugs, physicians seldom prescribe it today. The problem is that ephedrine mimics the effects of adrenaline and causes symptoms such as rapid heartbeat, high blood pressure, agitation, insomnia, nausea, and loss of appetite. The newer asthma drugs are much safer and easier to tolerate. This is a situation in which synthetic drugs are less dangerous than a natural one. Ma huang is not recommended for use in treating asthma.

OTHER PROPOSED NATURAL TREATMENTS

Other herbs and supplements. In a double-blind trial, thirty-two people with steroid-dependent asthma were given either placebo or essential oil of eucalyptus for twelve weeks. The results showed that people using eucalyptus were more able to gradually reduce their steroid dosage than those taking placebo.

Two double-blind, placebo-controlled studies enrolling more than eighty people with asthma suggest that oligomeric proanthocyanidins from pine bark might reduce symptoms. An extract made from ivy leaf has been advocated for the treatment of childhood asthma, but the meaningful supporting evidence is again limited to one placebo-controlled trial.

Another small, double-blind, placebo-controlled study evaluated the effects of four weeks of treatment with a Japanese herbal mixture traditionally called Saiboku-To. Researchers tested the tendency of the bronchial tubes to contract in response to an asthma-producing substance called methacholine. The results indicated that the use of Saiboku-To helped prevent such contractions, and it also reduced lung inflammation. Another study reportedly found benefit with a combination named Mai-Men-Dong-Tang.

Many studies have been conducted on the effects of vitamin C in treating asthma, but the evidence that it works remains inconsistent and highly incomplete. There is only weak and inconsistent evidence regarding whether two antioxidants in the carotenoid family, lycopene and beta-carotene, might help prevent exercise-induced asthma. One double-blind comparative study provides weak evidence that the Ayurvedic herbal combination called Astha might be helpful for mild asthma.

Vitamin B_6 is often mentioned as a treatment for asthma, but the evidence that it works is weak and contradictory at best. A double-blind study of seventy-six children with asthma found significant benefit from vitamin B_6 after the second month of usage. Children in the treated group were able to reduce their doses of bronchodilators and steroids. However, a recent double-blind study of thirty-one adults who also used either inhaled or oral steroids did not show any benefit. Supplementation with vitamin B_{12} is also often said to be effective for asthma. However, the scientific evidence in its favor consists almost entirely of open studies that did not attempt to eliminate the placebo effect.

Ajwain and Asthma

The spice ajwain (also known as ajowan, *Trachyspermum ammi*, and *Carum copticum*) has a long history of use in Indian cooking. In addition, it is said to have medicinal effects. Test-tube studies have provided support for some its traditional uses. Based on these findings, a preliminary human trial has been performed, with promising results.

This trial enrolled people with asthma. Researchers compared two different doses of ajwain with the outdated asthma drug theophylline and with placebo. Participants were given initial pulmonary function tests and then given either theophylline, one of the two doses of ajwain, or placebo. Repeat pulmonary function tests were done at stated intervals for the next three hours. The results from this preliminary trial suggest that ajwain was less effective than theophylline but more effective than placebo.

Ajwain is thought to act by dilating the bronchial tubes in the lungs. This is no longer the primary approach used for treating any but the mildest asthma. Nonetheless, the herb could be a source of a novel way to accomplish this. However, considerably more study is necessary before ajwain could be considered an effective (or safe) treatment for asthma.

Steven Bratman, M.D.

Preliminary evidence hints that the herb butterbur may be helpful for asthma. Another study found potential benefit with the spice *Carum copticum*.

Essential fatty acids, such as gamma-linolenic acid and those found in fish oil, as well as flaxseed oil, may inhibit inflammatory responses such as those that occur in asthma. However, of the studies that tried fish oil as a treatment for asthma, most failed to find significant clinical benefit; one study found that fish oil can worsen aspirin-related asthma. Nonetheless, there is some evidence from one research group that fish oil might be helpful for exercise-induced asthma. There is also some preliminary evidence that women who take fish oil during late pregnancy may reduce the risk of asthma in their children for up to sixteen years after birth.

A study of seventy-two children with moderate, persistent asthma found that combined or single supplementation with omega-3 oils, zinc, or vitamin C improved their symptoms and lung function. Combined supplementation was associated with the greatest improvement. The reliability of these results should be questioned, however, because about 20 percent of the children dropped out before the end of the thirty-eight-week study.

A preliminary double-blind, placebo-controlled trial suggests that green-lipped mussel extract might be helpful for allergic asthma. Another study suggests that the natural substance hyaluronic acid might be helpful for asthma when taken by inhalation.

Natural medicine practitioners frequently recommend the flavonoid quercetin as a treatment for asthma. However, the only basis for this recommendation consists of a few older, preliminary test-tube studies that suggest it might inhibit the release of inflammatory substances from special cells called mast cells. The asthma drugs Intal (cromolyn) and Tilade (nedocromil) are believed to work in this way. However, there is significant direct evidence from human trials that Tilade and Intal taken by inhalation actually work. In contrast, no such evidence exists for quercetin taken in any manner; and it is highly unlikely that oral intake of quercetin could produce levels in the body similar to the levels used in those test-tube studies.

Alternative medical literature frequently mentions magnesium as a treatment for asthma. However, this idea seems to be based primarily on the use of intravenous magnesium as an emergency treatment for asthma. (Taking something by mouth is very different from having it injected into the veins.) Studies of oral magnesium for asthma have shown more negative than positive results, but some evidence exists that intravenous or inhaled magnesium may be beneficial. Also, preliminary evidence, far too weak to be relied upon, has been used to suggest that the supplement coenzyme Q_{10} (CoQ_{10}) might be helpful for asthma.

Other natural products commonly recommended for asthma include the herbs aloe, brahmi (*Bacopa monniera*), chamomile, damiana, elecampane, garlic, grindelia, horehound, hyssop, licorice, marshmallow, mullein, onion, reishi, and yerba santa, and the supplements adrenal extract and betaine hydrochloride. *Lobelia inflata* is sometimes recommended as an herbal treatment for asthma; according to traditional directions, though, it should be taken to the point of vomiting. None of these treatments has any meaningful supporting evidence.

Antioxidants, such as vitamin E, beta-carotene, and selenium, are frequently recommended for asthma on the grounds that they may protect inflamed lung tissue. Although one study found that asthmatics placed on a low antioxidant diet for ten days experienced a worsening of their symptoms, there is no direct scientific evidence that antioxidant supplementation improves asthma. A rather theoretical study found evidence that the use of vitamin E might decrease the inflammatory response in children with asthma exposed to ozone. However, a far more meaningful double-blind, placebo-controlled study found vitamin E (as 500 mg of natural vitamin E) ineffective for asthma. Similarly, a large (almost two-hundred-participant) study failed to find selenium helpful for asthma.

The herb picrorhiza has been advocated as a treatment for asthma, based primarily on two studies conducted in the 1970s. However, none of these studies reached modern scientific standards. Two subsequent, and better-designed, studies of picrorhiza failed to find the herb more effective than placebo.

One study failed to find a mixture of probiotics (friendly bacteria) helpful for asthma in children. Another study, though, found that a mixture of probiotic *Bifidobacterium breve* and the prebiotic galacto- and fructo-oligosaccharide may help reduce wheezing in infants with eczema.

Children with asthma may have reduced growth, possibly from the use of inhaled steroids. One study failed to find protective benefits with a multivitamin that contained vitamin D. The tested supplement did not contain calcium. Other studies have found that combination treatment with both calcium and vitamin D may protect bone density in people taking oral corticosteroids (for various reasons, including asthma).

Two preliminary studies reported by one research group have led to publicized concerns that the use of the insomnia supplement melatonin may worsen night-time asthma. However, one double-blind study of melatonin in people with asthma found evidence of improved sleep without the worsening of asthma symptoms.

Acupuncture. Although there have been numerous reports on acupuncture treatment for asthma, the results have been contradictory. A team of three researchers analyzed thirteen trials on acupuncture in the treatment of asthma. These studies were scored on the basis of design quality, with a maximum possible score of 100 points. Criteria for assigning points included size of the study population, randomization procedure, description of treatment, measurement of effects, and follow-up. Eight studies earned more than 50 points, and the highest score was 72 points.

Probiotics for Asthma in Children

Probiotics are friendly bacteria, so-called because they promote health rather than harm it. They are most often used to restore the normal intestinal balance of bacteria when it has been altered by the use of antibiotics. Bacteria are constantly at war with one another; if friendly bacteria can be encouraged to grow, they will in turn inhibit or destroy unhelpful bacteria, which might otherwise cause diarrhea or other gastrointestinal problems. For this reason, probiotics have been extensively studied for the treatment of intestinal disorders.

Probiotics also have shown promise for other conditions. For example, the ecology of microorganisms in the digestive tract can influence the function of the immune system, and there is some evidence that deliberate colonization of the digestive tract by certain bacteria might prove beneficial for disorders related to the immune system, including forms of asthma.

Allergic asthma and allergic rhinitis (hay fever) are categories of immune disorder for which probiotics have been advocated. To test the hypothesis that probiotics can help these conditions, Italian researchers conducted a study that was published in 2007 in *Pediatric Research*. This double-blind, placebo-controlled trial enrolled 187 children age two to five years. All the participants in this trial had allergic rhinitis, allergic asthma, or both. Over the one-year study period, participants were given either ordinary milk or milk enriched with the probiotics *Lactobacillus casei, L. bulgaricus,* and *Streptococcus thermophilus.* The results showed that the use of the probiotic-enriched milk significantly reduced the severity of hay fever but did not significantly affect the severity of asthma. (Use of the probiotic mixture also reduced episodes of diarrhea, but this was not a new finding.)

Note that the foregoing word "significantly" refers to statistical significance. This means that the benefits seen were unlikely to have been caused by chance. It does not mean that these benefits were particularly marked. In fact, probiotics only very slightly reduced hay fever symptoms.

Steven Bratman, M.D.

However, the overall quality of studies was judged to be mediocre; in any case, the results were contradictory. The conclusion was that "claims that acupuncture is effective in the treatment of asthma are not based on the results of well-performed clinical trials." A more recent review of acupuncture for asthma came to identical conclusions.

Other alternative therapies. Sublingual immunotherapy, a form of "allergy shot" that involves drops under the tongue rather than injections, has shown promise for asthma. Some people with asthma may also have food allergies. One way to discover a food allergy is to eliminate potentially allergenic foods from the diet, then to systematically reintroduce them to the diet to see if a reaction occurs. This elimination diet should be done only under the care of a doctor because of the risk of severe allergic reaction. Other ways to diagnose a food allergy include the skin scratch test and blood tests (such as RAST or ELISA). Persons with a food allergy who eliminate the offending food from the diet might reduce their asthma symptoms.

A special breathing technique called Buteyko breathing may reduce medication use and subjective symptoms, though it does not appear to actually improve lung function. Hypnosis, massage, yoga, and some other forms of relaxation therapy may offer modest benefits for asthma. The same is true of standard aerobic exercise.

In two controlled studies, chiropractic spinal manipulation has failed to prove more effective than fake manipulation for treatment of asthma. One study of osteopathic manipulation reportedly found benefits, but the study's design was flawed.

HOMEOPATHIC REMEDIES

In a double-blind, placebo-controlled study of forty people with asthma severe enough to require corticosteroid treatment, the use of an injected homeopathic remedy consisting of *Asclepias vincetoxicum* and sulphur significantly improved symptoms.

EBSCO CAM Review Board

FURTHER READING

Biltagi, M. A., et al. "Omega-3 Fatty Acids, Vitamin C and Zn Supplementation in Asthmatic Children." *Acta Paediatrica* 98 (2009): 737-742.

Campos, F. L., et al. "Melatonin Improves Sleep in Asthma." *American Journal of Respiratory Critical Care Medicine* 170 (2004): 947-951.

Cowie, R. L., et al. "A Randomised Controlled Trial of the Buteyko Technique as an Adjunct to Conventional Management of Asthma." *Respiratory Medicine* 102 (2008): 726-732.

Falk, B., et al. "Effect of Lycopene Supplementation on Lung Function After Exercise in Young Athletes Who Complain of Exercise-Induced Bronchoconstriction Symptoms." *Annals of Allergy, Asthma, and Immunology* 94 (2005): 480-485.

Giovannini, M., et al. "A Randomized Prospective Double Blind Controlled Trial on Effects of Long-Term Consumption of Fermented Milk Containing *Lactobacillus casei* in Pre-school Children with Allergic Asthma and/or Rhinitis." *Pediatric Research* 62 (2007): 215-220.

Gontijo-Amaral, C., et al. "Oral Magnesium Supplementation in Asthmatic Children." *European Journal of Clinical Nutrition* 61 (2006): 54-60.

Guiney, P. A., et al. "Effects of Osteopathic Manipulative Treatment on Pediatric Patients with Asthma." *Journal of the American Osteopathic Association* 105 (2005): 7-12.

Gvozdjakova, A., et al. "Coenzyme Q10 Supplementation Reduces Corticosteroids Dosage in Patients with Bronchial Asthma." *Biofactors* 25 (2006): 235-240.

Hsu, C. H., et al. "Efficacy and Safety of Modified Mai-Men-Dong-Tang for Treatment of Allergic Asthma." *Pediatric Allergy and Immunology* 16 (2005): 76-81.

Huntley, A., A. R. White, and E. Ernst. "Relaxation Therapies for Asthma." *Thorax* 57 (2002): 127-131.

Matusiewicz, R. "The Homeopathic Treatment of Corticosteroid-Dependent Asthma." *Biomedical Therapy* 15 (1997): 117-122.

Mickleborough, T. D., et al. "Protective Effect of Fish Oil Supplementation on Exercise-Induced Bronchoconstriction in Asthma." *Chest* 129 (2006): 39-49.

Mihrshahi, S., et al. "Eighteen-Month Outcomes of House Dust Mite Avoidance and Dietary Fatty Acid Modification in the Childhood Asthma Prevention Study (CAPS)." *Journal of Allergy and Clinical Immunology* 111 (2003): 162-168.

Olsen, S. F., et al. "Fish Oil Intake Compared with Olive Oil Intake in Late Pregnancy and Asthma in the Offspring." *American Journal of Clinical Nutrition* 88 (2008): 167-175.

Ram, F. S., S. M. Robinson, and P. N. Black. "Effects of Physical Training in Asthma." *British Journal of Sports Medicine* 34 (2000): 162-167.

Sabina, A. B., et al. "Yoga Intervention for Adults with Mild-to-Moderate Asthma." *Annals of Allergy, Asthma, and Immunology* 94 (2005): 543-548.

Schubert, R., et al. "Effect of N-3 Polyunsaturated Fatty Acids in Asthma After Low-Dose Allergen Challenge." *International Archives of Allergy and Immunology* 148 (2009): 321-329.

Sienra-Monge, J. J., et al. "Antioxidant Supplementation and Nasal Inflammatory Responses Among Young Asthmatics Exposed to High Levels of Ozone." *Clinical and Experimental Immunology* 138 (2004): 317-322.

Sutherland, E. R., et al. "Elevated Serum Melatonin Is Associated with the Nocturnal Worsening of Asthma." *Journal of Allergy and Clinical Immunology* 112 (2003): 513-517.

Van der Aa, L. B., et al. "Synbiotics Prevent Asthma-Like Symptoms in Infants with Atopic Dermatitis." *Allergy* (June 17, 2010).

Vempati, R., R. L. Bijlani, and K. K. Deepak. "The Efficacy of a Comprehensive Lifestyle Modification Programme Based on Yoga in the Management of Bronchial Asthma." *BMC Pulmonary Medicine* 9 (2009): 37.

See also: Allergies; Boswellia; Bronchitis; Colds and flu; *Coleus forskohlii*; Echinacea; Ephedra; Tylophora.

Aston-Patterning

CATEGORY: Therapies and techniques

RELATED TERMS: Arthrokinetics, Aston kinetics, bodywork, ergonomics, fitness training, massage, movement education, myofascial release, myokinetics, Rolfing

DEFINITION: A bodywork system involving massage, exercise, movement education, and ergonomics to improve health and well-being.

PRINCIPAL PROPOSED USES: Boost strength and endurance; dissipate stress and tension; ease movements; improve alignment, balance, posture, and mobility; relaxation

OTHER PROPOSED USES: Backaches, chronic pain, headaches, neck pain, sports and repetitive stress injuries

OVERVIEW

Aston-Patterning was developed in 1977 by Judith Aston, a dancer and movement instructor, to promote mind/body health and well-being. Aston-Patterning uses a combination of bodywork and massage, myokinetics and arthrokinetics, movement education, fitness training, and ergonomics to build strength and endurance and to improve alignment, posture, and mobility. Aston-Patterning is designed to teach awareness to help a person discover easier ways of performing daily activities.

Mechanism of Action

Aston-Patterning is based on Rolfing, a method of soft tissue manipulation and of movement education, but focuses on the asymmetry of the body instead of linear symmetry. Aston-Patterning treats each body as a uniquely curved structure that moves in three-dimensional spiral patterns. Aston-Patterning encourages cooperation among body parts and decreases accumulated tension through numerous bodywork techniques.

Uses and Applications

Aston-Patterning is used to solve body movement, posture, and alignment issues. It is useful in improving balance and coordination and for relieving chronic pain from sports and repetitive stress injury, accidents, illness, and surgery. It may alleviate headaches, muscle tension, and neck and back pain and may aid in stress reduction and in relaxation.

Scientific Evidence

As with other complementary and alternative therapies, there is limited scientific research that documents the benefits of Aston-Patterning. Most of the evidence supporting its effectiveness is anecdotal.

Some research suggests that Aston-Patterning improves posture and balance while easing bodily movements. However, its claims have not been proven by Western standards through randomized, double-blind, placebo-controlled clinical trials. Bodywork therapies are difficult to study because of flaws in methodology.

Aston-Patterning has become an appealing treatment option and may be beneficial for some conditions because of its relaxation effects. However, more research is needed to properly assess the clinical effectiveness of Aston-Patterning.

Choosing a Practitioner

Because Aston-Patterning involves various forms of bodywork, treatments should be performed by skilled practitioners to avoid injury. A list of certified practitioners is available from the Aston Training Center in Incline Village, Nevada.

Safety Issues

Aston-Patterning is considered safe with relatively few side effects; feelings of pain and exhaustion are an indication of an unusually harsh treatment. Aston-Patterning may be physically demanding and should not be performed on persons with heart or respiratory issues, diabetes, osteoporosis, bleeding or bruising disorders, or varicose veins, or on persons taking anticoagulants, steroids, or medications that disrupt balance.

Rose Ciulla-Bohling, Ph.D.

Further Reading

Aston Kinetics. "What Is Aston Kinetics?" Available at http://www.astonkinetics.com.

Hannon, John C. "A Review of Aston Patterning." *Journal of Bodywork and Movement Therapies* 9 (2005): 260-269.

Pelletier, Kenneth R. *The Best Alternative Medicine.* New York: Simon & Schuster, 2002.

Servid, Laura. "Dimensions of Alignment: An Aston-Patterning Perspective." *Massage and Bodywork* 4 (January/February, 2009): 64-73. Also available at http://massagebodywork.idigitaledition.com/issues/4.

See also: Alexander technique; Applied kinesiology; Dance movement therapy; Exercise; Exercise-based therapies; Feldenkrais method; Fibromyalgia: Homeopathic remedies; Manipulative and body-based practices; Massage therapy; Pain management; Progressive muscle relaxation; Reflexology; Rolfing; Soft tissue pain.

Astragalus

Category: Herbs and supplements
Related term: *Astragalus membranaceus*
Definition: Natural plant product used as a dietary supplement for specific health benefits.
Principal proposed use: Strengthen immunity against colds, flu, and other illnesses
Other proposed uses: Acquired immunodeficiency syndrome, atherosclerosis, chemotherapy side effects, chronic active hepatitis, diabetes, genital herpes, hypertension, hyperthyroidism, insomnia

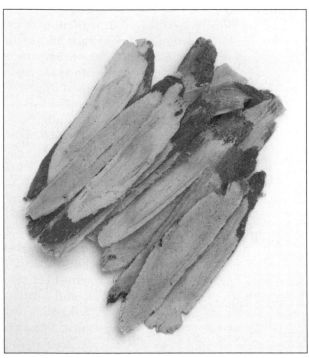

In the United States, astragalus has been presented as an immune stimulant useful for treating colds and flu. (©Lcc54613/Dreamstime.com)

OVERVIEW

Dried and sliced thin, the root of the astragalus plant is a common component of Chinese herbal formulas. According to tradition, astragalus, among other effects, strengthens organs such as the spleen, strengthens the blood, and strengthens qi, the energy or vital force of the body. The traditional understanding of the way astragalus works is different from the way it tends to be presented today.

USES AND APPLICATIONS

In the United States, astragalus has been presented as an immune stimulant useful for treating colds and flu. Many people have come to believe that they should take astragalus, like the commonly used herb *Echinacea*, at the first sign of a cold.

The belief that astragalus can strengthen immunity has a partial basis in traditional Chinese medicine, which says that the root creates a shield against infection. However, also according to tradition, astragalus formulas should not be taken during the early stage of infections. To do so is said to cause the infection to be "driven deeper." Rather, astragalus is thought to be appropriate only for use when a person is healthy. Its purpose is to prevent illness.

SCIENTIFIC EVIDENCE

Although Chinese herbal tradition suggests that astragalus should generally be used in combination with other herbs, modern Chinese investigators have found various intriguing effects when astragalus is taken by itself. Extracts of astragalus have been found to stimulate parts of the immune system in mice and humans and to increase the survival time of mice infected with various diseases. Astragalus has also been shown to enhance diuresis (urine output) by encouraging the kidneys to release more sodium into the urine. Other preliminary research suggests that astragalus might be useful in treating atherosclerosis, hyperthyroidism, hypertension, insomnia, diabetes, chronic active hepatitis, genital herpes, and acquired immunodeficiency syndrome, and to increase the efficacy and reduce the side effects of cancer chemotherapy. However, none of these possibilities has been proven.

DOSAGE

A typical daily dosage of astragalus involves boiling 9 to 30 grams (g) of dried root to make tea. Newer products use an alcohol-and-water extraction method to produce an extract standardized to astragaloside content, although there is no consensus on the proper percentage.

SAFETY ISSUES

Astragalus appears to be relatively nontoxic. High one-time doses, and long-term administration, have not caused significant harmful effects. Side effects are rare and generally limited to the usual mild gastrointestinal distress or allergic reactions. However, some Chinese herb manuals suggest that astragalus at 15 g or lower per day can raise blood pressure, whereas doses above 30 g may lower blood pressure.

Traditional Chinese medicine warns against using astragalus in cases of acute infections. Other traditional contraindications include "deficient yin patterns with heat signs" and "exterior excess heat patterns." Because understanding what these phrases mean would require an extensive education in traditional Chinese herbal medicine, one should use astragalus only under the supervision of a qualified Chinese herbalist. Finally, the safety of astragalus use in young children, pregnant or nursing women, or those with severe liver or kidney disease has not been established.

EBSCO CAM Review Board

FURTHER READING

Ai, P., et al. "Aqueous Extract of *Astragali radix* Induces Human Natriuresis Through Enhancement of Renal Response to Atrial Natriuretic Peptide." *Journal of Ethnopharmacology* 2007.

McCulloch, M., et al. "Astragalus-Based Chinese Herbs and Platinum-Based Chemotherapy for Advanced Non-Small-Cell Lung Cancer." *Journal of Clinical Oncology* 24 (2006): 419-430.

Yook, T., et al. "Comparing the Effects of Distilled *Rehmannia glutinosa*, Wild Ginseng, and *Astragali radix* Pharmacopuncture with Heart Rate Variability (HRV)." *Journal of Acupuncture and Meridian Studies* 2 (2009): 239-247.

See also: Atherosclerosis and heart disease prevention; Cancer chemotherapy support: Homeopathic remedies; Colds and flu; Diabetes; Hepatitis, viral; Herpes; Hypertension; Hyperthyroidism; Immune support; Insomnia.

Atherosclerosis and heart disease prevention

CATEGORY: Condition

RELATED TERMS: Coronary artery disease, coronary heart disease

DEFINITION: Prevention and treatment of diseases of the heart, including hardening of the arteries.

PRINCIPAL PROPOSED NATURAL TREATMENTS: Lifestyle changes, omega-3 fatty acids

OTHER PROPOSED NATURAL TREATMENTS: Antioxidants, astragalus, beta-carotene, bilberry fruit and leaf, chocolate, chromium, coenzyme Q_{10}, copper, flaxseed, garlic, genistein, ginger, ginkgo, grass pollen, green tea or black tea, hawthorn, lipoic acid, lutein, magnesium, mesoglycan, oligomeric proanthocyanidins, red yeast rice, resveratrol, sea buckthorn, selenium, trimethylglycine, turmeric, vitamin C, vitamin E

INTRODUCTION

Atherosclerosis, often known as hardening of the arteries, leads to cardiovascular disease and is the leading cause of death in men age thirty-five years and older and of all people older than age forty-five years. Most heart attacks and strokes are caused by atherosclerosis. Although the origin of this condition is not completely understood, it is known that atherosclerosis is accelerated by factors such as hypertension (high blood pressure), high cholesterol, diabetes and milder forms of impaired glucose tolerance, smoking, physical inactivity, and obesity. Chronic inflammation in the body (of various types) is also hypothesized to play a role.

Theories suggest that atherosclerosis begins with injury to the lining of the arteries. High blood pressure physically stresses this lining, while circulating substances such as low-density lipoprotein (LDL) cholesterol, homocysteine, free radicals, and nicotine chemically damage it. White blood cells then attach to the damaged wall and take up residence. Then, for reasons that are not entirely clear, the artery lining begins to accumulate cholesterol and other fats. Platelets also latch on, releasing substances that cause the

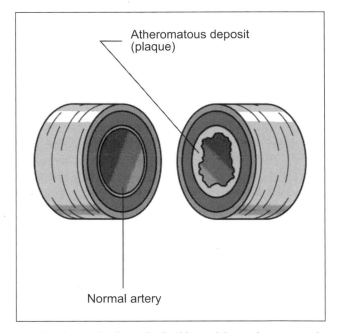

Atheromatous deposit (plaque)

Normal artery

Arteriosclerosis leads to the buildup of fatty plaques on the walls of arteries, which inhibits blood flow and may lead to obstructions resulting in stroke, heart attack, and other life-threatening events.

formation of fibrous tissue. The overall effect is a thickening of the artery wall called a fibrous plaque.

Over time, the thickening increases, narrowing the bore of the artery. When blockage of the coronary arteries (the arteries supplying the heart) reaches 75 to 90 percent, symptoms of angina develop. In the lower legs, blockage of the blood flow leads to leg pain with exercise, a condition called intermittent claudication.

Blood clots can develop on the irregular surfaces of arteries and may become detached and block downstream blood flow. Fragments of plaque can also detach. Heart attacks are generally caused by such blood clots, whereas strokes are more often caused by plaque fragments or gradual obstruction. Furthermore, atherosclerotic blood vessels are weak and can burst.

With a disease as serious and progressive as atherosclerosis, the best treatment is prevention. Conventional medical approaches focus on lifestyle changes, such as increasing aerobic exercise, reducing the consumption of saturated fats, and quitting smoking. The regular use of aspirin also appears to be quite helpful by preventing platelet attachment and blood clot formation. If necessary, drugs may be used to lower cholesterol levels or blood pressure.

PRINCIPAL PROPOSED NATURAL TREATMENTS

This section presents some promising and not-so-promising natural approaches for preventing cardiovascular disease by fighting atherosclerosis. Two classes of treatments have been omitted from this discussion: those that reduce elevated cholesterol and blood pressure and those that reduce levels of homocysteine.

Omega-3 fatty acids. Omega-3 fatty acids are healthy fats, found in certain foods such as cold-water fish. Some evidence suggests that fish or fish oil might help fight atherosclerosis. However, study results on fish or fish oil for cardiovascular disease have yielded contradictory results. A 2002 review (technically a meta-analysis) of many studies on the subject concluded that when all the evidence is put together, it appears that fish or fish oil can slightly reduce overall mortality, heart disease mortality, and sudden cardiac death (heart stoppage caused by arrhythmia). However, a subsequent comprehensive review published in 2004 included additional studies and came to a more pessimistic conclusion. According to the authors, "It is not clear that dietary or supplemental omega-3 fats

alter total mortality, combined cardiovascular events or cancers in people with, or at high risk of, cardiovascular disease or in the general population."

A large study (more than eighteen thousand participants) published in 2007 was widely described in the media as finally proving that fish oil helps prevent heart problems. This study, however, lacked a placebo group and therefore failed to provide reliable evidence.

If it does provide benefit for atherosclerosis, fish oil is thought to do so primarily by reducing serum triglycerides. Like cholesterol, triglycerides are a type of fat in the blood that tends to damage the arteries, leading to heart disease. According to most studies, fish oil can modestly reduce triglyceride levels. However, the standard drug, gemfibrozil, appears to be more effective than fish oil for this purpose. The most important omega-3 fatty acids found in fish oil are eicosapentaenoic acid (EPA) and docosahexaenoic acid (DHA). EPA and DHA may have different effects on triglycerides, but as is typical for studies involving marginally effective treatments, study results are not consistent; some found EPA more effective than DHA, while others did not find a difference. Similarly, some studies also suggest that fish, fish oil, or EPA or DHA separately can modestly raise levels of HDL (good) cholesterol.

Flaxseed oil (another source of omega-3 fatty acids) has been suggested as an alternative to fish oil. While fish oil is much better studied, there is some evidence, including two double-blind studies, that flaxseed oil or whole flaxseed may reduce LDL (bad) cholesterol, perhaps slightly reduce hypertension, and slow down atherosclerosis. Finally, while it is commonly stated that people require a certain optimum ratio of omega-3 to omega-6 fatty acids in the diet, there is no real evidence that this is true and some evidence that it is false.

Lifestyle approaches. There is no doubt that quitting smoking will significantly reduce heart disease risk. Increasing exercise and losing weight (if one is overweight) will most likely help too. Although for years there has been an emphasis on reducing fat in the diet, the balance of evidence indicates that it is more useful to substitute healthy fats (such as the monounsaturated fats in olive oil) for saturated fats than to try to reduce total fat intake. Evidence suggests that any low calorie diet, whether low-carbohydrate, low-fat, or in between, will result in weight loss and reduced cardiac risk.

Sources of Omega-3 Fatty Acids

Fatty fish is the main source of omega-3 fatty acids. Eating a lot of fish also takes the place of eating foods high in saturated fats. A good target for omega-3 consumption is 5 grams daily. One should be aware, however, that some fish contain significant amounts of mercury and may be harmful if eaten in excess.

Canned light tuna and crab, pollock, flounder, oysters, and shrimp are relatively low in mercury and provide good levels of omega-3 fatty acids in a 6- to 7-ounce serving. Omega-3s are also found in soybean and canola oils, flaxseed, flaxseed oil, walnuts, and leafy green vegetables.

The following is a list of food products and their respective amounts of omega-3 content in a 4-ounce serving (in grams):

- Chinook salmon (3.6)
- Sockeye salmon (2.3)
- Albacore tuna (2.6)
- Mackerel (1.8-2.6)
- Herring (1.2-2.7)
- Rainbow trout (1.0)
- Whiting (0.9)
- King crab (0.6)
- Shrimp (0.5)
- Cod (0.3)
- Tofu (0.4)
- Spinach (0.9)
- English walnuts (6.8)
- Wheat germ and oat germ (0.7-1.4)

Karen Schroeder Kassel, M.S., M.Ed., RD; reviewed by Brian Randall, M.D.

However, while it may not be important to cut down on total fat, accumulating evidence hints that trans-fatty acids, a type of fatty acid found in margarine and other hydrogenated oils, increase risk of cardiovascular disease. In July 2002, the Institute of Medicine of the U.S. National Academy of Sciences concluded that there is no safe intake level of trans-fatty acids and recommended that overall consumption be kept as low as possible.

The moderate use of alcohol is thought to help reduce cardiovascular risk, but the evidence regarding this subject is both inherently unreliable (because it is based on observational studies) and self-contradictory. According to the best evidence available, it appears to be the alcohol in alcoholic drinks that provides benefits rather than, as previously thought, particular substances found in wine. The optimal intake appears to be about one drink per day for women and one to two drinks per day for men. However, all of these statements are subject to revision, because they are based on problematic evidence.

OTHER PROPOSED NATURAL TREATMENTS

Several natural products have shown some promise for helping to prevent atherosclerosis.

Garlic. Garlic is generally said to produce several effects that together reduce atherosclerosis risk. Although garlic is no longer believed to strongly reduce cholesterol levels, it may improve cholesterol profiles to a modest extent; in addition, it may (mildly) lower blood pressure levels, protect against free radicals, and reduce the tendency of the blood to coagulate. However, the actual evidence for benefit is incomplete.

Garlic preparations have been shown to slow the development of atherosclerosis in rats and rabbits and in human blood vessels, reducing the size of plaque deposits by nearly 50 percent. Furthermore, in a double-blind, placebo-controlled study that followed 152 persons for four years, standardized garlic powder at a dosage of 900 milligrams (mg) per day significantly slowed the development of atherosclerosis as measured by ultrasound. This study, however, had some significant statistical problems.

An observational study of two hundred people suggests that garlic protects the arteries in other ways too. The study measured the flexibility of the aorta, the main artery exiting the heart. Participants who took garlic showed less evidence of damage to their arteries.

However, observational studies are notoriously unreliable.

Finally, in another study, 432 people who had experienced a heart attack were given either garlic oil extract or no treatment over a period of three years. The results showed a significant reduction of second heart attacks and an approximately 50 percent reduction in the death rate among those taking garlic. The researcher's failure to use a placebo in this trial greatly decreases the meaningfulness of the results.

Other potentially beneficial treatments. The substance red yeast rice has shown promise for reducing cholesterol levels. A double-blind study in China compared red yeast rice with placebo in almost five thousand people with heart disease. Over a four-year study period, the use of the supplement reportedly reduced the heart attack rate by about 45 percent compared with placebo and reduced total mortality by about 35 percent. However, these levels of reported benefit are so high that they raise questions about the study's reliability.

Mesoglycan is a substance obtained from the intestines of pigs. In one study, 200 mg per day of mesoglycan significantly slowed the rate of thickening of arteries. After eighteen months of treatment, the additional layering of the inside vessel lining was 7.5 times less in the group receiving mesoglycan than in the group that did not receive any treatment. However, because this was not a double-blind, placebo-controlled trial, the results cannot be taken as truly reliable. Preliminary evidence suggests that this supplement may work in several ways: supplying material for repair of arteries, "thinning" the blood, and improving cholesterol levels.

Magnesium also appears to be helpful. In a six-month, double-blind, placebo-controlled study, 187 persons with angina were given either 365 mg of magnesium daily or placebo. The results showed that the use of magnesium significantly improved exercise capacity, lessened exercise-induced chest pain, and improved general quality of life. Additionally, magnesium may reduce the atherosclerosis risk caused by hydrogenated oils, the margarine-like fats found in many junk foods.

Mildly impaired responsiveness to insulin (excluding diabetes) is a fairly common condition that appears to increase the risk of heart disease. Chromium supplementation might restore normal insulin responsiveness, aid in weight loss, and possibly improve cholesterol levels. The net result might be decreased risk of heart disease. In support of this theory, an observational trial found associations between higher chromium intake and reduced risk of heart attack.

Some observational studies suggest that green tea might help prevent heart disease. Black tea has shown inconsistent promise. Chocolate contains some of the same active ingredients as tea, and on this basis, it is sometimes mentioned as a potentially heart-healthy food.

Many herbs and supplements, including bilberry, feverfew, ginger, ginkgo, policosanol, and hawthorn, appear to decrease platelet stickiness. Whether this translates into an actual benefit for preventing atherosclerosis remains unknown.

Indirect evidence suggests that dehydroepiandrosterone might help prevent heart disease, especially in men. Also, frequent consumption of nuts may reduce the risk of heart disease, probably because the monounsaturated fats in nuts reduce cholesterol levels.

Whole grain oats may help prevent heart disease, but the supporting evidence is almost entirely limited to studies conducted by manufacturers of whole grain oat products. There is little to no evidence of benefit for other whole grains because studies have not been performed.

Chelation therapy, a technique that involves intravenous administration of the substance EDTA, is widely promoted in some alternative medicine circles as a treatment for atherosclerosis. However, there is no meaningful evidence that it works, and there is growing evidence that it does not work.

ANTIOXIDANTS

The body is in constant battle with damaging chemicals called free radicals, or pro-oxidants. These highly reactive substances are believed to play a major role in atherosclerosis, cancer, and aging in general. To counter the harmful effects of free radicals, the body manufactures antioxidants to chemically neutralize them. However, the natural antioxidant system may not always be equal to the task. Sources of free radicals, such as cigarette smoke and smoked meat, may overwhelm this defense mechanism.

Certain dietary nutrients augment the body's natural antioxidants and may be able to help when the primary system is under stress. Vitamins E and C and beta-carotene are the best known, but many other substances found in fruits and vegetables are also strong antioxidants. For years it was believed that anti-oxidant supplements might offer considerable protection against heart disease, especially vitamin E. However, later evidence appears to counter this theory.

Before presenting this information, it is necessary to explain the weaknesses of the observational studies that raised the hopes of the researchers looking into the effectiveness of antioxidants. Observational studies are relatively inexpensive and are often used to evaluate the potential health benefits of nutrients such as antioxidants. This type of study follows large groups of people for years and keeps track of a great deal of information about them, including diet. Researchers then examine the data closely and try to identify what dietary factors are associated with better health and longer life.

However, the results can be misleading. For example, if an observational study finds that people who take vitamin supplements live longer, it is not necessarily the vitamins that deserve the credit. Vitamin users also tend to exercise more and to eat more healthful foods, habits that may play a more important role than the vitamins. It is impossible to know for sure simply by evaluating the results of such a study.

Similarly, several observational studies have found that men who consume more foods that are rich in lycopene are less likely to develop prostate cancer. This does not necessarily mean, however, that taking lycopene supplements will reduce prostate cancer risk. Such foods contain many other nutrients, which may be more important than lycopene.

A more reliable kind of study is the intervention trial. In these studies, some people are given a specific substance, such as a vitamin, and are then compared with others who are given a placebo (or sometimes no treatment). The best intervention trials use a double-blind, placebo-controlled design. The results of intervention trials are far more conclusive than those of observational studies. In examinations of antioxidant therapy for preventing atherosclerosis, observational studies raised hopes, but intervention trials dashed them.

Vitamin E. Most observational studies have found associations between high intake of vitamin E and reduced risk of cardiovascular disease. Intervention trials, however, have failed to find vitamin E supplements effective.

The Heart Outcomes Prevention Evaluation (HOPE)

trial found that natural vitamin E (d-alpha-tocopherol) at a dose of 400 international units (IU) daily did not reduce the number of heart attacks, strokes, or deaths from heart disease any more than placebo. The details of this well-designed double-blind trial were published in the January 20, 2000, issue of the *New England Journal of Medicine*. The trial followed more than nine thousand men and women who had existing heart disease or were at high risk for it.

In addition, a large open trial compared the effectiveness of aspirin and vitamin E for the prevention of heart attacks, strokes, and other diseases related to atherosclerosis. Although aspirin treatment proved somewhat helpful, vitamin E produced little to no benefit.

Negative results have been seen in other large trials. A few trials have even found weak indications that the use of vitamin E may worsen certain outcomes.

When the results of these studies began to come in, some antioxidant proponents suggested that the persons enrolled in these trials already had too advanced disease for vitamin E to help. However, a large trial found vitamin E ineffective for slowing the progression of heart disease in healthy people. Moreover, in an extremely large placebo-controlled trial involving more than fourteen thousand American male physicians at low risk for heart disease, 400 IU of vitamin E every other day failed to lower the risk of major cardiovascular events or mortality in a period of eight years. On the contrary, vitamin E was associated with a slightly increased risk of stroke.

On balance, the evidence strongly suggests that vitamin E in the form used in these studies (alpha-tocopherol) is not helpful for preventing heart disease. It has been suggested that another form of vitamin E, gamma-tocopherol, might be more helpful than alpha-tocopherol. Gamma-tocopherol is present in the diet much more abundantly than alpha-tocopherol, and it could be that the studies showing benefits with dietary vitamin E actually tracked the influence of gamma-tocopherol. However, an observational study specifically looking to see if gamma-tocopherol levels were associated with risk of heart attack found no relationship between the two.

Beta-carotene. Beta-carotene is one member of a large category of substances in foods known as carotenoids, which are found in high levels in yellow, orange, and dark green vegetables. Many studies suggest that eating foods high in carotenoids can prevent atherosclerosis. However, isolated beta-carotene in supplement form may not help and could actually increase risk, especially if one consumes too much alcohol.

A huge double-blind intervention trial involving Finnish male smokers found 11 percent more deaths from heart disease and 15 to 20 percent more strokes in those participants taking beta-carotene supplements.

Similar poor results with beta-carotene were seen in another large double-blind study of smokers. Furthermore, beta-carotene supplementation was also found to increase the incidence of angina in smokers.

Smoking presents a challenge to antioxidants. However, the question remains: Why should beta-carotene not only fail to help but actually worsen the situation? One possible explanation is that beta-carotene in the diet always appears with other naturally occurring carotenes. It is likely that other carotenoids in the diet are at least as important as beta-carotene alone. Taking beta-carotene supplements may actually promote deficiencies of other natural carotenes, and overall, this may hurt more than it helps.

Other antioxidants. A single double-blind study suggests that the antioxidant coenzyme Q_{10} may help prevent the progression of atherosclerosis after a heart attack. Many other antioxidant vitamins, supplements, and herbs (including selenium, oligomeric proanthocyanidins from grape seed or pine bark, lipoic acid, turmeric, and resveratrol from red wine and grape skins) have been suggested as preventive treatments for atherosclerosis. However, although a number of studies have suggested that these substances may be beneficial, the state of the evidence is too preliminary to draw any conclusions.

Like other berries, sea buckthorn contains high levels of natural antioxidants. It has been widely advertised as effective for preventing heart disease, but the studies upon which this claim is based are far too preliminary to prove anything. Also, one large double-blind study explored the potential benefit of vitamin C for preventing cardiovascular problems in women at high risk for them, but it failed to find benefit.

Combined antioxidants. It has been suggested that the best approach is to use a combination of antioxidants. This makes sense theoretically because, for example, vitamin E fights free radicals that dissolve in fats while vitamin C fights those that dissolve in water.

However, evidence for benefit with such combinations comes only from observational studies.

A three-year, double-blind, placebo-controlled study of 160 persons found no benefit with combined antioxidant treatment providing vitamin E (800 IU), vitamin C (1,000 mg), beta-carotene (25 mg), and selenium (100 micrograms). Similarly, a three-year, double-blind, placebo-controlled study of 423 menopausal women with coronary artery disease found no benefit with combined vitamin E (800 IU daily) and vitamin C (1,000 mg daily). Furthermore, a seven-year, double-blind, placebo-controlled study of more than thirteen thousand French men and women failed to find any significant reduction of cardiovascular disease rates through the use of a daily supplement containing 120 mg of vitamin C, 30 mg of vitamin E, 6 mg of beta-carotene, 100 micrograms of selenium, and 20 mg of zinc.

HERBS AND SUPPLEMENTS TO USE ONLY WITH CAUTION

Various herbs and supplements may interact adversely with drugs used to treat atherosclerosis, so one should be cautious when considering the use of herbs and supplements.

EBSCO CAM Review Board

FURTHER READING

Anderson, T. J., et al. "Effect of Chelation Therapy on Endothelial Function in Patients with Coronary Artery Disease." *Journal of the American College of Cardiology* 41 (2003): 420-425.

Berglund, L., et al. "Comparison of Monounsaturated Fat with Carbohydrates as a Replacement for Saturated Fat in Subjects with a High Metabolic Risk Profile: Studies in the Fasting and Postprandial States." *American Journal of Clinical Nutrition* 86 (2007): 1611-1620.

Cook, N. R., et al. "A Randomized Factorial Trial of Vitamins C and E and Beta Carotene in the Secondary Prevention of Cardiovascular Events in Women: Results from the Women's Antioxidant Cardiovascular Study." *Archives of Internal Medicine* 167 (2007): 1610-1618.

Dansinger, M. L., et al. "Related Articles, Links, Abstract Comparison of the Atkins, Ornish, Weight Watchers, and Zone Diets for Weight Loss and Heart Disease Risk Reduction." *Journal of the American Medical Association* 293 (2005): 43-53.

Eidelman, R. S., et al. "Randomized Trials of Vitamin E in the Treatment and Prevention of Cardiovascular Disease." *Archives of Internal Medicine* 164 (2004): 1552-1556.

Gronbaek, M. "Alcohol, Type of Alcohol, and All-Cause and Coronary Heart Disease Mortality." *Annals of the New York Academy of Sciences* 957 (2002): 16-20.

Hooper, L., et al. "Omega 3 Fatty Acids for Prevention and Treatment of Cardiovascular Disease." *Cochrane Database of Systematic Reviews* (2004): CD003177. Available through *EBSCO DynaMed Systematic Literature Surveillance* at http://www.ebscohost.com/dynamed.

Howard, B. V., et al. "Low-Fat Dietary Pattern and Risk of Cardiovascular Disease: The Women's Health Initiative Randomized Controlled Dietary Modification Trial." *Journal of the American Medical Association* 295 (2006): 655-666.

Kelly, S., et al. "Wholegrain Cereals for Coronary Heart Disease." *Cochrane Database of Systematic Reviews* (2007): CD005051. Available through *EBSCO DynaMed Systematic Literature Surveillance* at http://www.ebscohost.com/dynamed.

Kleemola, P., et al. "Coffee Consumption and the Risk of Coronary Heart Disease and Death." *Archives of Internal Medicine* 160 (2000): 3393-3400.

Larmo, P., et al. "Effects of Sea Buckthorn Berries on Infections and Inflammation." *European Journal of Clinical Nutrition* 62 (2008): 1123-1130.

Lee, I. M., et al. "Vitamin E in the Primary Prevention of Cardiovascular Disease and Cancer: The Women's Health Study." *Journal of the American Medical Association* 294 (2005): 56-65.

Lichtenstein, A. H. "Dietary Fat and Cardiovascular Disease Risk: Quantity or Quality?" *Journal of Women's Health* 12 (2003): 109-114.

O'Keefe, J. H., K. A. Bybee, and C. J. Lavie. "Alcohol and Cardiovascular Health: The Razor-Sharp Double-Edged Sword." *Journal of the American College of Cardiology* 50 (2007): 1009-1014.

Ong, H. T., and J. S. Cheah. "Statin Alternatives or Just Placebo: An Objective Review of Omega-3, Red Yeast Rice, and Garlic in Cardiovascular Therapeutics." *Chinese Medical Journal* 121 (2008): 1588-1594.

Pelkman, C. L., et al. "Effects of Moderate-Fat (From Monounsaturated Fat) and Low-Fat Weight-Loss Diets on the Serum Lipid Profile in Overweight and Obese Men and Women." *American Journal of Clinical Nutrition* 79 (2004): 204-212.

Schecter, M., et al. "Effects of Oral Magnesium Therapy on Exercise Tolerance, Exercise-Induced Chest Pain, and Quality of Life in Patients with Coronary Artery Disease." *American Journal of Cardiology* 91 (2003): 517-521.

Sesso, H. D., et al. "Vitamins E and C in the Prevention of Cardiovascular Disease in Men." *Journal of the American Medical Association* 300 (2008): 2123-2133.

Stone, P. H., et al. "Effect of Intensive Lipid Lowering, with or Without Antioxidant Vitamins, Compared with Moderate Lipid Lowering on Myocardial Ischemia in Patients with Stable Coronary Artery Disease." *Circulation* 111 (2005): 1747-1755.

Vinson, J. A. "Black and Green Tea and Heart Disease." *Biofactors* 13 (2001): 127-132.

Vivekananthan, D. P., et al. "Use of Antioxidant Vitamins for the Prevention of Cardiovascular Disease." *The Lancet* 361 (2003): 2017-2023.

See also: Angina; Cholesterol, High; Hypertension; Congestive heart failure; Fish oil; Garlic; Heart attack; Intermittent claudication; Stroke; Vitamin E.

Athlete's foot

CATEGORY: Condition

RELATED TERMS: Fungal infection, foot, onychomycosis, ringworm, tinea pedis

DEFINITION: Treatment of fungal infections of the foot.

PRINCIPAL PROPOSED NATURAL TREATMENT: Tea tree oil

OTHER PROPOSED NATURAL TREATMENTS: *Ageratina pichinchensis* (snakeroot), essential oils, garlic, ozonized vegetable oil, *Solanum chrysotrichum* (sosa), various tropical/traditional medicinal plants

INTRODUCTION

Athlete's foot is the common name for a fungal infection of the foot, often called ringworm (although there is no "worm" involved). The three fungi most commonly implicated in athlete's foot (*Trichophyton rubrum*, *T. mentagrophytes*, and *Epidermophyton floccosum*) favor the warm, moist areas between the toes and tend to flare up during warm weather. Similar infections can occur in the nails, scalp, groin, and beard.

Infection with these fungi generally causes mild

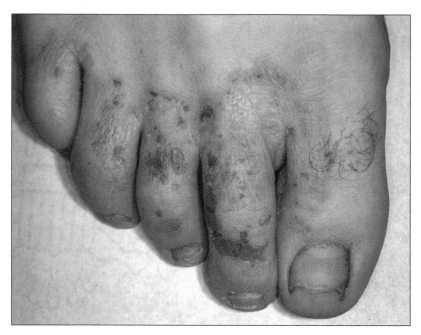

Athlete's foot is caused by a fungal infection. (CMSP/Getty Images)

scaling between the toes, but it can also cause more severe scaling, an itchy red rash, or blisters that cover the toes and the sides of the feet. Because the fungus may also cause the skin to crack, it can lead to bacterial infections, especially in older people or those with poor circulation in their feet. If the infection takes root under the toenails, it is called onychomycosis; it can be difficult, if not impossible, to eradicate.

Because the fungi that cause athlete's foot thrive in warm, moist areas, it is important to keep the feet clean and dry. Over-the-counter or prescription topical antifungal treatments containing miconazole, clotrimazole, econazole, or ketoconazole can generally cure athlete's foot, but treatment may have to be continued for one month or more for full results. In severe cases, oral antifungal medications may be necessary.

PRINCIPAL PROPOSED NATURAL TREATMENTS

Preliminary evidence suggests that tea tree oil might be helpful for athlete's foot.

Tea tree oil. Tea tree oil (*Melaleuca alternifolia*) has a long traditional use in Australia for the treatment of skin and other infections. This use is supported by evidence that tea tree oil is an effective antiseptic, active against many bacteria and fungi. Three double-blind

studies suggest it may be helpful for athlete's foot.

In a double-blind, placebo-controlled trial, 158 people with athlete's foot were treated with placebo, 25 percent tea tree oil solution, or 50 percent tea tree oil solution, applied twice daily for four weeks. The results showed that the two tea tree oil solutions were more effective than placebo at eradicating infection. In the 50 percent tea tree oil group, 64 percent were cured; in the 25 percent tea tree oil group, 55 percent were cured; in the placebo group, 31 percent were cured. These differences were statistically significant. A few people developed dermatitis in response to the tea tree oil and had to drop out of the study, but most people did not experience any significant side effects.

Another double-blind, placebo-controlled trial followed 104 people given either a 10 percent tea tree oil cream, the standard drug tolnaftate, or placebo. The results showed that tea tree oil reduced the symptoms of athlete's foot more effectively than placebo but less effectively than tolnaftate.

A third double-blind study followed 112 people with fungal infections of the toenails, comparing 100 percent tea tree oil to a standard topical antifungal treatment, clotrimazole. The results showed equivalent benefits; however, because topical clotrimazole is not regarded as a particularly effective treatment for this condition, the results mean little.

OTHER PROPOSED NATURAL TREATMENTS

Vegetable oils treated with ozone have antifungal properties. A double-blind (but not placebo-controlled) study of two hundred people with athlete's foot found that ozonized sunflower oil was as effective as the drug ketoconazole cream.

Solanum chrysotrichum (sosa) is an herb used in Mexico for the treatment of athlete's foot and related infections. In a double-blind study of 101 people, four weeks of application of a special extract made from this herb produced benefits equivalent to those of the drug ketoconazole (as 2 percent cream). However, because the study lacked a placebo group, these results cannot be taken as fully reliable. A similar study found potential benefit with the Mexican herb *Ageratina pichinchensis* (snakeroot).

Garlic has known topical antifungal properties. Preliminary evidence suggests that cream containing ajoene, a compound derived from garlic, might help treat athlete's foot.

Besides tea tree oil, other essential oils may be helpful as well, but the evidence remains weak. One study hinted that oil of bitter orange, a flavoring agent made from dried bitter orange peel, might have some effectiveness against athlete's foot when applied topically. Test tube studies indicate that the aromatic constituents of other essential oils, such as peppermint and eucalyptus, also have antifungal activity, but they have yet to be tested on people.

More than 120 plants traditionally used to treat skin diseases in Mexico, Palestine, British Columbia, and Guatemala have demonstrated antifungal properties in test-tube studies. Further research is needed to determine if these plant products are safe and effective for athlete's foot or other fungal infections.

EBSCO CAM Review Board

FURTHER READING

Herrera-Arellano, A., et al. "Effectiveness and Tolerability of a Standardized Phytodrug Derived from *Solanum chrysotrichum* on Tinea Pedis." *Planta Medica* 69 (2003): 390-395.

Ledezma, E., et al. "Efficacy of Ajoene in the Treatment of Tinea Pedis: A Double-Blind and Comparative Study with Terbinafine." *Journal of the American Academy of Dermatology* 43 (2000): 829-832.

May, J., et al. "Time-Kill Studies of Tea Tree Oils on Clinical Isolates." *Journal of Antimicrobial Chemotherapy* 45 (2000): 639-643.

Menendez, S., et al. "Efficacy of Ozonized Sunflower Oil in the Treatment of Tinea Pedis." *Mycoses* 45 (2002): 329-332.

Pattnaik, S., et al. "Antibacterial and Antifungal Activity of Aromatic Constituents of Essential Oils." *Microbios* 89 (1997): 39-46.

Romero-Cerecero, O., et al. "Effectiveness and Tolerability of a Standardized Extract from *Ageratina pichinchensis* on Patients with Tinea Pedis: An Explorative Pilot Study Controlled with Ketoconazole." *Planta Medica* 72 (2006): 1257-1261.

Satchell, A. C., et al. "Treatment of Interdigital Tinea Pedis with 25 Percent and 50 Percent Tea Tree Oil

Solution." *Australasian Journal of Dermatology* 43 (2002): 175-178.

See also: Eczema; Tea tree.

Attention deficit disorder

CATEGORY: Condition

RELATED TERMS: AADD, ADD, ADHD, adult attention-deficit disorder, attention deficit hyperactivity disorder, hyperkinetic syndrome

DEFINITION: Treatment of attention-deficit disorders.

PRINCIPAL PROPOSED NATURAL TREATMENTS: 2-dimethylaminoethanol, zinc

OTHER PROPOSED NATURAL TREATMENTS: Bach flower remedies, blue-green algae, calcium, combined amino acids, combined polysaccharides (galactose), food allergen avoidance and other dietary changes, fucose, glucose, glycine, inositol, iron, L-glutamine, L-phenylalanine, L-tyrosine, magnesium, mannose, massage, melatonin, N-acetylgalactosamine, N-acetylglucosamine, N-acetylneuraminic acid, St. John's wort, taurine, trace minerals, xylose

PROBABLY NOT EFFECTIVE TREATMENTS: Essential fatty acids (fish oil); evening primrose oil

INTRODUCTION

Originally, children who simply were incapable of concentrating at school were thought to have attention-deficit disorder (ADD). Hyperkinesia was used somewhat synonymously as a descriptive term for children who could not sit still. The definition has broadened to include adults and has been refined into two conditions: ADD and ADHD (attention deficit hyperactivity disorder). Characteristics include difficulty sustaining attention or completing tasks, easy distractibility, impulsive behavior, and, in the case of ADHD, an excessive inclination to fidget and move about. These problems make it difficult to succeed at work or at school.

Conventional treatment focuses on stimulants, such as amphetamine, dextroamphetamine, and methylphenidate (Ritalin, Concerta), and the newer drug atomoxetine (Strattera). Certain antidepressants may also be useful.

PROPOSED NATURAL TREATMENTS

2-Dimethylaminoethanol. There is some evidence that the supplement 2-dimethylaminoethanol (DMAE) may be helpful for ADD, according to studies performed in the 1970s. Two such studies were reported in a review article. Fifty children age six to twelve years who had been diagnosed with hyperkinesia participated in a double-blind study comparing DMAE to placebo. The dose was increased from 300 milligrams (mg) daily to 500 mg daily by the third week and continued for ten weeks. Evaluations revealed statistically significant test-score improvements in the treatment group compared with the placebo group.

Another double-blind study compared DMAE with both Ritalin and placebo in seventy-four children with learning disabilities. (Today, the participants likely would have been given a diagnosis of ADD.) The study found significant test-score improvement for both treatment groups over a ten-week period.

Zinc. The mineral zinc has shown some promise for treatment of ADHD. In a large double-blind, placebo-controlled study (approximately four hundred participants), the use of zinc at a dose of 35 mg daily produced statistically significant benefits compared with placebo. This dose of zinc is higher than nutritional needs, but not so high as to be unsafe. However, the benefits seen were quite modest: About 28 percent of the participants given zinc showed improvement, but so did 20 percent in the placebo group.

Another, much smaller study evaluated whether zinc at 15 mg per day could enhance the effect of Ritalin. Again, modest benefits were seen. Finally, exceedingly weak evidence hints that zinc might enhance the effectiveness of evening primrose oil for ADHD.

Essential fatty acids. Essential fatty acids (EFAs) are "good fats," substances as important to general health as vitamins. Based on evidence that essential fatty acids are necessary for the proper development of brain function in growing children, EFAs found in fish oil and evening primrose oil have been used for the treatment of ADHD and related conditions. The results, however, have been less than impressive.

A double-blind, placebo-controlled trial of seventy-five children with ADHD found that daily supplementation with omega-3 and omega-6 fatty acids may reduce ADHD symptoms in some children. However, in a similarly designed study of fifty such children, the use of essential fatty acids from fish oil and evening primrose oil failed to provide any consistent, significant benefit above and beyond the placebo effect. (The placebo effect, incidentally, was considerable.) In a slightly smaller trial, weak evidence of benefit was seen, but the results are difficult to interpret because of the high number of people who dropped out of the study.

In a double-blind, placebo-controlled trial of children already using stimulant therapy, the addition of the essential fatty acid docosahexaenoic acid (DHA, found in fish oil) for four months failed to further improve symptoms.

Evening primrose oil alone failed to prove effective for ADD in a small, double-blind, placebo-controlled trial. In a placebo-controlled comparative trial, evening primrose oil proved less effective than standard medical treatment. However, a close look at the data in this last trial hinted that evening primrose oil might have been more effective in people with adequate zinc levels. This suggests that combination therapy with zinc and evening primrose oil should be tested, but thus far, this approach has not undergone meaningful study.

Other natural treatments. A small, double-blind, placebo-controlled crossover trial evaluated the possible efficacy of the supplement carnitine for ADD in boys age thirteen years and younger. Approximately 50 percent of the participants responded to carnitine, a significantly higher percentage than responded to placebo. These promising results suggest that a larger trial is warranted.

A combination of American ginseng and *Ginkgo biloba* has shown some promise for treatment of ADHD. Vitamin B_3 (niacin), vitamin B_6, and multivitamin-multimineral supplements have been recommended for the treatment of ADD. However, a review of the literature found no meaningful evidence to indicate that these treatments are effective. One study reportedly proves that magnesium is helpful for ADD, but this study's design was too inadequate to prove much of anything.

Other supplements that are sometimes recommended for ADD include calcium, iron, inositol, trace minerals, blue-green algae, combinations of amino acids (usually gamma-aminobutyric acid, glycine, taurine, L-glutamine, L-phenylalanine, and L-tyrosine), and combinations of the polysaccharides galactose, glucose, mannose, N-acetylneuraminic acid, fucose, N-acetylgalactosamine, N-acetylglucosamine, and xylose. St. John's wort has also become popular, but unlike its effectiveness in depression, there is no convincing evidence for its effectiveness against ADD. St. John's wort interacts with many medications and could conceivably impair the effectiveness of conventional treatments for ADD.

One study hints that massage might be helpful for ADD. Also, it is commonly said that sugar, food allergens, and food additives, such as artificial colors, contribute to ADD symptoms. However, published evidence regarding these therapies remains incomplete and contradictory. The best evidence regards artificial colors and food additives. In a double-blind, placebo-controlled study of 153 persons without ADD, the use of certain food additives significantly increased hyperactivity compared with placebo.

A double-blind study reported in 2005 failed to find benefits for ADD with a treatment known as Bach flower remedies. Another study found that the supplement melatonin may be helpful for improving sleep in children with ADHD who are also taking stimulant medications. However, melatonin does not appear to be helpful for ADHD symptoms per se.

HOMEOPATHIC REMEDIES

In a double-blind study of sixty-two children with ADD, the use of constitutional, or classical, homeopathic remedies proved more effective than placebo. However, a similar study of forty-three children, again using constitutional remedies, failed to find statistically significant benefits.

EBSCO CAM Review Board

FURTHER READING

Arnold, L. E., S. M. Pinkham, and N. Votolato. "Does Zinc Moderate Essential Fatty Acid and Amphetamine Treatment of Attention-Deficit/Hyperactivity Disorder?" *Journal of Child and Adolescent Psychopharmacology* 10 (2000): 111-117.

Bilici, M., et al. "Double-Blind, Placebo-Controlled Study of Zinc Sulfate in the Treatment of Attention Deficit Hyperactivity Disorder." *Progress in Neuro-Psychopharmacology and Biological Psychiatry* 28 (2004): 181-190.

Breakey, J. "The Role of Diet and Behaviour in Childhood." *Journal of Paediatrics and Child Health* 33 (1997): 190-194.

Field, T. M., et al. "Adolescents with Attention Deficit Hyperactivity Disorder Benefit from Massage Therapy." *Adolescence* 33 (1998): 103-108.

Frei, H., et al. "Homeopathic Treatment of Children with Attention Deficit Hyperactivity Disorder." *European Journal of Pediatrics* 164 (2005): 758-767.

Jacobs, J., et al. "Homeopathy for Attention-Deficit/Hyperactivity Disorder." *Journal of Alternative and Complementary Medicine* 11 (2005): 799-806.

Johnson, M., et al. "Omega-3/Omega-6 Fatty Acids for Attention Deficit Hyperactivity Disorder: A Randomized Placebo-Controlled Trial in Children and Adolescents." *Journal of Attention Disorders* 12 (2009): 394-401.

Krummel, D. A., F. H. Seligson, and H. A. Guthrie. "Hyperactivity: Is Candy Causal?" *Critical Reviews in Food Science and Nutrition* 36 (1996): 31-47.

Lyon, M. R., et al. "Effect of the Herbal Extract Combination *Panax* Quinquefolium and *Ginkgo biloba* on Attention-Deficit Hyperactivity Disorder." *Journal of Psychiatry and Neuroscience* 26 (2001): 221-228.

McCann, D., et al. "Food Additives and Hyperactive Behaviour in Three-Year-Old and Eight/Nine-Year-Old Children in the Community." *The Lancet* 370 (2007): 1560-1567.

Pintov, S., et al. "Bach Flower Remedies Used for Attention Deficit Hyperactivity Disorder in Children." *European Journal of Paediatric Neurology* 9, no. 6 (2005): 395-398.

Rapp, D. J. "Does Diet Affect Hyperactivity?" *Journal of Learning Disabilities* 11 (1978): 383-389.

Richardson, A. J., and B. K. Puri. "A Randomized Double-Blind, Placebo-Controlled Study of the Effects of Supplementation with Highly Unsaturated Fatty Acids on ADHD-related Symptoms in Children with Specific Learning Difficulties." *Progress in Neuro-Psychopharmacology and Biological Psychiatry* 26 (2002): 233-239.

Schab, D. W., and N. H. Trinh. "Do Artificial Food Colors Promote Hyperactivity in Children with Hyperactive Syndromes?" *Journal of Developmental and Behavioral Pediatrics* 25 (2004): 423-434.

Stevens, L., et al. "EFA Supplementation in Children with Inattention, Hyperactivity, and Other Disruptive Behaviors." *Lipids* 38 (2003): 1007-1021.

Van der Heijden, K. B., et al. "Effect of Melatonin on Sleep, Behavior, and Cognition in ADHD and Chronic Sleep-Onset Insomnia." *Journal of the American Academy of Child and Adolescent Psychiatry* 46 (2007): 233-241.

Weber, W., et al. "Hypericum Perforatum (St John's Wort) for Attention-Deficit/Hyperactivity Disorder in Children and Adolescents." *Journal of the American Medical Association* 299 (2008): 2633-2641.

Weiss, M. D., et al. "Sleep Hygiene and Melatonin Treatment for Children and Adolescents with ADHD and Initial Insomnia." *Journal of the American Academy of Child and Adolescent Psychiatry* 45, no. 5 (2006): 512-519.

Wolraich, M. L., D. B. Wilson, and J. W. White. "The Effect of Sugar on Behavior or Cognition in Children." *Journal of the American Medical Association* 274 (1995): 1617-1621.

See also: DMAE; Fish oil; Zinc.

Atypical antipsychotics

CATEGORY: Drug interactions
DEFINITION: Drug used to treat schizophrenia.
INTERACTIONS: Ginkgo, glycine, St. John's wort
DRUGS IN THIS FAMILY: Olanzapine (Zyprexa), risperidone (Risperdal), clozapine (Clozaril), quetiapine (Seroquel), ziprasidone (Geodon), aripiprazole (Abilify)

ST. JOHN'S WORT

Effect: Possible Harmful Interaction

The herb St. John's wort might reduce levels of these medications in the blood. This could lead to an increase in the severity of psychotic symptoms.

Perhaps even more dangerously, if medication levels are adjusted for an individual already taking St. John's wort, stopping the herb could cause these levels to rise, potentially causing dangerous toxic symptoms.

GLYCINE

Effect: Possible Benefits and Risks

A few studies suggest that the amino acid glycine may augment the action of phenothiazine antipsychotic drugs. It might also augment the action of olanzapine and risperidone, but whether it augments or decreases the effectiveness of clozapine remains unclear.

GINKGO

Effect: Possible Helpful Interaction

Highly preliminary evidence suggests that ginkgo might reduce the side effects and increase the efficacy of various antipsychotic medications, including atypical antipsychotic drugs.

EBSCO CAM Review Board

FURTHER READING

Buchanan, R. W., et al. "The Cognitive and Negative Symptoms in Schizophrenia Trial (CONSIST): The Efficacy of Glutamatergic Agents for Negative Symptoms and Cognitive Impairments." *American Journal of Psychotherapy* 164 (2007): 1593-1602.

De Smet, P. A., and D. J. Touw. "Safety of St. John's Wort." *The Lancet* 355 (2000): 575-576.

Diaz, P., et al. "Double-Blind, Placebo-Controlled, Crossover Trial of Clozapine Plus Glycine in Refractory Schizophrenia Negative Results." *Journal of Clinical Psychopharmacology* 25 (2005): 277-278.

Evins, A. E., et al. "Placebo-Controlled Trial of Glycine Added to Clozapine in Schizophrenia." *American Journal of Psychiatry* 157 (2000): 826-828.

Heresco-Levy, U., et al. "High-Dose Glycine Added to Olanzapine and Risperidone for the Treatment of Schizophrenia." *Biological Psychiatry* 55 (2004): 165-171.

Potkin, S. G., et al. "Effect of Clozapine and Adjunctive High-Dose Glycine in Treatment-Resistant Schizophrenia." *American Journal of Psychiatry* 156 (1999): 145-147.

See also: Food and Drug Administration; Supplements: Introduction.

Autism spectrum disorder

CATEGORY: Condition
RELATED TERMS: Autism, autism disorder, atypical autism, infantile autism
DEFINITION: Treatment of behaviors associated with autism spectrum disorder.
PRINCIPAL PROPOSED TREATMENTS: None
OTHER PROPOSED TREATMENTS: Carnosine, food allergen avoidance, massage therapy, multivitamin-multimineral supplements, vitamin B_6 (alone or with magnesium), vitamin C

INTRODUCTION

Autism spectrum disorder (ASD, previously called autism) is a poorly understood family of related conditions. People with ASD generally lack normal social interaction skills and engage in a variety of unusual and often characteristic behaviors, such as repetitive movements. There is no specific medical treatment for ASD and its cause remains unclear. Anecdotal evidence of remarkable cures with the use of the substance secretin had raised hopes, but these hopes faded when numerous formal research trials found secretin ineffective. Also, despite public concerns that the measles, mumps, and rubella (MMR) vaccine may cause autism spectrum disorder, the balance of the evidence strongly suggests that this is not true.

Proposed Natural Treatments

Nutrients. Some physicians involved with natural medicine believe that ASD and many other illnesses are caused by genetic defects in the body that interfere with the metabolism of certain nutrients. For example, there is some evidence that children with ASD may have trouble metabolizing vitamin B_6. Based on this theory, various supplements have been advocated for treatment. However, despite a number of favorable anecdotal reports, there is no reliable supporting evidence from meaningful studies. As the secretin example shows, anecdotes can easily be misleading.

One ten-week, double-blind, placebo-controlled, crossover study of eighteen autistic children evaluated high doses of vitamin C for its effects on behavior. Participants received 8 grams (g) of vitamin C for every 70 kilograms (kg) of body weight. In this rather complex study, all participants received vitamin C for ten weeks. After that, half received vitamin C and the other half received placebo for another ten weeks. During the third and final ten-week period, the vitamin C and placebo groups were switched. (At this level of vitamin C intake, many people experience diarrhea.) The results indicated that the use of vitamin C caused significant improvements in behavior when compared with the use of placebo. This study, however, was small and had various design problems. Nonetheless, it does suggest that further research into using vitamin C for ASD might be advisable.

Another double-blind, placebo-controlled, crossover study found indications that high doses of vitamin B_6 may produce beneficial effects in the treatment of ASD. Again, however, this study was small and poorly designed; furthermore, it used a dose of vitamin B_6 so high that it could cause toxicity.

It has been suggested that combining magnesium with vitamin B_6 could offer additional benefits, such as reducing side effects or allowing a reduced dose of the vitamin. However, the two reasonably well-designed studies using combined vitamin B_6 and

---

Dietary Interventions in Treating ASD

Dietary interventions are based on the idea that food allergies exacerbate symptoms of autism (ASD) and that an insufficiency of a specific vitamin or mineral may trigger some symptoms of autism. If parents decide to try a special diet for a given period of time, they should be sure that the child's nutritional status is measured carefully.

A diet that some parents have found helpful is a gluten-free, casein-free diet. Gluten is a casein-like substance that is found in the seeds of various cereal plants—wheat, oat, rye, and barley. Casein is the principal protein in milk. Because gluten and milk are found in many foods, following a gluten-free, casein-free diet is difficult.

A supplement that some parents feel is beneficial for their child with autism is vitamin B_6, taken with magnesium (which makes the vitamin effective). The result of research studies is mixed; some children respond positively, some negatively, some not at all or very little.

In the search for treatment for autism, there has been discussion about the use of secretin, a substance approved by the U.S. Food and Drug Administration for a single dose normally given to aid in the diagnosis of a gastrointestinal problem. Anecdotal reports have shown improvement in autism symptoms, including sleep patterns, eye contact, language skills, and alertness. Several clinical trials have found no significant improvements in symptoms between patients who received secretin and those who received a placebo.

---

magnesium have failed to find benefits. Therefore, it is not possible to recommend vitamin B_6 with or without magnesium as a treatment for ASD.

One small study found that the use of a multivitamin-multimineral supplement improved sleep and gastrointestinal problems in people with ASD to a greater extent than placebo.

Other natural approaches. An eight-week, double-blind, placebo-controlled trial of thirty-one children found preliminary evidence that the supplement carnosine at a dose of 400 milligrams twice daily might be helpful for ASD. Massage therapy might also be helpful for ASD, according to one small controlled study.

It has been suggested that food additives, food

allergies, or other dietary factors may play a role in ASD, but meaningful supporting evidence for this theory has not been presented. One small but well-designed study failed to find benefit through eliminating gluten and casein from the diet. The study followed a double-blind design; parents generally thought they saw improvement, but perceived improvements were equally divided between the treatment group and the placebo group. A 2008 review of all published randomized trials on the subject found no convincing evidence that the elimination of gluten or casein (or both) from the diet of autistic children led to any significant improvement.

EBSCO CAM Review Board

FURTHER READING

Adams, J. B., and C. Holloway. "Pilot Study of a Moderate Dose Multivitamin/Mineral Supplement for Children with Autistic Spectrum Disorder." *Journal of Alternative and Complementary Medicine* 10 (2005): 1033-1039.

Chez, M. G., et al. "Double-Blind, Placebo-Controlled Study of L-carnosine Supplementation in Children with Autistic Spectrum Disorders." *Journal of Child Neurology* 17 (2002): 833-837.

Elder, J. H., et al. "The Gluten-Free, Casein-Free Diet in Autism." *Journal of Autism and Developmental Disorders* 36 (2006): 413-420.

Field, T., et al. "Brief Report: Autistic Children's Attentiveness and Responsivity Improve After Touch Therapy." *Journal of Autism and Developmental Disorders* 27 (1997): 333-338.

Madsen, K. M., et al. "A Population-Based Study of Measles, Mumps, and Rubella Vaccination and Autism." *New England Journal of Medicine* 347 (2002): 1477-1482.

Millward, C., et al. "Gluten- and Casein-Free Diets for Autistic Spectrum Disorder." *Cochrane Database of Systematic Reviews* (2008): CD003498. Available through *EBSCO DynaMed Systematic Literature Surveillance* at http://www.ebscohost.com/dynamed.

Molloy, C. A., et al. "Lack of Benefit of Intravenous Synthetic Human Secretin in the Treatment of Autism." *Journal of Autism and Developmental Disorders* 32 (2002): 545-551.

Nye, C., and A. Brice. "Combined Vitamin B6-Magnesium Treatment in Autism Spectrum Disorder." *Cochrane Database of Systematic Reviews* (2002): CD003497. Available through *EBSCO DynaMed Systematic Literature Surveillance* at http://www.ebscohost.com/dynamed.

See also: Adolescent and teenage health; Attention-deficit disorder; Children's health; Mental health.

Autogenic training

CATEGORY: Therapies and techniques
RELATED TERMS: Autosuggestion, hypnosis, relaxation
DEFINITION: A method of self-control therapy that teaches a person to use specific phrases to enter a state of deep relaxation and to achieve healing.
PRINCIPAL PROPOSED USES: Anxiety, chronic pain, depression, fatigue, sleep disorders, stress
OTHER PROPOSED USES: Constipation and diarrhea, gastritis, headaches, high blood pressure, infertility, irregular and accelerated heartbeat, irritable bowel syndrome, Raynaud's phenomenon, respiratory disorders, ulcers

OVERVIEW

Autogenic ("generated from within") training, or AT, is one of the oldest biobehavioral methods used in clinical psychology and stress management. Developed in the 1920s by Johannes H. Schultz as a self-hypnotic procedure, it drew on the observation that under hypnosis, persons often reported a sensation of heaviness (muscle relaxation) and warmth (vascular dilation) in their limbs.

A firm believer in the self-regulatory capacities of the human body, Schultz considered that hypnosis occurred not only because the patient allowed it but also because he or she induced it. Consequently, Schultz looked for an autogenic "trigger," or formula, that could be used to enter this state. Ultimately, he perfected a series of simple mental exercises that allow the mind to calm itself by turning off the body's stress responses.

The technique uses autosuggestion to establish a new mind/body balance through changes in the autonomic nervous system. Unlike progressive muscular relaxation and biofeedback, AT does not involve a conscious attempt to relax the muscles or control physiological functions. Rather, through passive self-suggestion ("observing" concentration and nonforcing), the person tries to render specific body regions warm and heavy. The training process involves focusing on, and subvocally repeating, one of six basic autogenic phrases, or orientations, several minutes each day, for one week or more. These phrases (with many possible variations) are "My arms and legs are heavy," "My arms and legs are warm," "My heartbeat is calm and regular," "My lungs are breathing for me," "My abdomen is warm," and "My forehead is cool." The words can be changed without altering the effectiveness of the method, to suit the practitioner's mind and circumstances. Within months of training, achieving a state of deep relaxation and beneficial physiological changes will take only seconds.

MECHANISM OF ACTION

The AT verbal suggestions represent a form of self-hypnosis, very powerful in inducing deep relaxation. Autogenic training uses selective awareness (SA), which represents the receptivity of the conscious mind to receive and acknowledge specific thoughts. Under SA circumstances, the censorship exerted by the ego should be annihilated, and thoughts should be allowed to travel freely from the conscious to the unconscious realm. The absence of censorship can improve dramatically the mind's ability to influence physiological processes as desired. In this receptive state, pain sensations are also significantly reduced.

Worldwide, abundant anecdotal reports of persons accomplishing daunting physical tasks while severely injured bear witness to the power of this phenomenon. Still insufficiently understood, the interplay between conscious and unconscious can nevertheless play important roles in maintaining physiological and psychological homeostasis. The method appears to exert a balancing effect upon the two branches of the autonomic nervous system (sympathetic and parasympathetic, fight-or-flight and rest-and-digest, respectively).

During AT training sessions, sudden physical and emotional reactions, such as numbness, muscle twitching, or tears, may result from the release of unconscious thoughts. The manifestation, considered normal and even beneficial, is called autogenic discharge.

USES AND APPLICATIONS

Autogenic training is most commonly used to reduce anxiety, fatigue, chronic pain, and stress. The sensations of warmth and heaviness can induce sleep, thus rendering the method useful in persons with insomnia.

Additional proposed uses for the method include constipation and diarrhea, gastritis, ulcers, headaches, high blood pressure, hyperventilation, asthma, irregular and rapid heartbeat, and Raynaud's phenomenon (episodic vasospasm of fingers and toes). Evidence also suggests that AT may enhance mental well-being and clinical outcome in persons with Ménière's disease (an inner-ear disorder that affects hearing and balance).

SCIENTIFIC EVIDENCE

Thousands of studies have been conducted on the effects and clinical applications of AT, both in Europe since the introduction of the method and in the United States beginning in the 1980s. A wealth of data remains in languages other than English.

Ample experimental support exists for the hypothesis that AT affects sympathetic tone and even parasympathetic function (that is, increased cardiac parasympathetic tone, with beneficial results). There is considerable difficulty in standardizing the technique, selecting participants, and measuring outcomes, so rigorous clinical studies are notoriously difficult to perform. Many studies have serious methodological flaws. Nevertheless, randomized-controlled trials have been conducted, with significant results indicating AT effectiveness in reducing anxiety and chronic pain, improving the symptoms of migraine headaches, and alleviating the symptoms of irritable bowel syndrome and other conditions.

CHOOSING A PRACTITIONER

AT is more popular in Europe and Japan than in North America. The British Autogenic Society offers therapist training courses and maintains a directory of practitioners in the United Kingdom and abroad. These practitioners have various backgrounds and may be doctors, nurses, psychotherapists, psychologists, complementary therapists, social workers, or teachers. Interested persons can learn the technique from numerous books, Web sites, or, preferably, from AT therapists. A specialist can confirm the quality of the practice, monitor progress, provide feedback, and implement variations from the standard.

SAFETY ISSUES

AT is generally safe and can be used by most people, except children younger than school age and persons with severe psychiatric disorders. Before implementing the technique, however, persons should undergo a physical examination and should discuss potential effects with a health care practitioner. It has been suggested that rapid autonomic rebound can lead to dizziness, disorientation, anxiety, panic, and even hallucinations in certain persons. Finally, persons with cardiovascular diseases, diabetes, or other severe disorders should use AT under medical supervision only.

Mihaela Avramut, M.D., Ph.D.

FURTHER READING

British Autogenic Society. http://www.autogenic-therapy. org.uk.

Edlin, Gordon, and Eric Golanty. *Health and Wellness.* 10th ed. Sudbury, Mass.: Jones and Bartlett, 2010. Covers multiple aspects of health and discusses stress management techniques, including AT.

Linden, Wolfgang. "The Autogenic Training Method of J. H. Schultz." In *Principles and Practice of Stress Management*, edited by Paul M. Lehrer, Robert L. Woolfolk, and Wesley E. Sime. 3d ed. New York: Guilford Press, 2009. A clear and authoritative discussion of AT, written for health practitioners and dedicated general readers.

Seaward, Brian L. *Managing Stress: Principles and Strategies for Health and Well-Being.* 6th ed. Sudbury, Mass.: Jones and Bartlett, 2009. An excellent work on stress management that includes a discussion of AT.

See also: Biofeedback; Hypnotherapy; Meditation; Mind/body medicine; Progressive muscle relaxation; Relaxation response; Relaxation therapies; Self-care; Stress; Transcendental Meditation.

Avicenna

CATEGORY: Biography

IDENTIFICATION: Persian physician and philosopher who developed chromotherapy

BORN: August or September, 980; Afshena, Transoxiana Province of Bukhara, Persian Empire (now in Uzbekistan)

DIED: 1037; Hamadhan, Persia (now in Iran)

ALSO KNOWN AS: Abū Alī al-Husayn ibn `Abd Allāh ibn Sīnā, Sharaf al-Mulk, Hujjat al-Haq, Sheikh al-Rayees

OVERVIEW

Avicenna, a Persian physician and writer, was a deeply influential philosopher-scientist of the Islamic world. He developed chromotherapy, or color therapy, an alternative healing method that uses color and light to balance a person's energy, particularly when clinical symptoms are present. He founded what came to be called Avicennism, a school of early Persian Islamic philosophy rooted in various metaphysical ideologies.

In his early life, Avicenna was an academic prodigy, exemplifying an aptitude for many subjects. He studied under a physician named Koushyar before establishing his own career in medicine (around the age of eighteen years) and in academia. During this career, he wrote about 450 pieces of work, about two-thirds of which were focused on philosophy and the other one-third on medicine. In particular, he discussed chromotherapy in his multivolume encyclopedic work *Qānūn* (1025; partial translation, *A Treatise on the Canon of Medicine*, 1930), in which he presented the idea that color is a symptom of disease and introduced a color chart for diagnostic purposes. This work, which was reportedly inspired by some principles of Galen and Hippocrates, was used as a textbook for medical students in Europe and the Islamic world up to around 1650. The work discussed a wide spectrum of early medical principles, including the ideas of causation, diagnosis, and treatment of various contagious diseases.

In *A Treatise on the Canon of Medicine*, Avicenna offered a theory based on a matrix of what he called humours and temperaments, a theory that served as a type of medical diagnosis tool. He also is credited for first reporting the makeup of the human eye and for describing many eye-related afflictions.

Importantly, *A Treatise on the Canon of Medicine* focused on both the theoretical and the practical components of medicine—making it an especially relevant piece in the context of complementary and alternative medicine. In particular, Avicenna emphasized the importance of exercise, diet, hygiene, psychology, and physical therapy—in addition to the many standard aspects of medicine—in maintaining or improving one's health.

Avicenna also wrote *al-Shifa'* (c. 1020; "The Healing"), a vast encyclopedia that included both scientific and philosophical topics and in which he discussed many aspects of the earth sciences and speculated about the evolution of geological features (such as mountain formation). He also developed elaborate theories in the realm of physics, especially regarding mechanics and optics. In addition, he supplied insights into various aspects of astronomy, chemistry, geology, mathematics, theology, science and research, and many other fields.

Avicenna is thought to have died of complications of colic at around the age of fifty-seven years. He continues to be regarded as one of the most influential thinkers and medical scholars, especially within the Muslim community. Accordingly, his name is acknowledged in many modern-day medical colleges and other institutions around the world.

Brandy Weidow, M.S.

Further Reading

Goodman, Lenn E. *Avicenna.* Updated ed. Ithaca, N.Y.: Cornell University Press, 2006.

Langermann, Y. T., ed. *Avicenna and His Legacy: A Golden Age of Science and Philosophy.* Turnhout, Belgium: Brepols, 2010.

See also: Color therapy; Spirituality.

Ayurveda

Category: Therapies and techniques

Related term: Ayurvedic herbs

Definition: A holistic medical system in which treatment is highly individualized and a wide range of methods are incorporated.

Principal proposed uses:

- *Acne:* Fixed combination containing oral and topical *Aloe barbadensis, Azardirachta indica, Curcuma longa, Hemidesmus indicus, Terminalia chebula, T. arjuna,* and *Withania somnifera*
- *Allergies:* Septilin, a fixed combination containing *Commiphora mukul, Tinospora cordifolia, Rubia cordifolia, Emblica officinalis, Moringa pterygosperma,* and *Glycyrrhiza glabra*
- *Angina:* Alba, a fixed herbal combination containing *T. arjuna* and approximately forty other herbs; *T. arjuna*
- *Asthma:* Boswellia, *Tylophora*
- *Bed-wetting:* Mentat, a fixed herbal combination containing *Bacopa monniera* and approximately thirty other ingredients

- *Colds and flus:* Andrographis
- *Diabetes:* Diabecon, a fixed herbal combination containing *Gymnema sylvestre, Eugenia jambolana, T. cordifolia, Pterocarpus marsupium, Ficus glomerata, Momordica charantia,* and *Ocimum sanctum;* pancreas tonic: fixed herbal combination containing *Aegle marelose, Azardirachta indica,* cinnamon, fenugreek, *F. racemosa, G. sylvestre, M. charantia, P. marsupeum, Syzigium cumini,* and *T. cordifolia;* fenugreek; *Gymnema*
- *Enhancing immunity:* Septilin
- *Enhancing memory:* *B. monniera,* mentat
- *Hemorrhoids:* Pilex, a fixed combination oral and topical herbal treatment
- *Hepatitis:* Kamalahar, a fixed combination containing *Tecoma undulate, Phyllanthus urinaria, Embelia ribes, Taraxacum officinale, Nyctanthes arbortistis,* and *T. arjuna; Phyllanthus; Picrorhiza kurroa*
- *Nausea:* Ginger
- *Osteoarthritis:* Articulin-F, a fixed combination containing *Boswellia serrata, W. somnifera, C. longa,* and zinc; RA-11 (similar constituents)
- *Rheumatoid arthritis:* Boswellia
- *Rotator cuff injury:* Rumalaya, a fixed oral and topical combination containing nearly fifteen herbs
- *Stress and fatigue:* Mentat
- *Varicose veins:* Gotu kola
- *Weight loss and cholesterol reduction:* Three fixed herbal combinations

Other proposed uses:

- *Aging:* Geriforte, a fixed herbal combination containing approximately forty herbs
- *Asthma:* Astha-15, a fixed herbal combination containing fifteen herbal ingredients
- *Atherosclerosis:* Garlic
- *Attention deficit disorder:* Mentat
- *Depression:* Mentat
- *Dyspepsia:* Turmeric
- *Epilepsy:* Mentat
- *Fluid retention:* Dandelion
- *Heart disease:* Garlic
- *Hypertension:* Alba, *Eclipta alba*
- *Febrile seizures:* Mentat
- *Improving immunity:* DefensePlus, a fixed combination containing *T. cordifolia, W. somnifera, O. sanctum,* and *E. officinalis*
- *Reducing cholesterol:* *E. alba,* garlic, *Commiphora wightii*

- *Rheumatoid arthritis:* RA-1, a fixed combination containing ashwagandha, boswellia, ginger, and turmeric
- *Stroke:* Mentat

OVERVIEW

Ayurveda, the ancient healing system of India, is one of the great healing traditions of the world. Like traditional Chinese medicine, with which it has many historical connections, Ayurveda is a holistic medical system grounded in a comprehensive philosophical/spiritual view of life.

Ayurvedic treatment is highly individualized and incorporates a wide range of methods, including dietary changes, herbal therapy, exercise, massage, meditation, and numerous special procedures such as cleansing of the nasal passages. Although the scientific base for Ayurveda is not strong, some of its methods have undergone meaningful scientific evaluation, and worldwide interest continues to increase.

One should note, however, that the presence of heavy metals in some Ayurvedic products makes them potentially harmful. Studies have found detectable levels of lead, mercury, and arsenic. Labeled as "Indian" or "South Asian," these products are sold on the Web and in stores. The U.S. Food and Drug Administration (FDA) does not review or approve Ayurvedic products, which can be especially harmful to children.

History of Ayurveda. The roots of Ayurveda lie in the ancient Sankhya school of Indian philosophy, developed many thousands of years ago. The first major classic of Ayurveda, the Caraka Samhita, was written between the second and fourth centuries B.C.E., but it is believed to be based on a much older oral tradition. This early text sets,out all the fundamental principles of Ayurveda but concentrates most of its attention on digestion (described as internal fire, or *agni*). Another early classic, the Susruta Samhita, focuses on surgical techniques. The Astanga Hridayam, written in about 500 C.E., sets out most of the detailed principles of Ayurveda, including the *dosha* and sub-*dosha*.

Ayurvedic thinking exerted a strong influence during the formation of traditional Chinese medicine, which in turn influenced Ayurveda's further development. The Ayurvedic technique of pulse-taking may have been derived from Chinese medical theory. Furthermore, translations of Ayurvedic texts influenced Islamic and European medicine.

In modern India, Ayurveda is one of three widely available forms of medicine, along with homeopathy and conventional medicine. It has become increasingly popular in the West as well, largely through the work of Deepak Chopra, Vasant Lad, and Maharishi Mahesh Yogi (the founder of Transcendental Meditation).

Principles of Ayurveda. In Ayurvedic theory, the body is said to contain three primal forces (*tridosha*) that work in tandem: *vata*, *pitta*, and *kapha*. These *dosha*, in turn, are formed from combinations of five elements that control the universe: space, air, fire, water, and earth. The *dosha vata* includes space and air; it controls movement. *Pitta* is made of fire and water; it controls digestion and metabolism. *Kapha* is composed of earth and water; it forms the body's structures. Each person can be said to be dominated by one or two of these *dosha* and may therefore be called a *vata*, *pitta*, *kapha*, *vata-pitta*, *vata-kapha*, or *pitta-kapha* type.

There are many other aspects of the body considered in Ayurveda. These include twenty attributes, five sub-*doshas*, seven tissues, four states of *agni*, and fourteen bodily systems. Health exists when all aspects of the body are in proper balance; disease occurs when that balance is disturbed. Excess *vata*, for example, might lead to arthritis, anxiety, and fatigue. Excess *kapha* is said to cause obesity and diabetes.

Practice of Ayurveda. The practice of Ayurveda is intrinsically holistic and preventive in intent. Perfect health in the Ayurvedic system involves not only physical wellness but also emotional, mental, and spiritual perfection. Treatment aims to promote and maintain balance to prevent or, when necessary, cure disease.

One of the primary methods of healing in Ayurveda involves diet. Foods are thought specifically to strengthen or weaken various *doshas*; therefore, people are prescribed a diet according to their constitutions. This method is different from the dietary approaches used in conventional medicine or the natural medicine systems that arose in the West (such as naturopathy). Westerners tend to consider certain foods healthy and others unhealthy; in Ayurveda, what is good for one person is bad for another, and vice versa. For example, a person tending toward an excess of *vata* might be advised to avoid raw vegetables but to consume nuts and seeds in abundance; someone with an excess of *kapha* would be given the opposite recommendation. To make matters more complex, dietary recommendations may vary from season to season,

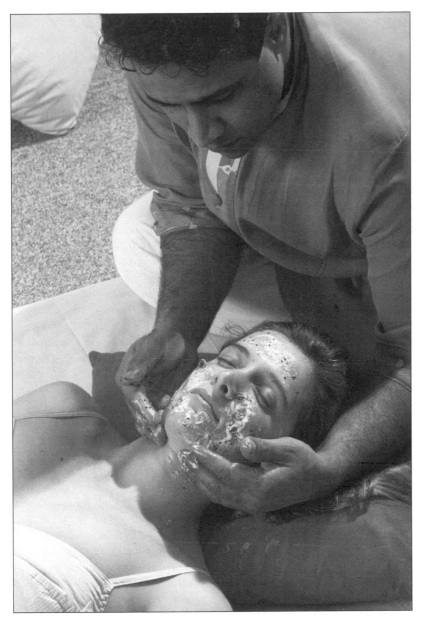

Woman receiving an Ayurveda massage. (Mauro Fermariello/Photo Researchers, Inc.)

healthy for a person with a different constitution.

In addition to spices for cooking, Ayurveda also uses purely medicinal herbs, which include andrographis, ashwagandha, *B. monnieri* (brahmi), *B. serrata*, *Coleus forskohlii*, dandelion, gotu kola, *Gymnema*, *C. wightii* (guggul), neem, *Phyllanthus*, *P. kurroa*, *Salacia oblonga*, and *Tylophora*. Minerals such as silver, mercury, and lead may be used too.

Ayurvedic therapy also has an exercise component known as hatha yoga. In general, the practice of yoga is believed to promote good health; in addition, certain postures are believed to offer assistance in specific medical conditions.

Like the acupuncture needles of Chinese medicine, Ayurveda has additional characteristic methods. One set of its therapies is collectively called *panchakarma*. This is a method of purification that may involve massage, *shirodhara* (extended pouring of warm oil on the "third eye" point in the center of the forehead), emetics, purgatives, enemas, cleansing of the nasal passages with various substances, and bloodletting. Additionally, the drinking of urine is recommended in certain situations.

SCIENTIFIC EVIDENCE

It is true that all people are different, and that the ideal form of medicine should take such differences into account. Ayurveda's strength in this regard is one of its sources of appeal. However, the mere fact that medicine ought to treat people individually does not imply that Ayurveda's individualized treatment techniques are actually grounded in reality. They could be wishful thinking rather than an insight into the truth.

It is very difficult to scientifically validate entire systems of health. In medicine, only double-blind, placebo-controlled trials produce scientifically reliable

and they frequently include numerous details about the optimal ways to prepare and consume foods.

Herbs (both culinary and medicinal) are another mainstay of Ayurvedic treatment. For example, people with a *vata* constitution are thought to benefit from turmeric, cumin, coriander, ginger, garlic, and fenugreek. However, some of these herbs might not be

results. However, there is really no way to fit Ayurvedic medicine into such a format.

One study did attempt to test the effectiveness of whole-person Ayurvedic treatment. In this trial, sixty people with diabetes were randomly assigned either to standard diabetes education classes or to a course of care involving exercise, Ayurvedic diet, meditation, and Ayurvedic herbal treatment. As it happened, the results failed to show much in the way of statistically significant benefits with the Ayurvedic treatment. However, even if results had been seen, they would be of minimal validity because to receive a complex, exciting course of treatment usually results in improvement, regardless of what treatment is used.

It is very difficult, if not impossible, to make a scientifically grounded statement regarding the effectiveness of Ayurveda as a whole. However, there exists some evidence for a subset of Ayurveda: its herbal therapies.

Many Ayurvedic herbs taken alone have undergone varying levels of study. These herbs include andrographis (for colds and flus), ashwagandha, boswellia (for rheumatoid arthritis, asthma), *C. forskohlii* (for asthma), dandelion (as a diuretic, to help treat fluid retention), fenugreek (for diabetes), garlic (for high cholesterol, heart disease), gymnema (for diabetes), ginger (for nausea), gotu kola (for varicose veins), guggul (for high cholesterol), neem, *Phyllanthus* (for hepatitis), turmeric (for dyspepsia), and *Tylophora* (for asthma).

Many other Ayurvedic herbal combinations have been studied in trials of lower quality, but because only double-blind, placebo-controlled studies can actually prove the effectiveness of a treatment, those studies are not reported here. Even the double-blind, placebo-controlled studies discussed here fall far short of modern scientific standards, and independent confirmation of results is usually lacking. Nonetheless, the results described here are somewhat encouraging.

A couple of studies have begun the process of examining classic Ayurvedic diagnosis to determine whether or not it has a relationship to physical reality. One study failed to find an expected correlation between Ayurvedic diagnosis and severity of symptoms in ankylosing spondylitis and low back pain. Another small study found that different Ayurvedic practitioners did in fact independently come up with similar diagnosis and treatment plans in three people with rheumatoid arthritis.

SINGLE HERBS

T. arjuna. In a double-blind study, fifty-eight men with chronic stable angina received either *T. arjuna* (500 milligrams [mg] every eight hours), the drug isosorbide mononitrate (40 mg daily), or a matching placebo for one week each. The results indicated that the use of *T. arjuna* was more effective than placebo for angina and approximately as effective as the medication.

In another study, 105 men with coronary heart disease received either placebo, vitamin E, or *T. arjuna* (500 mg daily) for thirty days. The results indicated that the herb reduced cholesterol levels. However, the researchers inexplicably decided to make this an "open label" study, meaning that participants and researchers knew which treatment was which. Because of this, the results are essentially meaningless.

P. kurroa. In a double-blind trial of thirty-three people with acute viral hepatitis, the use of the herb *P. kurroa* at a dose of 375 mg three times daily significantly speeded recovery time compared with placebo.

B. monniera (brahmi). The Ayurvedic herb *B. monniera* (brahmi) has a traditional reputation for improving memory. However, a twelve-week, double-blind, placebo-controlled trial of seventy-six people that tested the potential memory-enhancing benefits of brahmi generally failed to find much evidence of benefit. The only significant improvement seen among the many measures used was in one that evaluated the retention of new information. Although this may sound somewhat positive, in fact, it means little. When a study uses many different techniques to assess improvement, mere chance ensures that at least one of them will come up with results. Properly designed studies should focus on one test of benefit alone (the primary outcome measure) that is selected before running the trial. The use of multiple tests is sometimes called "fishing for results," and it is frowned upon.

If several independent studies use multiple tests of improvement, and the pattern of response is reliably maintained, then the results begin to appear more significant. This does not seem to be the case with brahmi. In a previous double-blind, placebo-controlled study enrolling forty-six people, the use of brahmi for two weeks produced quite a different pattern of benefits. In another double-blind, placebo-controlled study of thirty-eight people, short-term use of brahmi failed to produce any measurable improvements in memory. Other studies have failed to find benefit using a combination of *Ginkgo biloba* and brahmi, whether in the short term or over a period of several weeks.

COMBINATION THERAPIES

Septilin. Septilin is a fixed combination containing *C. mukul, T. cordifolia, R. cordifolia, E. officinalis, M. pterygosperma,* and *G. glabra.* This combination therapy has shown promise for the treatment of allergic rhinitis. In a double-blind study, 190 people were given either the herbal combination or a standard antihistamine (chlorpheniramine). The results over seven days indicated that the two treatments were equally effective.

Another study found general evidence for an antihistamine-like effect. In this double-blind, placebo-controlled trial of thirty-two healthy people, the use of septilin for four weeks significantly reduced the allergic reaction caused by injection of histamine under the skin.

Septilin has also been tried as a treatment for improving immunity. In a double-blind, placebo-controlled study of forty children with persistent low-grade infections (such as chronic sore throat or sinus infection), the use of septilin for one month led to significant improvement compared with placebo.

Mentat. The proprietary Ayurvedic mixture mentat, which is a fixed herbal combination containing *B. monniera* and almost thirty other ingredients, has been studied for numerous brain-related conditions. For example, in a three-month, double-blind, placebo-controlled study of fifty adult students, the use of mentat appeared to improve memory and attention and reduce stress. Similarly, in a three-month, double-blind, placebo-controlled trial of forty-two people in high-stress jobs who complained of fatigue, the use of mentat decreased symptoms.

In several double-blind, placebo-controlled trials, mentat has shown promise for normalizing the behavior of children with attention-deficit disorder, developmental disabilities, or brain damage. Other double-blind, placebo-controlled trials found evidence that this combination therapy might be helpful for depression, epilepsy, decreasing amnesia caused by electroconvulsive therapy, reducing frequency of febrile seizures (seizures caused by fever), enhancing recovery from aphasia (loss of speech caused by stroke), and improving memory in people with anxiety. Mentat has also shown promise for bed-wetting.

Kamalahar. Kamalahar is a fixed combination containing *T. undulate, P. urinaria, E. ribes, T. officinale, N. arbortistis,* and *T. arjuna.* In a double-blind, placebo-controlled study, fifty-two people with acute hepatitis were randomly assigned to receive placebo or this combination herbal therapy at a dose of 500 mg three times daily for fifteen days. The results indicate that the herbal combination improved liver function to a significantly greater extent than placebo.

Liv.52. Liv.52 is a fixed combination containing *Capparis spinosa, Cichorium intybus, Solanum nigrum, T. arjuna, Cassia occidentalis, Achillea millefolium,* and *Tamarix gallica.* In a poorly reported five-week, double-blind, placebo-controlled study of thirty children with hepatitis A, the use of this combination formula apparently improved the rate of recovery compared with placebo. Benefits were also seen in a six-week study of thirty-four people with acute hepatitis A.

Another double-blind, placebo-controlled study evaluated the effectiveness of Liv.52 in a variety of liver conditions. A total of 104 people were enrolled in this trial and were divided into three groups depending on the liver condition they had: cirrhosis, acute hepatitis, or chronic hepatitis (type not stated). Participants with cirrhosis were treated for twenty-four months, those with chronic active hepatitis were treated for twelve months, and participants with hepatitis A were treated for only six weeks. The use of Liv.52 was associated with substantially better outcomes than placebo. Apparent benefits were also seen in a six-month, double-blind, placebo-controlled study of thirty-six people with cirrhosis. However, in a six-month, double-blind study of eighty people with alcoholic liver disease (alcoholic hepatitis or cirrhosis), Liv.52 failed to provide any benefits.

Rumalaya. In a placebo-controlled trial of one hundred people with rotator-cuff injury (frozen shoulder), the use of the tablet and cream combination rumalaya, a fixed oral and topical combination containing almost fifteen herbs, significantly improved results compared with little improvement in the placebo group.

Weight loss and cholesterol reduction. In a three-month, double-blind, placebo-controlled study, seventy overweight people were divided into four groups and given one of the following treatments: placebo; triphala guggul (a mixture of five Ayurvedic ingredients) plus gokshuradi guggul (a mixture of eight Ayurvedic ingredients); triphala guggul plus sinhanad guggul (a mixture of six Ayurvedic herbs); or triphala guggul plus chandraprabha vati (a mixture of thirty-six Ayurvedic ingredients). Reportedly, all three Ayurvedic ingredients produced significant weight loss and improvements in cholesterol relative to placebo; furthermore, the improvements produced by all of the treatments were close to identical.

Articulin-F and RA-11. Articulin-F is a fixed combination containing *B. serrata, W. somnifera, C. longa,* and zinc. In a three-month, double-blind, placebo-controlled trial of forty-two people with osteoarthritis, the use of this combination therapy significantly improved pain and disability compared with placebo. Another double-blind study found benefit with RA-11, a combination therapy containing most of the same ingredients as articulin-F, but substituting ginger for zinc.

Diabecon. Diabecon is a fixed herbal combination containing *G. sylvestre, E. jambolana, T. cordifolia, P. marsupium, F. glomerata, M. charantia,* and *O. sanctum.* In a six-month, double-blind, placebo-controlled trial, forty people with type 2 diabetes who had failed to respond fully to oral drugs received either this combination of Ayurvedic herbal therapy or placebo. The results indicated that the herbal therapy was modestly helpful.

Pancreas tonic. Pancreas tonic is a fixed herbal combination of herbs with an antidiabetic reputation containing *A. marelose, A. indica,* cinnamon, fenugreek, *F. racemosa, G. sylvestre, M. charantia, P. marsupeum, S. cumini,* and *T. cordifolia.* Several animal studies had indicated that this traditional herbal formula might offer benefits in diabetes. Based on this, a three-month, double-blind study of thirty-six people with type 2 diabetes was undertaken. The results appeared to indicate that use of pancreas tonic can improve blood sugar control

Fixed topical and oral combination. A fixed topical and oral combination for the treatment of acne contains *A. barbadensis, A. indica, C. longa, H. indicus, T. chebula, T. arjuna,* and *W. somnifera.* In a four-week, double-blind study, fifty-three people with acne received one of four therapies: real herb in oral tablets and as topical cream; real herb in oral tablets and as topical gel; real herb in oral tablets with placebo gel; or placebo tablet with placebo topical treatment. The results appear to indicate that while oral herb alone is not helpful, oral herb plus topical herb can improve acne symptoms.

DefensePlus. DefensePlus is a fixed combination containing *T. cordifolia, W. somnifera, O. sanctum,* and *E. officinalis.* Test tube and animal trials suggest that this combination product may strengthen the immune response. Promising results have also been seen in two unpublished human trials. One was a double-blind, placebo-controlled trial of children age five to eighteen who experienced recurring bouts of tonsillitis. The results showed that participants taking the herbal combination were less likely to require surgical treatment (tonsillectomy) for the condition. The other double-blind, placebo-controlled study found that the use of this herbal combination along with standard therapy improved recovery from eye conditions requiring antibiotics.

RA-1. RA-1 is a fixed combination containing extracts of ashwagandha, boswellia, ginger, and turmeric. A sixteen-week, double-blind, placebo-controlled trial of 182 people with rheumatoid arthritis evaluated the potential effectiveness of this formula. Participants in both groups improved significantly; however, according to most measures of disease severity, the benefits of the herbal combination were no greater than those of placebo.

PILEX. The fixed combination oral and topical herbal treatment PILEX was evaluated in a double-blind, placebo-controlled trial of one hundred people with hemorrhoids. The results indicated that the benefits were seen in 50 percent of those using the herbal treatment compared with only 20 percent in the placebo group.

Alba. In a double-blind study of forty-three men and women with hypertension, the use of the proprietary herbal combination alba (*T. arjuna* and approximately forty other herbs) proved almost as effective for controlling blood pressure as the drug methyldopa. Additionally, in a double-blind, placebo-controlled trial of twenty-five people with angina, the use of this combination therapy reduced chest pain and improved heart function.

One study of somewhat questionable reliability reported that the herb *E. alba* (also known as Bhringraja or Keshraja) can improve blood pressure when taken by itself at a dose of 3 grams daily. This study also claimed to find reductions in cholesterol levels.

Geriforte. Geriforte, a fixed herb combination containing approximately forty Ayurvedic herbs, has been marketed as a general tonic for the elderly. Several poorly designed or incompletely reported placebo-controlled trials suggest that this herbal combination might possibly improve cholesterol levels, general well-being, and mood in the elderly.

Astha 15. One double-blind comparative study provides weak evidence that the herbal combination called Astha 15, a fixed herb combination containing fifteen herbs, might be helpful for mild asthma.

CHOOSING A PRACTITIONER

There is no widely accepted licensure for the practice of Ayurvedic medicine. However, several schools offer extensive training. These schools generally require from 500 to 3,500 hours of training. Some of the better-known schools are the Ayurvedic Institute in Albuquerque, New Mexico; the California College of Ayurveda in Grass Valley; and the American Institute of Vedic Studies in Santa Fe, New Mexico.

SAFETY ISSUES

Ayurvedic therapy presents numerous potential safety concerns. One serious problem is that many Ayurvedic herbs have never undergone a formal safety evaluation, and those that have been evaluated have not necessarily been proven harmless.

Most of the proprietary herbal formulas discussed in the foregoing have undergone a certain amount of safety testing by the manufacturer and were found nontoxic; however, verification of safety by independent laboratories that apply modern standards remains limited. Some traditional Ayurvedic formulas may contain toxic levels of heavy metals, especially lead, mercury, and arsenic. According to one study, approximately one in five American- and Indian-produced Ayurvedic medicines contained detectable amounts of a minimum of one of these heavy metals. In one particularly dramatic and tragic case report, a brain-damaged child born to a woman using an Ayurvedic formula was found to have the highest blood levels of lead ever recorded in a living newborn. Analysis of the formula revealed a high lead content, along with toxic levels of mercury.

There are other concerns too. For example, oral silver, a traditional Ayurvedic remedy, can cause permanent gray-black staining of the skin and mucous membranes. The dietary recommendations made within the context of Ayurvedic theory could conceivably lead to inadequate intake of essential nutrients,

and hence malnutrition. However, most reputable Ayurvedic practitioners are aware of modern nutrition knowledge and take care to make reasonable recommendations within that context.

Various traditional Ayurvedic techniques, such as bloodletting and drinking urine, clearly suggest possible health risks. Most modern Ayurvedic practitioners shun the most worrisome of these methods.

In a case report, a patient taking the antidepressant sertraline had two relapses of depression soon after taking an Ayurvedic herbal mixture containing *T. chebula* and *C. wightii.* The authors interpreted this as likely to have been caused by an adverse drug-herb interaction. Finally, one study found that an Ayurvedic herbal formula called trikatu (a mixture of black pepper and ginger) can reduce the effectiveness of the standard anti-inflammatory drug diclofenac. This finding was somewhat surprising because black pepper is generally thought to enhance the absorption and activity of various medications through a number of known chemical interactions.

EBSCO CAM Review Board

FURTHER READING

Chopra, A., et al. "A Thirty-Two-Week Randomized, Placebo-Controlled Clinical Evaluation of RA-11, an Ayurvedic Drug, on Osteoarthritis of the Knees." *Journal of Clinical Rheumatology* 10 (2006): 236-245.

Elder, C., et al. "Randomized Trial of a Whole-System Ayurvedic Protocol for Type 2 Diabetes." *Alternative Therapies in Health and Medicine* 12 (2006): 24-30.

Hsia, S. II., et al. "Effect of Pancreas Tonic (An Ayurvedic Herbal Supplement) in Type 2 Diabetes Mellitus." *Metabolism* 53 (2004): 1166-1173.

Huseini, H. F., et al. "The Efficacy of Liv-52 on Liver Cirrhotic Patients." *Phytomedicine* 12 (2005): 619-624.

Nathan, P. J., et al. "Effects of a Combined Extract of *Ginkgo biloba* and *Bacopa monniera* on Cognitive Function in Healthy Humans." *Human Psychopharmacology* 19 (2004): 91-96.

Prlic, H. M., et al. "Agreement Among Ayurvedic Practitioners in the Identification and Treatment of Three Cases of Inflammatory Arthritis." *Clinical and Experimental Rheumatology* 21 (2003): 747-752.

Rangineni V, Sharada D, Saxena S. "Diuretic, Hypotensive, and Hypocholesterolemic Effects of *Eclipta alba* in Mild Hypertensive Subjects." *Journal of Medicinal Food* 10 (2007): 143-148.

Roodenrys, S., et al. "Chronic Effects of Brahmi (*Bacopa monnieri*) on Human Memory." *Neuropsychopharmacology* 27 (2002): 279-281.

Saper, R. B., et al. "Lead, Mercury, and Arsenic in U.S.- and Indian-Manufactured Ayurvedic Medicines Sold via the Internet." *Journal of the American Medical Association* 300 (2008): 915-923.

See also: Alternative versus traditional medicine; Chinese medicine; Folk medicine; Herbal medicine; Home health; Naturopathy; Traditional Chinese herbal medicine; Traditional healing.

B

Bach flower remedies

CATEGORY: Therapies and techniques
RELATED TERM: Rescue Remedy
DEFINITION: A treatment that uses flower extracts.
PRINCIPAL PROPOSED USES: Anxiety, grief, shyness, stress
OTHER PROPOSED USE: Attention deficit disorder

OVERVIEW

In the early part of the twentieth century, a British physician named Edward Bach developed a system of healing based on flowers. Numerous additional remedies were added to the original repertory proposed by Bach, and this form of treatment is widely used today.

MECHANISM OF ACTION

Each of these Bach flower remedies was created by dipping a particular type of flower in water and then preserving the fragrant liquid with brandy. Bach flower remedies are sometimes compared to homeopathy, but they differ because they do not use extreme dilutions.

USES AND APPLICATIONS

According to Bach, the appropriately chosen flower could be used to treat emotional problems, such as shyness, anxiety, and grief.

SCIENTIFIC EVIDENCE

There is no scientific evidence that any Bach flower remedy produces a medicinal effect, and there is some evidence that the method does not work. In 2001, a double-blind, placebo-controlled study tested whether a particular combination of Bach flower remedies could relieve the anxiety that students experience while taking exams. The trial used a mixture containing ten flower extracts: impatiens, mimulus, gentian, chestnut bud, rock rose, larch, cherry plum, white chestnut, scleranthus, and elm. (An expert in the use of Bach flower remedies suggested this partic-ular combination.) Sixty-one students were enrolled in the study; fifty-five completed it. Each participant received either the Bach flower remedy or placebo for two weeks leading up to an exam. Participants answered a questionnaire to assess their anxiety levels before starting treatment and just before the test. The use of Bach flower remedies did not measurably reduce anxiety levels compared with placebo.

A previous study also evaluated the use of a Bach flower remedy (Rescue Remedy) for treating test anxiety and found no benefit. However, more than 50 percent of the participants dropped out, making the results of that trial unreliable. Another study of Rescue Remedy for situational anxiety also failed to find that it was more effective than placebo. However, after the study was concluded, researchers then explored the data and found a relative benefit in one subgroup of participants. This may appear to support the use of Rescue Remedy. However, such "post-hoc" statistical analyses are notoriously unreliable: Based on the laws of chance alone, it is almost always possible to find some subgroup that showed benefit in a study. The process of doing this is called data dredging. Such investigatory analyses of data can provide fodder for future studies, but they make no positive statement about the results of a study already conducted. Researchers must state in advance what measurement they plan to look at (the primary outcome measure) and base their conclusion on the results of that measurement. From that perspective, this was a negative trial.

Finally, a double-blind study reported in 2005 failed to find Bach flower remedies more effective than placebo for the treatment of attention deficit disorder.

SAFETY ISSUES

At the very least, Bach flower remedies should be harmless because they are sufficiently diluted to minimize the presence of any active ingredients.

EBSCO CAM Review Board

FURTHER READING

Armstrong, N. C., and E. Ernst. "A Randomized, Double-Blind Placebo-Controlled Trial of a Bach Flower Remedy." *Complementary Therapies in Nursing and Midwifery* 7 (2001): 215-221.

Halberstein, R. A., A. Sirkin, and M. M. Ojeda-Vaz. "When Less Is Better: A Comparison of Bach Flower Remedies and Homeopathy." *Annals of Epidemiology* 20 (2010): 298-307.

Pintov, S., et al. "Bach Flower Remedies Used for Attention Deficit Hyperactivity Disorder in Children." *European Journal of Paediatric Neurology* 9 (2005): 395-398.

Rilling, and U. Engelke. "Efficacy of Bach-Flower Remedies in Test Anxiety." *Journal of Anxiety Disorders* 15 (2001): 359-366.

Thaler, K., et al. "Bach Flower Remedies for Psychological Problems and Pain." *BMC Complementary and Alternative Medicine* 9 (2009): 16.

See also: Anxiety and panic attacks; Attention deficit disorder; Homeopathy; Mental health; Stress.

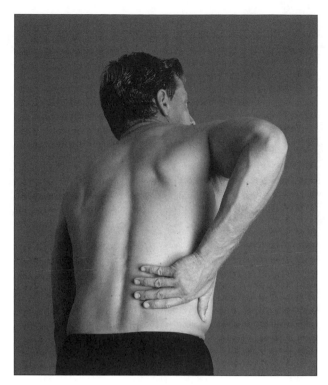

A man suffering from pain in his lower back. (Richard Luria/Photo Researchers, Inc.)

Back pain

CATEGORY: Condition

RELATED TERMS: Acute back pain, backache, back sprain, back strain, chronic back pain, lower back pain

DEFINITION: Treatment of acute and chronic pain of the back.

PRINCIPAL PROPOSED NATURAL TREATMENTS: Acupuncture, chiropractic, white willow

OTHER PROPOSED NATURAL TREATMENTS: Balneotherapy (spa therapy), boswellia, butterbur, chondroitin, comfrey (topical cream), devil's claw, ginger, glucosamine, magnet therapy, osteopathic manipulation, prolotherapy, proteolytic enzymes, relaxation therapies, turmeric, yoga

INTRODUCTION

Low back pain is one of the most common health conditions today. According to some estimates, each year nearly 15 to 20 percent of the population of the United States experiences low back problems, and as many as 80 percent of all adults experience significant low back pain at some point during their lives. Back pain is the second most common reason why adults age forty-five years and younger miss days from work (after the common cold). The cost of back pain has been estimated to reach $25 billion per year in the United States.

When back pain occurs suddenly (after lifting a heavy object, for example), it is called acute back pain or sprain. In most cases, acute back pain eventually improves by itself, but there may be weeks of discomfort, time lost from work, and impaired function at home.

When back pain persists over months or years, it is called chronic back pain. In the majority of cases, the cause of chronic back pain is unknown. Identifiable causes include osteoarthritis, fracture, or injury to the discs between the vertebrae.

Conventional treatment of acute back pain involves anti-inflammatory drugs, muscle relaxants, and the passage of time. Chronic back pain requires a medical examination to make sure there are no serious underlying causes. Evidence suggests that, in most cases, X rays are not necessary.

Treatment may also include physical therapy and a graded exercise program. However, there is little reliable evidence that these treatments actually provide much benefit. Surgery may be recommended in certain cases, such as when there are severe disc problems, but most forms of back surgery also lack reliable supporting evidence.

PRINCIPAL PROPOSED NATURAL TREATMENTS

Extract of the herb white willow appears to be helpful for acute and chronic back pain, presumably because of its similarity to aspirin. The little-known injection technique known as prolotherapy also may be effective for back pain. Lesser evidence supports the use of chiropractic and acupuncture.

White willow. Willow bark, which has been used as a treatment for pain and fever in China since 500 B.C.E., contains the substance salicin, which is chemically related to aspirin. Another ingredient of white willow, tremulacin, may also be important.

In a four-week, double-blind, placebo-controlled study of 210 persons with chronic back pain, two different doses of willow bark extract were compared with placebo. The higher-dose group received extract supplying 240 milligrams (mg) of salicin daily; in this group, 39 percent were pain-free for at least the last five days of the study. In the lower-dose group (120 mg of salicin daily), 21 percent became pain-free. In contrast, only 6 percent of those given placebo became pain-free. Stomach distress did not occur in this study. The only significant side effect seen was an allergic reaction in one participant given willow. White willow should not be combined with standard anti-inflammatory drugs, such as ibuprofen.

Chiropractic. Chiropractic spinal manipulation is one of the most popular treatments for acute and chronic back pain in the United States, and it may provide at least modest benefit; however, research evidence has failed to find chiropractic manipulation convincingly more effective than standard medical care.

Chiropractic does seem to be more effective than placebo, if not by a great deal. For example, a single-blind controlled study of eighty-four people with low back pain compared manipulation to treatment with a diathermy machine (a physical therapy machine that uses microwaves to create heat beneath the skin) that was not actually functioning. The researchers asked the participants to assess their own pain levels within fifteen minutes of the first treatment, then three and seven days after treatment. The only statistically significant difference between the two groups was within fifteen minutes of the manipulation. (Chiropractic had better results at that point.)

In another single-blind, placebo-controlled study, researchers assigned 209 persons to one of three groups: a high-velocity, low-amplitude spinal manipulation group; a sham manipulation group; or a back education-program group. Though this has been reported as a positive study, most of the differences seen between the groups were too small to be statistically significant.

Unimpressive results were also seen in a well-designed study of 321 people with back pain, comparing chiropractic manipulation, a special form of physical therapy (the Mackenzie method), and the provision of an educational booklet on treating low back pain. All groups improved to about the same extent. Several studies evaluated the effectiveness of chiropractic manipulation combined with a different kind of treatment called mobilization, but these studies too found little to no benefit.

On a positive note, one study of one hundred people with back pain and sciatica symptoms (pain down the leg caused by disc protrusion) found that chiropractic manipulation was significantly more effective at relieving symptoms than was sham chiropractic manipulation.

For low back pain, several studies have found that chiropractic is at least as helpful as other commonly used therapies, such as muscle relaxants, soft-tissue massage, and physical therapy. Furthermore, in one well-designed study, two months of chiropractic spinal manipulation produced somewhat greater pain relief than exercise therapy, and this relative superiority endured to the one-year follow-up point.

Acupuncture. The ancient technique of acupuncture has become increasingly popular as a treatment for pain and other conditions. However, research has not produced clear evidence of acupuncture's effectiveness for back pain. In a review of twenty-three randomized trials involving more than six thousand persons with chronic low back pain, researchers concluded that acupuncture is more effective than no treatment for short-term pain relief, but there was no significant difference between the effects of genuine treatment and sham treatment.

A six-month double-blind trial of 1,162 people with

back pain compared real acupuncture, fake acupuncture, and conventional therapy. Both real and fake acupuncture were twice as effective as conventional therapy, according to the measures used. However, there was only a minimal difference between real and fake acupuncture. This result does not indicate that acupuncture is effective per se; rather, it shows the significant power of acupuncture as a placebo.

Similarly, in a single-blind, sham-acupuncture, and no-treatment controlled study of 298 people with chronic back pain, the use of real acupuncture failed to prove significantly more effective than sham acupuncture. Also, in a fairly large randomized trial involving 638 adults with chronic back pain, there was no difference in pain at one year in persons receiving real versus fake acupuncture (with neither group improving significantly over standard care). Both real and simulated acupuncture were, however, associated with improved function at one year. Other studies have failed to find benefit; in several controlled studies enrolling more than three hundred people, real acupuncture again failed to prove more effective than sham acupuncture or other placebo treatments.

One study compared the effects of acupuncture, massage, and education (such as videotapes on back care) for 262 people with chronic back pain over a ten-week period. The exact type of acupuncture and massage was left to practitioners, but only ten visits were permitted. At the ten-week point, evaluations showed benefit with massage but not with acupuncture. One year later, massage and education were nearly equivalent, and both were superior to acupuncture.

Low level laser therapy (LLLT) is a technique similar to electro-acupuncture that uses precision laser energy instead of electricity conducted through a needle. In a detailed review of seven randomized trials, researchers were unable to draw any conclusions regarding the effectiveness of LLLT for nonspecific low back pain.

Many other studies have compared acupuncture to such treatments as transcutaneous electrical nerve stimulation (TENS), physical therapy, chiropractic care, and massage. In many of these trials, acupuncture provided benefits comparable to the other options tested. However, because TENS, physical therapy, and so forth have not been proven effective for back pain, studies of this type cannot be taken as evidence that acupuncture is effective. One study did find acupressure massage more effective than standard physical therapy; however, it was performed in a Chinese population that may have had more faith in this traditional approach than in physical therapy.

OTHER PROPOSED NATURAL TREATMENTS

Herbal treatments. In a double-blind, placebo-controlled study enrolling 215 people with back pain, the use of a topical cream made from the herb comfrey produced statistically significant benefits compared with placebo. The herb devil's claw, which is used for the treatment of osteoarthritis, has been tried for back pain too. However, the results have been less than impressive. A double-blind, placebo-controlled study of 197 persons with chronic back pain found devil's claw only marginally effective at best. Similarly poor results were seen in an earlier four-week, double-blind, placebo-controlled study of 118 persons with acute back pain. However, a four-week, double-blind, placebo-controlled study of 63 people with mild to moderate chronic muscular tension in the neck, back, and shoulders did find some benefit.

The herb cayenne contains capsaicin, a substance that produces an immediate burning sensation but later reduces pain. One double-blind study found a topical cayenne treatment more effective than placebo in 320 people with low back pain. However, upon closer inspection, one finds it difficult to believe that this study was truly double-blind. When cayenne is applied to the skin, it causes such an intense sensation that participants would hardly fail to notice it. When people in a study know whether they are getting real treatment or placebo treatment, the validity of the study's results is greatly decreased.

Other herbs and supplements sometimes recommended for back pain, but with no real supporting evidence, include boswellia, butterbur, chondroitin, ginger, glucosamine, and turmeric.

Manual therapies. Osteopathic manipulation (OM) is a form of treatment related to chiropractic manipulation, but it tends to use gentle, extended movements (low velocity, high amplitude) rather than the quick, short, cracking movements of chiropractic. Although OM has shown some promise for the treatment of back pain, one of the best-designed trials failed to find it a superior alternative to conventional medical care. In this twelve-week study of 178 persons, osteopathic manipulation proved no more effective than standard treatment for back pain. Another study failed to find OM more effective than sham manipulation.

In a review of thirteen randomized trials, researchers concluded that massage may be effective for nonspecific low back pain, and the beneficial effects can last for up to one year in persons with chronic pain. The researchers also noted that exercise and education appear to enhance the effectiveness of massage.

The Alexander technique (AT) is a special method of postural training popular among dancers and other performers. A review of the literature found no more than weak preliminary evidence that AT may help with back pain, but it concluded that further research is warranted. A subsequent controlled trial involving 579 persons with chronic or recurrent low back pain found that AT lessons, particularly when combined with exercise, were more effective than normal care or massage after one year.

Prolotherapy. The use of prolotherapy to treat back pain has had mixed results in clinical studies.

Invented in the 1950s by George Hackett, prolotherapy is based on the theory that chronic pain is often caused by laxness of the ligaments that are responsible for keeping a joint stable. When ligaments and associated tendons are loose, the body is said to compensate by using muscles to hold the joint stable. The net result, according to prolotherapy theory, is muscle spasms and pain.

Prolotherapy treatment involves injections of chemical irritant solutions into the area around such ligaments. These solutions are believed to cause tissue to proliferate (grow), increasing the strength and thickness of ligaments. This presumably serves to tighten up the joint and allow the associated muscles to stop having spasms. In the case of arthritic joints, increased ligament strength would allow the joint to function more efficiently, reducing pain.

Although two studies have suggested prolotherapy may be effective, two more recent studies found prolotherapy to be ineffective. In a review of five studies, three found prolotherapy to be no more effective than control treatments for treating low back pain. The other two studies suggested that prolotherapy was more effective than control treatments when used with therapies such as spinal manipulation and exercise. Another review suggested prolotherapy may be effective when used with other therapies, but not when used alone.

What can one make of this contradictory evidence? When used alone, prolotherapy is probably no more effective than a placebo injection for the treatment of chronic low back pain. However, there is some evidence that the technique may be beneficial when combined with other therapies.

Other therapies. Biofeedback, balneotherapy, hatha yoga, magnet therapy, and relaxation therapies have also shown some promise for treating back pain. Though for some of these, there have been as many negative as positive studies, and for many of them only short-term benefits were shown.

In one study, 444 people with acute low back pain were randomly assigned to receive either usual care or usual care plus a choice of alternative therapies (chiropractic, acupuncture, or massage). The results showed that while the use of alternative therapies improved patient satisfaction, it did not significantly improve symptoms. Finally, preliminary evidence suggests that proteolytic enzymes might be helpful for back pain.

HERBS AND SUPPLEMENTS TO USE ONLY WITH CAUTION

Various herbs and supplements may interact adversely with drugs used to treat back pain, so persons should be cautious when considering the use of herbs and supplements.

EBSCO CAM Review Board

FURTHER READING

Andersson, G. B., et al. "A Comparison of Osteopathic Spinal Manipulation with Standard Care for Patients with Low Back Pain." *New England Journal of Medicine* 341 (1999): 1426-1431.

Assendelft, W. J. J., et al. "Spinal Manipulative Therapy for Low Back Pain: A Meta-analysis of Effectiveness Relative to Other Therapies." *Annals of Internal Medicine* 138 (2003): 871-881.

Aure, O. F., et al. "Manual Therapy and Exercise Therapy in Patients with Chronic Low Back Pain." *Spine* 28 (2003): 525-531.

Brinkhaus, B., et al. "Acupuncture in Patients with Chronic Low Back Pain." *Archives of Internal Medicine* 166 (2006): 450-457.

Cherkin, D. C., Sherman, K. J., et al. "A Randomized Trial Comparing Acupuncture, Simulated Acupuncture, and Usual Care for Chronic Low Back Pain." *Archives of Internal Medicine* 169 (2009): 858-866.

Dagenais, S., et al. "Evidence-Informed Management

of Chronic Low Back Pain with Prolotherapy." *Spine Journal* 8 (2008): 203-212.

Frerick, H., W. Keitel, and U. Kuhn. "Topical Treatment of Chronic Low Back Pain with a Capsicum Plaster." *Pain* 106 (2003): 59-64.

Furlan, A. D., et al. "Massage for Low-Back Pain." *Cochrane Database of Systematic Reviews* (2008): CD001929. Available through *EBSCO DynaMed Systematic Literature Surveillance* at http://www.ebsco-host.com/dynamed.

Hayden, J. A., et al. "Exercise Therapy for Treatment of Non-specific Low Back Pain." *Cochrane Database of Systematic Reviews* (2005): CD000335. Available through *EBSCO DynaMed Systematic Literature Surveillance* at http://www.ebscohost.com/dynamed.

Hoiriis, K. T., et al. "A Randomized Clinical Trial Comparing Chiropractic Adjustments to Muscle Relaxants for Subacute Low Back Pain." *Journal of Manipulative and Physiological Therapeutics* 27 (2004): 388-398.

Hsieh, L. L., et al. "Treatment of Low Back Pain by Acupressure and Physical Therapy." *British Medical Journal* 332 (2006): 696-700.

Kucera, M., et al. "Topical Symphytum Herb Concentrate Cream Against Myalgia." *Advances in Therapy* 22 (2005): 681-692.

Little, P., et al. "Randomised Controlled Trial of Alexander Technique Lessons, Exercise, and Massage (ATEAM) for Chronic and Recurrent Back Pain." *British Medical Journal* 337 (2008): 884.

Morone, N. E., C. M. Greco, and D. K. Weiner. "Mindfulness Meditation for the Treatment of Chronic Low Back Pain in Older Adults." *Pain* 134 (2007): 310-319.

Pittler, M. H., et al. "Spa Therapy and Balneotherapy for Treating Low Back Pain." *Rheumatology* (Oxford) 45 (2006): 880-884.

Tekur, P., et al. "Effect of Short-Term Intensive Yoga Program on Pain, Functional Disability, and Spinal Flexibility in Chronic Low Back Pain." *Journal of Alternative and Complementary Medicine* 14 (2008): 637-644.

Wilkey, A., et al. "A Comparison Between Chiropractic Management and Pain Clinic Management for Chronic Low-Back Pain in a National Health Service Outpatient Clinic." *Journal of Alternative and Complementary Medicine* 14 (2008): 465-473.

Yuan, J., et al. "Effectiveness of Acupuncture for Low Back Pain." *Spine* 33 (2008): 887-900.

See also: Acupressure; Acupuncture; Balenotherapy; Bone and joint health; Chiropractic; Fibromyalgia: Homeopathic remedies; Massage therapy; Neck pain; Osteopathic manipulation; Pain management; Progressive muscle relaxation; Prolotherapy; Rolfing; Shiatsu; Soft tissue pain; Therapeutic touch; White willow.

Balneotherapy

CATEGORY: Therapies and techniques
RELATED TERMS: Bath therapy, hot springs immersion, hydrotherapy, spa therapy
DEFINITION: Treatment using hot and cold baths, saunas, mud packs, and other therapies.
PRINCIPAL PROPOSED USES: Arthritis (rheumatoid arthritis, osteoarthritis, and ankylosing spondylitis), low back pain
OTHER PROPOSED USES: Eczema, fibromyalgia, Parkinson's disease, psoriasis, varicose veins

OVERVIEW

The use of hot and cold baths for treating illnesses goes back to the dawn of civilization. In later centuries, the use of hot springs and water in other forms was popularized by early practitioners of what later would become naturopathy. From these practices developed a formal system of medicine known as hydropathy. Today, mud packs, saunas, and steam baths are often included along with water baths under the general name of "balneotherapy."

Certain types of water are often particularly prized by practitioners of balneotherapy. These include sulfur springs and the concentrated salty water of drying lake beds, such as the Dead Sea (in Israel). Hot springs that are high in the radioactive substance radon are also said by some proponents to possess particular healing properties.

SCIENTIFIC EVIDENCE

Although various forms of balneotherapy have undergone some scientific study, none of this evidence is reliable. There are many causes of the inadequacies in the research record, but one is intrinsic and probably not correctable. This is the problem of blinding.

For the results of a study to be reliable, participants and researchers must be kept in the dark ("blind") regarding who received the treatment under study (the active group) and who received a placebo treatment (the control group). If practitioners and researchers know who is in which group, numerous confounding factors take over and produce misleading results. These factors include observer bias, reporting bias, and the placebo effect. To briefly summarize this complex issue, one could say that unblinded studies usually mean little to nothing.

It is difficult, though, to keep study participants from knowing they have taken a hot bath. Some researchers have used ordinary tap water as a comparison with special mineral water. If, as was the case in some studies, the active treatment smelled of sulfur or (as in other studies) it was so dense with minerals that it made the skin tingle and the body float high in the water, participants would have been able to determine what group they were in. This would effectively destroy blinding and would fundamentally compromise the study results. Given these caveats, there is some evidence that balneotherapy of various kinds might be helpful for conditions such as ankylosing spondylitis, fibromyalgia, low back pain, osteoarthritis, psoriasis, rheumatoid arthritis, and varicose veins. Balneotherapy is also said to be helpful for eczema, Parkinson's disease, and numerous other conditions, but for these conditions the therapy lacks even unreliable supporting evidence. If indeed it does work, balneotherapy could act both locally (on muscles, joints, and skin) through the effects of heat, and systemically, through absorption of substances, such as sulfur through the skin.

SAFETY ISSUES

Excessive immersion in hot baths can be dangerous for pregnant women, young children, those with a heart condition or other serious medical illness, and people under the influence of alcohol or other intoxicating substances. There are concerns also that hot springs high in radon might present a cancer risk, though this has not been proven.

EBSCO CAM Review Board

FURTHER READING

Carpentier, P. H., and B. Satger. "Randomized Trial of Balneotherapy Associated with Patient Education in Patients with Advanced Chronic Venous Insufficiency." *Journal of Vascular Surgery* 49 (2009): 163-170.

Codish, S., et al. "Mud Compress Therapy for the Hands of Patients with Rheumatoid Arthritis." *Rheumatology International* 25 (2005): 49-54.

Cozzi, F., et al. "Mud-Bath Treatment in Spondylitis Associated with Inflammatory Bowel Disease." *Joint, Bone, Spine* 74 (2007): 436-439.

Dawe, R. S., et al. "A Randomized Controlled Comparison of the Efficacy of Dead Sea Salt Balneophototherapy vs. Narrowband Ultraviolet B Monotherapy for Chronic Plaque Psoriasis." *British Journal of Dermatology* 153 (2005): 613-619

McVeigh, J. G., et al. "The Effectiveness of Hydrotherapy in the Management of Fibromyalgia Syndrome." *Rheumatology International* 29 (2008): 119-130.

Pittler, M. H., et al. "Spa Therapy and Balneotherapy for Treating Low Back Pain." *Rheumatology* 45 (2006): 880-884.

Yurtkuran, M., et al. "Balneotherapy and Tap Water Therapy in the Treatment of Knee Osteoarthritis." *Rheumatology International* 27 (2006): 19-27.

See also: Back pain; Fibromyalgia: Homeopathic remedies; Hydrotherapy; Osteoarthritis; Pain management; Rheumatoid arthritis.

Barberry

CATEGORY: Herbs and supplements
RELATED TERM: *Berberis vulgaris*
DEFINITION: Natural plant product used to treat specific health conditions.
PRINCIPAL PROPOSED USES: None
OTHER PROPOSED USES: Allergies, constipation, diarrhea, dyspepsia, eczema, heartburn, high blood pressure, high cholesterol, psoriasis, minor wounds

OVERVIEW

Barberry (*Berberis vulgaris*) is a bush that grows wild in Europe and North America. It is closely related to Oregon grape (*B. aquifolium*). The root, stem, bark, and fruit of barberry are all used medicinally. Barberry was traditionally used as a treatment for digestive problems, including constipation, diarrhea, dyspepsia (stomach upset), heartburn, and loss of appetite. It was said to work by increasing the flow of bile, and on this basis it has also been used for liver and gallbladder problems. Topical preparations of

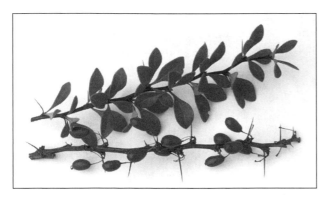

Fruit and leaves of the barberry plant. (TH Foto-Werbung/ Photo Researchers, Inc.)

barberry have been recommended for the treatment of eczema, psoriasis, and minor wounds.

THERAPEUTIC DOSAGES

Barberry is traditionally used at a dose of 2 grams three times daily, or an equivalent amount in extract form. For treatment of psoriasis and other skin conditions, barberry is used in the form of a 10 percent cream, applied to the skin three times daily.

THERAPEUTIC USES

Berberine inhibits the growth of many microorganisms, including fungi, protozoa, and bacteria. In one placebo-controlled study, berberine effectively reduced lung injury among persons with lung cancer receiving radiation therapy.

Berberine has been proposed as topical antiseptic for use in minor wounds and vaginal infections. Berberine has also shown potential as a treatment for various heart-related conditions, including high cholesterol and high blood pressure, and for preventing heart arrythmias. However, it is not clear that barberry provides enough berberine to produce any of these potential benefits.

Topical formulations of the related plant Oregon grape have shown some promise for psoriasis, and barberry also has been marketed for this condition. However, there is no direct evidence that it works.

SCIENTIFIC EVIDENCE

There are no medically established uses of barberry. Only double-blind, placebo-controlled studies can establish a treatment to be effective, and none have been performed on barberry. Weak evidence, too weak to be relied upon, hints that barberry root extracts may have anti-inflammatory, fever-reducing, and analgesic (pain-reducing) effects. Similarly weak evidence hints that barberry fruit may have antihypertensive and antihistaminic effects.

Barberry, like goldenseal and Oregon grape, contains the chemical berberine. There have been some studies of purified berberine that might also apply to barberry.

SAFETY ISSUES

One study suggests that topical use of berberine could cause photosensitivity, an increased tendency to react to sun exposure. Berberine-containing herbs should not be used by pregnant women because berberine may increase levels of bilirubin, potentially damaging the fetus, and might also cause genetic damage. Persons who already have elevated levels of bilirubin (jaundice) or any other form of liver disease should also avoid berberine-containing herbs.

Safety in young children and nursing women has not been established. One study hints that berberine may decrease the efficacy of the drug tetracycline.

EBSCO CAM Review Board

FURTHER READING

Bae, E. A., et al. "Anti-*Helicobacter pylori* Activity of Herbal Medicines." *Biological and Pharmaceutical Bulletin* 21 (1998): 990-992.

Doggrell, S. A. "Berberine: A Novel Approach to Cholesterol Lowering." *Expert Opinion on Investigational Drugs* 14 (2005): 683-685.

Inbaraj, J. J., et al. "Photochemistry and Photocytotoxicity of Alkaloids from Goldenseal (*Hydrastis canadensis* L.) Berberine." *Chemical Research in Toxicology* 14 (2001): 1529-1534.

Kong, W., et al. "Berberine Is a Novel Cholesterol-Lowering Drug Working Through a Unique Mechanism Distinct from Statins." *Nature Medicine* 10 (2004): 1344-1351.

Kupeli, E., et al. "A Comparative Study on the Anti-inflammatory, Antinociceptive and Antipyretic Effects of Isoquinoline Alkaloids from the Roots of Turkish *Berberis* Species." *Life Sciences* 72 (2002): 645-657.

Lau, C. W., et al. "Cardiovascular Actions of Berberine." *Cardiovascular Drug Reviews* 19 (2001): 234-244.

See also: Goldenseal; Herbal medicine; Oregon grape.

Barrett, Stephen

CATEGORY: Biography
IDENTIFICATION: American psychiatrist, writer, and health fraud activist
BORN: September 6, 1933; New York, New York

OVERVIEW

Stephen Barrett, a retired American psychiatrist and writer, cofounded the National Council Against Health Fraud, a nonprofit organization that investigates and reports on health misinformation, fraud, and quackery (that is, fraudulent medical practices). By his own definition, "quackery" refers to "anything involving overpromotion in the field of health." He claims to reserve the word "fraud" only for deliberate deception. Barrett also is the founder of Quackwatch, a Web-based network covering health fraud and related issues. Because he is a leading voice in questioning complementary and alternative medical practices, such as chiropractic, acupuncture, and herbal medicine, he has gained much media attention.

The mission of NCAHF is, in part, to protect consumers from fraudulent health-related practices and products, promote medical ethics, and explore scientific skepticism. Barrett has argued that alternative practices should be further classified as either questionable, experimental, or genuine, based on existing scientific evidence. He is a vocal proponent of the "HON-code," a code of conduct developed by the nonprofit Health on the Net Foundation to improve the reliability and clarity of medical information on the Web.

Barrett received his medical degree from Columbia University College of Physicians and Surgeons in 1957, and he completed his psychiatry residency in 1961. He was a practicing physician in Allentown, Pennsylvania, until his retirement in 1993. Barrett has received numerous awards for his work in consumer protection in medicine. In 1984, he received a special award for public service from the U.S. Food and Drug Administration recognizing his contribution to combating quackery in nutrition. In addition, he was profiled in *Time* magazine in 2001. The site Quackwatch also has received various honors.

Barrett is a consulting editor for the Prometheus Books series Consumer Health Library, a peer reviewer for various medical journals, an adviser to the American Council on Science and Health, and a Fellow of the Committee for Skeptical Inquiry. He has reportedly authored more than two thousand articles and delivered more than three hundred lectures and talks.

Brandy Weidow, M.S.

FURTHER READING

Barrett, Steven, et al. *Consumer Health: A Guide to Intelligent Decisions.* 8th ed. Columbus, Ohio: McGraw-Hill, 2006.

_____. "Stephen Barrett, M.D." Interview by Marjorie Rosen. *Biography*, October, 1998. Also available at http://www.quackwatch.org/10Bio/biography.html.

Jaroff, Leon. "The Man Who Loves to Bust Quacks." *Time*, April 30, 2001. Also available at http://www.time.com/time/magazine/article/0,9171,1101010430-107254,00.html.

See also: Clinical trials; Dawkins, Richard; Internet and CAM, The; Pseudoscience; Regulation of CAM; Sampson, Wallace; Scientific method.

Bates method

CATEGORY: Therapies and techniques
RELATED TERMS: Iridology, natural vision, pinhole glasses
DEFINITION: The improvement of vision using eye exercises.
PRINCIPAL PROPOSED USES: Astigmatism, hyperopia, myopia, presbyopia
OTHER PROPOSED USES: Amblyopia, glaucoma, strabismus

OVERVIEW

In the early twentieth century, ophthalmologist William H. Bates proposed an alternative method for improving eyesight. Through his work, he concluded that most vision problems were caused by habitual tension and strain of the eyes.

MECHANISM OF ACTION

Bates claimed that the eyeball changes shape to maintain focus. He maintained that relaxation of the eye muscles using basic exercises removed the habitual tension that caused poor eyesight and helped preserve the correct shape of the eyeball.

Perfect Sight Without Glasses: The Fundamental Principle

In his book Perfect Sight Without Glasses *(1920), ophthalmologist William H. Bates outlines the basic premise of his method.*

Do you read imperfectly? Can you observe then that when you look at the first word, or the first letter, of a sentence you do not see best where you are looking; that you see other words, or other letters, just as well as or better than the one you are looking at? Do you observe also that the harder you try to see the worse you see?

Now close your eyes and rest them, remembering some color, like black or white, that you can remember perfectly. Keep them closed until they feel rested, or until the feeling of strain has been completely relieved. Now open them and look at the first word or letter of a sentence for a fraction of a second. If you have been able to relax, partially or completely, you will have a flash of improved or clear vision, and the area seen best will be smaller.

After opening the eyes for this fraction of a second, close them again quickly, still remembering the color, and keep them closed until they again feel rested. Then again open them for a fraction of a second. Continue this alternate resting of the eyes and flashing of the letters for a time, and you may soon find that you can keep your eyes open longer than a fraction of a second without losing the improved vision.

If your trouble is with distant instead of near vision, use the same method with distant letters. In this way you can demonstrate for yourself the fundamental principle of the cure of imperfect sight by treatment without glasses. If you fail, ask someone with perfect sight to help you.

USES AND APPLICATIONS

Proponents of the Bates method claim that proper use of the method can help to eliminate conditions, such as nearsightedness, farsightedness, and astigmatism, for which corrective lenses are normally prescribed. More serious conditions of the eye, such as cataracts and glaucoma, have been improved by employing the Bates method.

SCIENTIFIC EVIDENCE

In his writings, Bates discusses several techniques of visual training that can help improve eyesight. He claims that covering the eyes gently with the palms of the hands (palming), forming mental images (visualization), moving the eyes back and forth rapidly while closed (shifting or swinging), and exposure of the eyes to sunlight (sunning) are the basic exercises necessary for maintaining good vision and correcting poor vision. It was later decided that sunning must be done with the eyelids closed.

In 1942, British writer Aldous Huxley reported that although his vision was far from normal, it had been improved by using the Bates method. In 1983, a randomized controlled trial using the Bates method with myopic children in India over a period of six months did not yield any significant improvement of vision, although eye strain was relieved in many of the children.

Bates's main physiological proposition, that the eyeball changes shape to maintain focus, has been contradicted by numerous laboratory tests. In 2004, the American Academy of Ophthalmology published its review of research involving the Bates method of visual training and found no evidence that such techniques objectively benefit eyesight. In some of the investigated cases, the visual acuity of nearsighted persons was affected, but it was affected both positively and negatively. Based on further research, this change in nearsightedness is not caused by any change in refractive error, but is best explained by the improvement in interpreting blurred images and by the contact-lens effect, which is produced by changing amounts of moisture in the eye because of increased tear action.

SAFETY ISSUES

As long as one does not expose his or her eyes directly to sunlight, the exercises making up the Bates method are generally safe. In some cases, application of the Bates method may keep persons from seeking needed medical advice for sight-threatening conditions, such as glaucoma or "lazy eye" (amblyopia and strabismus) in children, that need prompt treatment. Discarding corrective lenses, or wearing weaker lenses than those prescribed, poses safety hazards during the operation of motor vehicles and heavy equipment.

Alvin K. Benson, Ph.D.

FURTHER READING

Association of Vision Educators. http://www.vision-educators.org.

Bates, William H. *The Bates Method for Better Eyesight Without Glasses*. Reprint. London: Thorsons, 2000.

Carrington, Hereward. *Your Eyesight: An Outline of the Bates Method of Treatment Without Glasses*. Whitefish, Mont.: Kessinger, 2010.

Kaufman, Paul L., and Albert Alm. *Adler's Physiology of the Eye: Clinical Application*. 10th ed. St. Louis, Mo.: Mosby, 2003.

"Natural Vision Correction: Does It Work?" http://www.webmd.com/eyehealth/featuresnatural-vision-correction-does-it-work.

Quackenbush, Thomas R. *Relearning to See: Improve Your Eyesight, Naturally!* Berkeley, Calif.: North Atlantic Books, 2000.

See also: Iridology; Night vision, impaired.

Beano

CATEGORY: Herbs and supplements
RELATED TERMS: Alpha-galactosidase, *Aspergillus niger*
DEFINITION: Natural substance used as a dietary supplement for specific health benefits.
PRINCIPAL PROPOSED USE: Intestinal gas

OVERVIEW

Many foods, including beans (legumes), broccoli, cabbage, onions, and whole grains, can cause gassiness. This occurs because these foods contain complex carbohydrates that are not entirely broken down in the digestive tract; instead, they serve as food for intestinal bacteria. These bacteria produce hydrogen and carbon dioxide gas as they digest the carbohydrates. While everyone develops intestinal gas to some extent, certain people have an intolerance of complex carbohydrates and develop relatively more severe symptoms.

The use of alpha-galactosidase (trade name Beano) has been advocated as a treatment for both complex carbohydrate intolerance and ordinary gassiness. This enzyme helps break down complex carbohydrates. When taken as a supplement, it may enhance the digestive process and thereby deprive gas-producing bacteria of fuel to work on.

REQUIREMENTS AND SOURCES

Alpha-galactosidase is ordinarily manufactured by the body and is not a nutrient. It is found in particularly high quantities in the yeast *Aspergillus niger*, the source of commercial products that treat intestinal gas.

THERAPEUTIC DOSAGES

A typical supplemental dosage of alpha-galactosidase provides 450 GalU (galactosidase units) per meal.

THERAPEUTIC USES

Although alpha-galactosidase is widely marketed as an over-the-counter treatment to prevent intestinal gas, there is only limited evidence that it really works. In two preliminary double-blind, controlled trials enrolling thirty-nine people, the use of alpha-galactosidase along with a meal of beans significantly reduced symptoms of excess gas. Two other relevant trials were also small, and they had significant design flaws. Larger and more strictly designed studies are necessary to determine whether alpha-galactosidase is truly an effective treatment for reducing intestinal gas.

SAFETY ISSUES

Although alpha-galactosidase appears to be safe for people in normal health, there are potential concerns involving persons with diabetes or with a rare genetic condition called galactosemia. Alpha-galactosidase breaks down complex carbohydrates into easily absorbed sugars. This may raise blood sugar levels in people with diabetes. Drugs that block alpha-galactosidase (alpha-galactosidase inhibitors) have proven benefit for people with diabetes. One study found that the use of alpha-galactosidase supplements reduced the effectiveness of the diabetes drug acarbose, an alpha-galactosidase inhibitor. For this reason, people with diabetes who are using alpha-galactosidase inhibitors should avoid alpha-galactosidase supplements. In addition, it is theoretically possible that alpha-galactosidase might increase blood sugar levels in people with diabetes who are not taking alpha-galactosidase inhibitors, but this has not been thoroughly evaluated.

People with galactosemia should also avoid alpha-galactosidase, as it could, in theory, worsen symptoms of the disease. Finally, the safety of alpha-galactosidase in young children, pregnant or nursing women, and people with severe liver or kidney disease has not been established.

IMPORTANT INTERACTIONS

Alpha-galactosidase may decrease the effectiveness of the drugs acarbose (Precose) and miglitol (Glyset), which are treatments for diabetes.

EBSCO CAM Review Board

FURTHER READING

Ganiats, T. G., et al. "Does Beano Prevent Gas? A Double-Blind Crossover Study of Oral Alpha-Galactosidase to Treat Dietary Oligosaccharide Intolerance." *Journal of Family Practice* 39 (1994): 441-445.

Lettieri, J. T., and B. Dain. "Effects of Beano on the Tolerability and Pharmacodynamics of Acarbose." *Clinical Therapeutics* 20 (1998): 497-504.

Levine, B., and S. Weisman. "Enzyme Replacement as an Effective Treatment for the Common Symptoms of Complex Carbohydrate Intolerance." *Nutrition in Clinical Care* 7 (2004): 75-81.

See also: Diabetes; Fructo-oligosaccharides; Functional foods: Overview; Gas, intestinal; Low-carbohydrate diet.

Bed-wetting

CATEGORY: Condition
RELATED TERMS: Enuresis, nocturnal enuresis, primary nocturnal enuresis, secondary nocturnal enuresis
DEFINITION: Treatment of unintended urination while sleeping.
PRINCIPAL PROPOSED NATURAL TREATMENTS: None
OTHER PROPOSED NATURAL TREATMENTS: Acupuncture, bach flower remedies, Chinese herbal medicine, food allergies, hypnosis, juniper, lobelia, magnet therapy, marshmallow root, parsley root, uva ursi

INTRODUCTION

Nocturnal enuresis, or bed-wetting, is defined as unintended nighttime urination in a child who is older than five years of age. In most cases, there is no underlying medical cause, in which case the condition is called primary nocturnal enuresis (PNE). When enuresis occurs as a result of another illness, it is called secondary nocturnal enuresis.

The adult bladder that becomes full during the night signals to the brain that this has occurred; in turn, the brain informs the bladder not to empty and also begins the process leading to wakefulness. The ability to carry out this process is not present at birth, but most children gradually develop this capacity and achieve it in full by age six years. However, as many as 7 percent of ten-year-olds and 1 to 2 percent of fifteen-year-olds continue to have trouble. Nearly all children with primary nocturnal enuresis will cease bed-wetting by the time they reach puberty. However, PNE remains a problem for up to 1 percent of adults.

Enuresis occurs more commonly in boys than in girls. In addition, there is a strong genetic predisposition: If both parents have enuresis, there is a 75 percent chance that a child will; this decreases to 40 percent if only one parent has enuresis.

Nocturnal enuresis is not a disease, but it can lead to significant embarrassment and limitation of activities, and for this reason treatment may be desired. The first step is a medical examination to rule out rare underlying causes, such as infection. Common-sense steps follow, such as not drinking much liquid near bedtime and urinating just before going to bed. More specific treatment can be delayed as long as desired, because in the great majority of cases, nocturnal enuresis will eventually disappear. For older children who wish to accelerate the process, nighttime alarm systems that wake the child in response to moisture in the child's underwear are often highly effective. Other methods include bladder exercises and a schedule of planned nighttime waking. If these behavioral methods fail, the use of various medications may be considered.

PROPOSED NATURAL TREATMENTS

Many parents turn to alternative medicine for the treatment of nocturnal enuresis if behavioral methods do not work. However, no alternative therapies have been proven effective for this condition.

Hypnosis has shown some promise for nocturnal enuresis. In one study, fifty children were given the drug imipramine or given hypnotherapy for three months. The results showed substantial and approximately equal benefits in the two groups. Subsequently, children in the hypnosis group practiced self-hypnosis for another six months, while those in the imipramine group did not utilize any special therapy. At the end of the six months, children practicing self-hypnosis had maintained their benefits to a much greater extent than those in the imipramine group. Other studies found benefits with hypnosis too; however, these studies had significant design limitations. Overall, the evidence supporting hypnosis for nocturnal enuresis is not strong.

It has been suggested that food allergies may play a role in nocturnal enuresis. However, there is only incomplete evidence that allergen avoidance or any other dietary approaches can help.

Herbs used for miscellaneous bladder problems are often recommended for nocturnal enuresis, on general principles. These herbs include juniper, lobelia, marshmallow root, parsley root, and uva ursi. However, there is no evidence that these herbs help the condition, and some, such as uva ursi, may have toxic properties, especially when given for the long term.

Acupuncture, bach flower remedies, and Chinese herbal medicine are also sometimes recommended for nocturnal enuresis, but there is no reliable evidence that they are effective. One reasonably well-designed study found evidence that a special form of chiropractic (the activator technique) is not effective for bed-wetting. A small preliminary study suggested that the use of pulsed magnetic stimulation day and night for two months may be helpful in girls.

HERBS AND SUPPLEMENTS TO USE ONLY WITH CAUTION

Various herbs and supplements may interact adversely with drugs used to treat nocturnal enuresis, so persons should be cautious when considering the use of herbs and supplements.

EBSCO CAM Review Board

FURTHER READING

Banerjee, S., A. Srivastav, and B. M. Palan. "Hypnosis and Self-Hypnosis in the Management of Nocturnal Enuresis: A Comparative Study with Imipramine Therapy." *American Journal of Clinical Hypnosis* 36 (1993): 113-119.

But, I., and N. M. Varda. "Functional Magnetic Stimulation: A New Method for the Treatment of Girls with Primary Nocturnal Enuresis?" *Journal of Pediatric Urology* 2 (2006): 415-418.

Egger, J., et al. "Effect of Diet Treatment on Enuresis in Children with Migraine or Hyperkinetic Behavior." *Clinical Pediatrics* 31 (1992): 302-307.

Mellon, M. W., and M. L. McGrath. "Empirically Supported Treatments in Pediatric Psychology: Nocturnal Enuresis." *Journal of Pediatric Psychology* 25 (2000): 193-214.

Reed, W. R., et al. "Chiropractic Management of Primary Nocturnal Enuresis." *Journal of Manipulative and Physiological Therapeutics* 17 (1994): 596-600.

See also: Bladder infection; Children's health; Uva ursi.

Bee pollen

CATEGORY: Herbs and supplements
DEFINITION: Natural substance used as a supplement to treat specific health conditions.
PRINCIPAL PROPOSED USES: None
OTHER PROPOSED USES: Allergies, enhancing memory, enhancing sports performance, respiratory infections

OVERVIEW

Bee pollen is the pollen collected by bees as they gather nectar from flowers for making honey. Like honey, bee pollen is used as a food by the hive. The pollen granules are stored in pollen sacs on the bees' hind legs. Beekeepers who wish to collect bee pollen place a screen over the hive with openings just large enough for the bees to pass through. As the bees enter the hive, the screen compresses their pollen sacs, squeezing the pollen from them. The beekeepers can then collect the pollen from the screen.

Bee pollen is very high in protein and carbohydrates, and it contains trace amounts of minerals and vitamins. It is used in a number of traditional Chinese herbal formulas and is sold as a nutritional supplement in the United States and other countries. Although it has been recommended for a variety of uses, particularly for improving sports performance and relieving allergies, little to no scientific evidence backs up any of the claims about the therapeutic value of bee pollen.

REQUIREMENTS AND SOURCES

Bee pollen is not typically found in a person's everyday diet, unless the person regularly eats the snack bars that include it. Tablets and some snack products containing bee pollen are available in pharmacies and health food stores.

THERAPEUTIC DOSAGES

Athletes using bee pollen report consuming five to ten tablets per day. Tablets can contain variable amounts of bee pollen, usually from 200 to 500 milligrams. The manufacturer's recommendations may provide more guidance.

THERAPEUTIC USES

Bee pollen has been touted as an energy enhancer and is sometimes used by athletes in the belief that it will enhance performance during competitions. However, there is no real evidence that bee pollen is effective and some evidence that it is not.

Bee pollen is also commonly taken to try to prevent hay fever on the theory that eating pollens will help persons build up resistance to them. When used for this purpose, locally grown bee pollen is usually recommended; however, it is possible to have a severe allergic reaction to the bee pollen itself. Other proposed uses of bee pollen include combating age-related memory loss and other effects of aging, as well as treating respiratory infections, endocrine disorders, and colitis. No scientific evidence supports any of these uses.

SCIENTIFIC EVIDENCE

A few clinical trials have tested bee pollen's ability to increase energy, such as in sports performance, or to improve memory.

Sports performance. According to a 1977 article in *The New York Times,* two studies on the use of bee pollen to improve sports performance found it to be of no significant benefit. Both trials were said to be double-blind and placebo-controlled. The first, performed in 1975, involved thirty members of a university swim team. Participants were divided into three groups and given a daily dose of either ten tablets of bee pollen, ten placebo tablets, or five bee pollen and five placebo tablets. In 1976, the same experimental protocol was used, but this time with sixty participants: thirty swimmers, and thirty long-distance runners. Bee pollen did not significantly improve performance in

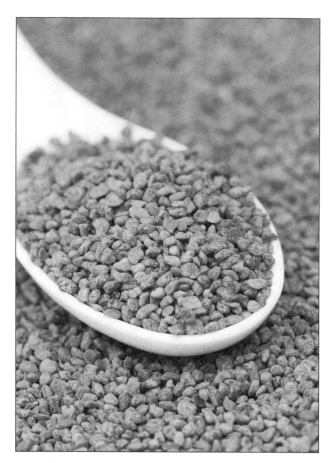

Bee pollen has been touted as an energy enhancer; however, there is no real evidence to support this claim and some evidence discredits it. (©Pittapitta/Dreamstime.com)

either trial. A third study on bee pollen's effects on sports performance, also difficult to obtain, reportedly found that breathing, heart rate, and perspiration returned to normal levels more quickly in track team members taking pollen than in those taking a placebo. However, reviewers criticized the methods used in this study. The runners may have known who was taking placebo and who was taking pollen, and this could have influenced the results.

Memory. The effects of pure bee pollen on memory have not been investigated, but clinical trials of a Chinese herbal medicine containing bee pollen have been conducted in China and Denmark. The improvements in memory seen in the Chinese study were not significant, and in the more recent double-blind, placebo-controlled crossover study in Denmark, no improvements were found. The formula tested was only 14 percent bee pollen, so the results may not reveal very much about bee pollen's effectiveness.

SAFETY ISSUES

Several cases of serious allergic reactions to bee pollen, including anaphylaxis, an acute allergic response that can be life-threatening, have been reported in the medical literature. The anaphylactic reactions occurred within twenty to thirty minutes of ingesting fairly small amounts of bee pollen—in one case, less than a teaspoon. The majority of these case reports involved people with known allergies to pollen.

EBSCO CAM Review Board

FURTHER READING

Blustein, P. "Pollinated Presidents Aside, Experts Doubt Value of Bee Pick-me-up." *Wall Street Journal,* February 12, 1981.

Cohen, S. H., et al. "Acute Allergic Reaction After Composite Pollen Ingestion." *Journal of Allergy and Clinical Immunology* 64 (1979): 270-274.

Geyman, J. P. "Anaphylactic Reaction After Ingestion of Bee Pollen." *Journal of the American Board of Family Practice* 7 (1994): 250-252.

Iverson, T., et al. "The Effect of NaO Li Su on Memory Functions and Blood Chemistry in Elderly People." *Journal of Ethnopharmacology* 56 (1997): 109-116.

Montgomery, P. L. "Bee Pollen: Wonder Drug or Humbug?" *The New York Times,* February 6, 1977, pp. 1, 7.

See also: Bee propolis; Bee venom therapy; Herbal medicine; Memory and mental function impairment; Sports and fitness support: Enhancing performance.

Bee propolis

CATEGORY: Herbs and supplements
RELATED TERMS: Bee glue, bee putty, propolis
DEFINITION: Natural substance used as a supplement to treat specific health conditions.
PRINCIPAL PROPOSED USES: None
OTHER PROPOSED USES:
- *Topical:* Genital herpes, oral surgery, skin wounds, tooth decay, vaginal infections
- *Oral:* Cancer prevention, giardiasis

OVERVIEW

Although honey is perhaps the most famous bee product of interest to humans, bees also make propolis, another substance that humans have used for thousands of years. Bees coat their hives with propolis in much the same way humans use paint and caulking on their homes. People began using propolis more than twenty-three hundred years ago for many purposes, the foremost of which was applying it to wounds to fight infection. It is a resinous compound made primarily from tree sap, and it contains biologically active compounds called flavonoids, which come from its plant source. Propolis does indeed have antiseptic properties; the flavonoids in propolis may be responsible for its antimicrobial effects as well as other alleged health benefits.

REQUIREMENTS AND SOURCES

Propolis is available in a wide assortment of products found in pharmacies and health food stores, including tablets, capsules, powders, extracts, ointments, creams, lotions, and other cosmetics.

THERAPEUTIC DOSAGES

Topical propolis ointments, creams, lotions, balms, and extracts are usually applied directly to the area being treated. However, applying bee propolis directly to the eyes is not recommended.

Propolis intended for oral use comes in a wide variety of forms, including tablets, capsules, and extracts. Products vary so much that the proper dosage is best determined by following the directions on the label.

THERAPEUTIC USES

Test tube studies have found propolis to be active against a variety of microorganisms, including bacteria, viruses, and protozoans. These findings have been the basis for most propolis research in humans and animals. The results of a small controlled study suggest that propolis cream might cause attacks of genital herpes to heal faster.

A preliminary controlled study found that propolis mouthwash following oral surgery significantly speeded healing time compared with a placebo. Propolis extracts may also have value in treatment of severe periodontal disease, according to a study that evaluated the use of propolis extracts as part of an irrigation procedure performed twice weekly by dentists.

In one study, rats given propolis in their drinking water developed fewer cavities than rats given regular water. However, no human studies have been performed. Animal studies also suggest that topical propolis may be of benefit in healing wounds.

One group of researchers compared a propolis extract against the standard antiprotozoal drug tinidazole in 138 people infected with the parasite giardiasis. The extract appeared to work about as well as the drug therapy.

A number of clinical trials have tested the use of propolis for eye infections and vaginal infections. However, these were poorly designed; better trials are necessary before propolis can be determined to be effective for treating any of these conditions.

One isolated study, published only in abstract form, tested bee propolis in women with mild endometriosis and infertility. Reportedly, researchers found that use of bee propolis at a dose of 500 milligrams twice daily resulted in a pregnancy rate of 60 percent compared with 20 percent in the placebo group, a difference that was statistically significant. It is not clear why propolis should have this effect.

Finally, test-tube studies suggest that propolis has antioxidant, anti-inflammatory, and cancer-preventing properties. Again, without actual human studies, these results suggest the need for future research but do not prove propolis to be effective for any particular condition.

SAFETY ISSUES

Propolis is an ingredient commonly consumed in small quantities in honey. Safety studies have found it to be essentially nontoxic when taken orally; propolis also appears to be nonirritating when applied to the skin. However, allergic reactions to propolis are relatively common; it is a known "sensitizing agent," meaning it tends to induce allergies to itself when it is taken for an extended time.

EBSCO CAM Review Board

FURTHER READING

Ali, A. F. M., and A. Awadallah. "Bee Propolis Versus Placebo in the Treatment of Infertility Associated with Minimal or Mild Endometriosis." *Fertility and Sterility* 80 (2003): S32.

Burdock, G. A. "Review of the Biological Properties and Toxicity of Bee Propolis." *Food and Chemistry Toxicology* 36 (1998): 347-363.

Gebaraa, E. C., et al. "Propolis Extract as an Adjuvant to Periodontal Treatment." *Oral Health and Preventative Dentistry* 1 (2005): 29-35.

Trevelyan, J. "Spirit of the Beehive." *Nursing Times* 93 (1997): 72-74.

Vynograd, N., I. Vynograd, and Z. Sosnowski. "A Comparative Multi-centre Study of the Efficacy of Propolis, Acyclovir, and Placebo in the Treatment of Genital Herpes." *Phytomedicine* 7 (2000): 1-6.

See also: Bee pollen; Bee venom therapy; Herbal medicine.

Bee venom therapy

CATEGORY: Therapies and techniques
RELATED TERM: Apitherapy
DEFINITION: The use of bee venom to treat specific health conditions.
PRINCIPAL PROPOSED USES: None
OTHER PROPOSED USES: Burns bursitis, chronic fatigue syndrome, fibromyalgia, gout, hay fever, scar tissue, shingles, tendonitis

OVERVIEW

Most people associate bees with honey or pollen. Another bee product, bee venom, is used to treat certain illnesses. The medicinal effects of bee honey are well known. Indeed, tea with honey has long been a remedy of choice for sore throats, and some nutritionists consider bee pollen to be a near perfect source of protein.

Bee venom, however, is looked upon with some trepidation, given that most people's only experience with the venom is with a painful bee sting. For thousands of years, though, the medicinal benefits of bee venom have been touted throughout the world. While these medicinal effects have not been scientifically proven, the use of bee venom (a practice called apitherapy) to treat various ailments is actively being studied.

USES AND APPLICATIONS

The medicinal use of bee venom apparently dates back to ancient Egypt and is reported in various histories of Europe and Asia. Charlemagne and Ivan the Terrible, for example, reportedly used bee venom to treat joint ailments. In more modern times, interest in the effects of bee venom was renewed in the 1860s with the publication of a clinical study conducted in Europe on bee venom's effect on rheumatism. Since then, interest in bee venom treatment has ebbed and flowed.

With the increasing advent and acceptance of natural medicines, interest in the therapeutic value of bee venom has grown. However, there is conflicting evidence that bee venom is a useful therapy. For example, a small randomized trial did not show any effectiveness for bee venom in the treatment of multiple sclerosis. However, a review of studies did find that the venom may help treat arthritis.

Despite these contradictory findings, there are numerous conditions that bee venom has been proposed to treat. These conditions include chronic injuries such as bursitis and tendonitis, hay fever, scar tissue, gout, shingles, burns, fibromyalgia, and chronic fatigue syndrome. Again, not much evidence exists to show that bee venom is an effective therapy.

MECHANISM OF ACTION

Before the invention of the syringe, bee venom was administered directly from bees. Today, in some cases, it is still administered in this way. The live bee is held (with tweezers or some other small instrument) by the person administering the bee venom, who then places the bee on the part of the body to be treated, at which point the bee reflexively stings. Depending on the condition, the treatment schedule can vary. The venom also can be given via a syringe, rather than directly from the bee.

SCIENTIFIC EVIDENCE

Scientists do not definitively understand how bee venom, which is a complex mixture of numerous compounds, acts on the human body. However, the components of bee venom that have been identified and studied include mellitin, adolapin, and apamine. Rather than these individual components having an effect, it may be more likely that the body has an immune reaction to bee venom that proves beneficial in certain circumstances.

CHOOSING A PRACTITIONER

Persons considering bee venom therapy should recognize that such therapy is a natural treatment for which there is no rigorous scientific evidence proving its medicinal effectiveness. Before trying this therapy, one should consult a doctor.

SAFETY ISSUES

The greatest risk of bee venom therapy is the risk of an anaphylactic allergic reaction, including anaphylactic shock, which can cause a person to stop breathing. If not treated immediately, anaphylactic shock can result in death. Though only a small percentage of the population is allergic to bee venom, it is important that the person be tested for a bee sting allergy before the treatment.

Rick Alan; reviewed by Brian Randall, M.D.

FURTHER READING

American Apitherapy Society. http://www.apitherapy. org.

Cuende, E., et al. "Beekeeper's Arthropathy." *Journal of Rheumatology* 26 (1999): 2684.

Lee, J. D., et al. "An Overview of Bee Venom Acupuncture in the Treatment of Arthritis." *Evidence Based Complementary and Alternative Medicine* 2 (2005): 79-84.

Novella, S. "Bee Venom Therapy: Grassroots Medicine." Available at http://www.sciencebasedmedicine.org/ ?p=296.

Wesselius, T., et al. "A Randomized Crossover Study of Bee Sting Therapy for Multiple Sclerosis." *Neurology* 65 (2005): 1764-1768.

See also: Bee pollen; Bee propolis; Honey; Insect bites and stings.

Bell's palsy

CATEGORY: Condition
RELATED TERMS: Facial nerve palsy, facial palsy, facial paralysis, idiopathic facial paralysis
DEFINITION: Treatment of facial paralysis.
PRINCIPAL PROPOSED NATURAL TREATMENTS: None
OTHER PROPOSED NATURAL TREATMENTS: Acupuncture, biofeedback, hyperbaric oxygen therapy, vitamin B_{12} injections

INTRODUCTION

Bell's palsy is the common name for a condition in which paralysis strikes the seventh cranial nerve, which controls much of the face. Only one side of the face is affected. Symptoms usually appear suddenly and painlessly and are first noticed as a droop in one corner of the mouth, with an inability to smile properly. Other symptoms include drooling, an inability to close the eye on the drooping side, tearing, impairment of taste, and pain. Although anyone can develop Bell's palsy, it occurs most often in pregnant women and people who have diabetes, hypertension, or a respiratory infection.

Conventional treatment for Bell's palsy involves corticosteroid drugs (such as prednisone) and sometimes the antiviral drug acyclovir. However, according to a review published in 2002, there is no reliable evidence that either treatment provides any benefit. A later published study did show a slight benefit with early, high-dose corticosteroid treatment.

Useful supportive measures for Bell's palsy include patching the affected eye at night and using artificial tears. Surgery or electrical stimulation of the nerve are used rarely. Medical evaluation is essential because, in rare cases, Bell's palsy may be caused by an underlying condition that requires specific treatment, such as a tumor.

Proposed Natural Treatments

Hyperbaric oxygen therapy involves breathing 100 percent oxygen at increased pressure. It is used by both conventional and alternative practitioners. A placebo-controlled study found hyperbaric oxygen more effective than prednisone. In this trial, seventy-nine people with Bell's palsy were randomly assigned to receive either prednisone or hyperbaric oxygen (one hour twice daily, five days per week, for thirty sessions or up to full recovery). Placebo pills were given with hyperbaric therapy, and fake hyperbaric therapy was given with prednisone. The results showed a significantly greater speed of recovery and a higher percentage of full recovery in the hyperbaric oxygen group compared with the prednisone group.

Many alternative practitioners recommend the use of injected vitamin B_{12} for Bell's palsy. However, the only scientific support for this approach comes from one study that was not double-blind. Other treatments that are sometimes recommended for Bell's palsy, but with inadequate supporting evidence, include acupuncture and biofeedback.

EBSCO CAM Review Board

Further Reading

Jalaludin, M. A. "Methylcobalamin Treatment of Bell's Palsy." *Methods and Findings in Experimental and Clinical Pharmacology* 17 (1995): 539-544.

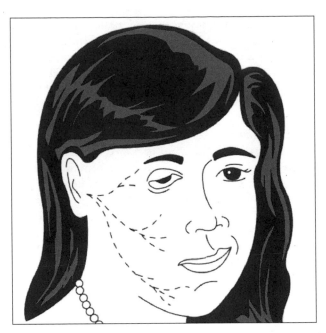

Bell's palsy results in a temporary sagging and paralysis of one side of the face; dashed lines show the main neural pathways affected.

Lagalla, G., et al. "Influence of Early High-Dose Steroid Treatments on Bell's Palsy Evolution." *Neurological Sciences* 23 (2002): 107-112.

Racic, G., et al. "Hyperbaric Oxygen as a Therapy of Bell's Palsy." *Undersea and Hyperbaric Medicine* 24 (1997): 35-38.

Salinas, R. A., et al. "Corticosteroids for Bell's Palsy (Idiopathic Facial Paralysis)." *Cochrane Database of Systematic Reviews* (2002): CD001942. Available through *EBSCO DynaMed Systematic Literature Surveillance* at http://www.ebscohost.com/dynamed.

See also: Acupuncture; Biofeedback; Corticosteroids; Vitamin B_{12}.

Benign prostatic hyperplasia

Category: Condition
Related terms: Enlarged prostate, prostate enlargement
Definition: Treatment of enlarged prostate not caused by cancer.

Principal proposed natural treatments: Beta-sitosterol, grass pollen, nettle root, pygeum, saw palmetto

Other proposed natural treatments: Antioxidants, *Bixa orellana* (annatto), flaxseed, flaxseed oil, green tea, maca, oat straw, pumpkin seeds, zinc

INTRODUCTION

Any man who lives long enough will almost certainly develop benign prostatic hyperplasia (BPH). Ninety percent of all men show signs of such prostatic enlargement by the age of eighty years. Symptoms include difficulty in starting urination, a diminished force of urinary stream, a sensation of fullness in the bladder after urination, and the need to urinate many times at night. Ultimately, the obstruction can become so severe that urination is impossible.

The most common treatment for BPH is surgery that removes most of the prostate gland. Medications such as Cardura, Flomax, Hytrin, and Proscar can relieve symptoms of BPH. In addition, Proscar has been shown to shrink the prostate and reduce the need for surgery. However, all of these medications can cause significant side effects.

PRINCIPAL PROPOSED NATURAL TREATMENTS

Men who suspect they may have BPH should consult a physician to rule out prostate cancer. Many natural options are available that have good scientific backing. Indeed, there are few other conditions for which so many natural therapies have good supporting evidence for efficacy. However, there is one potential advantage for standard medications: Some have been shown sufficiently effective at slowing the progression of BPH to help men avoid surgery, while this has not been shown to be true of any natural options.

Saw palmetto. The best-documented herbal treatment for BPH is the oil of the berry of the saw palmetto tree. This herb is so well accepted in Europe that synthetic pharmaceuticals are considered alternative therapy for BPH. Saw palmetto offers two potential advantages over conventional drug treatment. The most obvious is that it usually causes no side effects. Another advantage is that saw palmetto does not change protein-specific antigen (PSA) levels. Laboratory tests that measure PSA are used to screen for prostate cancer. The widely used drug Proscar can artificially lower PSA levels, which may have the unintended effect of masking prostate cancer.

Despite its popularity, the scientific evidence that saw palmetto is effective for prostate enlargement is inconsistent. A number of double-blind, placebo-controlled studies involving about nine hundred participants compared the benefits of saw palmetto with placebo over a period of one to twelve months. In all but three of these studies, the herb significantly improved urinary flow rate and most other measures of prostate disease. However, in the most recent and perhaps best designed of these studies, a one-year trial of 225 men, saw palmetto product failed to prove more effective than placebo. Furthermore, a large review of fourteen trials with 5,222 men found that saw palmetto did not improve urinary symptom scores or peak urine flow compared with placebo. Subjects taking saw palmetto reported more overall symptom improvement than those taking placebo, but this result is questionable because of a lack of consistency among the studies.

A double-blind study followed 1,098 men who received either saw palmetto or the drug Proscar over a period of six months. According to the results, the two treatments were about equally successful at reducing noticeable symptoms, and none produced much in the way of side effects. However, Proscar lowered PSA levels, presenting a risk of masking prostate cancer. Saw palmetto did not cause this problem. On the other hand, careful measurements showed that Proscar caused men's prostates to shrink by 18 percent, while saw palmetto caused only a 6 percent decrease in size. Although prostate size does not correlate well with severity of symptoms, such a decrease in size might indicate a reduced likelihood of need for surgery. This is a potential advantage for the drug.

A fifty-two-week double-blind study of 811 men compared saw palmetto to a standard drug for BPH in another class: the alpha-blocker tamsulosin. Once again, both treatments proved equally effective. However, saw palmetto caused fewer side effects than the drug. In addition, the herb caused some prostate shrinkage, while the drug allowed a slight prostate enlargement.

Although there are many theories about how saw palmetto works, none have been conclusively established. The best evidence suggests that the herb affects male hormones.

Pygeum. The pygeum tree is a tall evergreen native to central and southern Africa. Its bark has been used since ancient times for urinary problems.

Benign Prostatic Hyperplasia: Its Possible Causes

The cause of benign prostatic hyperplasia (BPH) is not well understood. No definite information on risk factors exists. For centuries, it has been known that BPH occurs mainly in older men and that it does not develop in men whose testes were removed before puberty. For this reason, some researchers believe that factors related to aging and the testes may spur the development of BPH.

Throughout their lives, men produce testosterone, an important male hormone, and small amounts of estrogen, a female hormone. As men age, the amount of active testosterone in the blood decreases, leaving a higher proportion of estrogen. Studies done on animals suggest that BPH may occur because the higher amount of estrogen within the gland increases the activity of substances that promote cell growth.

Another theory focuses on dihydrotestosterone (DHT), a substance derived from testosterone in the prostate, which may help control its growth. Most animals lose their ability to produce DHT as they age. However, some research has indicated that even with a drop in the blood's testosterone level, older men continue to produce and accumulate high levels of DHT in the prostate. This accumulation of DHT may encourage the growth of cells. Scientists have also noted that men who do not produce DHT do not develop BPH.

Some researchers suggest that BPH may develop as a result of "instructions" given to cells early in life. According to this theory, BPH occurs because cells in one section of the gland follow these instructions and "reawaken" later in life. These reawakened cells then deliver signals to other cells in the gland, instructing them to grow or making them more sensitive to hormones that influence growth.

At least seventeen double-blind trials, ranging in length from forty-five to ninety days, of pygeum for BPH have been performed, involving almost one thousand men. Many of these studies were poorly reported or designed. Nonetheless, overall, the results do suggest that pygeum can reduce symptoms such as nighttime urination, urinary frequency, and residual urine volume.

The best of these trials was conducted at eight sites in Europe and included 263 men between fifty and eighty-five years of age. Participants received 50 milligrams (mg) of a pygeum extract or placebo twice daily. The results showed significant improvements in various measures of BPH severity.

It is not known how pygeum works. Unlike the standard drug finasteride, it does not appear to work by affecting the conversion of testosterone to dihydrotestosterone. Rather, it is thought to reduce inflammation in the prostate and to inhibit prostate growth factors, substances implicated in inappropriate pros-

tate enlargement. It is not known whether pygeum can reduce the need for prostate surgery or whether it affects PSA levels.

Nettle root. Persons who live in a locale where nettle grows wild will likely discover the powers of this dark green plant. Depending on the species, the fine hairs on its leaves and stem cause burning pain that lasts from hours to weeks. Both its leaves and roots can be used as medicine. The root is a popular treatment in Europe for BPH, but it has not been as well studied as saw palmetto or pygeum.

In a double-blind, placebo-controlled study in Iran, 558 men were given either placebo or nettle root for six months. The results indicated that nettle root is significantly more effective than placebo on all major measures of BPH severity. Benefits were seen in three other double-blind studies as well, enrolling more than 150 men.

Beta-sitosterol. Numerous plants contain cholesterol-like compounds called sitosterols and their close relatives sitosterolins. A special mixture of these, called beta-sitosterol, is used for the treatment of BPH.

A review of the literature, published in 1999, found four randomized, double-blind, placebo-controlled studies on beta-sitosterol for BPH, enrolling 519 men. All but one of these studies found significant benefits in both perceived symptoms and objective measurements, such as urine flow rate. The largest trial followed two hundred men with BPH for six months. After the study was completed, many of the participants were followed for an additional year, during which the benefits continued. Similar results were seen in a six-month double-blind trial of 177 men with BPH.

Grass pollen. Grass pollen is also used to treat BPH. The grasses used for this preparation are 92 percent rye, 5 percent timothy, and 3 percent corn. Related grass pollen extracts are used for allergy shots. However, the grass pollen extracts described here are different in that they have their allergenic components removed. Grass pollen is also an entirely different product from bee pollen.

Two double-blind, placebo-controlled studies found that grass pollen extract can improve symptoms of prostate enlargement. There have also been open studies that compared grass pollen to different treatments for BPH.

In the first double-blind, placebo-controlled study, 103 men with BPH were assigned to take either placebo or two capsules of a standardized grass pollen extract three times daily for twelve weeks. At the end of the study, 69 percent of the participants who had been taking the grass pollen had reduced the number of trips they had to make to the toilet at night. In the placebo group, only 37 percent reported improvement in this symptom. The amount of urine remaining in the bladder following urination was reduced in the treatment group by 24 milliliters (ml) and by 4 ml for the placebo group. Both of these were statistically significant improvements for those taking grass pollen.

The second double-blind, placebo-controlled study lasted longer but enrolled fewer participants. Fifty-seven men with prostate enlargement were enrolled in the study, with thirty-one taking 92 mg of the grass pollen extract daily for six months and the remaining twenty-six taking placebo. As with the foregoing study, statistically significant improvements in nighttime frequency of urination and emptying of the bladder were found with the use of grass pollen extract. Additionally, 69 percent of the participants receiving treatment reported overall improvement, while only 29 percent of the group taking the placebo felt they had improved, another statistically significant difference. An important finding in this study was that the prostates of the men taking grass pollen significantly decreased in size according to ultrasound measurements taken.

No one is certain how the grass pollen extract causes the beneficial results seen in the studies. One theory is that it inhibits the body's manufacturing of prostaglandins and leukotrienes, which might relieve prostate congestion by reducing inflammation.

Combination treatment. A forty-eight-week double-blind trial of 543 men with early BPH compared combined saw palmetto and nettle root with Proscar and found equal benefits. The same combination proved superior to placebo in a twenty-four-week double-blind study of 257 men. In a three-month, double-blind, placebo-controlled study of 144 men with BPH,

the use of a combination product containing saw palmetto, grass pollen extract, beta-sitosterol, and vitamin E significantly reduced symptoms.

A six-month, double-blind, placebo-controlled trial of forty-four men given a saw palmetto herbal blend (with nettle root and pumpkin seed oil) found shrinkage in prostate tissue. No significant improvement in symptoms was seen, but the authors pointed out that the study size was too small to statistically detect such improvements if they did occur. Another small study failed to find significant benefit with a combination of pygeum and nettle root.

OTHER PROPOSED NATURAL TREATMENTS

One study provides weak evidence that green tea extracts taken orally might reduce symptoms of BPH. Pumpkin seeds are approved for use in BPH in Germany. The mineral zinc is also commonly recommended in both Europe and the United States as a treatment for prostate disease, as are both whole flaxseed and flaxseed oil, along with the herbs maca (*Lepidium meyenii*) and oat straw (*Avena sativa*). However, there is no meaningful evidence to indicate that any of these proposed options are effective.

In a large study investigating the influence of dietary patterns and supplement use on the risk of BPH, researchers followed 4,770 men, initially with normal-sized prostates, for seven years. Researchers found that antioxidant supplements did not significantly reduce BPH risk and that lycopene, zinc, and vitamin D supplementation had only a modest beneficial effect.

In a twelve-month, double-blind, placebo-controlled study of 136 men with BPH of moderate severity, the use of *Bixa orellana* (annatto) at a dose of 250 mg three times daily failed to improve symptoms. In a preliminary double-blind trial of seventy-eight older men, flaxseed extract modestly improved the urinary symptoms associated with benign prostatic hyperplasia (prostate enlargement) after four months of treatment.

EBSCO CAM Review Board

FURTHER READING

Bent, S., et al. "Saw Palmetto for Benign Prostatic Hyperplasia." *New England Journal of Medicine* 354 (2006): 557-566.

Bettuzzi, S., et al. "Chemoprevention of Human Prostate Cancer by Oral Administration of Green Tea Catechins in Volunteers with High-Grade Prostate

Intraepithelial Neoplasia." *Cancer Research* 66 (2006): 1234-1240.

Debruyne, F., et al. "Comparison of a Phytotherapeutic Agent (Permixon) with an Alpha-Blocker (Tamsulosin) in the Treatment of Benign Prostatic Hyperplasia." *European Urology* 41 (2002): 497-507.

Gerber, G. S., et al. "Randomized, Double-Blind, Placebo-Controlled Trial of Saw Palmetto in Men with Lower Urinary Tract Symptoms." *Urology* 58 (2001): 960-964.

Kristal, A. R., et al. "Dietary Patterns, Supplement Use, and the Risk of Symptomatic Benign Prostatic Hyperplasia: Results from the Prostate Cancer Prevention Trial." *American Journal of Epidemiology* 167 (2008): 925-934.

Lopatkin, N., et al. "Long-Term Efficacy and Safety of a Combination of Sabal and Urtica Extract for Lower Urinary Tract Symptoms." *World Journal of Urology* 23 (2005): 139-146.

McConnell, J. D., et al. "The Long-Term Effect of Doxazosin, Finasteride, and Combination Therapy on the Clinical Progression of Benign Prostatic Hyperplasia." *New England Journal of Medicine* 349 (2003): 2387-2398.

Melo, E. A., et al. "Evaluating the Efficiency of a Combination of *Pygeum africanum* and Stinging Nettle (*Urtica dioica*) Extracts in Treating Benign Prostatic Hyperplasia (BPH)." *International Brazilian Journal of Urology* 28 (2005): 418-425.

Preuss, H. G., et al. "Randomized Trial of a Combination of Natural Products (Cernitin, Saw Palmetto, B-sitosterol, Vitamin E) on Symptoms of Benign Prostatic Hyperplasia (BPH)." *Int Urol Nephrol.* 33 (2001): 217-225.

Safarinejad, M. R. "*Urtica dioica* for Treatment of Benign Prostatic Hyperplasia." *Journal of Herbal Pharmacotherapy* 5 (2006): 1-11.

Tacklind, J., et al. "*Serenoa repens* for Benign Prostatic Hyperplasia." *Cochrane Database of Systematic Reviews* (2009): CD001423. Available through *EBSCO DynaMed Systematic Literature Surveillance* at http://www.ebscohost.com/dynamed.

Wilt, T., et al. "*Pygeum africanum* for Benign Prostatic Hyperplasia." *Cochrane Database of Systematic Reviews* (2002): CD001044. Available through *EBSCO DynaMed Systematic Literature Surveillance* at http://www.ebscohost.com/dynamed.

Zegarra, L., et al. "Double-Blind Randomized Placebo-Controlled Study of *Bixa orellana* in Patients with Lower Urinary Tract Symptoms Associated to Benign Prostatic Hyperplasia." *International Brazilian Journal of Urology* 33 (2007): 493-501.

Zhang, W., et al. "Effects of Dietary Flaxseed Lignan Extract on Symptoms of Benign Prostatic Hyperplasia." *Journal of Medicinal Food* 11 (2008): 207-214.

See also: Beta-sitosterol; Grass pollen extract; Nettle; Pygeum; Saw palmetto.

Benzodiazepines

CATEGORY: Drug interactions
DEFINITION: Medications used as muscle relaxants, sedatives, and anticonvulsants.
INTERACTIONS: Grapefruit juice, hops, kava, melatonin, passionflower, pregnenolone, valerian
DRUGS IN THIS FAMILY: Alprazolam (Xanax), chlordiazepoxide hydrochloride (Libritabs, Librium, Limbitrol, Lipoxide, Mitran, Reposans-10, Sereen), clonazepam (Klonopin), clorazepate dipotassium (Gen-XENE, Tranxene-T, Tranxene-SD), diazepam (Diastat, Valium, Valrelease, Vazepam), estazolam (ProSom), flurazepam hydrochloride (Dalmane, Durapam), halazepam (Paxipam), lorazepam (Ativan), oxazepam (Serax), quazepam (Doral), temazepam (Razepam, Restoril, Temaz), triazolam (Halcion)

GRAPEFRUIT JUICE
Effect: Possible Harmful Interaction

Grapefruit juice slows the body's normal breakdown of several drugs, including some benzodiazepines, allowing them to build up to potentially dangerous levels in the blood. A recent study indicates that this effect can last for three days or more following the last glass of juice. Because of this risk, if one takes benzodiazepines, the safest approach is to avoid grapefruit juice altogether.

HOPS, KAVA, PASSIONFLOWER, VALERIAN
Effect: Possible Harmful Interaction

The herb kava (*Piper methysticum*) has a sedative effect and is used for anxiety and insomnia. Combining kava with drugs in the benzodiazepine family, which possess similar effects, could result in "add-on" or excessive physical depression, sedation, and impairment. In one case report of a fifty-four-year-old man hospitalized for lethargy and disorientation, these side effects were attributed to his having taken the combination of kava and alprazolam for three days.

Experimental studies suggest that kava, similarly to benzodiazepines, exerts its sedative effects at binding sites in the brain called GABA receptors.

Other herbs with a sedative effect that might cause problems when combined with benzodiazepines include ashwagandha (*Withania somnifera*), calendula (*Calendula officinalis*), catnip (*Nepeta cataria*), hops (*Humulus lupulus*), lady's slipper (*Cypripedium*), lemon balm (*Melissa officinalis*), passionflower (*Passiflora incarnata*), sassafras (*Sassafras officinale*), skullcap (*Scutellaria lateriflora*), valerian (*Valeriana officinalis*), and yerba mansa (*Anemopsis californica*). Because of the potentially serious consequences, one should avoid combining these herbs with benzodiazepines or other drugs that also have sedative or depressant effects unless advised by one's physician.

MELATONIN

Effect: Supplementation Possibly Helpful

Melatonin is a natural hormone that regulates sleep. Many people who take conventional sleeping pills (most of which are in the benzodiazepine family) find it difficult to quit. The reason is that when one tries to stop the medication, one may experience severe insomnia or interrupted sleep. A double-blind, placebo-controlled study of thirty-four people who regularly used such medications found that melatonin at a dose of 2 milligrams (mg) nightly (in a controlled-release formulation) could help them discontinue the use of the drugs.

Warning: It can be dangerous to stop using benzodiazepines if one has taken them for a while. Consult a physician before trying melatonin to help handle benzodiazepine withdrawal or before trying to stop benzodiazepine medication under any conditions.

PREGNENOLONE

Effect: Supplementation May Decrease Effectiveness of the Drug

The hormone pregnenolone is widely sold as a kind of "fountain of youth." However, the only direct evidence that pregnenolone supplements have any effect relates to a potential interaction between the hormone and benzodiazepine drugs. In a carefully designed clinical trial, regular use of pregnenolone was found to greatly decrease the sedative effects of diazepam (Valium). The reasons for this interaction are not known. However, people who rely upon benzodiazepine drugs may find them less effective if pregnenolone is added into the mix.

KAVA

Effect: Possibly Helpful

Although they are highly effective for anxiety, benzodiazepine drugs can cause unpleasant and dangerous withdrawal symptoms when they are discontinued.

A six-week, double-blind, placebo-controlled trial of forty people who had been taking benzodiazepines found that use of kava significantly reduced withdrawal symptoms and helped maintain control of anxiety.

This trial involved close medical supervision and very gradual tapering of benzodiazepine dosages. Persons should not discontinue anti-anxiety medications except on the advice of a physician, as withdrawal symptoms can be life-threatening.

EBSCO CAM Review Board

FURTHER READING

Almeida, J. C., and E. W. Grimsley. "Coma from the Health Food Store: Interaction Between Kava and Alprazolam." *Annals of Internal Medicine* 125 (1996): 940-941.

Malsch, U., and M. Kieser. "Efficacy of Kava-Kava in the Treatment of Non-psychotic Anxiety, Following Pretreatment with Benzodiazepines." *Psychopharmacology* 157 (2001): 277-283.

Meieran, S. E., et al. "Chronic Pregnenolone Effects in Normal Humans: Attenuation of Benzodiazepine-Induced Sedation." *Psychoneuroendocrinology* 29 (2004): 486-500.

Takanaga, H., et al. "Relationship Between Time After Intake of Grapefruit Juice and the Effect on Pharmacokinetics and Pharmacodynamics of Nisoldipine in Healthy Subjects." *Clinical Pharmacology and Therapeutics* 67 (2000): 201-214.

See also: Food and Drug Administration; Supplements: Introduction.

Beta-blockers

CATEGORY: Drug interactions

DEFINITION: Medications used to treat hypertension and a variety of heart conditions.

INTERACTIONS: Chromium, coenzyme Q_{10}, *Coleus forskohlii*

DRUGS IN THIS FAMILY: Acebutolol hydrochloride (Sectral), atenolol (Tenormin), alprenolol, Betaxolol hydrochloride (Kerlone), bisoprolol fumarate (Zebeta), carteolol (Cartrol), carvedilol (Coreg), esmolol hydrochloride (Brevibloc), labetalol hydrochloride (Normodyne, Trandate), metoprolol (Lopressor, Toprol XL), nadolol (Corgard), penbutolol (Levatol), pindolol (Visken), propranolol hydrochloride (Betachron E-R, Inderal, Inderal LA), sotalol (Betapace), timolol maleate (Blocadren)

COENZYME Q_{10} (CoQ_{10})

Effect: Supplementation Possibly Helpful

There is some evidence that beta-blockers (specifically propranolol, metoprolol, and alprenolol) might impair the body's ability to utilize the substance CoQ_{10}. This is particularly of concern, because CoQ_{10} appears to play a significant role in normal heart function. Depletion of CoQ_{10} might be responsible for some of the side effects of beta-blockers. In one study, CoQ_{10} supplements reduced side effects caused by the beta-blocker propranolol. The beta-blocker timolol may interfere with CoQ_{10} production to a lesser extent than other beta-blockers.

CHROMIUM

Effect: Possible Helpful Interaction

Beta-blockers have been known to reduce levels of HDL (good) cholesterol. According to one study, chromium supplementation can offset this adverse effect.

Coleus forskohlii

Effect: Theoretical Interaction

The herb *Coleus forskohlii* relaxes blood vessels and might have unpredictable effects on blood pressure if combined with beta-blockers.

EBSCO CAM Review Board

FURTHER READING

Folkers, K. "Basic Chemical Research on Coenzyme Q10 and Integrated Clinical Research on Therapy of Diseases." In *Coenzyme Q: Biochemistry, Bioenergetics, and Clinical Applications of Ubiquinone*, edited by G. Lenaz. New York: John Wiley & Sons, 1985.

Hamada, M., et al. "Correlation Between Serum Coq10 Level and Myocardial Contractility in Hypertensive Patients." In *Biomedical and Clinical Aspects of Coenzyme Q*, Vol. 4, edited by K. Folkers. Amsterdam: Elsevier Science, 1984.

Roeback, J. R., et al. "Effects of Chromium Supplementation on Serum High-density Lipoprotein Cholesterol Levels in Men Taking Beta-blockers." *Annals of Internal Medicine* 115 (1991): 917-924.

See also: Cholesterol, high; Chromium; Coenzyme Q_{10}; *Coleus forskohlii*; Food and Drug Administration; Heart attack; Herbal medicine; Hypertension; Supplements: Introduction.

Beta-carotene

CATEGORY: Herbs and supplements

DEFINITION: Natural substance promoted as a dietary supplement for specific health benefits.

PRINCIPAL PROPOSED USE: Nutritional vitamin A

OTHER PROPOSED USES: Alcoholism, cataract prevention, depression, enhancing mental function, epilepsy, exercise-induced asthma, female infertility, headaches, heartburn, human immunodeficiency virus support, macular degeneration prevention, male infertility, osteoarthritis, Parkinson's disease, photosensitivity, psoriasis, rheumatoid arthritis, schizophrenia, sunburn prevention

PROBABLY INEFFECTIVE USES: Cancer prevention, diabetes, heart disease prevention

OVERVIEW

All the significant positive evidence for beta-carotene applies to beta-carotene from food sources, not supplements. Beta-carotene belongs to a family of natural chemicals known as carotenoids. Widely found in plants, carotenoids (along with another group of chemicals, bioflavonoids), give color to fruits, vegetables, and other plants.

Beta-carotene is a particularly important carotenoid from a nutritional standpoint, because the body easily transforms it to vitamin A. While vitamin A supplements themselves can be toxic when taken to excess, it is believed (although not proven) that the body will make only as much vitamin A out of beta-carotene as it needs. Assuming this is true, this built-in safety feature makes beta-carotene the best way for a person to get vitamin A.

Beta-carotene is also often recommended for another reason: it is an antioxidant, like vitamin E and vitamin C. In observational studies, a high intake of carotenoids from food has been associated with reduced risk of various illnesses (including heart disease and cancer). However, observational studies are inherently unreliable, as described below. In intervention trials, beta-carotene supplements have not been found to offer any benefits; in fact, when taken in high doses for a long period of time, beta-carotene supplements might slightly increase the risk of heart disease and some forms of cancer.

REQUIREMENTS AND SOURCES

Although beta-carotene is not a required nutrient, vitamin A is essential for health, and beta-carotene is converted into vitamin A in the body. The exact conversion factor varies with the circumstances; in general, 2 micrograms (mcg) of beta-carotene in supplement form is thought to be equivalent to 1 mcg of vitamin A. Plant sterols, used to treat high cholesterol, may impair absorption of beta-carotene.

Dark green and orange-yellow vegetables are good sources of beta-carotene. These include carrots, sweet potatoes, squash, spinach, romaine lettuce, broccoli, apricots, and green peppers.

THERAPEUTIC DOSAGES

It has not been determined whether it is advisable to take dosages of beta-carotene supplements much higher than the recommended allowance for nutritional purposes, which is about 1.5 to 1.8 milligrams (mg) daily in adults. Rather than taking doses higher than this, people should probably increase their intake of fresh fruits and vegetables.

THERAPEUTIC USES

There are no well-documented therapeutic uses of beta-carotene, beyond supplying nutritional doses of vitamin A. Numerous observational studies have found that a high intake of foods rich in carotenoids is associated with a lower incidence of lung cancer, other forms of cancer, and heart disease. However, beta-carotene supplements have not been found to be

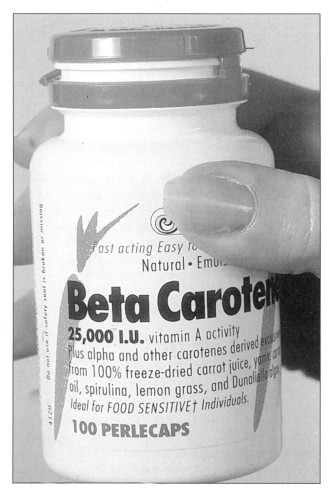

Dietary supplements such as these beta carotene pills have become increasingly popular in the United States, despite a lack of government regulation regarding safety and claims. (SIU School of Medicine)

helpful for preventing these conditions. In fact, when all major beta-carotene studies are statistically combined through a process called meta-analysis, some evidence appears to suggest that long-term usage of beta-carotene at high doses might increase the overall death rate, for reasons that are unclear.

Similarly, observational evidence links high dietary intake of carotenoids to a lower incidence or slowed progression of cataracts, macular degeneration, and osteoarthritis, but again there is no reliable evidence that beta-carotene supplements are helpful for these conditions. In fact, a twelve-year study of more than twenty-two thousand male physicians failed to find that beta-carotene had any effect on the incidence of macular degeneration.

Preliminary evidence raised hopes that beta-carotene supplements might increase or preserve immune function or decrease symptoms among people with human immunodeficiency virus (HIV) infection. However, other studies found no benefit, and some evidence hints that too much beta-carotene might actually be harmful.

Beta-carotene supplements may be helpful for protecting the skin from sunburn, particularly in people with extreme sensitivity to the sun, but the evidence regarding this potential use is somewhat contradictory. One double-blind trial found that faithful daily use of sunscreen was more effective at preventing sun damage to the skin than oral beta-carotene plus sunscreen used as needed.

One preliminary study found evidence that beta-carotene might be helpful for cystic fibrosis, by helping prevent lung infections. Another preliminary study suggests that beta-carotene might help prevent exercise-induced asthma. Weak evidence culled from a large double-blind, placebo-controlled study hints that use of beta-carotene over many years might enhance mental function.

Beta-carotene has been proposed as a treatment for alcoholism, asthma, depression, epilepsy, headaches, heartburn, male infertility, female infertility, Parkinson's disease, psoriasis, rheumatoid arthritis, and schizophrenia, but there is little to no evidence that it works. There is some evidence that beta-carotene is not effective for cervical dysplasia or intermittent claudication.

SCIENTIFIC EVIDENCE

Cancer prevention. The story of beta-carotene and cancer prevention is full of apparent contradictions. It starts in the early 1980s, when the cumulative results of many studies suggested that people who eat a lot of fruits and vegetables are significantly less likely to get cancer. A close look at the data pointed to carotenoids as the active ingredients in fruits and vegetables. It appeared that a high intake of dietary carotene might significantly reduce the risk of lung, bladder, breast, esophageal, and stomach cancers.

However, observational studies cannot prove cause and effect. It is always possible that persons who consume a great deal of carotenoids in their diet are different in other ways; for example, they might exercise more or have healthier lifestyles in other regards.

This is not a purely theoretical issue. For example, based primarily on observational studies, hormone replacement therapy was promoted as a heart-protective treatment for postmenopausal women. However, when placebo-controlled studies were performed, hormone replacement therapy was shown to slightly increase the risk of heart disease. One possible explanation for this discrepancy is that the apparent benefits of hormone replacement therapy were due to the fact that women who used it tended to belong to a higher socioeconomic class than those who did not. (For a variety of reasons, some of which are not known, higher income is associated with improved health.)

Something similar appears to be the case with beta-carotene. Although persons who consume foods high in beta-carotene appear to obtain some protection from heart disease and cancer, when researchers gave beta-carotene supplements to study participants, there was no protective effect. Most studies enrolled people in high-risk groups, such as smokers, because it is easier to see results when researchers look at people who are more likely to develop cancer.

The anticancer bubble burst for beta-carotene in 1994 when the results of the Alpha-Tocopherol, Beta-Carotene (ATBC) study became available. These results showed that beta-carotene supplements did not prevent lung cancer but actually increased the risk of getting it by 18 percent. This trial followed 29,133 male smokers in Finland who took supplements of about 50 international units (IU) of vitamin E (alpha-tocopherol), 20 mg of beta-carotene (more than ten times the amount necessary to provide the daily requirement of vitamin A), both, or placebo daily for five to eight years. (In contrast to the results for beta-carotene, vitamin E was found to reduce the risk of cancer, especially prostate cancer.)

In January 1996 researchers monitoring the Beta-Carotene and Retinol Efficacy Trial (CARET) confirmed the prior bad news with more of their own: the beta-carotene group had 46 percent more cases of lung cancer deaths. This study involved smokers, former smokers, and workers exposed to asbestos. Alarmed, the National Cancer Institute ended the $42 million CARET trial twenty-one months before it was planned to end.

At about the same time, the twelve-year Physicians' Health Study of twenty-two thousand male physicians was finding that 50 mg of beta-carotene (about twenty-five times the amount necessary to provide the daily requirement of vitamin A) taken every other day had no effect, good or bad, on the risk of cancer or heart disease. In this study, 11 percent of the participants were smokers, and 39 percent were former smokers.

Similarly, another study of beta-carotene supplements failed to find any effect on the risk of cancer in women. Also, in a final indictment of beta-carotene's safety and effectiveness, researchers, who combined the results of twelve recent placebo-controlled trials investigating the association between antioxidant supplementation and cancer, found that beta-carotene use was associated with an increased incidence of cancer among smokers. However, the story does not end there. In yet another careful analysis of four randomized trials involving 109,394 smokers and former smokers, researchers found that current smokers who consumed between 20 and 30 mg of beta-carotene were at a significantly greater risk of developing lung cancer. There was no such risk among former smokers.

There are several possible explanations for these apparently contradictory findings. As noted above, it is possible that intake of carotenoids as such is unrelated to cancer and that some unrelated factor common to individuals with a high carotene diet is the cause of the benefits seen in observational trials.

Another possibility is that beta-carotene alone is not effective, and the other carotenoid found in fruits and vegetables may be more important for preventing cancer than beta-carotene. One researcher has suggested that taking beta-carotene supplements depletes the body of these other beneficial carotenoids and thereby causes a harmful effect. In support of this theory, a large study found that consumption of fruits and vegetables is generally associated with lower lung cancer risk, but when beta-carotene is taken, this preventive effect disappears.

Heart disease prevention. The situation with beta-carotene and heart disease is rather similar to that of beta-carotene and cancer. Numerous studies suggest that carotenoids as a whole can help prevent heart disease. However, isolated beta-carotene may not help prevent heart disease and could actually increase a person's risk.

The same double-blind intervention trial involving 29,133 Finnish male smokers (mentioned under the discussion of cancer and beta-carotene) found 11 percent more deaths from heart disease and 15 to 20 percent more strokes in those participants taking beta-carotene supplements.

Similar poor results with beta-carotene were seen in another large, double-blind study of smokers. Beta-carotene supplementation was also found to increase the incidence of angina in smokers.

Osteoarthritis. A high dietary intake of beta-carotene is associated with a significantly slower progression of osteoarthritis, according to a study in which researchers followed 640 individuals over a period of eight to ten years. However, as with heart disease and cancer, it is not known if beta-carotene is responsible for this effect.

HIV support. One small, double-blind study suggested that beta-carotene supplements might raise white blood cell count in people with HIV. However, two subsequent, larger controlled trials found no significant differences between those taking beta-carotene or placebo in white blood cell count, CD4+ count, or other measures of immune function.

Evidence from observational studies suggests that higher intakes of vitamin A or beta-carotene may be helpful; however, caution is in order regarding dosage. Researchers generally linked higher intake of vitamin A or beta-carotene to lower risk of AIDS and lower death rates, with an important exception: people with the highest intake of either nutrient (more than 11,179 IU per day of beta-carotene or more than 20,268 IU per day of vitamin A) did worse than those who took somewhat less.

Macular degeneration and cataracts. Despite promising results from observational studies, intervention trials of beta-carotene for these eye conditions have generally not shown benefit. Beta-carotene proved ineffective for preventing cataracts in one large study, and in another large study, beta-carotene supplements combined with vitamin E and C failed to prevent either macular degeneration or cataracts. On a more positive note, one large study found that beta-carotene supplements helped prevent cataracts in study participants who smoked; nonetheless, no benefit was seen in the group as a whole.

Cervical dysplasia. According to a two-year, double-blind, placebo-controlled study of 141 women with mild cervical dysplasia (a precancerous condition of the cervix), beta-carotene, taken at a dosage of 30 mg daily along with 500 mg of vitamin C, does not help to reverse the dysplasia. Negative results were seen in other trials of beta-carotene as well.

Intermittent claudication. A double-blind, placebo-controlled trial of 1,484 individuals with intermittent claudication found no benefit from beta-carotene (20 mg daily), vitamin E (50 mg daily), or a combination of the two.

Diabetes. In a very large study involving more than twenty-nine thousand male smokers, researchers failed to find benefits from beta-carotene (20 mg/day), alpha-tocopherol (50 IU/day), or the two taken together for the prevention of type 2 diabetes over a five-to eight-year period.

SAFETY ISSUES

At recommended dosages, beta-carotene is believed to be very safe. The only side effects reported from beta-carotene overdose are diarrhea and a yellowish tinge to the hands and feet. These symptoms disappear once a person stops taking beta-carotene or reduces the dose.

However, long-term use of beta-carotene supplements, especially at doses considerably above the amount necessary to supply adequate vitamin A, might slightly increase the risk of heart disease and certain forms of cancer and raise overall death rate. A large study following 77,126 adults over age fifty suggested that long-term use of beta-carotene, lutein, or retinol supplements may increase lung cancer risk. Long-term supplement use was determined by subjects' memory of the previous ten years, so the results of this study should be interpreted with some caution. If the risk of long-term supplementation is a concern, one solution would be to eat plenty of fresh fruits and vegetables to obtain beta-carotene. In addition, some evidence suggests that beta-carotene supplements might cause alcoholic liver disease to develop more rapidly in individuals who abuse alcohol.

EBSCO CAM Review Board

FURTHER READING

Bardia, A., et al. "Efficacy of Antioxidant Supplementation in Reducing Primary Cancer Incidence and Mortality: Systematic Review and Meta-analysis." *Mayo Clinic Proceedings* 83 (2008): 23-34.

Frieling, U. M., et al. "A Randomized, Twelve-Year Primary-Prevention Trial of Beta Carotene Supplementation for Nonmelanoma Skin Cancer in the Physicians' Health Study." *Archives of Dermatology* 136 (2000): 179-184.

Gallicchio, L., et al. "Carotenoids and the Risk of Developing Lung Cancer: A Systematic Review." *American Journal of Clinical Nutrition* 88 (2008): 372-383.

Kataja-Tuomola, M., et al. "Effect of Alpha-tocopherol and Beta-carotene Supplementation on the Incidence of Type 2 Diabetes." *Diabetologia* 51, no. 1 (2008): 47-53.

Keefe, K. A, et al. "A Randomized, Double Blind, Phase III Trial Using Oral Beta-carotene Supplementation for Women with High-Grade Cervical Intraepithelial Neoplasia." *Cancer Epidemiology, Biomarkers and Prevention* 10 (2001): 1029-1035.

Neuhouser, M. L., et al. "Fruits and Vegetables Are Associated with Lower Lung Cancer Risk Only in the Placebo Arm of the Beta-carotene and Retinol Efficacy Trial (CARET)." *Cancer Epidemiology, Biomarkers and Prevention* 12 (2003): 350-358.

Tanvetyanon, T., and G. Bepler. "Beta-carotene in Multivitamins and the Possible Risk of Lung Cancer Among Smokers Versus Former Smokers: A Meta-analysis and Evaluation of National Brands." *Cancer* 113, no. 1 (2008): 150-157.

See also: Cartenoids; Herbal medicine; Vitamin A.

Beta-glucan

CATEGORY: Herbs and supplements
RELATED TERM: Oat bran
DEFINITION: Natural plant product used to treat specific health conditions.
PRINCIPAL PROPOSED USE: High cholesterol
OTHER PROPOSED USE: Immune support

OVERVIEW

The term "beta-glucan" refers to a class of soluble fibers found in many plant sources. The best documented use of beta-glucan involves improving heart health; the evidence for benefit is strong enough that the U.S. Food and Drug Administration (FDA) has allowed a "heart healthy" label claim for food products containing substantial amounts of beta-glucan. Much weaker evidence supports the potential use of certain beta-glucan products for modifying the activity of the immune system.

REQUIREMENTS AND SOURCES

Beta-glucan is not an essential nutrient. It is found in whole grains (especially oats, wheat, and barley) and fungi such as baker's yeast, *Coriolus versi-*

color, and the medicinal mushrooms maitake and reishi.

Different food sources contain differing amounts of the various chemical constituents collectively called beta-glucan. Grains primarily contain beta-1,3-glucan and beta-1,4-glucan. Fungal sources contain a mixture of beta-1,3-glucan, and purified products containing only the 1,3 form are also available.

THERAPEUTIC DOSAGES

For improving total and LDL cholesterol, studies have found benefit with beta-glucan at doses ranging from 3 to 15 grams (g) daily. However, benefits have been seen more consistently at the higher end of this range, and one carefully designed study found no benefit at 3 g daily.

Beta-glucan products can contain molecules of various average lengths (molecular weight). Some manufacturers claim superior benefits with either high or low molecular weight versions. However, one study failed to find any difference between high molecular weight and low molecular weight beta-glucan for normalizing cholesterol and blood sugar levels.

THERAPEUTIC USES

A substantial, if not entirely consistent, body of evidence indicates that beta-glucan, or foods containing it (especially oats), can modestly improve a person's cholesterol profile. The most reliable benefits have been seen regarding levels of total cholesterol and LDL (low-density lipoprotein, or bad) cholesterol. Modest improvements of up to 10 percent have been seen in studies. Possible improvements in HDL (high-density lipoprotein, or good) cholesterol have been seen only inconsistently. It is thought that beta-glucan reduces cholesterol levels by increasing excretion of cholesterol from the digestive tract. This affects two forms of cholesterol: cholesterol from food, and, more important, cholesterol from the blood "recycled" by the liver through the intestines. However, virtually all studies involved oats and were conducted by manufacturers of oat products; independent confirmation remains minimal.

Beta-glucan may also modestly improve blood pressure levels, though not all studies agree. In addition, beta-glucan may help limit the rise in blood sugar that occurs after a meal. This could, in theory, offer heart-healthy benefits, especially in people with diabetes.

The other primary proposed use of beta-glucan products involves effects on the immune system. Test tube, animal, and a few controlled studies in humans suggest that beta-glucans can alter various measurements of immune function. In the alternative medicine literature, these effects are commonly summarized as indicating that beta-glucan is an "immune stimulant." This description, however, is an oversimplification. The immune system is extraordinarily complicated and, as yet, incompletely understood. At the current level of scientific understanding, it is not possible to characterize the effects of beta-glucan more specifically than to say that it has "immunomodulatory" actions, or that it is a "biological response modifier." These intentionally unsensational terms indicate that it is known that beta-glucan affects (modulates) immune function, not that it improves immune function. Some of the immune-related effects seen in studies include alterations in the activity of certain white blood cells and changes in the levels or actions of substances, called cytokines, that modulate immune function.

Based on these largely theoretical findings, as well a small number of very preliminary human trials, various beta-glucan products have been advocated for the treatment of conditions as diverse as allergic rhinitis, cancer, infections, and sepsis (overwhelming infection following major trauma, illness, or surgery). However, the evidence for actual clinical benefit remains highly preliminary.

One study failed to find that beta-1,3-glucan (in topical gel form) was helpful for treatment of actinic keratosis, a form of sun-induced precancerous changes seen in aging skin. Another study found that it had no significant effect on periodontal disease (gingivitis), an inflammation of the gums caused by bacteria found in dental plaques.

SAFETY ISSUES

Beta-glucan, as a substance widely present in foods, is thought to have a high margin of safety. However, if it really does activate the immune system, harmful effects are at least theoretically possible in people with conditions in which the immune system is overactive. These include multiple sclerosis, lupus, rheumatoid arthritis, asthma, inflammatory bowel disease, and hundreds of others conditions. In addition, people taking immunosuppressant drugs following organ transplantation surgery could, in theory, increase their risk of organ rejection. However, there are no reports as yet to indicate that any of these hypothetical problems have actually occurred. Maximum safe doses in young children, pregnant or nursing women, or people with severe liver or kidney disease have not been established.

EBSCO CAM Review Board

FURTHER READING

Davy, B. M., et al. "Oat Consumption Does Not Affect Resting Casual and Ambulatory 24-H Arterial Blood Pressure in Men with High-Normal Blood Pressure to Stage I Hypertension." *Journal of Nutrition* 132 (2002): 394-398.

Jenkins, A. L., et al. "Depression of the Glycemic Index by High Levels of Beta-glucan Fiber in Two Functional Foods Tested in Type 2 Diabetes." *European Journal of Clinical Nutrition* 56 (2002): 622-628.

Jenkins, D. J., et al. "Soluble Fiber Intake at a Dose Approved by the U.S. Food and Drug Administration for a Claim of Health Benefits: Serum Lipid Risk Factors for Cardiovascular Disease Assessed in a Randomized Controlled Crossover Trial." *American Journal of Clinical Nutrition* 75 (2002): 834-839.

Keogh, G. F., et al. "Randomized Controlled Crossover Study of the Effect of a Highly Beta-glucan-Enriched Barley on Cardiovascular Disease Risk Factors in Mildly Hypercholesterolemic Men." *American Journal of Clinical Nutrition* 78 (2003): 711-718.

Kirmaz, C., et al. "Effects of Glucan Treatment on the Th1/Th2 Balance in Patients with Allergic Rhinitis." *European Cytokine Network* 16 (2005): 128-134.

Onning, G., et al. "Consumption of Oat Milk for Five Weeks Lowers Serum Cholesterol and LDL Cholesterol in Free-Living Men with Moderate Hypercholesterolemia." *Annals of Nutrition and Metabolism* 43 (2000): 301-309.

Pins, J. J., et al. "Do Whole-Grain Oat Cereals Reduce the Need for Antihypertensive Medications and Improve Blood Pressure Control?" *Journal of Family Practice* 51 (2002): 353-359.

See also: Cholesterol, high; Herbal medicine; Oat straw.

Betaine hydrochloride

CATEGORY: Herbs and supplements
DEFINITION: Natural substance used to treat specific health conditions.

PRINCIPAL PROPOSED USES: None
OTHER PROPOSED USES: Asthma, digestive problems, excess *Candida*, food allergies, hay fever, heartburn, lupus, rheumatoid arthritis, ulcers

OVERVIEW

When taken as a supplement, betaine hydrochloride, an acidic form of betaine (a natural substance that is found in foods, such as grains), provides extra hydrochloric acid in the stomach. A major branch of alternative medicine known as naturopathy has long held that low stomach acid is a widespread problem that interferes with digestion and the absorption of nutrients. Betaine hydrochloride is one of the most common recommendations for this proposed condition, along with apple cider vinegar, a folk remedy.

Betaine without the hydrochloride molecule attached is also sold as a supplement. In this chemically different form, it is called trimethylglycine; it is not acidic, and it has completely different properties.

REQUIREMENTS AND SOURCES

Betaine hydrochloride is not an essential nutrient, and no food sources exist.

THERAPEUTIC DOSAGES

Betaine hydrochloride is typically taken in pill form at dosages ranging from 325 to 650 milligrams (mg) with each meal.

THERAPEUTIC USES

Based on theories about the importance of stomach acid to overall health, betaine hydrochloride has been recommended for a wide variety of problems, including asthma, digestive problems, excess *Candida*, food allergies, hay fever, lupus, and rheumatoid arthritis. When one sees such broadly encompassing uses, it is not surprising to find that there is no real scientific research on its effectiveness for any of these conditions.

Many naturopathic physicians also believe that betaine hydrochloride can heal ulcers and esophageal reflux (heartburn). This sounds paradoxical, because conventional treatment for those conditions involves reducing stomach acid, while betaine hydrochloride increases it. However, according to one theory, lack of stomach acid leads to incomplete digestion of proteins, and these proteins cause allergic reactions and other responses that lead to digestive problems, which in turn cause ulcers and heartburn. Again, scientific evidence is lacking.

SAFETY ISSUES

Betaine hydrochloride should not be used by those with ulcers or esophageal reflux (heartburn) except on the advice of a physician. This supplement seldom causes any obvious side effects, but it has not been put through rigorous safety studies. In particular, safety for young children, pregnant or nursing women, or those with severe liver or kidney disease has not been established.

EBSCO CAM Review Board

FURTHER READING

Pereira, R. S. "Regression of Gastroesophageal Reflux Disease Symptoms Using Dietary Supplementation with Melatonin, Vitamins, and Amino Acids: Comparison with Omeprazole." *Journal of Pineal Research* 41, (2006): 195-200.

See also: Gastroesophageal reflux disease; Gastrointestinal health; Herbal medicine; Naturopathy; Proton pump inhibitors; Ulcers.

Beta-sitosterol

CATEGORY: Herbs and supplements
DEFINITION: Natural plant product used to treat specific health conditions.
PRINCIPAL PROPOSED USE: Benign prostatic hyperplasia
OTHER PROPOSED USES: Immune support, sports and fitness support

OVERVIEW

Numerous plants contain cholesterol-like compounds called sitosterols and their close relatives, sitosterolins. A special mixture of these called beta-sitosterol is used for the treatment of benign prostatic hyperplasia (BPH).

THERAPEUTIC USES

For whatever reason, there seem to be more useful herbal treatments for BPH than for almost any other disease. Beta-sitosterol joins saw palmetto, pygeum,

nettle, and grass pollen as a moderately well-documented treatment for BPH.

Based on highly preliminary evidence, it has been suggested that sitosterols may also help strengthen the immune system. In particular, one study suggests that beta-sitosterol can help prevent the temporary immune weakness that typically occurs during recovery from endurance exercise and can lead to a post-race infection.

SCIENTIFIC EVIDENCE

A review of the literature, published in 1999, found a total of four double-blind placebo-controlled studies on beta-sitosterol for BPH, enrolling a total of 519 men. All but one of these studies found significant benefits in both perceived symptoms and objective measurements, such as urine flow rate.

The largest study followed 200 men with BPH for a period of six months. After the trial was completed, many of the participants were followed for an additional year, during which the benefits continued. Similar results were seen in a six-month, double-blind trial of 177 individuals.

Beta-sitosterol binds to prostate tissue and affects the metabolism of prostaglandins, substances found in the body that affect pain and inflammation. However, it is not clear whether this is the correct explanation for how beta-sitosterol might help in BPH.

SAFETY ISSUES

Although detailed safety studies have not been performed, beta-sitosterol is believed to be safe. No significant side effects or drug interactions have been reported.

EBSCO CAM Review Board

FURTHER READING

Berges, R. R., A. Kassen, and T. Senge. "Treatment of Symptomatic Benign Prostatic Hyperplasia with Beta-sitosterol: An Eighteen-Month Follow-up." *British Journal of Urology International* 85 (2000): 842-846.

Bouic, P. J. D., et al. "The Effects of B-sitosterol (BSS) and B-sitosterol Glucoside (BSSG) Mixture on Selected Immune Parameters of Marathon Runners: Inhibition of Post Marathon Immune Suppression and Inflammation." *International Journal of Sports Medicine* 20 (1999): 258-262.

Wilt, T. J., R. MacDonald, and A. Ishani. "Beta-sitosterol for the Treatment of Benign Prostatic Hyperplasia."

British Journal of Urology International 83 (1999): 976-983.

See also: Grass pollen extract; Herbal medicine; Nettle; Pygeum; Saw palmetto.

Bilberry

CATEGORY: Herbs and supplements
RELATED TERMS: European blueberry, *Vaccinium myrtillus*
DEFINITION: Natural plant product used to treat specific health conditions.
PRINCIPAL PROPOSED USES: None
OTHER PROPOSED USES: Diabetes, diabetic retinopathy, easy bruising, hemorrhoids, minor injuries, surgery support, varicose veins
Probably not effective use: Poor night vision

OVERVIEW

Often called European blueberry, bilberry is closely related to American blueberry, cranberry, and huckleberry. Its meat is creamy white instead of purple, but it is traditionally used, like blueberries, in the preparation of jams, pies, cobblers, and cakes.

Bilberry fruit also has a long medicinal history. In the twelfth century, Abbess Hildegard of Bingen wrote of bilberry's usefulness for inducing menstruation. Over subsequent centuries, the list of uses for bilberry grew to include a bewildering variety of possibilities, from bladder stones to typhoid fever.

THERAPEUTIC DOSAGES

The standard dosage of bilberry is 120 to 240 milligrams (mg) twice daily of an extract standardized to contain 25 percent anthocyanosides.

Selected Alternate Names for Bilberry

Arándano, bilberry fruit, bilberry leaf, black whortles, bleaberry, blueberry, brimbelle, burren myrtle, dwarf bilberry, dyeberry, European bilberry, fruit de myrtille, huckleberry, hurtleberry, mauret, myrtille, *Myrtilli fructus*, raisin des bois, Swedish bilberry, trackleberry, *Vaccinium myrtillus*, whortleberry, wineberry

THERAPEUTIC USES

The modern use of bilberry dates back to World War II, when British Royal Air Force pilots reported that a good dose of bilberry jam just prior to a mission improved their night vision, often dramatically. Subsequent investigation showed that bilberry contains biologically active substances known as anthocyanosides. Some evidence suggests that anthocyanosides may benefit the retina, as well as strengthen the walls of blood vessels, reduce inflammation, and stabilize tissues containing collagen (such as tendons, ligaments, and cartilage).

However, neither anecdote nor basic scientific evidence of this type can prove a treatment effective. Only double-blind, placebo-controlled studies can do that. Regarding night vision, the balance of the evidence suggests that bilberry is not helpful. Slight evidence hints that bilberry might be helpful for diabetic retinopathy. One double-blind study suggests that bilberry might be helpful for hemorrhoids.

Finally, because the anthocyanosides in bilberry resemble the oligomeric proanthocyanidin complexes (OPCs) found in grape seed and pine bark, bilberry has been recommended for all the same uses as those substances, including easy bruising, varicose veins, minor injuries, and surgery support. Animal studies also suggest that bilberry leaves (rather than the fruit) may be helpful for improving blood sugar control in diabetes and also in lowering blood triglycerides.

SCIENTIFIC EVIDENCE

Night vision. A double-blind crossover trial of fifteen individuals found no short- or long-term improvements in night vision attributable to bilberry. Similarly negative results were seen in a double-blind, placebo-controlled crossover trial of eighteen subjects and another of sixteen subjects.

In contrast, two much earlier controlled, but not double-blind, studies of bilberry found that the herb temporarily improved night vision. However, the effect was not found to persist with continued use. A later double-blind, placebo-controlled study on forty healthy subjects found that a single dose of bilberry extract improved visual response for two hours. Visual benefits have also been reported in other small trials, but these studies did not use a placebo control group and are therefore not valid as evidence.

Hemorrhoids. In a four-week, double-blind, placebo-controlled study of forty people with hemorrhoids, oral use of bilberry extract significantly reduced hemorrhoid symptoms compared with a placebo.

Diabetic retinopathy. A double-blind, placebo-controlled trial of bilberry extract in fourteen people with diabetic retinopathy or hypertensive retinopathy (damage to the retina caused by diabetes or hypertension, respectively) found significant improvements in the treated group. However, the small size of this study makes the results less than fully reliable. Other studies are also cited as indicating benefits, but they were not double-blind and therefore mean little.

SAFETY ISSUES

Bilberry fruit is a food and, as such, is quite safe. Enormous quantities have been administered to rats without toxic effects. One study of 2,295 people given bilberry extract found a 4 percent incidence of side effects such as mild digestive distress, skin rashes, and drowsiness. Although safety in pregnancy has not been proven, clinical trials have enrolled pregnant women. Safety in young children, nursing women, or those with severe liver or kidney disease is not known. There are no known drug interactions. Bilberry does not appear to interfere with blood clotting.

Little is known about the safety of bilberry leaf. Based on animal evidence that it can reduce blood sugar levels in people with diabetes, it is possible that use of bilberry leaf by people with diabetes could require a reduction in drug dosage. Those taking medications to reduce blood sugar may find that bilberry leaf (not fruit) amplifies the effect, and they may need to reduce their dose of medication.

EBSCO CAM Review Board

FURTHER READING

Bone, K. "Bilberry: The Vision Herb." *MediHerb Professional Review* 59 (1997): 1-4.

Levy, Y., and Y. Glovinsky. "The Effect of Anthocyanosides on Night Vision." *Eye* 12 (1998): 967-969.

Muth, E. R., J. M. Laurent, and P. Jasper. "The Effect of Bilberry Nutritional Supplementation on Night Visual Acuity and Contrast Sensitivity." *Alternative Medicine Review* 5 (2000): 164-173.

Zadok, D., et al. "The Effect of Anthocyanosides on Night Vision Tests." *Investigative Ophthalmology and Visual Science* 38 (1997): 633.

See also: Cranberry; Herbal medicine; Night vision, impaired.

Bile acid sequestrant drugs

CATEGORY: Drug interactions
DEFINITION: A drug used to lower levels of cholesterol.
INTERACTION: Many nutrients
DRUGS IN THIS FAMILY: Colestipol hydrochloride (Colestid), cholestyramine resin (Locholest, Prevalite, Questran, Questran Light)

NUTRIENTS

Effect: Supplementation Likely Helpful

Bile acid sequestrants have been reported to impair the absorption of numerous nutrients, including calcium, folate, iron, vitamin A, vitamin B_{12}, and vitamin E. It appears, however, that only folate supplementation may be needed by persons on long-term therapy with bile acid sequestrants. Although the bile acid sequestrant used in the studies interfered with the absorption of the other nutrients, their levels remained in the normal range. Just to be safe, though, one should be sure to get enough vitamin E and vitamin A (in the form of beta-carotene).

EBSCO CAM Review Board

FURTHER READING

West, R. J., and J. K. Lloyd. "The Effect of Cholestyramine on Intestinal Absorption." *Gut* 16 (1975): 93-98.

See also: Calcium; Cholesterol, high; Folate; Food and Drug Administration; Iron; Supplements: Introduction; Vitamin A; Vitamin B_{12}; Vitamin E; Vitamins and minerals.

Biochemic tissue salt therapy

CATEGORY: Therapies and techniques
RELATED TERMS: Cell salts, mineral salts, tissue salts
DEFINITION: A treatment that uses inorganic mineral salts.
PRINCIPAL PROPOSED USES: Allergies, anxiety, cold symptoms, depression, headaches, minor skin conditions, muscle aches, stomach upset
OTHER PROPOSED USES: Blisters, chronic cold feet, dandruff, dizziness, dry skin, earache, fatigue, hemorrhoids, hiccups, irritability, nervous asthma, pimples, sinusitis, sleeplessness, swollen glands, tonsillitis

OVERVIEW

Biochemic tissue salts are minerals discovered in the 1870s by Wilhelm Heinrich Schüssler, a German scientist and homeopathic doctor. Schüssler believed that a proper balance of these salts is essential in maintaining normal organ, tissue, muscle, and cell function. Any disruption in this balance weakens the body, making it more susceptible to illness. Biochemic tissue salts include calcium fluoride, calcium phosphate, calcium sulfate, potassium chloride, potassium phosphate, potassium sulfate, sodium phosphate, sodium sulfate, sodium chloride, ferric pyrophosphate, magnesium phosphate, and silica.

MECHANISM OF ACTION

Biochemic tissue salt therapy is used to diagnose and treat minor ailments. Each salt in the therapy has its own properties and produces unique symptoms when deficient. Replenishing the deficient salt or salts eliminates the symptoms and reestablishes balance, good health, and optimal bodily functioning.

USES AND APPLICATIONS

Biochemic tissue salt therapy is used to treat cold symptoms (coughs, congestion, sore throat), allergies (hay fever), headaches, anxiety, stomach upsets (indigestion, heartburn, cramps), depression, muscle aches, and minor skin conditions. It can be used alone or in combination with conventional or alternative and complementary therapies.

SCIENTIFIC EVIDENCE

Biochemic tissue salt therapy has been used for many years to treat a multitude of ailments. However, most of the evidence supporting its effectiveness is anecdotal (as "provings") and has not been scientifically validated by Western standards.

Proving was developed in the nineteenth century by Samuel Hahnemann, the founder of homeopathy, as a method of testing the efficacy of a substance by observing what symptoms occurred after that substance's use. Although these observations suggest some beneficial aspects of biochemic tissue salt therapy, no randomized, double-blind, placebo-controlled clinical trials exist to support the therapy as an effective treatment for any specific condition.

Studying the effectiveness of biochemic tissue salt therapy is difficult using current Western scientific methods. Efficacy data are frequently unavailable be-

cause of flaws in study design; these flaws include inadequate "blinding" procedures, control groups, treatment length, and enrollment. Furthermore, the high dilution of these tissue salts can cause problems with reliably measuring effects and with duplicating studies.

Regardless, biochemic tissue salt therapy remains an appealing treatment option for a variety of ailments. However, rigorous research is needed to determine its clinical effectiveness.

CHOOSING A PRACTITIONER

Biochemic tissue salts should be prescribed by qualified homeopaths, naturopaths, and herbalists.

SAFETY ISSUES

Biochemic tissue salts are widely available, nonhabit forming, and safe at typical-use levels. However, one should consult a health care professional before beginning treatment.

Rose Ciulla-Bohling, Ph.D.

FURTHER READING

Boericke, William, and Willis A. Dewey. *The Twelve Tissue Remedies of Schüssler.* 6th ed. New Delhi, India: B. Jain, 2005.
Card, David R. *Twelve Essential Minerals for Cellular Health: An Introduction to Cell Salts.* Prescott, Ariz.: Hohm Press, 2007.
Lennon, Nigey, and Lionel Rolfe. *Homeopathic Cell Salt Remedies: Healing with Nature's Twelve Mineral Compounds.* Garden City Park, N.Y.: Square One, 2004.

See also: Balneotherapy; Chelation therapy; Homeopathy; Hydrotherapy; Naturopathy.

Bioenergetics

CATEGORY: Therapies and techniques
DEFINITION: The study of energy transfer between all living systems.

OVERVIEW

Bioenergetics uses the electromagnetic energy fields of the body to determine discrepancies and weakness in the electrical facet of the human cell and tissue in effort to repair the concern before physiological damage can occur. The process uses energy from the body itself to facilitate the healing process.

Mechanism of Action

The main challenge in disease is over-acidification during trauma and injury, causing a lack of blood flow and oxygen to the area, resulting in swelling and changes in the pH and polarity of the tissue. Bioenergetic therapy using magnets can increase oxidation and overall reduce the amount of acid in the body, allowing it to heal itself rapidly.

Magnets can have a direct effect on acidity and alkalinity on tissues, specifically the pH. As the pH increases or decreases, the area is said to be alkalotic or acidic, respectively. In an acidic environment, the areas affected can become solid and smaller and eventually degenerate. During times of increased pH, bodies can swell. Using the methods of bioenergetics, magnets can cancel out the charges and return the body to a steady state and allow the body to heal itself in a swift manner.

Uses and Applications

Bioenergetics can assist the body in the healing in many diseases, among them lower respiratory infections, HIV, malaria, diarrhea, tuberculosis, measles, pertussis, meningitis, and syphilis.

Scientific Evidence

In 1988, Richard Broeringmeyer spoke of a "short leg phenomenon," in which he noticed that when astronauts from the National Aeronautics and Space Administration returned from space, one of their limbs was shorter than the other. Their bodies being away from the earth's magnetic influence caused a disruption in the polarity of the organs. Using magnets and returning the body to a normal state allowed the body to heal itself and bring the affected limb back to standard length. Organs and tissues can be magnetically polarized; leaving a magnet on muscle tissue will lead to depolarization.

Robert O. Becker observed that when an injury occurs, the injured area conveys a magnetically positive charge as a signal of damage and a negative charge as a measure of healing. When using magnets, these processes can be quickened, and the amount of time needed for healing is vastly reduced.

Isaac Goiz stated that magnets organize and stabilize cells so that the body can heal itself. He noticed that bacteria and viruses apparently travel within the body along magnetic lines. For example, the rabies virus consistently prefers to migrate to the axilla, *Clostridium tetani* to the kidneys, and anthrax bacilli to the brain. Using magnets, each pathogen then can be eradicated or greatly weakened by the body.

Safety Issues

In contrast to pharmaceutical drugs and other medical treatments, bioenergetics therapy and treatment apparently have no adverse effects.

Vibu Varghese, M.S.

Further Reading

Kahn, Sherry. *Healing Magnets: A Guide for Pain Relief, Speeding Recovery, and Restoring Balance*. New York: Three Rivers Press, 2000.

Philpot, William H., et al. *Magnet Therapy: An Alternative Medicine Definitive Guide*. Tiburon, Calif.: Alternative Medicine Books, 2000.

See also: Energy medicine; Magnet therapy.

Biofeedback

Category: Therapies and techniques
Definition: Complementary and alternative therapy involving control over bodily processes through mental suggestion.
Principal proposed use: High blood pressure
Other proposed uses: Anxiety, back pain, constipation, female stress incontinence, insomnia, migraine headaches, pain in general, Raynaud's phenomenon, rehabilitation from strokes, stress, tension headaches

Overview

Some functions in the body, such as heart rate and blood pressure, occur automatically, outside conscious control. Biofeedback is a method of making those involuntary processes something a person can do at will.

The basic method is quite simple. In biofeedback, a machine provides direct information regarding the bodily process in question (the "feedback" part of the term "biofeedback"). Given this information, a person can find a way to control the bodily process, just like

Neurofeedback

Neurofeedback, also called electroencephalogram (EEG) feedback, is the most controversial form of biofeedback therapy, largely because so few controlled clinical trials have been able to assess its efficacy. Neurofeedback is the "retraining" of brain-wave patterns. Although controversial, it is experiencing a resurgence of interest in the treatment of a variety of disorders, including depression, attention deficit hyperactivity disorder (ADHD), and alcoholism.

In a neurofeedback training session, several sensors that measure the brain's electrical activity are attached to a participant's scalp. The person relaxes and plays a video game, which is controlled just by the brain waves and responds favorably to brain waves of the desired pattern. As one plays the game, the trainer observes the participant's EEG, transmitted to a separate video terminal. Most practitioners recommend a minimum of twenty sessions to obtain significant, long-lasting results, although improvement is usually noted early on if the treatment protocol is right. Because the field is new, many practitioners have little or no experience beyond a week-long training session, so one should consult a primary care provider before embarking on a treatment program.

Reviewed by Brian Randall, M.D.

some can learn to wiggle their ears if they try hard enough.

For example, in biofeedback, a person's blood pressure might be displayed on a screen. Blood pressure naturally goes up and down from time to time. A person will notice when the pressure goes down and will feel pleased; when the pressure goes up, the person will feel displeased. Pleasure and displeasure act like the reward and punishment technique used for training animals. When a rat in a maze is rewarded with food for going the right way and is given an electric shock for going the wrong way, it will soon learn to go the right way. Similarly, the unconscious parts of the nervous system figure out a way to get a "reward" instead of "punishment." In the case just described, the way to get a reward is to reduce one's blood pressure.

The display screen provides the feedback because normally a person cannot detect his or her own blood pressure. Using a machine to provide that information allows the person to achieve conscious control. This process generally works. After a number of sessions, most people reach a place where they can lower their blood pressure simply by thinking "I want my blood pressure to fall." In addition to measuring blood

pressure and heart rate, there are biofeedback machines in fairly common use that measure muscle tension, skin temperature, skin resistance to electricity, and brain wave activity.

USES AND APPLICATIONS

Probably the most common use of biofeedback is to treat stress and stress-related conditions, including anxiety, insomnia, high blood pressure, fibromyalgia, muscle pain, migraine headaches, and tension headaches.

SCIENTIFIC EVIDENCE

Although many studies have evaluated biofeedback, most of them are inadequately designed. Only one form of study can truly prove that a treatment is effective: the double-blind, placebo-controlled trial. However, it is somewhat tricky to fit biofeedback into a study design of this type. The main problem is finding a placebo for biofeedback treatment.

In the best-designed studies of biofeedback, people in the placebo group practice biofeedback with a machine that produces carefully garbled information. Study participants in this group believe they are practicing biofeedback, but in fact they are not learning any conscious control over the body process in question.

Many biofeedback studies do not use placebo biofeedback; they compare biofeedback to no treatment. Studies of this type cannot provide reliable evidence about the efficacy of a treatment. If a benefit is seen, there is no way to determine whether biofeedback caused it or whether it was caused generically by attention. (Attention alone will almost always produce some reported benefit.)

Other trials used intentionally neutral therapies, such as the use of a home diary. These are better than studies with a no-treatment control group. However, when the placebo is so different in form than the treatment under study, any apparent differences in outcome could simply represent differences in the power of suggestion in each approach.

Still other studies simply involved giving people

biofeedback and seeing whether they improved. Such trials are almost completely meaningless; numerous studies have shown that both participants and examining physicians will frequently think they observe improvement in people given a treatment, regardless of whether the treatment does anything on its own. For example, early studies of biofeedback for stroke rehabilitation that did not use blinding or a control group reported miraculous successes equivalent to the "throw down your crutches and walk" cliché. However, when controlled trials were performed, it turned out that biofeedback did not provide much more than marginal benefit, if any.

Possible effects of biofeedback. Of all the medical conditions for which biofeedback has been advocated, the best studied is hypertension. However, a review of the literature published in 2003, which found twenty-two controlled trials of acceptable quality, concluded that real biofeedback is not more effective than fake biofeedback. A study published subsequent to this review did report benefits, but the study was poorly designed. In addition, a 2010 review of thirty-six trials involving 1,660 persons found no consistent evidence that biofeedback's effectiveness for hypertension compared with the effectiveness of other behavioral therapies, drug therapy, placebo, or no intervention.

Biofeedback also has been studied for other medical conditions. A minimum of one controlled study supports the use of biofeedback for each of the following: anxiety, chronic low-back pain, female stress incontinence, incontinence associated with radical prostatectomy, insomnia, and, possibly, rehabilitation from strokes. The evidence of benefit with biofeedback is not definitive for any of these conditions, and in many cases there are also studies with negative outcomes.

There is mixed evidence for the effectiveness of biofeedback for recurrent headaches, both migraine and tension. In a detailed review of multiple controlled studies, however, researchers concluded that biofeedback is useful for tension headaches, particularly when combined with other relaxation therapies. In another review of ninety-four studies, researchers concluded that biofeedback is capable of significantly reducing the frequency of both migraine and tension-type headaches, among other benefits. However, it is important to note that not all of the studies they used to arrive at this conclusion were randomized, placebo-controlled trials.

The balance of the evidence suggests that biofeedback is not effective for asthma and is no more than marginally effective for Raynaud's phenomenon. Evidence is mixed regarding biofeedback's effectiveness for constipation and fecal incontinence. However, a number of small trials have found biofeedback to be more effective than standard therapies alone for constipation related to pelvic floor dysfunction.

WHAT TO EXPECT DURING TREATMENT

Biofeedback training involves the use of a machine that relays information about the aspect of the body that one wishes to control. In early stages, one has to find the "muscles" necessary to produce the desired effect. Typically, a biofeedback practitioner will teach a series of visualizations and other mental exercises in the hope that it will facilitate the process. For example, a person with high blood pressure might be asked to imagine the blood vessels in his or her body opening up and dilating.

CHOOSING A PRACTITIONER

As with all medical therapies, it is best to choose a licensed practitioner. Where licensure is not available, one should seek a referral from a qualified and knowledgeable health-care provider.

SAFETY ISSUES

There are no known safety risks with biofeedback.

EBSCO CAM Review Board

FURTHER READING

Dhanani, N. M., T. J. Caruso, and A. J. Carinci. "Complementary and Alternative Medicine for Pain." *Current Pain and Headache Reports* (November 10, 2010).

Greenhalgh, J., R. Dickson, and Y. Dundar. "Biofeedback for Hypertension." *Journal of Hypertension* 28 (2010): 644-652.

McGrady, A. "The Effects of Biofeedback in Diabetes and Essential Hypertension." *Cleveland Clinic Journal of Medicine* 77, suppl. 3 (2010): S68-S71.

Mariotti, G., et al. "Early Recovery of Urinary Continence After Radical Prostatectomy Using Early Pelvic Floor Electrical Stimulation and Biofeedback Associated Treatment." *Journal of Urology* 181 (2009): 1788-1793.

Nestoriuc, Y., W. Rief, and A. Martin. "Meta-analysis of Biofeedback for Tension-Type Headache: Efficacy,

Specificity, and Treatment Moderators." *Journal of Consulting and Clinical Psychology* 76 (2008): 379-396.

Tsai, P. S., et al. "Blood Pressure Biofeedback Exerts Intermediate-Term Effects on Blood Pressure and Pressure Reactivity in Individuals with Mild Hypertension." *Journal of Alternative and Complementary Medicine* 13 (2007): 547-554.

See also: Hypertension; Mind/body medicine.

Biofeedback for the headache

CATEGORY: Therapies and techniques
DEFINITION: Therapy involving the use of sensors attached to the body.

OVERVIEW

Biofeedback is the body's cued response to its physiologic state. These responses include scratching an itch, grabbing a snack when hungry, and using the toilet when feeling the urge.

With biofeedback training, however, a person is cued by sensors attached to the body. These sensors measure heart rate, the temperature of extremities, the muscle tension in specific muscle groups, or, in neurofeedback, the kinds of brainwaves a person is emitting. This information is conveyed by visual displays or sounds.

Using imagery and mental exercises, one learns to control these functions, using the feedback provided by the sensors as a gauge of success. With practice, a person can learn to "tune in" without instruments and to control these functions at will.

MODES OF ACTION

In a biofeedback training session for headache, temperature sensors are attached first to the hands, then to the feet, and finally to the forehead, if needed. The goal is to increase blood flow away from the brain by raising the temperature in the hands and feet and eventually lowering it in the temples. Other sensors might monitor a person's electrodermal or galvanic skin response, that is, how easily one sweats or gets goose bumps, because this affects a person's ability to alter his or her skin temperature.

In biofeedback, warming up one's hands and feet might involve imagining oneself basking in the sun on a beach while listening to a script such as "I feel warm. My hands are growing warm and heavy." Both the image and the script would be personally tailored to evoke a vivid and relaxing mental image. After the training session, the person would be sent home with this recorded script and with small thermometers to use in daily practice.

NEUROFEEDBACK

Neurofeedback, also called electroencephalogram (EEG) feedback, is the most controversial form of biofeedback therapy, largely because so few controlled clinical trials have been able to assess its efficacy. Neurofeedback is the "retraining" of brainwave patterns. Although controversial, it is experiencing a resurgence of interest in the treatment of a variety of disorders, including depression, attention deficit disorder (ADD), and alcoholism.

In a neurofeedback training session, several sensors that measure the brain's electrical activity are attached to the scalp. The person relaxes and plays a video game, which is controlled only by the brainwaves and which responds favorably to brainwaves of the desired pattern. As the person plays the game, the trainer observes the EEG, which is transmitted to a separate video terminal. Most practitioners recommend a minimum of twenty sessions to obtain significant, long-lasting results, although improvement is usually noted early on if the treatment protocol is right for the patient.

Linda H. Underhill; reviewed by Brian Randall, M.D.

FURTHER READING

Andrasik, F. "Biofeedback in Headache: An Overview of Approaches and Evidence." *Cleveland Clinic Journal of Medicine* 77, suppl. 3 (2010): S72-S76.

Association for Applied Psychophysiology and Biofeedback. http://www.aapb.org.

Biofeedback Certification Institute of America. http://www.bcia.org.

Walker, J. E. "QEEG-Guided Neurofeedback for Recurrent Migraine Headaches." *Clinical EEG and Neuroscience* 42, no. 1 (2011): 59-61.

See also: Guided imagery; Hypnotherapy; Mental health; Mind/body medicine.

Biologically based therapies

CATEGORY: Issues and overviews
RELATED TERMS: Herbs, natural therapies
DEFINITION: The use of natural substances for general well-being and for the prevention and treatment of illness.

OVERVIEW

Wellness and the allure of nature attract people to biologically based therapies, often known as herbs and herbal medicine. Biologically based products include a variety of natural substances, including herbs, vitamins, minerals, foods, and dietary supplements. Formulations include solids, liquids, or gels and are found in pills, powders, tablets, capsules, teas, syrups, and oils.

Clinical trials for prescription medications generate extensive lists of potential side effects. These lists often lead to apprehension about taking prescription medications. Natural substances, often mistakenly viewed as free of harmful side effects, can interact negatively with prescription medications or other natural substances. (Poison ivy, for example, is a natural substance, but most people experience negative skin rashes after contacting poison ivy.)

USES AND APPLICATIONS

Scientific evidence supports some biologically based therapies, including aromatherapy and milk thistle. Aromatherapies improve infections caused by viruses, bacteria, or fungi, and aromatherapies foster well-being, calm, and feelings of increased energy. Fragrant aromas from plants such as chamomile, lavender, cedar wood, and lemon help with infectious disease and can benefit persons being treated for cancer. Integrative medicine, the combination of alternative and conventional treatments, enables the effective use of many biologically based therapies. Aromatherapy lessens anxiety in persons with cancer who are treated with chemotherapy. Enhanced mood and an improved view of personal health can help persons who are receiving conventional treatment for illnesses such as cancer and infectious disease. Essential oils extracted from aromatic plants have been shown to improve problems associated with infectious agents such as the herpes simplex virus. Reported aromatherapy side effects include allergic reactions and skin rashes.

Milk thistle seeds contain a powerful antioxidant called silymarin, which regenerates diseased liver cells. Studies might demonstrate that milk thistle and its potent ingredient, silymarin, also can help with the treatment of hepatitis and liver cancers. The treatment of liver cancer presents another potential beneficial application for integrative medicine. The effective combined use of silymarin and chemotherapy may improve outcomes and enhance treatment.

The integration of biologically based therapies with conventional medicine can help to avoid problems associated with the use of amygdalin in cancer treatment. Amygdalin, which is found in the pits of fruits such as apricots, is used as an alternative treatment for cancer, but there is little scientific evidence to support its use in cancer treatment. Amygdalin metabolism produces cyanide, a poison that leads to blue skin in humans because it deprives the body of oxygen; it also can lead to liver injury, uncoordinated body movements, and hanging upper eyelids.

Although many persons with cancer are willing to try any available treatment, coordinated medical care can help to better assess the risk and benefits of alternative treatments and better direct efforts toward effective treatment and support.

Some biologically based therapies, such as the use of cranberries, have proven helpful in the prevention of urinary tract infections, but cranberries do not effectively treat existing infections. Sensible integrative medicine involves diagnosis and treatment of urinary tract infections with conventional medicine and the prevention of recurrences with cranberry preparations. Similarly, cranberries may prevent recurrence of stomach ulcers. Cranberries, however, also interact with blood-thinning drugs and with medications metabolized by the liver. Because of the potential for drug interactions, one should discuss the use of alternative therapies with a primary care provider.

No antibiotic treats cold or flu viruses. Colds and flu occur often, and many alternative treatments are available in attempts to treat these conditions. Peppermint, honey, elderberries, and ginseng are some of the biologically based treatments used to treat colds and flu. Although echinacea, zinc, and vitamin C have some scientific evidence supporting their use in decreasing the length of symptoms and in possibly preventing colds and flu, many other biologically based remedies lack scientific support for their routine use.

A reasoned approach to cold and flu prevention involves frequent hand-washing during cold and flu seasons. Consideration of alternatives such as echinacea, zinc, and vitamin C could be added to this preventive base. Research and health care consultation best optimize wellness.

PERSPECTIVES

The regulation of biologically based therapies is much less stringent than the regulation of prescription medications. Critical thinking skills enable effective and safe use of biologically based therapies. One should research alternative therapies using credible sources. One should discuss alternative therapies with conventional health-care providers and should consider one's overall health and potential medication interactions. One could broaden his or her knowledge and understanding of alternative medicine by supporting research initiatives that study alternative therapies. Active and reasoned involvement in available health-care options fosters well-being while enhancing peace of mind.

Richard P. Capriccioso, M.D.

FURTHER READING

Capriccioso, Richard P. "Alternative Therapies." In *Salem Health: Infectious Diseases and Conditions*, vol. 1, edited by H. Bradford Hawley. Pasadena, Calif.: Salem Press, 2011. A comprehensive overview of complementary and alternative categories and therapies with an emphasis on the treatment of infectious diseases.

_____. "Complementary and Alternative Therapies." In *Salem Health: Cancer*, vol. 1, edited by Jeffrey A. Knight. Pasadena, Calif.: Salem Press, 2008. This overview article in a four-volume set surveys complementary and alternative therapies, with an emphasis on cancer treatments.

Fontaine, K. L. *Complementary and Alternative Therapies for Nursing Practice*. 2d ed. Upper Saddle River, N.J.: Prentice Hall/Pearson, 2005. An informative complementary and alternative medicine (CAM) text integrating sections on nursing practice and CAM.

Mayoclinic.com. "Complementary and Alternative Medicine." Available at http://mayoclinic.com/health/alternative-medicine/pn00001. Mayo Clinic staff present useful resources on CAM.

National Center for Complementary and Alternative Medicine. http://nccam.nih.gov. An authoritative and comprehensive source for CAM information and resources. The National Center for Comple-

mentary and Alternative Medicine is part of the National Institutes of Health, serving as the U.S. government's main CAM portal.

Peters, David, and Anne Woodham. *Encyclopedia of Natural Healing*. London: Dorling Kindersley, 2000. A well-illustrated compilation of complementary and alternative medical therapies including information on CAM organizations and practitioners. An interesting CAM first-aid kit is detailed in this book.

See also: Anti-inflammatory diet; Diet-based therapies; Functional foods: Introduction; Functional foods: Overview; Herbal medicine; Macrobiotic diet; Raw foods diet; Vegan diet; Vegetarian diet; Vitamins and minerals.

Biorhythms

CATEGORY: Therapies and techniques
RELATED TERM: Chronobiology
DEFINITION: The theory that natural cycles regulate a person's body, mentation, and emotions.
PRINCIPAL PROPOSED USES: Physiological and psychological optimization
OTHER PROPOSED USES: Industrial safety, sports performance

OVERVIEW

Biorhythm theory was conceived by Wilhelm Fliess, a German physician, and Hermann Swoboda, an Austrian psychologist, in the late nineteenth century. The two believed that basic human functions occur in periods of twenty-three and twenty-eight days. Associating the latter figure with the menstrual cycle, Fliess called the twenty-eight-day cycle female, or emotional, and the twenty-three-day cycle male, or physical. In the 1920s, Alfred Teltscher, an engineering professor, perceived a thirty-three-day intellectual cycle based on observations of his students' performances.

Biorhythms did not claim wide popularity until the 1970s. Subsequently, additional cycles of thirty-eight, forty-three, and fifty-three days were proposed, as were cycles that combine two of the original three.

MECHANISM OF ACTION

Proponents of biorhythms have not identified specific mechanisms that produce them. Each person's biorhythms are said to begin at birth and are afterward regular, although some proponents claim that arrhythmia can occur.

In classic three-cycle theory, the twenty-three-day physical cycle governs coordination, strength, endurance, sexual vigor, metabolism, and resistance to illness. The twenty-eight-day emotional cycle regulates temperament, nervous reactions, fantasy, and desires. The thirty-three-day intellectual cycle affects reasoning, alertness, judgment, memory, and sense of purpose.

The cycles fluctuate like a sine wave (a mathematical function) with positive and negative polarities. The nadir of a cycle's negative polarity is called a critical (or transition) day because it is the least favorable day for an activity associated with the physiological or psychological states managed by a cycle; conversely, the acme of the positive polarity is the most favorable day for such an activity.

USES AND APPLICATIONS

Proponents insist that biorhythm cycles in themselves do not determine behavior because each person's environment influences his or her expression. Rather, biorhythms enable a person to prepare for the best and worst times for any given activity. For instance, a person should not participate in a sport or have surgery on the critical day of the physical cycle, should avoid proposing marriage on the critical day of the emotional cycle, and should not take an examination on the critical day of the intellectual cycle. During the cycles' positive polarities, these activities are more likely to turn out well.

SCIENTIFIC EVIDENCE

Studies supporting biorhythm theory exist but fall short of scientific rigor because they depend upon anecdotal evidence, have statistical or mathematical flaws, or are based on subjective assumptions and ad hoc hypotheses. Peer-reviewed studies and mathematical analyses demonstrate that the predictions of biorhythms are no more accurate than chance.

CHOOSING A PRACTITIONER

Persons wanting to discover their own cycles can do so without the help of a practitioner. Also, Web sites offer special calculators and calendars for this discovery process.

Roger Smith, Ph.D.

FURTHER READING

"Biorhythms." In *The Skeptics Dictionary.* Available at http://www.skepdic.com.

Gittelson, Bernard. *Biorhythm: A Personal Science, 1997-1999.* 10th ed. New York: Grand Central, 1996.

Hines, Terence. "Biorhythm Theory: A Critical Review." In *Paranormal Borderlands of Science,* edited by Kendrick Frazier. Amherst, N.Y.: Prometheus Books, 1991.

_____. *Pseudoscience and the Paranormal.* 2d ed. New York: Prometheus Books, 2003.

West, Peter. *Surf Your Biowaves: Use Your Biorhythms to Bring You Success.* London: Quantum, 1999.

See also: Bioenergetics; Biofeedback; Energy medicine; Pseudoscience; Relaxation therapies.

Biotin

CATEGORY: Herbs and supplements

RELATED TERM: Biocytin (brewer's yeast biotin complex)

DEFINITION: Natural substance used as a supplement to treat specific health conditions.

PRINCIPAL PROPOSED USE: Supplementation during pregnancy

OTHER PROPOSED USES: Brittle nails, cradle cap in children, diabetic neuropathy, improving blood sugar control in diabetes, support for individuals on anticonvulsants

OVERVIEW

Biotin is a water-soluble B vitamin that plays an important role in metabolizing the energy humans obtain from food. Biotin assists four essential enzymes that break down fats, carbohydrates, and proteins.

Biotin deficiency is rare, except, possibly, among pregnant women. All proposed therapeutic uses of biotin supplements are highly speculative.

REQUIREMENTS AND SOURCES

Although biotin is a necessary nutrient, humans usually get enough from bacteria living in the digestive tract. Severe biotin deficiency has been seen in people who frequently eat large quantities of raw egg whites. Raw egg whites contain a protein that blocks

effects of antiseizure drugs. Also, despite promising preliminary indications, a double-blind study failed to find that folate enhances the effect of the drug lithium. Lithium is sometimes sold as a mineral supplement for treating bipolar disorder. However, this proposed use is based on a misunderstanding. When lithium is used medically as treatment for bipolar disorder, it is taken at doses far above any possible nutritional need. No researcher has seriously suggested that lithium deficiency causes bipolar symptoms, and low doses of lithium are unlikely to have any effect.

HERBS AND SUPPLEMENTS TO USE ONLY WITH CAUTION

Antidepressant drugs may cause manic episodes in people with bipolar disorder. For this reason, herbs and supplements with antidepressant properties might also be risky. Case reports suggest that S-adenosylmethionine, St. John's wort, and inositol can trigger manic episodes.

The supplement L-glutamine, while not normally considered to have antidepressant properties, has reportedly triggered episodes of mania in two people not previously known to have bipolar disorder. A ginseng product has also been associated with an episode of mania.

The supplement chromium is often sold in the form of chromium picolinate. Picolinate can alter levels of neurotransmitters. This has led to concern among some experts that chromium picolinate might be harmful to people with bipolar disorder.

It has been suggested that the drug lithium works, in part, by reducing the body's level of vanadium. Persons with bipolar disorder should avoid using supplements that contain vanadium. Numerous herbs and supplements may interact adversely with drugs used to prevent or treat bipolar disorder. For example, people who use lithium should avoid herbal diuretics.

EBSCO CAM Review Board

FURTHER READING

Allan, S. J., et al. "The Effect of Inositol Supplements on the Psoriasis of Patients Taking Lithium." *British Journal of Dermatology* 150 (2004): 966-969.

Attenburrow, M. J., et al. "Chromium Treatment Decreases the Sensitivity of 5-HT(2A) Receptors." *Psychopharmacology* 159 (2002): 432-436.

Dolberg, O. T., et al. "Transcranial Magnetic Stimulation in Patients with Bipolar Depression." *Bipolar Disorders* 4 (2002): 94-95.

Frangou, S., et al. "Efficacy of Ethyl-Eicosapentaenoic Acid in Bipolar Depression." *British Journal of Psychiatry* 188 (2006): 46-50.

Giannini, A. J., et al. "Treatment of Acute Mania with Ambient Air Anionization: Variants of Climactic Heat Stress and Serotonin Syndrome." *Psychological Reports* 100 (2007): 157-163.

Keck, P. E., Jr, et al. "Double-Blind, Randomized, Placebo-Controlled Trials of Ethyl-Eicosapentanoate in the Treatment of Bipolar Depression and Rapid Cycling Bipolar Disorder." *Biological Psychiatry* 60 (2006): 1020.

Lin, P. Y., and K. P. Su. "A Meta-analytic Review of Double-Blind, Placebo-Controlled Trials of Antidepressant Efficacy of Omega-3 Fatty Acids." *Journal of Clinical Psychiatry* 68 (2007): 1056-1061.

Vazquez, I., and L. F. Aguera-Ortiz. "Herbal Products and Serious Side Effects: A Case of Ginseng-Induced Manic Episode." *Acta Psychiatrica Scandinavica* 105 (2002): 76-77.

Zhang, Z. J., et al. "Adjunctive Herbal Medicine with Carbamazepine for Bipolar Disorders." *Journal of Psychiatric Research* 41 (2005): 360-369.

See also: Depression, mild to moderate; Herbal medicine; Lithium; Mental health; Obsessive-compulsive disorder (OCD); Seasonal affective disorder; Tricyclic antidepressants.

Bitter melon

CATEGORY: Herbs and supplements
RELATED TERM: *Momordica charantia*
DEFINITION: Natural plant product used to treat specific health conditions.
PRINCIPAL PROPOSED USE: Diabetes

OVERVIEW

Widely sold in Asian groceries as food, bitter melon is also a folk remedy for diabetes, cancer, and various infections.

THERAPEUTIC DOSAGES

The typical dosage of bitter melon is one small, unripe, raw melon or about 50 to 100 milliliters (ml) of fresh juice, divided into two or three doses over the course of the day. The only problem is that bitter melon tastes extremely bitter.

THERAPEUTIC USES

Bitter melon continues to be advertised as an effective treatment for diabetes, especially of the type 2 variety. However, evidence used to support this claim is limited to animal studies, uncontrolled human trials, and other unreliable forms of evidence. Only double-blind, placebo-controlled studies can prove a treatment effective, and the single such study of bitter melon failed to find any benefit.

In test-tube studies, a protein in bitter melon called MAP-30 kills viruses and slows the growth of some cancer cells. However, it is a long way from the test tube to real people, and there have not as yet been any human trials of bitter melon or its constituents for the treatment of cancer or viral diseases.

SAFETY ISSUES

As a widely eaten food in Asia, bitter melon is often regarded as safe. However, it does appear to present some health risks. The most significant of these comes from the fact that it may work. Combining bitter melon with standard drugs may reduce blood sugar too well, possibly leading to dangerously low blood sugar levels. In fact, there are case reports of two children with diabetes who went into hypoglycemic comas after taking bitter melon. For this reason, persons taking drugs for diabetes should add bitter melon to their diet only with a physician's supervision. Also, one should not stop taking any medications and take bitter melon instead, as it is not as powerful as insulin or other conventional treatments.

Other possible risks include impaired fertility, liver inflammation, and spontaneous abortion. The safety of bitter melon use in young children, nursing women, or those with severe kidney disease has not been established. Those taking medications to reduce blood sugar should be aware that bitter melon might amplify the effect of those medications and that they may need to reduce the dosage.

EBSCO CAM Review Board

FURTHER READING

Ahmad, N., et al. "Effect of *Momordica charantia* (Karolla) Extracts on Fasting and Postprandial Serum Glucose Levels in NIDDM Patients." *Bangladesh Medical Research Council Bulletin* 25 (1999): 11-13.

Basch, E., S. Gabardi, and C. Ulbricht. "Bitter Melon (*Momordica charantia*): A Review of Efficacy and Safety." *American Journal of Health-System Pharmacy* 60 (2003): 356-359.

Dans, A. M., et al. "The Effect of *Momordica charantia* Capsule Preparation on Glycemic Control in Type 2 Diabetes Mellitus Needs Further Studies." *Journal of Clinical Epidemiology* 60 (2007): 554-559.

See also: Diabetes; Herbal medicine.

Black cohosh

CATEGORY: Herbs and supplements
RELATED TERM: *Cimicifuga racemosa*
PRINCIPAL PROPOSED USE: Menopausal symptoms
OTHER PROPOSED USES: Dysmenorrhea (painful menstruation), osteoporosis, premenstrual syndrome

OVERVIEW

Black cohosh is a tall perennial herb originally found in the northeastern United States. Native Americans used it primarily for women's health problems, but also as a treatment for arthritis, fatigue, and snakebite. European colonists rapidly adopted the herb for similar uses. In the late nineteenth century, black cohosh was the principal ingredient in the wildly popular Lydia E. Pinkham's Vegetable Compound for menstrual cramps.

Black cohosh's main use today is for the treatment of menopausal symptoms. Meaningful but far from definitive evidence indicates that black cohosh extract might reduce hot flashes as well as other symptoms of menopause.

THERAPEUTIC DOSAGES

The most commonly used dosage of black cohosh is one or two 20-mg tablets twice daily of a standardized extract, manufactured to contain 1 mg of 27-deoxyactein per tablet. An analysis of eleven available black cohosh products found that three of them contained an Asian herb related to black cohosh rather than the proper herb. Black cohosh should not be confused with the toxic herb blue cohosh (*Caulophyllum thalictroides*).

THERAPEUTIC USES

In the past, black cohosh was believed to be a phytoestrogen, a plant-based substance that has actions similar to estrogen. However, growing evidence indicates that black cohosh does not have general estrogen-like actions. Rather, it may act like estrogen only in certain areas of the body: the brain (reducing hot flashes), bone (potentially fighting osteoporosis), and vagina (reducing vaginal dryness).

Black cohosh has also been tried for reducing hot flashes in women who have undergone surgery for breast cancer, but it does not appear to be effective for this purpose. Finally, black cohosh is sometimes recommended as a kind of general women's herb, said to be effective for a variety of menstrual issues, such as dysmenorrhea, premenstrual syndrome (PMS), and irregular menstruation. However, there is no meaningful evidence that the herb is effective for these conditions.

SCIENTIFIC EVIDENCE

Menopausal symptoms. The body of evidence regarding black cohosh for menopausal symptoms remains incomplete and inconsistent. The best study was a two-week, double-blind, placebo-controlled trial of 304 women with menopausal symptoms. This study appeared to find that black cohosh was more effective than placebo. The best evidence was for a reduction in hot flashes. However, the statistical procedures used in the study were somewhat unusual and open to question.

Promising results were also seen in a three-month, double-blind study of 120 menopausal women. Participants were given either black cohosh or fluoxetine (Prozac). Over the course of the trial, black cohosh proved more effective than fluoxetine for hot flashes, but fluoxetine was more effective than black cohosh for menopause-related mood changes.

Previous smaller studies have found improvements not only in hot flashes but also in other symptoms of menopause. For example, in a double-blind, placebo-controlled study, ninety-seven menopausal women received black cohosh, estrogen, or placebo for three months. The results indicated that the herb reduced overall menopausal symptoms (such as hot flashes) to the same extent as the drug. In addition, microscopic analysis showed that black cohosh had an estrogen-like effect on the cells of the vagina. This is a positive result because it suggests that black cohosh might reduce vaginal thinning. However, black cohosh did not affect the cells of the uterus in an estrogen-like manner; this too is a positive result, as estrogen's effects on the uterus are potentially harmful. Finally, the study found hints that black cohosh might help protect bone. However, a great many of the study participants dropped out, making the results less than reliable.

One study, too small to have reliable results from a statistical point of view, found black cohosh as effective as 0.6 milligrams (mg) daily of conjugated estrogens. A study reported in 2006 found that black cohosh has weak estrogen-like effects on vaginal cells and possible positive effects on bone (specifically, stimulating new bone formation).

An earlier study also found multiple benefits with black cohosh, but its results are difficult to trust. This trial followed eighty women for twelve weeks and compared the effects of black cohosh, estrogen, and placebo. Again, black cohosh improved menopausal symptoms and vaginal cell health. However, in this study estrogen proved less effective than a placebo. This result is so difficult to believe that it casts serious doubt on the meaningfulness of the results.

Several other studies are also often cited as evidence that black cohosh is useful for various symptoms of menopause, but in reality they prove nothing. These trials lacked a placebo group. Although women reported improvements in symptoms, there is no way to know whether black cohosh was responsible. Women given placebo reliably report improvements in menopausal symptoms too; a 50 percent reduction in hot flashes is fairly typical. Thus, it is possible that the benefits seen in these studies had nothing to do with black cohosh.

A substantial (244-participant) double-blind study published in 2007 compared black cohosh against the synthetic hormone tibolone and found them equally effective for treating menopausal symptoms. Though not approved as a drug in the United States, tibolone does appear to be effective for menopausal symptoms; therefore, these results are somewhat promising. However, this study lacked a placebo group, and since the placebo effect is powerful for this condition, this omission significantly reduces the meaningfulness of the result.

One double-blind study evaluated a combination therapy containing black cohosh and St. John's wort in 301 women with general menopausal symptoms as

Black Cohosh for Menopausal Symptoms

The herb black cohosh is one of the prime candidates for a safe alternative treatment for menopausal symptoms. Some studies have found it helpful for a variety of menopausal symptoms. The strongest evidence regards hot flashes, but black cohosh has also shown some promise for stabilizing mood.

On the pharmaceutical side, the antidepressant drug fluoxetine (Prozac) has known antidepressant properties that are thought to help calm menopausal mood disorders. Despite fears raised when it was first released, Prozac has a good track record of safety. It also is recommended as an alternative to hormone replacement therapy.

Researchers have conducted a double-blind study comparing black cohosh and fluoxetine for the treatment of menopausal symptoms. A total of 120 women with menopausal symptoms were enrolled in this double-blind study. One-half received fluoxetine and the other one-half were given black cohosh. Participants kept symptom diaries. In addition, they were examined at the end of the first, second, third, and sixth months of the study. The results were, perhaps, predictable. Black cohosh proved more effective than Prozac for reducing hot flashes; conversely, Prozac was a better mood stabilizer.

Steven Bratman, M.D.

well as depression. The results showed that use of the combination treatment was significantly more effective than a placebo for both problems.

A smaller study using a combination of the same two herbs found improvements in overall menopausal symptoms as well as in cholesterol profile.

In contrast, several other studies failed to find any benefit. For example, in a twelve-month, double-blind, placebo-controlled study of 350 women, participants were given either black cohosh, a multibotanical containing ten herbs, the multibotanical plus soy, standard hormone replacement therapy, or placebo. The results showed that hormone replacement therapy was more effective than placebo, but the other treatments were not. In addition, a double-blind study of 122 women failed to find statistically significant benefits with black cohosh compared with placebo, as did

another study enrolling 132 women, as well as one that involved 124 women using a black cohosh/soy isoflavone combination. These negative outcomes were possibly due to the relatively small sizes of the black cohosh groups. In a condition such as menopausal symptoms, where the placebo effect is strong, and when the treatment is relatively weak, large numbers of participants are necessary to show benefit above and beyond the placebo effect. Nonetheless, this is an impressive number of negative studies, and some question remains about the efficacy of this herb.

Some information has developed regarding how black cohosh may work. In the past, the herb was described as a phytoestrogen, a plant-based chemical with estrogen-like effects. However, subsequent evidence indicates that black cohosh is not a general phytoestrogen, but may act like estrogen in only a few parts of the body: the brain (reducing hot flashes) and bone (potentially helping to prevent or treat osteoporosis), and perhaps to some extent in the vagina. It does not appear to act like estrogen in the breast or the uterus. If this theory is true then black cohosh is a selective-estrogen receptor modifier (SERM) somewhat like the drug raloxifen (Evista). However, more evidence is needed to establish the facts of the matter.

Female infertility. Because of its estrogenic properties, researchers investigated whether black cohosh might be helpful in women who were having difficulty conceiving. Women with unexplained infertility who were not responding to clomiphene, a commonly used medication to induce ovulation, were randomly divided into two groups. Both groups continued to receive clomiphene, but the women in one of the groups also received 120 mg of black cohosh. Pregnancy rates were significantly higher in the black cohosh plus clomiphene group compared with the clomiphene-only group.

Breast cancer. Women who have had treatment for breast cancer frequently experience hot flashes, often but not always because of the use of estrogen-antagonist medications like tamoxifen. Estrogen treatment is not an option for this problem, as it might increase risk of cancer recurrence. Because black cohosh does not seem to have estrogen-like actions in the breast, researchers felt safe to try it in eighty-five women who had undergone treatment for breast cancer. The results were not encouraging: in this two-month, double-blind, placebo-controlled trial, black cohosh did not reduce hot-flash symptoms.

Safety Issues

Black cohosh seldom produces any side effects other than occasional mild gastrointestinal distress. One rigorous study looked for possible deleterious effects on cholesterol levels, blood sugar, and blood coagulability but did not find any. Studies in rats have found no significant toxicity when black cohosh was given at ninety times the therapeutic dosage for a period of six months. Because six months of life in a rat corresponds to decades of life in a human, this study appears to make a strong statement about the long-term safety of black cohosh.

Unlike estrogen, black cohosh does not stimulate breast-cancer cells growing in a test tube. However, black cohosh has not yet been subjected to large-scale studies similar to those conducted for estrogen. For this reason, safety for those with previous breast cancer is not known. Also, because of potential hormonal activity, black cohosh is not recommended for adolescents or pregnant or nursing women.

There are a growing number of case reports in which it appeared that use of a black cohosh led to severe liver injury. However, it is not clear whether the cause was black cohosh itself, or a contaminant present in the product. One highly preliminary study found that black cohosh might reduce the effectiveness of the chemotherapy drug cisplatin. Safety in young children or those with severe liver or kidney disease is not known.

EBSCO CAM Review Board

Further Reading

Borrelli, F., and E. Ernst. "Black Cohosh (*Cimicifuga racemosa*) for Menopausal Symptoms: A Systematic Review of Its Efficacy." *Pharmacological Research* 58, no. 1 (2008): 8-14.

Hostanska, K., et al. "*Cimicifuga racemosa* Extract Inhibits Proliferation of Estrogen Receptor-Positive and Negative Human Breast Carcinoma Cell Lines by Induction of Apoptosis." *Breast Cancer Research and Treatment* 84 (2004): 151-160.

O'Connor, A. M., et al. "A Case of Autoimmune Hepatitis Associated with the Use of Black Cohosh." *American Journal of Gastroenterology* 98 (2003): S165.

Pockaj, B. A., et al. "Phase III Double-Blind, Randomized, Placebo-Controlled Crossover Trial of Black Cohosh in the Management of Hot Flashes." *Journal of Clinical Oncology* 24 (2006): 2836-2841.

Rockwell, S., Y. Liu, and S. Higgins. "Alteration of the

Effects of Cancer Therapy Agents on Breast Cancer Cells by the Herbal Medicine Black Cohosh." *Breast Cancer Research and Treatment* 90 (2005): 233-239.

Verhoeven, M. O., et al. "Effect of a Combination of Isoflavones and *Actaea racemosa Linnaeus* on Climacteric Symptoms in Healthy Symptomatic Perimenopausal Women." *Menopause* 12 (2005): 412-420.

Wuttke, W., C. Gorkow, and D. Seidlova-Wuttke. "Effects of Black Cohosh (*Cimicifuga racemosa*) on Bone Turnover, Vaginal Mucosa, and Various Blood Parameters in Postmenopausal Women: A Double-Blind, Placebo-Controlled, and Conjugated Estrogens-Controlled Study." *Menopause* 13 (2006): 185-196.

See also: Blue cohosh; Estrogen; Herbal medicine; Menopause; Women's health.

Black tea

CATEGORY: Functional foods

RELATED TERMS: *Camellia sinensis*, theanine

DEFINITION: Natural plant product consumed for specific health benefits.

PRINCIPAL PROPOSED USE: Heart disease prevention

OTHER PROPOSED USES: Cancer prevention, diabetes, high blood pressure, high cholesterol, osteoporosis prevention, sports and fitness, stress reduction

Overview

Black and green tea are made from the same plant, but in processing, black tea has been allowed to oxidize, which alters its constituents. Although green tea is high in catechins (especially epigallocatechin gallate), black tea contains relatively high levels of theaflavins, theanine, and thearubigens. Although green tea is more commonly presented as a healthful beverage, traditional black tea too might have health-promoting properties. However, there is no reliable evidence for any of black tea's proposed health benefits.

Uses and Applications

According to some observational studies, the high consumption of black tea is associated with reduced risk of heart disease and death from heart disease.

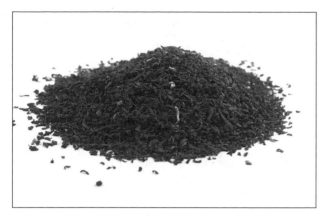

Black tea contains relatively high levels of theaflavins, theanine, and thearubigens. (©Ion Prodan/Dreamstime. com)

However, observational studies are notoriously unreliable for proving the efficacy of a treatment. Some additional support for black tea comes from animal studies that hint black tea may help prevent atherosclerosis, the primary cause of heart disease. However, only double-blind, placebo-controlled studies can actually prove a treatment effective, and few have been conducted on black tea.

One double-blind, placebo-controlled study found that black tea modestly improves cholesterol profile, but it enrolled too few participants (fifteen) to provide trustworthy results. Another study, about twice as large, failed to find benefit. A much larger study (more than two hundred participants) evaluated a form of green tea enriched with black tea theaflavin. In this substantial three-month study, the use of the tea product resulted in significant reductions in LDL (bad) cholesterol compared with placebo. However, these results might not apply to black tea itself.

Theanine, a component of black tea, has been advocated as a sports supplement. Physical activity causes elevation of the stress hormone cortisol, which could, in theory, interfere with the benefits of exercise by slowing muscle growth. One study widely reported by tea advocates tested a mixture of theanine and several other herbs and supplements (*Magnolia officinalis*, *Epimedium koreanum*, beta-sitosterol, and phosphatidylserine). The results appeared to indicate that the use of this combination could decrease the cortisol response to exercise. On this basis, theanine and the combination supplement are widely marketed as an aid to body building. However, this study has a number of limitations. Perhaps the most important of these limitations is that presumably the body releases cortisol during exercise for a reason; preventing this response may not produce health benefits. In addition, the study was not designed to look for particular benefits, such as improved muscle development. Other preliminary evidence from small trials suggests that the consumption of theanine in black tea may reduce the body's response to stress in general (physical or psychological), may lead to a more relaxed mental state, and may help reduce blood pressure.

Black tea might also help prevent cancer, though evidence from observational studies is thoroughly inconsistent. Weak observational study evidence additionally hints at benefits for osteoporosis. Though black tea has shown blood-sugar-lowering effects in healthy people, one study failed to find that a combined extract of black and green tea could help control blood sugar levels in people with type 2 diabetes.

DOSAGE

The optimal doses of black tea or its constituents are not known.

SAFETY ISSUES

As a widely consumed beverage, black tea is presumed to have a high safety factor. Its side effects would be expected to be similar to those of coffee: heartburn, gastritis, insomnia, anxiety, and heart arrhythmia (benign palpitations or more serious disturbances of heart rhythm). All drug interactions that can occur with caffeine would be expected to occur with black tea.

IMPORTANT INTERACTIONS

The caffeine in black tea could cause dangerous drug interactions in persons who are taking monoamine oxidase inhibitors. Also, the stimulant effects of black tea might be amplified in persons taking stimulant drugs such as ritalin. Black tea might interfere with the action of drugs taken to prevent heart arrhythmias or to treat insomnia, heartburn, ulcers, or anxiety. Finally, black tea may decrease the absorption of folic acid into the bloodstream.

EBSCO CAM Review Board

FURTHER READING

Bryans, J. A., P. A. Judd, and P. R. Ellis. "The Effect of Consuming Instant Black Tea on Postprandial

Plasma Glucose and Insulin Concentrations in Healthy Humans." *Journal of the American College of Nutrition* 26 (2007): 471-477.

Mackenzie, T., L. Leary, and W. B. Brooks. "The Effect of an Extract of Green and Black Tea on Glucose Control in Adults with Type 2 Diabetes Mellitus." *Metabolism* 56 (2007): 1340-1344.

Mukamal, K. J., et al. "A Six-Month Randomized Pilot Study of Black Tea and Cardiovascular Risk Factors." *American Heart Journal* 154 (2007): 724.

Nobre, A. C., A. Rao, and G. N. Owen. "L-Theanine, a Natural Constituent in Tea, and Its Effect on Mental State." *Asia Pacific Journal of Clinical Nutrition* 17, suppl. 1 (2008): 167-168.

Rogers, P. J., et al. "Time for Tea: Mood, Blood Pressure, and Cognitive Performance Effects of Caffeine and Theanine Administered Alone and Together." *Psychopharmacology* 195 (2008): 569-577.

Vinson, J. A., et al. "Green and Black Teas Inhibit Atherosclerosis by Lipid, Antioxidant, and Fibrinolytic Mechanisms." *Journal of Agricultural and Food Chemistry* 52 (2004): 3661-3665.

See also: Folk medicine; Functional beverages; Green tea; Herbal medicine; Hypertension; Kombucha tea; Red tea.

Bladder infection

CATEGORY: Condition
RELATED TERMS: Cystitis, urinary tract infection
DEFINITION: Treatment of infections of the bladder.
PRINCIPAL PROPOSED NATURAL TREATMENTS: Cranberry, uva ursi
OTHER PROPOSED NATURAL TREATMENTS: Buchu, cleavers, goldenseal, goldenrod, horseradish with nasturtium, juniper, lapacho, low-sugar diet, mannose, methionine, probiotics, sandalwood, vitamin C, zinc

INTRODUCTION

Bladder infections are a common problem for women, accounting for more than six million office visits each year. Men, because of the greater distance between their bladder and urethral opening, only rarely develop bladder infections.

The primary symptoms of a bladder infection are burning during urination, frequency of urination, and urgency to urinate, possibly accompanied by pain in the lower abdomen and cloudy or bloody urine. Occasionally, the infection spreads upward into the kidneys, producing symptoms such as intense back pain, high fever, chills, nausea, and diarrhea.

Conventional treatment for bladder infections consists of appropriate antibiotic treatment guided by urine culture. Women with frequent bladder infections may keep on hand a prescription for antibiotics to be used when symptoms arise. Some women may choose to take antibiotics continuously to prevent infection. Certain hygiene habits, such as showering before or urinating after oral sex or intercourse, are commonly said to be helpful, although this has not been proven.

PRINCIPAL PROPOSED NATURAL TREATMENTS

Women who do not want to use antibiotics may be able to find some help through the use of herbs. However, if symptoms do not improve or signs of a kidney infection develop, medical attention is essential to prevent serious complications.

Cranberry. Cranberry juice is commonly used to prevent bladder infections and to overcome low-level chronic infections. The cranberry plant is a close relative of the common blueberry. Native Americans used it both as food and as a treatment for bladder and kidney diseases. The pilgrims learned about cranberry from local tribes and quickly adopted it for their own use. Subsequent physicians used it for bladder infections, for "bladder gravel," and to remove "blood toxins."

In the 1920s, researchers observed that drinking cranberry juice makes the urine more acidic. Because common urine-infection bacteria, such as *Escherichia coli*, dislike acidic surroundings, physicians concluded that they had discovered a scientific explanation for the traditional uses of cranberry. This discovery led to widespread medical use of cranberry juice for bladder infections. Cranberry fell out of favor after World War II, only to return in the 1960s as a self-treatment for bladder infections.

Recent research has revised the conclusions reached by scientists in the 1920s. It appears that cranberry's acidification of the urine is not likely to play an important role in the treatment of bladder infections; later research has instead focused on cranberry's apparent ability to interfere with the bacteria

Cranberry for Bladder Infections: What the Science Says

There is some evidence that cranberry can help to prevent urinary tract infections; however, the evidence is not definitive, and more research is needed. Cranberry has not been shown to be effective as a treatment for an existing urinary tract infection.

Research shows that components found in cranberry may prevent bacteria, such as *Escherichia coli,* from clinging to the cells along the walls of the urinary tract and causing infection. There is also preliminary evidence that cranberry may reduce the ability of *Helicobacter pylori* bacteria to live in the stomach and cause ulcers.

Findings from a few laboratory studies suggest that cranberry may have antioxidant properties and may also be able to reduce dental plaque (a cause of gum disease).

The National Center for Complementary and Alternative Medicine is funding studies of cranberry, primarily to better understand its effects on urinary tract infection. The Office of Dietary Supplements and other agencies of the National Institutes of Health are also supporting research on cranberries. For example, the National Institute on Aging is funding a laboratory study of the potential anti-aging effects of cranberry.

establishing a foothold on the bladder wall. If the bacteria cannot "hold on," they will be washed out with the stream of urine. Studies suggest that in women who frequently develop bladder infections, bacteria have an especially easy time holding on to the bladder wall. Thus, when taken regularly, cranberry juice might break the cycle of repeated infection.

The best evidence for the use of cranberry juice for preventing bladder infections comes from a one-year, double-blind, placebo-controlled study of 150 sexually active women that compared placebo with both cranberry juice (eight ounces three times daily) and cranberry tablets. The results showed that both forms of cranberry significantly reduced the number of episodes of bladder infections.

A double-blind study of 376 hospitalized elderly adults attempted to determine whether a low dose of cranberry juice cocktail would help prevent acute infections. It failed to find benefit, most likely because of the minimal dosage of cranberry: only ten ounces daily of cranberry juice cocktail. Furthermore, because of the low rate of infections, it would necessarily have been more difficult for this study to produce statistically significant results.

Another double-blind study evaluated cranberry juice cocktail for treatment of chronic bladder infections. This trial followed 153 women with an average age of 78.5 years for six months. Many women of this age group have what are called chronic asymptomatic bladder infections: signs of bacteria in the urine without any symptoms. One-half of the participants were given ten ounces per day of a standard commercial cranberry cocktail drink, the other a placebo drink prepared to look and taste the same. Both treatments contained the same amount of vitamin C to eliminate the possible effect of that supplement. Despite the weak preparation of cranberry used, the results showed that the treatment significantly reduced bacteria and white blood cells in the urine.

In addition, a year-long open trial of 150 women found that regular use of a cranberry juice and lingonberry combination reduced the rate of urinary tract infection compared with a probiotic drink or no treatment. However, because this study was not double-blind, the results are unreliable.

A review of ten studies investigated the benefits of cranberry juice or tablets compared with a placebo control in persons susceptible to urinary tract infections. Among 1,049 participants, the researchers found the cranberry products reduced the incidence of urinary tract infections by 35 percent, a statistically significant amount, over a twelve-month period. The effect was most notable in those with recurrent infections. However, many subjects dropped out of the studies early, suggesting that continuous consumption of cranberries is not well tolerated.

On the negative side, three double-blind, placebo-controlled studies failed to find cranberry extract helpful for preventing bladder infection in people with bladder paralysis (neurogenic bladder). However, a subsequent study of forty-seven persons with neurogenic bladder from spinal cord injuries found that the use of cranberry extract tablets over six months significantly reduced the risk of urinary tract infection.

Uva ursi. Uva ursi has a long history of use for urinary conditions in both the Americas and in Europe.

Until the development of sulfa antibiotics, uva ursi's principal active component, arbutin, was frequently prescribed by physicians as a treatment for bladder and kidney infections. It appears that the arbutin contained in uva ursi leaves is broken down in the intestine to another chemical, hydroquinone. This chemical is altered a bit by the liver and then sent to the kidneys for excretion. Hydroquinone then acts as an antiseptic in the bladder. (It is, however, potentially toxic.)

The European Scientific Cooperative on Phytotherapy (ESCOP) is an organization assigned the task of harmonizing herb policy among European countries. ESCOP recommends uva ursi for "uncomplicated infections of the urinary tract such as cystitis when antibiotic treatment is not considered essential." Despite this recommendation, surprisingly little research has been done on uva ursi.

Two studies evaluated the antibacterial power of the urine of people who were taking uva ursi and found activity against most major bacteria that infect the urinary tract. What is needed, however, is a double-blind trial to discover whether the use of uva ursi actually helps people with urinary tract infections.

One study did evaluate uva ursi for prevention of bladder infections. This double-blind trial followed fifty-seven women for one year. One-half were given a standardized dose of uva ursi (with dandelion leaf, which is intended to promote urine flow), while the others received placebo. During the study, none of the women on uva ursi developed a bladder infection, whereas five of the untreated women did. However, this study is a bit of an aberration because most experts do not believe that continuous treatment with uva ursi is a good idea. Hydroquinone is toxic, and for this reason most experts recommend that uva ursi should not be used for more than a couple of weeks at a time.

OTHER PROPOSED NATURAL TREATMENTS

Probiotics (friendly bacteria) have shown some promise for preventing bladder infections. The best results have been seen with an unusual type of probiotic consisting of a harmless form of *E. coli*. This double-blind trial enrolled 453 women with an ongoing bladder infection at the beginning of the study. Participants received either the *E. coli* or placebo for ninety days, then went three months without treatment; they then received treatment again for the first

ten days in months seven, eight, and nine. The results showed that compared with placebo, the use of the probiotic led to a 34 percent reduction in urinary tract infections. However, other studies have failed to find benefit with the use of the more common *Lactobacillus* probiotics.

A single-blind study found suggestive evidence that the use of vitamin C during pregnancy at a dose of 100 milligrams daily could reduce incidence of bladder infections. A preliminary double-blind, placebo-controlled study published in 2007 tested a standardized combination of nasturtium and horseradish and found some evidence that it might help prevent new bladder infections among people with a history of frequently recurrent bladder infections. This study, however, had numerous problems in design and statistical analysis.

Extremely weak evidence, far too weak to rely upon, has been used to suggest that the use of the substance d-mannose might help prevent or treat bladder infections. The herb goldenseal too is widely recommended for bladder infections, based on the antibiotic properties of its ingredient berberine. However, it is unlikely that goldenseal taken by mouth provides enough berberine in the bladder wall to have any effect.

Many nutritionally oriented physicians believe that regularly taking zinc supplements and decreasing sugar in the diet will help improve immunity against bladder infections. Herbs such as buchu, dandelion, goldenrod, juniper, cleavers, and sandalwood may increase urine flow, which could be helpful for increasing the speed of recovery from an infection that has already occurred. The herb lapacho and the supplement methionine are also sometimes recommended for bladder infections, but there is no real evidence that they work.

EBSCO CAM Review Board

FURTHER READING

Albrecht, U., K. H. Goos, and B. Schneider. "A Randomised, Double-Blind, Placebo-Controlled Trial of an Herbal Medicinal Product Containing *Tropaeoli majoris herba* (Nasturtium) and *Armoraciae rusticanae radix* (Horseradish) for the Prophylactic Treatment of Patients with Chronically Recurrent Lower Urinary Tract Infections." *Current Medical Research and Opinion* 23 (2007): 2415-2422.

Barrons, R., and D. Tassone. "Use of *Lactobacillus* Probiotics for Bacterial Genitourinary Infections in Women." *Clinical Therapeutics* 30 (2008): 453-468.

Bauer, H. W., et al. "A Long-Term, Multicenter, Double-Blind Study of an *Escherichia coli* Extract (OM-89) in Female Patients with Recurrent Urinary Tract Infections." *European Urology* 47 (2005): 542-548.

Hess, M. J., et al. "Evaluation of Cranberry Tablets for the Prevention of Urinary Tract Infections in Spinal Cord Injured Patients with Neurogenic Bladder." *Spinal Cord* 46 (2008): 622-626.

Jepson, R., and J. Craig. "Cranberries for Preventing Urinary Tract Infections." *Cochrane Database of Systematic Reviews* (2008): CD001321. Available through *EBSCO DynaMed Systematic Literature Surveillance* at http://www.ebscohost.com/dynamed.

McMurdo, M. E., et al. "Does Ingestion of Cranberry Juice Reduce Symptomatic Urinary Tract Infections in Older People in Hospital?" *Age and Ageing* 34 (2005): 256-261.

Ochoa-Brust, G. J., et al. "Daily Intake of 100 mg Ascorbic Acid as Urinary Tract Infection Prophylactic Agent During Pregnancy." *Acta Obstetricia et Gynecologica Scandinavica* 86 (2007): 783-787.

See also: Horseradish; Uva ursi.

Bladder infection: Homeopathic remedies

CATEGORY: Homeopathy

DEFINITION: The use of highly diluted remedies to treat infections of the bladder.

Studied homeopathic remedies: Belladonna, *Berberis vulgaris*, *Cantharis*, *Equisetum*, staphysagria

INTRODUCTION

Bladder infections are a common problem for women, accounting for more than six million office visits each year. Bacteria from the skin or rectal area can easily move the short distance from a woman's urethral opening into the bladder, particularly after sexual intercourse. Men, because of the greater distance between their bladder and urethral opening, only rarely develop bladder infections.

The primary symptoms of a bladder infection are burning during urination, increased frequency of urination, and an urgent need to urinate, possibly accompanied by pain in the lower abdomen and cloudy or bloody urine. Occasionally, the infection spreads upward into the kidneys, producing symptoms such as intense back pain, high fever, chills, nausea, and diarrhea.

SCIENTIFIC EVALUATIONS OF HOMEOPATHIC REMEDIES

A one-month, single-blind, placebo-controlled study of two hundred women who had developed bladder infections after sexual intercourse evaluated the effectiveness of staphysagria at 30c (centesimal) dilution. The results were positive. In the treatment group, 90 percent of the participants stopped developing bladder-related symptoms, 8 percent were very much better, and 2 percent remained unchanged (a much better outcome than in the placebo group). However, because the study was single-blind rather than double-blind, it lacks credibility. (If the researchers were predisposed to find homeopathy effective, they would tend to bias the results.)

TRADITIONAL HOMEOPATHIC TREATMENTS

Classical homeopathy offers many possible homeopathic treatments for bladder infections. These therapies are chosen based on various specific details of the person seeking treatment. The symptom picture of homeopathic belladonna includes frequent and intense urges to urinate, cramping in the bladder, and dark yellow urine released in small amounts, accompanied by fever, flushing, and restless irritability.

A bladder infection with twinges of cutting pain or a burning feeling that extends to the urethra and its opening may indicate a need for the *Berberis vulgaris* remedy. The urinary passage may also burn at times when there is no attempt at urination. After emptying the bladder, the person feels as if some urine still remains inside, and the urge to urinate is often made worse by walking.

When the passage of urine is associated with sharp cutting pains, homeopathic *Cantharis* might be recommended. *Equisetum* is typically associated with sensations of pain and fullness in the bladder that are worsened rather than improved by emptying the bladder.

EBSCO CAM Review Board

FURTHER READING

Imanshahidi, M., and H. Hosseinzadeh. "Pharmaco-logical and Therapeutic Effects of *Berberis vulgaris* and Its Active Constituent, Berberine." *Phytotherapy Research* 22 (2008): 999-1012.

Josephson, Laura. *Homeopathic Handbook of Natural Remedies: Safe and Effective Treatment of Common Ailments and Injuries.* New York: Random House, 2002.

Ustianowski, P. A. "A Clinical Trial of Staphysagria in Postcoital Cystitis." *British Homeopathic Journal* 63 (1974): 276-277.

See also: Bladder infection; Homeopathy; Women's health.

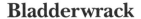

Bladderwrack

CATEGORY: Herbs and supplements

RELATED TERMS: Black tang, cut weed, *Fucus vesiculosus*, rockweed, rockwrack, seawrack

DEFINITION: Natural plant product used to treat specific health conditions.

PRINCIPAL PROPOSED USES: None

OTHER PROPOSED USES: Atherosclerosis, constipation, heartburn, hypothyroidism caused by iodine deficiency, immune support

OVERVIEW

Bladderwrack is a type of seaweed found on the coasts of the North Sea, the western Baltic Sea, and the Atlantic and Pacific Oceans. A common food in Japan, it is used as an additive and flavoring in various food products in Europe. Bladderwrack is commonly found as a component of kelp tablets or powders used as nutritional supplements. It is sometimes loosely called kelp, but that term technically refers to a different seaweed.

THERAPEUTIC DOSAGES

It is important not to take bladderwrack in dosages providing more than the recommended daily intake of iodine. Products that provide bladderwrack should state the amount of iodine they provide. Only products stating the amount of iodine should be used.

THERAPEUTIC USES

Bladderwrack contains high concentrations of

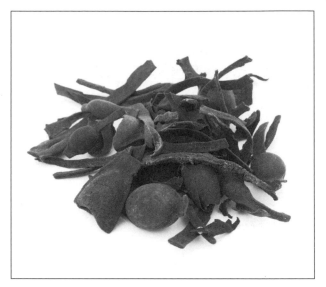

Bladderwrack contains high concentrations of iodine, and for this reason it has been recommended as a treatment for hypothyroidism (underactive thyroid gland). However, iodine will help only for the type of hypothyroidism caused by iodine deficiency, which is a relatively rare condition in the developed world. (Geoff Kidd/Photo Researchers, Inc.)

iodine, and for this reason it has been recommended as a treatment for hypothyroidism (underactive thyroid gland). However, iodine will help only for the type of hypothyroidism caused by iodine deficiency, which is a relatively rare condition in the developed world. If a person's iodine levels are not low, taking extra amounts of iodine can cause the thyroid gland to become either over- or underactive, causing hyperthyroidism or hypothyroidism, respectively. Furthermore, the amount of iodine supplied by bladderwrack is unpredictable.

A component of bladderwrack called alginic acid swells upon contact with water. When taken orally, it forms a type of seal at the mouth of the stomach and for this reason is used in over-the-counter preparations for heartburn. The same constituent gives bladderwrack laxative properties as well. Other proposed uses of bladderwrack include treating atherosclerosis and strengthening immunity, but there is no meaningful evidence at present that it works for these purposes.

SAFETY ISSUES

Studies have found that levels of iodine vary widely among bladderwrack products. Because of this, if a person uses bladderwrack as a regular supplement, the individual may receive an overdose of iodine and develop hyperthyroidism or hypothyroidism. Bladderwrack and other seaweed preparations can also worsen acne and decrease iron absorption.

Finally, bladderwrack, like other sea plants, can concentrate toxic heavy metals, such as arsenic, from the surrounding sea water. One report suggests that use of a bladderwrack product with a high heavy metal content is responsible for a case of kidney failure. Heavy metals present particular risks for pregnant or nursing women, children, individuals with kidney disease, or anyone using bladderwrack in high doses or over a long period of time.

EBSCO CAM Review Board

FURTHER READING

Conz, P. A., et al. "*Fucus vesiculosus*: A Nephrotoxic Alga?" *Nephrology Dialysis Transplantation* 13 (1998): 526-527.

Norman, J. A., et al. "Human Intake of Arsenic and Iodine from Seaweed-Based Food Supplements and Health Foods Available in the UK." *Food Additives and Contaminants* 5 (1987): 103-109.

See also: Herbal medicine; Hypothyroidism; Kelp.

Blepharitis

CATEGORY: Condition

DEFINITION: Treatment of irritation and inflammation of the eyelids and eyelashes.

PRINCIPAL PROPOSED TREATMENT: N-acetylcysteine

OTHER PROPOSED TREATMENTS: Barberry, bayberry, beta-carotene, bilberry, calendula, chamomile, citrus bioflavonoids, dandelion, evening primrose oil, eyebright, fish oil, goldenseal, lutein, passionflower, red clover, selenium, vitamin A, vitamin B complex (mixture of vitamins B_1, B_2, B_3, B_6, and B_{12}, and pantothenic acid, biotin, folate, inositol, and choline), vitamin C, vitamin E, zinc

INTRODUCTION

Blepharitis is a common eye disease that affects the edge of the eyelids and the eyelash hair follicles. Symptoms include red and swollen eyelids, crusting of the eyelashes on awakening, redness of the eye, sensitivity to light, excessive tearing, frothy tears, and an itching, burning, or foreign-body sensation in the eye.

There are two forms of blepharitis: anterior and posterior. Anterior blepharitis involves the portion of the eyelid where the eyelashes attach. It is caused either by a bacterial infection or by part of the same skin condition that causes dandruff (seborrheic dermatitis).

Posterior blepharitis occurs when the oil-secreting glands inside the eyelid (the meibomian glands) become inflamed and, eventually, cannot secrete properly. This leads to changes in the liquid bathing the eye (the tear film). Like anterior blepharitis, posterior blepharitis may occur as part of seborrheic dermatitis. Acne rosacea has also been associated with the condition.

Treatment of blepharitis primarily involves various methods to keep the eyelids clean and free of crusts. In some cases, antibiotic or steroid eye drops are used.

PRINCIPAL PROPOSED TREATMENTS

N-acetylcysteine (NAC) is a specially modified form of the dietary amino acid cysteine. When taken orally, NAC is thought to help the body make the important antioxidant enzyme glutathione. NAC is also thought to help loosen secretions, and for this reason, it has been tried as a treatment for loosening the thick crusty secretions that block the oil-secreting glands in posterior blepharitis.

In posterior blepharitis, the tear film becomes abnormal. A controlled but not blinded study evaluated the potential benefits of NAC in fifty people with chronic posterior blepharitis. All participants received standard eye care for blepharitis. In addition, about one-half the participants received NAC at a dose of 100 milligrams three times daily for eight weeks. Researchers used various methods to objectively evaluate the quality of the tear film and found that the use of NAC brought about significant improvements.

Further research, including double-blind, placebo-controlled trials, are necessary to determine whether these apparent benefits translate into meaningful improvement for people with chronic blepharitis.

OTHER PROPOSED TREATMENTS

For various theoretical reasons, other natural treatments have been recommended for blepharitis, including beta-carotene, citrus bioflavonoids, dandelion, evening primrose oil, fish oil, lutein, red clover, selenium, vitamin B complex (a mixture of vitamins B_1, B_2, B_3, B_6, and B_{12}, and pantothenic acid, biotin, and folate, possibly with inositol and choline), vitamins A, C, and E, and zinc. However, there is no meaningful scientific evidence to indicate that these treatments are helpful.

Certain herbs have been used, traditionally in the form of eye drops, to treat blepharitis and related conditions, including barberry, bayberry, bilberry, calendula, chamomile, eyebright, goldenseal, and passionflower. However, there is no meaningful evidence to indicate that they are effective. Furthermore, using herbal preparations in the eye is risky and should not be attempted except under the supervision of a qualified health-care provider. Natural treatments used for seborrheic dermatitis or acne rosacea may also be worth considering, as these conditions are closely related to blepharitis.

EBSCO CAM Review Board

FURTHER READING

Johnson, Gordon J., et al., eds. *The Epidemiology of Eye Disease.* 2d ed. New York: Oxford University Press, 2003.

National Institutes of Health, National Eye Institute. http://www.nei.nih.gov.

Sutton, Amy L., ed. *Eye Care Sourcebook: Basic Consumer Health Information About Eye Care and Eye Disorders.* 3d ed. Detroit: Omnigraphics, 2008.

Yalcin, E., et al. "N-acetylcysteine in Chronic Blepharitis." *Cornea* 21 (2002): 164-168.

See also: Conjunctivitis; N-acetylcysteine; Uveitis.

Blessed thistle

CATEGORY: Herbs and supplements
RELATED TERM: *Cnicus benedictus*
DEFINITION: Natural plant product used to treat specific health conditions.
PRINCIPAL PROPOSED USES: Dyspepsia, poor appetite

OVERVIEW

Blessed thistle has a long history of use in European herbal medicine. All parts of the above-ground plant are used medicinally. The herb was used primarily for digestive problems, including heartburn, gastritis, burping, constipation, and flatulence. Blessed thistle was also used for liver and gallbladder diseases.

THERAPEUTIC DOSAGES

A typical dose of blessed thistle is 2 grams two or three times daily.

THERAPEUTIC USES

Blessed thistle is also a component of the famous herbal combination therapy Essiac, widely used (though without scientific support) as a treatment for cancer. Also, blessed thistle has been approved by Germany's Commission E as a treatment for loss of appetite and nonspecific indigestion (dyspepsia). Blessed thistle contains the bitter constituent cnicin. Bitter substances are widely believed to promote appetite, though this has not been proven.

Cnicin does appear to have antimicrobial properties, killing bacteria and fungi in the test tube. These findings do not, however, indicate that blessed thistle can be used as an oral antibiotic. Antibiotics are substances that can be taken into the body at high enough doses to kill microbes throughout the system. In contrast, blessed thistle extracts, like those of many plants, appear to have antiseptic properties, meaning that they kill microbes on direct contact.

SAFETY ISSUES

Although comprehensive safety studies have not been performed, blessed thistle is believed to be safe. However, cross-reactions are possible among people allergic to plants in the daisy family. Safety in young children, pregnant or nursing women, or people with severe liver or kidney disease has not been established.

EBSCO CAM Review Board

FURTHER READING

Barrero, A. F., et al. "New Sources and Antifungal Activity of Sesquiterpene Lactones." *Fitoterapia* 71 (2000): 60-64.

Bruno, M., et al. "Antibacterial Evaluation of Cnicin and Some Natural and Semisynthetic Analogues." *Planta Medica* 69 (2003): 277-281.

See also: Dyspepsia; Herbal medicine.

Bloodroot

CATEGORY: Herbs and supplements

RELATED TERM: *Sanguinaria canadensis*

DEFINITION: Natural plant product used to treat specific health conditions.

PRINCIPAL PROPOSED USES: Cavity prevention, periodontal disease prevention, respiratory illnesses, warts

OVERVIEW

Bloodroot is a perennial flowering herb that was widely used by Native Americans both as a reddish-orange dye and as a medicine. Some tribes drank bloodroot tea as a treatment for sore throats, fevers, and joint pain, while others applied the somewhat caustic sap to skin cancers. European herbalists used bloodroot to treat respiratory infections, asthma, joint pain, warts, ringworm, and nasal polyps.

In the mid-nineteenth century, a doctor at Middlesex Hospital in London developed a treatment consisting of a paste of bloodroot, flour, water, and zinc chloride applied directly to breast tumors and other cancers. Similar formulations were used in various locales up through the turn of the century. Bloodroot remains a common constituent of folk-medicine drawing salves, said to pull tumors from the body.

THERAPEUTIC DOSAGES

For the treatment of warts, bloodroot can be made into a paste and applied directly to the involved area. However, it is important to start slowly. Excessive application can lead to severe burns. After a person has discovered his or her tolerance for bloodroot, the herb can be applied for a day or so; it should then be removed. A scab will develop and drop off. This process is repeated until the wart is gone. Bloodroot tea for internal use is made by boiling 1 teaspoon of powdered root in a cup of water, taken two or three times daily.

THERAPEUTIC USES

Herbalists frequently recommend bloodroot pastes and salves for the treatment of warts. Bloodroot is an escharotic, that is to say a scab-producing substance, and it functions much like commercial wart plasters containing salicylic acid. Although there has not been any real scientific study of the use of bloodroot for warts, based on its escharotic effects, it could be helpful.

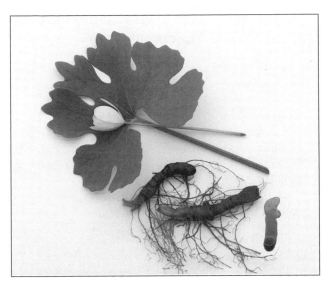

The flower, leaf, and roots of bloodroot, a perennial flowering herb. (Wally Eberhart/Getty Images)

One constituent of bloodroot, sanguinarine, appears to possess topical antibiotic properties. On this basis, the U.S. Food and Drug Administration has approved the use of bloodroot in commercially available toothpastes and oral rinses to inhibit the development of dental plaque and periodontal disease (gingivitis). However, the evidence that it really helps remains incomplete and inconsistent. On a similar note, one very preliminary study found suggestive evidence that use of a toothpaste containing sanguinaria plus fluoride is more effective for cavity prevention than one containing fluoride alone.

Bloodroot is also often combined with other herbs in cough syrups. Some herbalists recommend drinking bloodroot tea for respiratory ailments, but others consider the herb to be too unpredictable in its side effects.

SAFETY ISSUES

Oral bloodroot appears to be relatively safe and nontoxic. However, in large doses, it causes nausea and vomiting, and even at lower dosages, it has been reported to cause peculiar side effects in some people, such as tunnel vision and pain in the feet. For this reason, many herbalists recommend that it be used only under the supervision of a qualified practitioner.

Topical applications of bloodroot can cause severe burns if used too vigorously and for too long a time. Despite some reassuring evidence from animal studies, there are still theoretical concerns that bloodroot could be harmful during pregnancy. Safety in young children, nursing women, or those with severe liver or kidney disease has also not been established.

EBSCO CAM Review Board

FURTHER READING

Hong, S. J., et al. "Effects of *Sanguinaria* in Fluoride-Containing Dentifrices on the Remineralisation of Subsurface Carious Lesion In Vitro." *International Dental Journal* 55 (2005): 128-132.

See also: Herbal medicine; Warts.

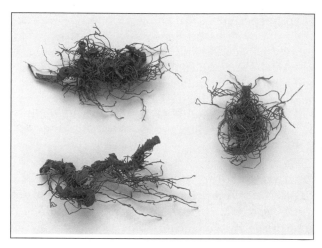

Blue cohosh is widely prescribed by herbalists and midwives. (Andy Crawford and Steve Gorton/Getty Images)

Blue cohosh

CATEGORY: Herbs and supplements
RELATED TERM: *Caulophyllum thalictroides*
DEFINITION: Natural plant product used to treat specific health conditions.
PRINCIPAL PROPOSED USES: None
OTHER PROPOSED USES: Inducing labor (not recommended), regulating menstrual cycle (not recommended)

OVERVIEW

Blue cohosh, a toxic, flowering herb that is native to North America, grows in forested areas from the southeastern United States to Canada. Sometimes known as squaw root or papoose root, the herb may have been used medicinally by Native Americans, although this belief is controversial. Other common names for the herb include yellow ginseng and blue ginseng. Blue cohosh should not be confused with the similarly named (but unrelated and much safer) black cohosh. Blue cohosh was used in the nineteenth century by European settlers and African Americans, primarily for gynecologic conditions. Blue cohosh also has a reputation as an herb that can induce abortions, although concerns regarding its efficacy and safety make this use extremely ill-advised. In addition, it has been used for the treatment of arthritis, cramps, epilepsy, inflammation of the uterus, hiccups, colic, and sore throat.

THERAPEUTIC DOSAGES

Blue cohosh is usually used as a tincture. Common dosages range from five to ten drops taken every two to four hours.

THERAPEUTIC USES

Blue cohosh is widely prescribed by herbalists and midwives. A 1999 survey published in the *Journal of Nurse-Midwifery* found that 64 percent of certified nurse-midwives who prescribe herbal medicines use blue cohosh to induce labor. It has also been used for a wide variety of menstrual problems, including several for which it would not be logical to believe that the same treatment could help. For example, blue cohosh has been used to start menstrual periods that were late in coming and yet also to stop excessive or ongoing menstrual flow.

There is no credible evidence that blue cohosh is effective for any of the conditions for which it has been used. Furthermore, several published reports cite cases of serious side effects to infants apparently caused by blue cohosh.

SAFETY ISSUES

There are many serious safety concerns with blue cohosh. Some of the compounds found in blue cohosh, such as caulophyllosaponin, methylcytosine, and caulosaponin, appear to constrict coronary vessels, limiting blood flow to the heart and reducing its ability to pump. One published case report documents profound heart failure in a child born to a woman who used blue cohosh to induce labor. Severe medical consequences also were seen in another child. Other blue cohosh constituents are known to interfere with the ability of a newly fertilized ovum to implant in the uterus, damage the uterus and thyroid, and cause severe birth defects in cattle and laboratory rats. Given these reports, the availability of safe alternatives for stimulating labor, and the lack of studies to document the herb's efficacy and safety, experts strongly advise against using blue cohosh.

EBSCO CAM Review Board

FURTHER READING

Irikura, B., and E. J. Kennelly. "Blue Cohosh: A Word of Caution." *Alternative Therapies in Women's Health* 1 (1999): 81-83.

Jones, T. K., and B. M. Lawson. "Profound Neonatal Congestive Heart Failure Caused by Maternal Consumption of Blue Cohosh Herbal Medication." *Journal of Pediatrics* 132 (1998): 550-552.

McFarlin, B. L., et al. "A National Survey of Herbal Preparation Use by Nurse-Midwives for Labor Stimulation: Review of the Literature and Recommendations for Practice." *Journal of Nurse-Midwifery* 44 (1999): 205-216.

See also: Black cohosh; Herbal medicine; Women's health.

Blue flag

CATEGORY: Herbs and supplements
RELATED TERMS: *Iris caroliniuna Watson, I. versicolor*
DEFINITION: Natural plant product used to treat specific health conditions.
PRINCIPAL PROPOSED USES: None
OTHER PROPOSED USE: Impetigo

OVERVIEW

Blue flag, a member of the iris family, is found throughout North America. It was widely used by Native Americans for digestive problems. In the nineteenth century, physicians of the Eclectic school of medicine also used blue flag for digestive problems and to treat thyroid enlargement, enhance immunity, stimulate the liver, and "detoxify" the body. Topical preparation of the herb was used for impetigo (a skin infection caused by *Streptococcus* bacteria). The rhizome (underground stem) is the part used medicinally.

Blue flag has undergone no meaningful scientific study. In view of the lack of documented benefits, the absence of toxicity studies, the toxicity of related species, and the known side effects, the use of this herb is not recommended.

THERAPEUTIC DOSAGES

A typical dosage is 1 to 2 grams three times daily.

THERAPEUTIC USES

Blue flag is used by some herbalists today to treat liver problems and skin diseases. However, there has been essentially no scientific evaluation of the efficacy of this herb. It is thought to contain isophtalic acid, iridin, and the volatile oil furfural.

SAFETY ISSUES

Blue flag has not undergone any meaningful scientific study. High doses of blue flag are known to cause severe gastrointestinal upset, including nausea, vomiting, and diarrhea, and related species are known to be toxic. The fresh herb can irritate the mouth and stomach. Blue flag is considered unsafe for use by pregnant or nursing women and young children.

EBSCO CAM Review Board

FURTHER READING

Felter, H. W. "Iris." *The Eclectic Materia Medica, Pharmacology and Therapeutics.* Available at http://www.ibiblio.org/herbmed/eclectic/felter/iris.html.

Newall, C., L. Anderson, and J. Phillipson. *Herbal Medicines: A Guide for Healthcare Professionals.* London: Pharmaceutical Press, 1996.

See also: Folk medicine; Herbal medicine; Traditional healing.

Boldo

CATEGORY: Herbs and supplements
RELATED TERM: *Peumus boldus*
DEFINITION: Natural plant product used to treat specific health conditions.
PRINCIPAL PROPOSED USES: None
OTHER PROPOSED USES: Constipation, dyspepsia, liver protection

OVERVIEW

Boldo (*Peumus boldus*) is an evergreen shrub that is native to South America. It grows about 6 to 20 feet high and has thick waxy leaves. Although boldo has a long history of use as a culinary spice and medicinal herb and is still one of the most common medicinal plants used in Chile, it has only recently become the subject of scientific research.

The leaves of the boldo plant have traditionally been used as a treatment for liver and bladder disorders as well as rheumatism. They have also been used for a wide variety of other ailments, including headache, earache, congestion, menstrual pain, and syphilis. Recent research suggests that boldo may protect the liver from toxins, stimulate the gallbladder, and reduce inflammation.

THERAPEUTIC DOSAGES

Germany's Commission E recommends 3 grams of the dried leaf or its equivalent per day for digestive complaints.

THERAPEUTIC USES

Germany's Commission E has approved boldo for "spastic gastrointestinal complaints and dyspepsia." Dyspepsia is a rather vague term that corresponds to the common word "indigestion," indicating a wide variety of digestive problems including stomach discomfort, lack of appetite, and nausea.

In Europe, dyspepsia is commonly attributed to inadequate flow of bile from the gallbladder. Although this connection has not been proven, boldo has been used as a treatment for dyspepsia based on how it affects the gallbladder. Boldo does not seem to increase bile production, but it may cause gallbladder contraction.

Boldo taken alone has not been well evaluated as a treatment for dyspepsia; however, a combination herbal treatment containing boldo (along with other herbs thought to stimulate the gallbladder) has been studied. In a double-blind, placebo-controlled trial, sixty people given either an artichoke leaf/boldo/celandine combination or placebo found improvements in symptoms of indigestion after fourteen days of treatment. How this combination might be effective for treating dyspepsia is unclear. Celandine may present significant risk of liver toxicity.

Studies on animals have found that boldo may have some ability to protect the liver from toxins, perhaps

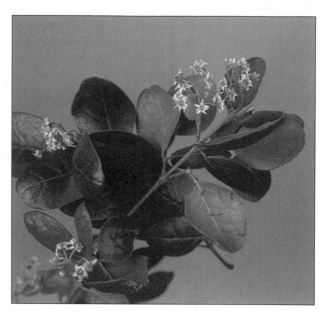

The leaves of the boldo plant have been used medicinally. (DEA/A. Moreschi/Getty Images)

due to the antioxidant effects of a boldo constituent called boldine. Boldo also has anti-inflammatory properties and, in addition, may act as a laxative. Finally, the essential oils found in boldo have antimicrobial properties; this is true of many essential oils, however, and does not indicate that boldo can act as an antibiotic.

SAFETY ISSUES

Although comprehensive safety studies have not been completed, boldo leaf appears to be safe at normal doses. No side effects were reported in any of the animal studies. However, the plant's essential oils are very toxic and can cause kidney damage if taken in purified form, or if very large amounts of the leaf are ingested. The safety of long-term use is also questionable.

Individuals with gallstones should take boldo only under a physician's supervision because of the risk of gallstones being expelled and becoming lodged in a bile duct or the intestines. Those with obstruction of the bile ducts should not use boldo because of the risk of rupture.

Animal studies suggest that boldo can cause birth defects and spontaneous abortion. For this reason, pregnant women should not use boldo. Safety in nursing women, young children, and individuals with severe liver or kidney disease has not been established.

EBSCO CAM Review Board

FURTHER READING

Benninger, J., et al. "Acute Hepatitis Induced by Greater Celandine (*Chelidonium majus*)." *Gastroenterology* 117 (1999): 1234-1237.

Jimenez, I., et al. "Protective Effects of Boldine Against Free Radical-Induced Erythrocyte Lysis." *Phytotherapy Research* 14 (2000): 339-343.

Jimenez, I., and H. Speisky. "Biological Disposition of Boldine: In Vitro and In Vivo Studies." *Phytotherapy Research* 14 (2000): 254-260.

Vila, R., L. Valenzuela, and H. Bello. "Composition and Antimicrobial Activity of the Essential Oil of *Peumus boldus* Leaves." *Planta Medica* 65 (1999): 178-179.

See also: Dyspepsia; Herbal medicine.

Bone and joint health

CATEGORY: Issues and overviews

RELATED TERMS: Osteoarthritis, osteoporosis, rheumatoid arthritis

DEFINITION: Complementary and alternative methods to prevent or treat disorders of the joints, which consist primarily of bones covered by cartilage that reduces friction, by tendons for stability, and by synovial membranes for lubrication.

OVERVIEW

Many diseases and conditions affect the bones and joints, yet the treatment of these diseases and conditions with complementary and alternative medicine (CAM) has yet to be evaluated extensively by clinical studies; thus, variability of results among studies is typical.

"Arthritis" is the general term for joint inflammation and is the primary distinguishing feature of joint disorders. CAM seeks to reduce inflammation regardless of the cause of arthritis. Osteoarthritis, also known as degenerative joint disease, is the most common disorder involving joint movement. Not limited to old age, osteoarthritis can result from a complex interaction of mechanical, biological, or genetic factors that result in the depletion of joint cartilage. Rheumatoid arthritis is an autoimmune disease in which the immune system attacks the tissues surrounding and cushioning the joint, eventually affecting the cartilage and bones of the joints. Gout and bursitis also affect the joint.

Some diseases affecting the joint also affect other tissues and organs. These diseases include systemic lupus erythematosus, fibromyalgia, and ankylosing spondylitis. Another disorder, osteoporosis, is the decrease in density of many different bones of the body and does not affect the joint. Osteoporosis is often confused with osteoarthritis, yet they are very different medical conditions with little in common.

OSTEOARTHRITIS

Osteoarthritis (OA) is distinguished by degeneration of joint cartilage and adjacent bone, leading to pain, difficulty in movement, and stiffness. OA can affect any joints in the body, including knees, hips, shoulders, vertebrae, fingers, toes, and the temporomandibular joint, which is in the jaw. Standard treatments consist of exercise or physical therapy programs, analgesic drugs or corticosteroids for pain, and, as a last resort, joint replacement surgery.

None of the standard treatments regenerate lost or damaged cartilage. Cartilage is composed of collagen and proteoglycan. Collagen is a large fibrous protein, whereas proteoglycan consists of a core protein with linkages to many long-chain carbohydrates known as glycosaminoglycans. Chondroitin sulfate is the glycosaminoglycan found in collagen. Because chondroitin sulfate is an integral part of collagen, and glucosamine is an essential metabolic intermediate in the formation of collagen, it was reasoned that providing these compounds to persons with joint disorders would serve as a stimulus for the formation of collagen.

Considerable research has been reported on the effectiveness of glucosamine and chondroitin sulfate in halting and reversing joint degeneration. Although earlier research did indeed seem to show effectiveness, there were some questions about research design and methodology. Recent studies were more rigorous in nature, involving larger numbers of persons and using the gold standard of clinical trials: randomized, double-blind, and placebo-controlled trials. Meta-analyses compile the data from many studies for overall statistical analyses. In the case of glucosamine

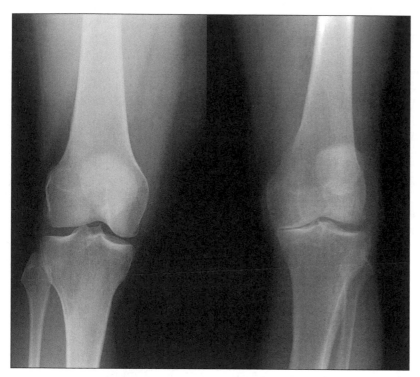

A normal knee (on the left) compared to the knee (on the right) with advanced osteoarthritis. (Living Art Enterprises/Photo Researchers, Inc.)

and chondroitin, recent analyses do not support much benefit from their use.

A review article in 1998 reported on studies that evaluated the effectiveness of glucosamine and chondroitin sulfate in reducing pain symptoms in OA. Most studies showed that persons receiving glucosamine had a reduction in pain score, compared with those receiving placebo. Fewer studies were reported on the effectiveness of chondroitin sulfate, but the compound appeared to produce what were called favorable outcomes. An analysis reported in 2003 found that glucosamine was significant in alleviating pain and in maintaining cartilage, while chondroitin was effective in some indices of pain reduction.

Another review in 2008 studied the results of twenty-five randomized controlled studies involving 4,963 persons. When all studies (including older studies) were analyzed, glucosamine improved pain more than did a placebo after six months. When the analysis was restricted to higher-quality studies with adequate blinding (in which neither the persons studied nor the researchers knew the identity of the treatments), no benefit was observed.

A meta-analysis was reported in 2007 on twenty trials evaluating the effectiveness of chondroitin sulfate for reducing symptoms of OA. Heterogeneity among the trials made analysis difficult, but when only large, methodologically sound trials were included in the analysis, no significant benefits of chondroitin were found.

A two-year study reported in 2006 evaluated the effectiveness of glucosamine and chondroitin sulfate on slowing structural damage of knee OA. Measurements of joint space width (cartilage depletion) were used as measures of structural damage. At the two-year stage of treatment, no statistical differences were found among the treatments, compared with the placebo control. The combination of glucosamine and chondroitin may be less active, compared with their individual effects. Persons with less severe OA at the beginning of the study tended to show less joint loss than those using a placebo.

A large glucosamine/chondroitin arthritis intervention trial (GAIT) involved 1,583 persons. After twenty-four weeks of treatment, glucosamine or chondroitin singly or in combination did not show the significant 20 percent reductions in knee pain, compared with placebo, although the groups did show numerical improvements over placebo. A subgroup of persons with moderate to severe pain at the beginning of the study showed a significant reduction in pain, compared with placebo.

A companion GAIT trial studied the effect of glucosamine and chondroitin singly or in combination on progressive loss of joint space width (JSW). At two years, no treatment achieved statistically significant differences in JSW loss, compared with placebo, although the placebo had less JSW loss than anticipated.

RHEUMATOID ARTHRITIS

Rheumatoid arthritis (RA) is an autoimmune disorder in which the immune system attacks the tissues lining the joints, causing swelling, pain, and stiffness. Rheumatoid arthritis can eventually affect the bones and cartilage in the joints.

CAM seeks to alleviate the symptoms of rheumatoid arthritis without attempting cures for the underlying causes. Mind/body techniques, such as relaxation, imagery, and biofeedback, can improve symptoms such as pain, psychological state, physical function, and ability to cope. In terms of dietary supplements, some clinical studies have shown that omega-3 fatty acids may be beneficial in reducing the inflammation of rheumatoid arthritis. Preliminary evidence suggests that gamma linolenic acid can have the same effect.

Tai Chi is a traditional martial art that combines slow and gentle movements with mental focus. A twelve-week study showed that Tai Chi improved muscle function in lower limbs in persons with RA. Persons using Tai Chi experienced improved psychosocial benefits such as less pain and improved posture, balance, and coordination.

OTHER JOINT DISEASES AND CONDITIONS

Gout. Gout is a recurrent, acute inflammation of peripheral joints, such as the big toe, instep, ankle, knee, wrist, and elbow. The condition is caused by deposits of monosodium urate crystals in cartilage, tendons, and ligaments and can become chronic with joint deformities. CAM focuses on the diet and includes recommendations such as avoiding foods with high purine content (such as beef, organ meats, sardines, and anchovies), eating cherries, taking fish oil supplements, minimizing alcohol consumption, and drinking eight glasses of water per day.

Systemic lupus erythematosus. Systemic lupus erythematosus (SLE) is an autoimmune disease in which antibodies attack connective tissue cells. Connective tissue serves to support and connect organs, muscles, joints, and other body parts. Because connective tissue is widespread, the organs affected and symptoms observed are also broad. The vast majority of persons with SLE experience joint pain and swelling.

A few studies have indicated that dehydroepiandiosterone (DHEA) may lead to decreased symptoms of lupus. Persons with lupus have abnormally high levels of estrogen metabolites and low levels of testosterone. DHEA may control these hormone abnormalities and may have effects on immune system components, such as a decrease in pro-inflammatory cytokines. Preliminary studies have also indicated a beneficial effect of omega-3 fatty acids in fish oils on reducing abnormal levels of the immune components cytokine and interleukin.

Fibromyalgia. Fibromyalgia (FM), or fibromyalgia syndrome, is a disorder characterized by chronic pain, tenderness, and stiffness in soft tissues, including muscles, tendons, and ligaments. FM most commonly affects women, and its cause is unknown. Some believe the disorder is triggered by physical or mental stress. Other symptoms of the disorder include severe fatigue, nonrestorative sleep, irritable bowel syndrome, depression, and cognitive difficulty (also called brain fog).

CAM seems to be particularly useful in treating FM because conventional therapies, namely drugs, are only partially effective and may have undesirable side effects. The treatments focus on the overall health of the person with FM, including his or her emotional state and nutritional health, and how these states can affect the condition. A review article found the largest improvements occurred with mind/body techniques, such as biofeedback, hypnosis, and cognitive behavioral therapy, especially when they were part of a multidisciplinary approach to treatment. Acupuncture was only moderately effective, while manipulative techniques such as chiropractic and massage were least effective. Another study, however, showed that just twenty minutes of moderate-pressure massage can lessen the flow of chemicals associated with pain and stress while increasing production of serotonin, a nerve transmitter that improves mood.

OSTEOPOROSIS

Osteoporosis (OP), or "porous bone," is the gradual weakening of bone structure caused by the depletion of calcium and other minerals. The condition can lead to bone fractures. Fractures are most common in the arm bone, vertebrae, and hip. Women are more subject to OP than men, but before menopause, estrogen secretion provides a protective effect against OP. For both prevention and treatment of OP, emphasis is placed on consuming adequate calcium and vitamin D and engaging in weight-bearing exercises. Prevention is more successful than treatment.

Estrogen therapy was common practice for postmenopausal women because of the beneficial effects in preventing hot flashes and reducing OP. However, a large Women's Health Initiative Study concluded that the health risks of estrogen therapy exceeded its benefits. In the search for alternatives to estrogen therapy, attention has focused on the use of dietary isoflavones. Isoflavones are non-nutritive compounds found in relatively large amounts in soybeans. The most common isoflavones are genistein and daidzein. They are also known as phytoestrogens, because they are similar in structure to estrogens and have weak estrogenic activity. Researchers have shown that isoflavones bind to estrogen receptors in osteoblast (bone-forming) cells, although in a manner different from estrogen. As a result, isoflavones were characterized as selective estrogen receptor modulators that could provide some of the beneficial effects of estrogen without the negative effects. Isoflavones could also inhibit osteoclast (bone-breakdown) cells by decreasing acid secretion or regulatory enzyme activities.

A review article summarized the results of two double-blind, randomized-control studies and one case-control study. Those persons receiving isoflavone treatments showed improvements in bone mass and reductions in the loss of bone mass, compared with those persons in the control group.

Another study evaluated the effect of isoflavones on bone resorption. Subjects were provided with radioactive calcium and three levels of isoflavones in a double-blind, randomized-control study. Serum and urinary samples were taken and analyzed for radioactive calcium to determine the rate of bone resorption (loss). Isoflavones did not have any influence on bone resorption.

Another study compared the effect of isoflavones on bone mineral density (BMD) in men and women. The results showed that isoflavones had a modest benefit in preserving spine but not hip BMD in women.

David A. Olle, M.S.

FURTHER READING

Beers, Mark H., ed. *The Merck Manual of Medical Information, Second Home Edition.* Whitehouse Station, N.J.: Merck Research Laboratories, 2003. This is the layperson's version of professional *Merck Manual of Diagnosis and Therapy.* Provides an excellent discussion of bone and joint disorders.

Brynin, Rona. "Soy and Its Isoflavones: A Review of Their Effects on Bone Density." *Alternative Medicine Review* 7, no. 4 (2002): 317-326. Describes the nature of soy isoflavones and relevant studies to evaluate the effect of isoflavones on bone density.

Clegg, Daniel, et al. "Glucosamine, Chondroitin Sulfate, and the Two in Combination for Painful Knee Osteoarthritis." *New England Journal of Medicine* 354 (February 23, 2006): 795-808. Reports on the effect of glucosamine and chondroitin on pain alleviation in GAIT studies.

Kelly, Gregory. "The Role of Glucosamine Sulfate and Chondroitin Sulfates in the Treatment of Degenerative Joint Disease." *Alternative Medicine Review* 3, no. 1 (1998): 27-39. Describes the structure and metabolism of glucosamine and chondroitin and discusses relevant clinical trials.

National Center for Complementary and Alternative Medicine. "Rheumatoid Arthritis and CAM." Available at http://www.nccam.nih.gov/health/ra. Provides a summary of all CAM methods that treat symptoms of rheumatoid arthritis.

Reichenbach, Stephan, et al. "Meta-analysis: Chondroitin for Osteoarthritis of the Knee or Hip." *Annals of Internal Medicine* 146 (2007): 580-590. Concludes that chondroitin showed no benefit for osteoarthritis in those studies that were large and well designed.

Sawitzke, Allen, et al. " The Effect of Glucosamine and/or Chondroitin Sulfate on the Progression of Knee Osteoarthritis." *Arthritis and Rheumatism* 58, no. 10 (2008): 3183-3191. Reports on the effect of glucosamine and chondroitin on reducing cartilage loss in osteoarthritis in GAIT studies.

See also: Aging; Back pain; Bursitis; Calcium; Chondroitin; Fibromyalgia: Homeopathic remedies; Glucosamine; Gout; Lupus; Neck pain; Nonsteroidal anti-inflammatory drugs (NSAIDs); Osteoarthritis; Osteoporosis; Pain management; Rheumatoid arthritis; Soy; Temporomandibular joint syndrome (TMJ); Tendonitis; Vitamin D.

Boron

CATEGORY: Herbs and supplements
RELATED TERMS: Boron chelate, sodium borate
DEFINITION: Natural substance used as a supplement to treat specific health conditions.
PRINCIPAL PROPOSED USES: None
OTHER PROPOSED USES: Osteoarthritis, osteoporosis, prostate cancer prevention, rheumatoid arthritis, sports supplement

OVERVIEW

Plants need boron for proper health, but it is not known if humans likewise need boron. However, boron does seem to assist in the proper absorption of calcium, magnesium, and phosphorus from foods, and it slows the loss of these minerals through urination. Preliminary evidence suggests that boron supplements may be helpful for osteoarthritis and osteoporosis.

REQUIREMENTS AND SOURCES

No dietary or nutritional requirement for boron has been established, and boron deficiency is not known to cause any disease. Good sources include leafy vegetables, raisins, prunes, nuts, noncitrus fruits, and grains. A typical American daily diet provides 1.5 to 3 milligrams (mg) of boron.

THERAPEUTIC DOSAGES

When used as a treatment for osteoarthritis or osteoporosis, boron is often recommended at a dosage of 3 mg per day, an amount similar to the average daily intake from food, but food sources may be safer.

THERAPEUTIC USES

Boron aids in the proper metabolism of vitamins and minerals involved with bone development, such as calcium, copper, magnesium, and vitamin D. In addition, boron appears to affect estrogen and possibly testosterone as well, hormones that affect bone health. On this basis, boron has been suggested for preventing or treating osteoporosis. However, there have been no clinical studies to evaluate the potential benefits of boron supplements for any bone-related conditions. On the basis of similarly weak evidence, boron is often added to supplements intended for the treatment of osteoarthritis.

Boron has also been proposed as a sports supplement, based on its effects on hormones. However, studies have, as yet, failed to find evidence that it helps increase muscle mass or enhances performance.

One large observational study suggests that higher intake of boron may reduce the risk of prostate cancer. Finally, boron is sometimes recommended as a treatment for rheumatoid arthritis, but there is no evidence to support this use.

SCIENTIFIC EVIDENCE

Osteoarthritis. In areas of the world where people eat relatively high amounts of boron–between 3 and 10 mg per day–the incidence of osteoarthritis is below 10 percent. However, in regions where there is less boron in the diet–1 mg or less per day–the incidence of arthritis is much higher. In addition, the joints of people with osteoarthritis have been found to contain less boron than people without the condition. These observations have given rise to the hypothesis that boron supplements might be helpful for people who already have arthritis symptoms. However, the only direct evidence that it works comes from one highly preliminary study reported in 1990.

Osteoporosis. In one small study, thirteen postmenopausal women were first fed a diet that provided 0.25 mg of boron for 119 days; then they were fed the same diet with a boron supplement of 3 mg daily for 48 days. The results revealed that boron supplementation reduced the amount of calcium lost in the urine. This suggests (but certainly does not prove) that boron can help prevent osteoporosis. However, in a similar study, boron administration did not affect urine calcium loss. Another study found that boron fails to affect calcium loss among people who receive enough magnesium.

SAFETY ISSUES

Since the therapeutic dosage of boron is about the same as the amount a person can get from food, it is probably fairly safe. Unpleasant side effects, including nausea and vomiting, are only reported at about fifty times the highest recommended dose.

One potential concern with boron regards its effect on hormones. In at least two small studies, boron was found to increase the body's own estrogen levels, especially in women on estrogen-replacement therapy. Because elevated estrogen increases the risk of breast and uterine cancer in women past menopause, this may be a matter of concern for those who wish to take supplemental boron. Further research is necessary to discover whether boron's apparent effect on estrogen is a real problem or not. Experts recommend getting boron from fruits and vegetables: A large study found that high intake of boron from these sources did not affect breast cancer rates.

IMPORTANT INTERACTIONS

For persons undergoing hormone-replacement therapy, the use of boron may not be advisable because of the risk of elevating estrogen levels excessively.

EBSCO CAM Review Board

FURTHER READING

Benderdour, M., et al. "In Vivo and In Vitro Effects of Boron and Boronated Compounds." *Journal of Trace Elements in Medicine and Biology* 12 (1998): 2-7.

Kreider, R. B. "Dietary Supplements and the Promotion of Muscle Growth with Resistance Exercise." *Sports Medicine* 27 (1999): 97-110.

Naghii, M. R. "The Significance of Dietary Boron, with Particular Reference to Athletes." *Nutritional Health* 13 (1999): 31-37.

Samman, S., et al. "The Nutritional and Metabolic Effects of Boron in Humans and Animals." *Biological Trace Elements Research* 66 (1998): 227-235.

See also: Herbal medicine; Osteoarthritis; Osteoporosis; Sports and fitness support: Enhancing performance.

Boswellia

CATEGORY: Herbs and supplements
RELATED TERMS: *Boswellia serrata*, frankincense
DEFINITION: Natural plant product used to treat specific health conditions.
PRINCIPAL PROPOSED USES: Asthma, osteoarthritis, rheumatoid arthritis
OTHER PROPOSED USES: Bursitis, collagenous colitis, Crohn's disease, tendonitis, ulcerative colitis

OVERVIEW

The gummy resin of the boswellia tree has a long history of use in Indian herbal medicine as a treatment for arthritis, bursitis, respiratory diseases, and diarrhea.

THERAPEUTIC DOSAGES

A typical dose of boswellia is 300 to 400 mg three times a day of an extract standardized to contain 37.5 percent boswellic acids. Some studies have used dosages as high as 1,200 mg three times daily.

THERAPEUTIC USES

Growing evidence suggests that boswellia has antiinflammatory effects. On this basis, the herb has been tried for a number of conditions in which inflammation is involved, including painful conditions such as bursitis, osteoarthritis, rheumatoid arthritis, and tendonitis. For the same reason, it has also been tried for asthma and inflammatory bowel disease (ulcerative colitis or Crohn's disease). In addition, boswellia has shown promise for the relatively rare disease of the colon in which inflammation plays a role: collagenous colitis.

Furthermore, extracts of boswellia have been studied as an aid to standard care for malignant glioma (a type of incurable brain tumor). Use of boswellia appears to decrease symptoms, probably by decreasing inflammation in the brain (as well as through other mechanisms). However, this has not been proven, and individuals with cancer should not use boswellia (or any other herb or supplement) except on a physician's advice.

SCIENTIFIC EVIDENCE

Rheumatoid arthritis. According to a review of unpublished studies, preliminary double-blind trials have found boswellia effective in relieving the symptoms of rheumatoid arthritis. Two placebo-controlled studies, involving a total of eighty-one people with rheumatoid arthritis, reportedly found significant reductions in swelling and pain over the course of three months. In addition, a comparative study of sixty people over six months found that boswellia extract produced symptomatic benefits comparable to oral gold therapy. However, this review was rather sketchy on details.

A more recent double-blind, placebo-controlled study that enrolled seventy-eight people with rheumatoid arthritis found no benefit. However, about one-half of the patients dropped out, which seriously diminishes the significance of the results.

Asthma. A six-week double-blind, placebo-controlled study of eighty people with relatively mild asthma found that treatment with boswellia at a dose of 300 milligrams (mg) three times daily reduced the frequency of asthma attacks and improved objective measurements of breathing capacity.

Osteoarthritis. In a double-blind study of thirty people with osteoarthritis of the knee, researchers compared boswellia against placebo. Participants received either boswellia or placebo for eight weeks and were then switched over to the opposite treatment for an additional eight weeks. The results showed significantly greater improvement in knee pain, knee mobility, and walking distance with boswellia compared to a placebo.

Inflammatory bowel disease. An eight-week double-blind, placebo-controlled trial of 102 people with Crohn's disease compared a standardized boswellia extract against the drug mesalazine. Participants taking boswellia fared at least as well as those taking mesalazine, according to a standard score of Crohn's disease severity. A small, poorly designed trial found some indications that boswellia might also offer benefit in ulcerative colitis.

SAFETY ISSUES

In clinical trials of pharmaceutical grade standardized boswellia extract, no serious side effects have been reported. Crude herb preparations, however, may not be as safe as the specially manufactured extract. Safety in young children, pregnant or nursing women, and individuals with severe liver or kidney disease has not been established.

EBSCO CAM Review Board

FURTHER READING

Gerhardt, H., et al. "Therapy of Active Crohn Disease with *Boswellia serrata* Extract H 15." *Zeitschrift fur Gastroenterologie* 39 (2001): 11-17.

Glaser, T., et al. "Boswellic Acids and Malignant Glioma: Induction of Apoptosis but No Modulation of Drug Sensitivity." *British Journal of Cancer* 80 (1999): 756-765.

Janssen, G., et al. "Boswellic Acids in the Palliative Therapy of Children with Progressive or Relapsed Brain Tumors." *Klinische Padiatrie* 212 (2000): 189-195.

Kimmatkar, N., et al. "Efficacy and Tolerability of *Boswellia serrata* Extract in Treatment of Osteoarthritis of Knee." *Phytomedicine* 10 (2003): 3-7.

Madisch, A., et al. "*Boswellia serrata* Extract for the Treatment of Collagenous Colitis." *International Journal of Colorectal Disease* 22, no. 12 (2007): 1445-1451.

Safayhi, H., et al. "Concentration-Dependent Potentiating and Inhibitory Effects of *Boswellia* Extracts on 5-lipoxygenase Product Formation in Stimulated PMNL." *Planta Medica* 66 (2000): 110-113.

Winking, M., et al. "Boswellic Acids Inhibit Glioma Growth: A New Treatment Option?" *Journal of Neuro-Oncology* 46 (2000): 97-103.

See also: Asthma; Crohn's disease; Herbal medicine; Osteoarthritis.

Bowers, Edwin

CATEGORY: Biography
IDENTIFICATION: American medical critic and writer who was an early contributor to zone therapy, a precursor to the practice of reflexology
FLOURISHED: Early twentieth century

OVERVIEW

Edwin Bowers was an American medical critic and writer who, with William H. Fitzgerald in 1913, introduced zone therapy, an early form of the modern field of reflexology. Their book, *Zone Therapy* (1917), outlines treatments for a number of existing ailments and examines other clinical issues, including relieving pain by applying various forms of pressure to overcome hay fever, asthma, upset stomach, and pain associated with childbirth.

Reflexology was called zone therapy until the early 1960s. Modern-day reflexology is a complementary, alternative healing practice that involves the physical act of applying pressure to the feet and hands, often with the use of lotion or oil, to treat persons with various ailments.

Zone therapy in its infancy was somewhat less developed in its approach, and it was rooted in the idea that the body could be divided into zones that ran from the feet to the head. Bowers and Fitzgerald reportedly discovered that when a disturbance, or ailment, affected a particular "zone" of the body, then all of the organs and other anatomy in the same zone was also affected. Using this logic, they employed pegs and other devices to apply pressure to the affected zone in the hands or feet (or both) to attempt to remedy various health issues.

Bowers first presented on the subject of zone therapy in an article, "To Stop That Toothache, Squeeze Your Toe" (1915), which was published in *Everybody's Magazine*. The publication of this article likely marked the first time zone therapy was introduced to general readers. Bowers cited Fitzgerald as a source of inspiration for the article. It is thought that Bowers was initially skeptical of Fitzgerald's claims about the therapy, but Bowers would later reveal findings that led him to accept the validity of the practice.

The methods of Bowers and Fitzgerald were advocated by a number of esteemed colleagues during their lifetime, including by Benedict Lust (the founder of naturopathy in the United States), and

Pressure Therapy

In his article "'To Stop that Toothache, Squeeze Your Toe,'" (1915), Edwin Bowers, an early proponent of zone therapy, provides a simple example of the therapy involving direct pressure that was developed by his colleague William H. Fitzgerald.

The Hartford physician [William H. Fitzgerald] divides the body into ten perpendicular zones, including the line running up the middle of the body, and these zones correspond to the fingers of the hand, or the toes. One using his method must know what hand or foot to press, and how, in order to get a definite desired result.

If the first joint of the thumb is pressed firmly and steadily for three minutes, it will relieve and favorably influence pain in the stomach, the chest, the front teeth, the nose, the great toe, as well as everything else in this zone. But it will have not the slightest influence upon the tonsils, the liver, or the spleen, for they are in the fourth zone, and to affect them it is necessary to make pressure upon the fourth finger. Furthermore, pressure on the right hand will not have any effect on the left half of the body.

were further developed by other influential reflexologists, such as Eunice D. Ingham, who brought the field closer to its current state. The practice of reflexology has also been criticized by other clinicians, especially those rooted in more traditional modern medicine. Regardless, the ideas and practices that originated with Bowers and Fitzgerald continue to be used and expanded upon.

Brandy Weidow, M.S.

FURTHER READING

Bowers, Edwin Frederick. *Side-Stepping Ill Health.* Reprint. Charleston, S.C.: Nabu Press, 2010.

Fitzgerald, William H., and Edwin Frederick Bowers. *Zone Therapy: Or, Relieving Pain at Home.* Reprint. Whitefish, Mont.: Kessinger, 2007.

Marquardt, Hanne. *Reflex Zone Therapy of the Feet: A Textbook for Therapists.* Rochester, Vt.: Healing Arts Press, 1988.

See also: Acupressure; Fitzgerald, William H.; Lust, Benedict; Manipulative and body-based practices; Massage therapy; Pain management; Reflexology.

Brahmi

CATEGORY: Herbs and supplements
RELATED TERM: *Bacopa monnieri*
DEFINITION: Natural plant product used to treat specific health conditions.
PRINCIPAL PROPOSED USE: Enhancing memory and mental function
OTHER PROPOSED USES: Allergies, asthma, depression, hypothyroidism, narcotic addiction, ulcers

OVERVIEW

Bacopa monnieri is a creeping perennial with white or blue flowers that grows throughout much of South Asia. It has been used traditionally to treat epilepsy, depression, insomnia, and schizophrenia. In the traditional medicine of India, Ayurveda, *B. monnieri* is considered to fall in the "brahmi" category of herbs, a group of substances said to assist the mind and enhance awareness. From this comes *B. monnieri*'s common name of brahmi, despite the fact that many other herbs also fall into the brahmi category.

THERAPEUTIC DOSAGES

The proposed active ingredients in *B. monnieri* are substances called bacosides. A typical dose of *B. monnieri* used in the studies described below was 300 to 450 mg daily of a concentrated alcohol extract standardized to bacoside content, equivalent to about 6 to 9 grams of whole dried herb.

THERAPEUTIC USES

B. monnieri is widely marketed as a "brain tonic" for enhancing memory and mental function. However, as discussed in the next section, the evidence that it works remains weak at best.

Even weaker evidence, far too preliminary to rely upon, hints that *B. monnieri* might have potential value for allergies, asthma, narcotic addiction, hypothyroidism, depression, and ulcers. However, far more research is necessary before anyone could responsibly promote *B. monnieri* for these conditions.

SCIENTIFIC EVIDENCE

Although several double-blind, placebo-controlled studies have evaluated the potential value of *B. monnieri* for enhancing mental function, the results are far from conclusive. *B. monnieri* appears to have antioxidant properties in the brain, which could potentially lead to positive effects on mental function. However, a two-week, double-blind, placebo-controlled trial of seventy-six persons who tested the potential memory-enhancing benefits of *B. monnieri* generally failed to find much evidence of benefit. The only significant improvement seen among all the many measures used was in one that evaluated retention of new information. While this may sound at least somewhat promising, in fact it means almost nothing. When a study uses many different techniques to assess improvement, mere chance ensures that at least one of them will come up with results. Properly designed studies should focus on one test of benefit alone (the "primary outcome measure") that is selected prior to running the trial. "Fishing" for results among multiple tests is a highly suspect method. Similarly, a randomized trial involving forty-eight healthy elderly subjects found some memory enhancing effects of *B. monnieri* compared with placebo, but the outcomes measured were too numerous to be meaningful.

Nonetheless, if several independent studies use multiple tests of improvement, and the pattern of response is reliably maintained, then the results begin to appear more significant. This does not seem to be the case with *B. monnieri*. In a previous double-blind, placebo-controlled study enrolling forty-six individuals, use of *B. monnieri* over a two-week period again produced benefits, but in an entirely different pattern. In yet another double-blind, placebo-controlled study, this one involving thirty-eight people, short-term use of *B. monnieri* failed to produce any measurable improvements in memory. In addition, use of combined *Ginkgo biloba* (120 milligrams, or mg) and *B. monnieri* (300 mg) has also failed to improve mental function. This type of inconsistency suggests that the limited benefits seen in some studies were due to chance.

Slightly more promising results have been seen in studies of a proprietary Ayurvedic mixture containing *B. monnieri* and about thirty other ingredients. However, these studies are generally not up to modern scientific standards.

SAFETY ISSUES

There are no well-known significant side effects associated with the use of *B. monnieri*. However, comprehensive safety studies have not been reported. Safety in young children, pregnant or nursing women, and people with severe liver or kidney disease has not been established.

EBSCO CAM Review Board

FURTHER READING

Channa, S., et al. "Broncho-Vasodilatory Activity of Fractions and Pure Constituents Isolated from *Bacopa monniera*." *Journal of Ethnopharmacology* 86 (2003): 27-35

Maher, B. F., et al. "The Acute Effects of Combined Administration of *Ginkgo biloba* and *Bacopa monniera* on Cognitive Function in Humans." *Human Psychopharmacology* 17 (2002): 163-164.

Nathan, P. J., J. Clarke, et al. "The Acute Effects of an Extract of *Bacopa monniera* (*B. monnieri*) on Cognitive Function in Healthy Normal Subjects." *Human Psychopharmacology* 16 (2001): 345-351.

Nathan, P. J., S. Tanner, et al. "Effects of a Combined Extract of *Ginkgo biloba* and *Bacopa monniera* on Cognitive Function in Healthy Humans." *Human Psychopharmacology* 19 (2004): 91-96.

Roodenrys, S., et al. "Chronic Effects of *B. monnieri* (*Bacopa monnieri*) on Human Memory." *Neuropsychopharmacology* 27 (2002): 279-281.

Samiulla, D. S., D. Prashanth, and A. Amit. "Mast Cell Stabilising Activity of *Bacopa monnieri*." *Fitoterapia* 72 (2001): 284-285.

See also: Herbal medicine; Memory and mental function impairment.

Braid, James

CATEGORY: Biography

IDENTIFICATION: Scottish physician and surgeon who was a pioneer of hypnotism and hypnotherapy

BORN: June 19, 1795; Ryelaw House, Portmoak, Kinross, Scotland

DIED: March 25, 1860; Manchester, England

OVERVIEW

James Braid was a Scottish physician and surgeon who specialized in ocular and muscular conditions. He later pioneered hypnotism and hypnotherapy, and he coined the English words "neuro-hypnotism" ("nervous sleep") and "hypnotism," from which the term "hypnosis" was later derived. Braid is often regarded as the first genuine hypnotherapist.

The Human Eye in Hypnosis

In his 1843 work Neurypnology, James Braid outlines his theories on hypnotism. The following passage discusses his idea of why the eye is a central component of hypnosis.

[F]rom a careful analysis of the whole of my experiments, which have been very numerous, I have been led to the following conclusion: That it is a law in the animal economy, that by a continued fixation of the mental and visual eye, on any object which is not of itself of an exciting nature, with absolute repose of body, and general quietude, they become wearied; and, provided the patients rather favor than resist the feeling of stupor of which they will soon experience the tendency to creep upon them, during such experiments, a state of somnolency is induced, accompanied with that condition of the brain and nervous system generally, which renders the patient liable to be affected, according to the mode of manipulating, so as to exhibit the hypnotic phenomena.

In addition to being noted for his work in hypnosis, Braid was a practicing surgeon. He was an apprentice to a father-and-son pair of surgeons (both named Charles Anderson). He also attended the University of Edinburgh from 1812 to 1814. He obtained a diploma from the Licentiate of the Royal College of Surgeons of the City of Edinburgh in 1815, which promoted him from Fellow to a Member of the College. He became a surgeon in Leadhills, Lanarkshire, and later set up a private practice in Dumfries. Braid moved to Manchester, England, in 1828 and practiced medicine there until his death.

In 1841, after observing the work of traveling mesmerist Charles Lafontaine, Braid found that mesmerized persons demonstrated an altered physical state. Lafontaine was practicing Mesmerism, or "animal magnetism," which was based on the work of Franz Mesmer. Braid later claimed his own discovery of the psycho-physiological mechanism underlying the altered state and went on to give widespread public lectures on the subject.

Braid based his practice on Mesmerism, but his theory differed from the originators as to how the procedure worked. Braid later changed his sleep-based physiological theory to a psychological one that concentrated on a single item or idea. He thus renamed the theory monoideism in 1847.

During his lifetime, Braid published many articles, booklets, and other pieces of literature primarily focused on various aspects of hypnotism. In his first major publication, *Neurypnology: Or, the Rationale of Nervous Sleep, Considered in Relation with Animal Magnetism* (1843), he reported the importance of both visual and mental concentration for successful transition to the altered physiological state. He asserted that continued fixation of both aspects of concentration served to induce a natural physiological mechanism that existed in human beings.

Braid's career strongly influenced a number of medical figures. Also of note, the term "Braidism" has been used as a synonym for "hypnotism," although it is rarely used in modern times.

Brandy Weidow, M.S.

FURTHER READING

Braid, James. *Neurypnology: Or, the Rationale of Nervous Sleep, Considered in Relation with Animal Magnetism.* 1843. Reprint. New York: Classics of Psychiatry & Behavioral Sciences Library, 1994.

Kravis, N. M. "James Braid's Psychophysiology: A Turning Point in the History of Dynamic Psychiatry." *American Journal of Psychiatry* 145, no. 10 (1988): 1191-1206.

Robertson, Donald, and Michael Heap, eds. *The Discovery of Hypnosis: Complete Writings of James Braid, the Father of Hypnotherapy.* Studley, England: National Council for Hypnotherapy, 2008.

See also: Hypnotherapy; Mind/body medicine.

Branched-chain amino acids

CATEGORY: Herbs and supplements

RELATED TERMS: BCAAs, isoleucine, leucine, valine

DEFINITION: Natural substance of the human body used as a supplement to treat specific health conditions.

PRINCIPAL PROPOSED USES: Amyotrophic lateral sclerosis (Lou Gehrig's disease), loss of appetite (in persons with cancer)

OTHER PROPOSED USES: Muscular dystrophy, recovery from surgery, recovery from traumatic brain injury, severe liver disease such as cirrhosis, sports and fitness support, tardive dyskinesia

OVERVIEW

Branched-chain amino acids (BCAAs) are naturally occurring molecules (leucine, isoleucine, and valine) that the body uses to build proteins. The term "branched chain" refers to the molecular structure of these particular amino acids. Muscles have a particularly high content of BCAAs. For reasons that are not entirely clear, BCAA supplements may improve appetite in cancer patients and slow the progression of amyotrophic lateral sclerosis (ALS, or Lou Gehrig's disease, a condition that leads to degeneration of nerves, atrophy of the muscles, and eventual death). BCAAs have also been proposed as a supplement to boost athletic performance.

REQUIREMENTS AND SOURCES

Dietary protein usually provides all the BCAAs needed. However, physical stress and injury can increase a person's need for BCAAs to repair damage, so supplementation may be helpful.

BCAAs are present in all protein-containing foods, but the best sources are red meat and dairy products. Chicken, fish, and eggs are excellent sources as well. Whey protein and egg protein supplements are another way to ensure that a person is getting enough BCAAs. Supplements may contain all three BCAAs together or simply individual BCAAs.

THERAPEUTIC DOSAGES

The typical dosage of BCAAs is 1 to 5 grams (g) daily.

THERAPEUTIC USES

Preliminary evidence suggests that BCAAs may improve appetite in people undergoing treatment for cancer. There is also some evidence that BCAA supplements may reduce symptoms of amyotrophic lateral sclerosis (ALS, or Lou Gehrig's disease); however, not all studies have had positive results.

Preliminary evidence from a series of small studies suggests that BCAAs might decrease symptoms of tardive dyskinesia, a movement disorder caused by long-term usage of antipsychotic drugs. BCAAs have also shown a bit of promise for enhancing recovery from traumatic brain injury.

Because of how they are metabolized in the body, BCAAs might be helpful for individuals with severe liver disease (such as cirrhosis). BCAAs have also been tried for aiding muscle recovery after bedrest, such as following surgery.

Although there is a little supportive evidence, on balance, current research does not indicate that BCAAs are effective for enhancing sports performance. One preliminary study hints that BCAAs might aid recovery from long-distance running. BCAAs have also as yet failed to prove effective for muscular dystrophy.

SCIENTIFIC EVIDENCE

Appetite in cancer patients. A double-blind study tested BCAAs on twenty-eight people with cancer who had lost their appetites because of either the disease itself or its treatment. Appetite improved in 55 percent of those taking BCAAs (4.8 g daily) compared with only 16 percent of those taking a placebo.

Amyotrophic lateral sclerosis (Lou Gehrig's disease). A small double-blind study found evidence that BCAAs might help protect muscle strength in people with Lou Gehrig's disease. Eighteen individuals were given either BCAAs (taken four times daily between meals) or a placebo and followed for one year. The results showed that people taking BCAAs declined much more slowly than those receiving a placebo. In the placebo group, five of nine participants lost their ability to walk, two died, and another required a respirator. Only one of the nine participants receiving BCAAs became unable to walk during the study period. This study is too small to provide conclusive evidence, but it does suggest that BCAAs might be helpful for this disease. However, other studies found no effect, and one actually found a slight increase in deaths during the study period among those treated with BCAAs compared with those treated with a placebo.

Muscular dystrophy. One double-blind, placebo controlled study found leucine (one of the amino acids in BCAAs) ineffective at the dose of 0.2 g per kilogram body weight (for example, 15 g daily for a 75-kilogram woman) in 96 individuals with muscular dystrophy. Over the course of one year, no differences were seen between the effects of leucine and a placebo.

SAFETY ISSUES

BCAAs are believed to be safe; when taken in excess, they are simply converted into other amino acids. However, like other amino acids, BCAAs may interfere with medications for Parkinson's disease. They may reduce the effectiveness of medications for Parkinson's disease (such as levodopa).

EBSCO CAM Review Board

FURTHER READING

Aquilani, R., et al. "Branched-Chain Amino Acids Enhance the Cognitive Recovery of Patients with Severe Traumatic Brain Injury." *Archives of Physical Medicine and Rehabilitation* 86 (2005): 1729-1735.

Charlton, M. "Branched-Chain Amino Acid Enriched Supplements as Therapy for Liver Disease." *Journal of Nutrition* 136 (2005): 295S-298S.

Crowe, M. J., et al. "Effects of Dietary Leucine Supplementation on Exercise Performance." *European Journal of Applied Physiology* 97 (2006): 664-671.

Marchesini, G., et al. "Nutritional Treatment with Branched-Chain Amino Acids in Advanced Liver Cirrhosis." *Journal of Gastroenterology* 35 (2000): 7-12.

Richardson, M. A., et al. "Branched Chain Amino Acid Treatment of Tardive Dyskinesia in Children and Adolescents." *Journal of Clinical Psychiatry* 65 (2004): 92-96.

Richardson, M. A., et al. "Efficacy of the Branched-Chain Amino Acids in the Treatment of Tardive Dyskinesia in Men." *American Journal of Psychiatry* 160 (2003): 1117-1124.

Stein, T. P., et al. "Branched Chain Amino Acid Supplementation During Bed Rest: Effect on Recovery." *Journal of Applied Physiology* 94 (2003): 1345-1352.

Watson, P., et al. "The Effect of Acute Branched-Chain Amino Acid Supplementation on Prolonged Exercise Capacity in a Warm Environment." *European Journal of Applied Physiology* 93 (2004): 306-314.

See also: Amyotrophic lateral sclerosis; Herbal medicine; Sports and fitness support: Enhancing recovery.

Breast engorgement: Homeopathic remedies

CATEGORY: Homeopathy
DEFINITION: The use of highly diluted remedies to treat pain and swelling from swollen breasts during lactation.
STUDIED HOMEOPATHIC REMEDIES: Belladonna; *Bryonia*; homeopathic remedy containing *Apis Mellifica* and *Bryonia*

INTRODUCTION

Women who choose not to nurse their infants often experience breast pain and swelling until milk production stops. Although this condition is not dangerous, the discomfort can be quite severe. Similar symptoms occur when a woman weans her baby. Homeopathic remedies have a long history of use for easing this transition, and there is preliminary support for the belief that they are effective. Breast engorgement should not be confused with mastitis, however, an infection or inflammation of the nursing breast.

SCIENTIFIC EVALUATIONS OF HOMEOPATHIC REMEDIES

A double-blind trial of seventy-one women tested a homeopathic remedy consisting of *Apis mellifica* and *Bryonia*, both at 9c (centesimal) potency. The results showed that, compared with placebo, the use of homeopathic treatment significantly reduced pain and tension sensations in the breast. Spontaneous milk flow also decreased.

TRADITIONAL HOMEOPATHIC TREATMENTS

Classical homeopathy offers many possible homeopathic treatments for breast engorgement. These therapies are chosen based on various specific details of the person seeking treatment.

The symptom picture for homeopathic *Bryonia* includes breast pain and fullness without redness and pain in the left breast, especially when raising the arm. Pain is said to be increased by motion and touch or by deep breathing, and is reduced when pressure is applied. Homeopathic belladonna might be recommended when breasts are inflamed, warm, reddened, and hard to the touch, and when these symptoms are accompanied by fever. These symptoms also could indicate infection.

EBSCO CAM Review Board

FURTHER READING

Kraft, K. "Complementary/Alternative Medicine in the Context of Prevention of Disease and Maintenance of Health." *Preventive Medicine* 49 (2009): 88-92.

Mangesi, L., and T. Dowswell. "Treatments for Breast Engorgement During Lactation." *Cochrane Database of Systematic Reviews* (2010): CD006946. Available through *EBSCO DynaMed Systematic Literature Surveillance* at http://www.ebscohost.com/dynamed.

See also: Breast-feeding support; Breast pain, cyclic; Women's health.

Breast enhancement

RELATED TERM: Breast augmentation
CATEGORY: Therapies and techniques
DEFINITION: The use of herbs and supplements, phytoestrogen, and progesterone to increase breast size.
PRINCIPAL PROPOSED USE: Increasing breast size

OVERVIEW

Each year, as many as one-quarter million women in the United States utilize surgery to increase their breast size. Many other women purchase natural products touted to achieve the same goal without surgery. However, there is no meaningful evidence that any of these herbs and supplements actually have this effect, and no theoretical evidence to suppose that they would.

CLINICALLY PROVEN PRODUCTS

Many manufacturers of breast enhancement products claim that their treatments are clinically proven. A typical Web site may quote a study that states something like "One hundred women were given this product, and after 6 months their breast size increased by 10 percent!" However, while this may sound promising, it actually shows nothing.

The problem lies in a deeply rooted feature of human perception: When people expect to observe something, they usually do observe it, whether or not it actually occurred. In the foregoing hypothetical breast enhancement study, researchers would find it almost impossible not to "discover" an improvement. Measurement of breast size is an inexact art that allows for considerable leeway. Human nature would inevitably incline researchers to err on the side of finding improvement when they make their measurements at the end of the study. This would be the case even if the researchers were completely impartial, and it is even more of a problem if they are paid by the product's manufacturer (which is usually the case).

To avoid this problem, medical researchers use a special type of study: the double-blind, placebo-controlled trial. In these trials, some participants receive real treatment, others receive fake treatment, and neither the participants nor the researchers know which is which (until the study is over). When performed correctly, double-blind, placebo-controlled studies eliminate the influence of bias (and other confounding fac-

tors), and for this reason they are the accepted source of reliable knowledge regarding medical treatments.

There are no published double-blind, placebo-controlled studies of breast enhancement products. Until breast enhancement products are subjected to this form of study, it is not possible to take any of them as evidence-based. In lieu of clinical evidence, one might possibly be encouraged to try breast enhancement products if they had a reasonable theoretical likelihood of increasing breast size. However, these products fall short.

There are three basic categories of herbs and supplements found in breast enhancement products: phytoestrogens, herbs and supplements said to raise progesterone levels, and miscellaneous herbs and supplements that have no real relationship to breast enhancement.

Phytoestrogens. The hormone estrogen, if taken in high enough doses, increases breast size by stimulating the growth of breast tissue. However, it is not safe to use estrogen in this way because when breast cells are stimulated to grow, they are more likely to turn cancerous. A woman who takes enough estrogen to enlarge her breasts will greatly increase her risk of breast cancer.

Many herbs and supplements provided in breast enhancement products are included in these products because they act somewhat like estrogen in the body. These substances are called phytoestrogens, meaning "plant-based estrogens," and include alfalfa, fennel, flaxseed, hops, isoflavones, licorice, lignans, red clover, sage, soy, and verbena. Other herbs and supplements that are not phytoestrogens, but are widely promoted as if they were, are added to breast enhancement products. These include black cohosh, chasteberry, dong quai, ginseng, and Mexican yam. Black cohosh may have estrogen-like actions in some parts of the body, but probably not in breast tissue; the other herbs are probably not phytoestrogenic.

According to manufacturers of breast enhancement products, phytoestrogens can enlarge the breasts, like estrogen, but without the user incurring estrogen's risks. There are several problems with this hypothesis. Perhaps the most important is that phytoestrogens generally act to decrease the estrogen-related functions of the body, rather than to increase them. They do so because natural human estrogen exerts its effects in the body by latching on to special sites on cells called estrogen receptors. Phytoestrogens also latch

Foods with High Phytoestrogen Content, Micrograms per 100 Grams

Food Source	Phytoestrogen Content
Flax seed	379,380
Soy beans	103,920
Tofu	27,150
Soy yogurt	10,275
Sesame seeds	8,008
Flax bread	7,540
Multigrain bread	4,798
Soy milk	2,957
Hummus	993
Garlic	603
Mung bean sprouts	495
Dried apricots	444
Alfalfa sprouts	441
Dried dates	329
Sunflower seeds	216
Chestnuts	210
Olive oil	180
Almonds	131
Green beans	105
Peanuts	34
Onion	32
Blueberry	17
Corn	9
Coffee (regular)	6
Watermelon	2
Milk (cow's)	1

trogens should decrease breast size, not increase it. Furthermore, studies indicate that many breast enhancement products do not even contain substantial amounts of phytoestrogens.

In any case, if a breast enhancement product were to contain a powerful phytoestrogen in sufficient quantities to actually stimulate the growth of breast cells, it would also increase the risk of breast cancer. A person cannot get one effect without the other. The measurement of estrogenic breast-cell stimulation is one way of determining the breast cancer risk posed by a substance under study, whether it is a supplement or an environmental contaminant. Thus, there is no particular reason to believe that phytoestrogens can enhance breast size, or, if they did, that they would produce such an effect safely.

Raising progesterone levels. Other constituents of breast enhancement products are used because of their supposed effect on the hormone progesterone. This approach does have a certain logic to it. When taken as a pill, progesterone does increase breast size, and it is fairly safe. However, it does so by stimulating the growth and development of milk-producing cells, an effect that most nonnursing women would wish to avoid.

The herb chasteberry, added to breast enhancement products, might increase progesterone levels in some women. However, there is no evidence that it increases breast size. Another herb added to breast enhancement products as a source of progesterone, Mexican yam, does not raise levels of progesterone. The widespread belief that it does so is based on a misconception.

Other herbs and supplements. Numerous herbs and supplements are added to breast enhancement formulas merely on the basis that they have been used for some condition that affects women. Some of the

on to estrogen receptors. However, when they do so, they only produce a partial effect. In addition, they block the ability of real estrogen to bind to those receptors. The net effect in women of menstrual age is to reduce the action of estrogen. This may be a very useful effect because, in theory, it could decrease a woman's chance of developing breast cancer. However, the same line of reasoning suggests that phytoes-

more commonly mentioned include damiana (an unproven herbal treatment for sexual dysfunction in women), saw palmetto (an unproven herbal treatment for problems with nursing), fish oil (possibly helpful for painful menstruation), and calcium (probably helpful for premenstrual syndrome), among literally hundreds of others. However, there is no reason to believe that an herb or supplement used to treat an unrelated women's health condition will enhance breast size.

EBSCO CAM Review Board

FURTHER READING

Coldham, N. G., and M. J. Sauer. "Identification, Quantitation, and Biological Activity of Phytoestrogens in a Dietary Supplement for Breast Enhancement." *Food and Chemical Toxicology* 39 (2001): 1211-1224.

Fugh-Berman, A. "'Bust Enhancing' Herbal Products." *Obstetrics and Gynecology* 101 (2003): 1345-1349.

Kurzer, M. S. "Phytoestrogen Supplement Use by Women." *Journal of Nutrition* 133 (2003): 1983-1986.

Patisaul, H. B., and W. Jefferson. "The Pros and Cons of Phytoestrogens." *Frontiers in Neuroendocrinology* 31 (2010): 400-419.

Setchell, K. D., et al. "Bioavailability of Pure Isoflavones in Healthy Humans and Analysis of Commercial Soy Isoflavone Supplements." *Journal of Nutrition* 131 (2001): 362-375.

See also: Breast engorgement: Homeopathic remedies; Breast pain, cyclic; Estrogen; Herbal medicine; Progesterone; Women's health.

Breast-feeding support

CATEGORY: Therapies and techniques

RELATED TERMS: Breast engorgement, enhancing breast milk, milk production, nursing support, weaning

DEFINITION: Treatments to aid in the production of nutritional breast milk and to aid in breast-feeding.

PRINCIPAL PROPOSED NATURAL TREATMENTS: None

OTHER PROPOSED NATURAL TREATMENTS

- *Enhancing milk production:* Acupuncture, fenugreek, milk thistle
- *Weaning/breast engorgement:* Proteolytic enzymes, sage

- *Nipple pain:* Peppermint
- *Preventing allergies in children:* Probiotics, reducing saturated fats
- *General nutritional support:* Calcium, multivitamin-multimineral supplement, omega-3 fatty acids

INTRODUCTION

It was one of the more shameful chapters of conventional medicine when, for many decades, physicians discouraged women from breast-feeding. By the 1970s, the poor judgment inherent in this recommendation had become abundantly clear. There is no longer any doubt regarding what should have been obvious from the beginning: that human breast milk is the ideal food for a human infant.

Not only does breast milk contain all the necessary nutrients, it also contains additional substances such as colostrum that provide important health benefits. In addition, human breast milk lacks allergenic substances found in infant formulas based on cow or soy milk. For this reason, breast-feeding, as opposed to formula feeding, may reduce the risk of the infant developing allergy-related diseases such as eczema.

Nursing can also cause difficulties for the mother of a newborn. Milk flow may be insufficient, the breasts may become inflamed or infected, and when it comes time to stop nursing, there may be an interval of severe discomfort. Medical treatments are available for some of these conditions, although in many cases these treatments are more traditional and "low-tech" than modern.

The constituents of human breast milk can be affected in both positive and negative ways by the mother's diet. On the one hand, herbs and supplements, like drugs, should be considered risky in breast-feeding until demonstrated otherwise. On the other hand, certain supplements for the mother might benefit the baby. There is considerable overlap in this subject between conventional and alternative medicine, and only the more "alternative" of the relevant information is presented here.

PROPOSED NATURAL TREATMENTS

Weaning/breast engorgement. Sage leaf tea traditionally has been recommended to dry up milk supply and reduce breast engorgement for the purpose of weaning, but supporting scientific studies are lacking. One early double-blind, placebo-controlled trial did find some benefit for breast engorgement with the

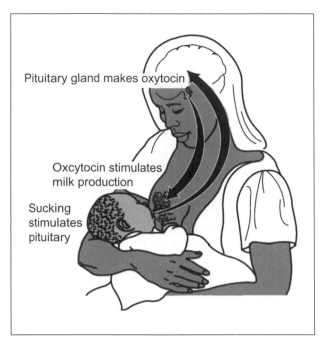

Pituitary gland makes oxytocin

Oxcytocin stimulates
milk production

Sucking
stimulates
pituitary

Breast-feeding involves a hormonal feedback loop that encourages milk production.

use of proteolytic enzymes, but considerably more evidence would be necessary before it could be considered an effective treatment.

According to traditional wisdom, the application of cabbage leaves to the breast can reduce the discomfort of breast engorgement during weaning, but controlled studies indicated that they are not effective for this purpose.

Nipple pain. Pain and irritation in the nipples can cause a nursing mother to cease breast-feeding earlier than she might otherwise wish to. A double-blind study performed in Iran found that applying peppermint water (essentially, lukewarm peppermint tea) directly to the nipples helped prevent nipple and aureola cracks.

Promoting milk supply. The herbs milk thistle and fenugreek have been used historically to promote milk supply, but no studies have been performed to establish whether or not they actually provide any benefit. The herb chasteberry has also been used traditionally for this purpose, but it is not recommend.

Acupuncture has also been proposed for increasing milk supply. However, no benefits were seen in a well-designed and reasonably large (almost 180-participant) trial.

Preventing eczema and other allergic conditions in children. Double-blind, placebo-controlled trials suggest that nursing women may be able to help ward off eczema and other allergic conditions in their children by taking probiotics (friendly bacteria). Cutting down on saturated fat (animal fat) may be helpful too.

General nutritional support. Because breast-feeding requires a woman to supply nutrients to another human being, the use of a general multivitamin-multimineral supplement is advisable. However, such supplements seldom contain adequate amounts of calcium, so a separate calcium supplement should be taken. Calcium supplements offer the additional benefit of reducing lead levels in breast milk.

Essential fatty acids in the omega-3 family are thought to be essential for infant health, especially brain development, so it has been suggested that nursing women should supplement their diet with this nutrient.

Finally, while human breast milk supplies nearly all essential nutrients, it does not contain an adequate amount of iron. This problem is exacerbated by the modern practice of rapidly cutting the umbilical cord, which has the effect of reducing the infant's iron stores. For this reason, some physicians routinely recommend that breast-fed infants should receive iron supplements. However, some evidence suggests that this practice is warranted only if the infant is anemic; otherwise, supplementation may decrease growth rate.

HERBS AND SUPPLEMENTS TO AVOID

Virtually no medicinal herb has been established as safe in nursing, and even herbs that might seem safe because of their wide use in cooking could cause problems when they are taken in the form of highly concentrated extracts. There could even be problems with herbs traditionally recommended for use by nursing mothers. For example, the herb chasteberry is traditionally used to promote milk supply. However, it inhibits prolactin, a hormone that is vital to milk production.

Supplements that are essential nutrients, such as vitamins, generally have a maximum safe intake established for them by a governmental agency. However, other supplements that are not essential nutrients are in much the same position as herbs and could conceivably cause harm. This may even be the case for apparently safe supplements. For example, one double-blind, placebo-controlled study found that if a nursing woman consumes the supplement conjugated linoleic acid, the fat content of her breast milk will be reduced with potentially harmful effects.

EBSCO CAM Review Board

FURTHER READING

Dewey, K. G., et al. "Iron Supplementation Affects Growth and Morbidity of Breast-Fed Infants: Results of a Randomized Trial in Sweden and Honduras." *Journal of Nutrition* 132 (2002): 3249-3255.

Hernandez-Avila, M., et al. "Dietary Calcium Supplements to Lower Blood Lead Levels in Lactating Women." *Epidemiology* 14 (2003): 206-212.

Hoppu, U., M. Kalliomaki, and E. Isolauri. "Maternal Diet Rich in Saturated Fat During Breastfeeding Is Associated with Atopic Sensitization of the Infant." *European Journal of Clinical Nutrition* 54 (2000): 702-705.

Isolauri, E., et al. "Probiotics in the Management of Atopic Eczema." *Clinical and Experimental Allergy* 30 (2000): 1604-1610.

Kalliomaki, M., et al. "Probiotics in Primary Prevention of Atopic Disease." *The Lancet* 357 (2001): 1076-1079.

Masters, N., et al. "Maternal Supplementation with CLA Decreases Milk Fat in Humans." *Lipids* 37 (2002): 133-138.

Sayyah, Melli M., et al. "Effect of Peppermint Water on Prevention of Nipple Cracks in Lactating Primiparous Women." *International Breastfeeding Journal* 2 (2007): 7.

See also: Allergies; Breast engorgement: Homeopathic remedies; Breast pain, cyclic; Children's health; Food allergies and sensitivities; Pain management; Pregnancy support; Premenstrual syndrome (PMS); Women's health.

Breast pain, cyclic

CATEGORY: Condition
RELATED TERMS: Breast tenderness, cyclic, cyclic mastalgia, cyclic mastitis, fibrocystic breast disease
DEFINITION: Treatment of breast pain most often associated with the menstrual cycle.
PRINCIPAL PROPOSED NATURAL TREATMENTS: Chasteberry, *Ginkgo biloba*
OTHER PROPOSED NATURAL TREATMENTS: Diindolyl-methane, evening primrose oil, iodine, red clover isoflavones, soy

INTRODUCTION

Some women's breasts are unusually tender and lumpy, with symptoms of pain and dull heaviness that vary with the menstrual cycle. This condition is called cyclic mastalgia or cyclic mastitis and is often associated with premenstrual syndrome (PMS). When the lumps become significant enough to be called cysts, the condition is called fibrocystic breast disease.

Besides discomfort, perhaps the worst problem of this condition is that it can mimic the appearance of breast cancer on mammograms, leading to false alarms. To make matters worse, fibrocystic changes can also hide true cancers, and some evidence hints that women with fibrocystic breast disease may also have a greater tendency toward breast cancer.

The cause of cyclic breast pain is unclear. One theory, popular in Europe, suggests that higher than normal levels of the hormone prolactin may be involved. Another theory attributes the condition to an imbalance of essential fatty acids. Conventional treatment for cyclic mastalgia involves anti-inflammatory medications and, sometimes, hormonal treatments.

PRINCIPAL PROPOSED NATURAL TREATMENTS

Cyclic mastalgia often occurs in connection with PMS.

Chasteberry. In Germany, the herb chasteberry is frequently used to treat cyclic mastalgia and other symptoms of PMS because of its effect on the pituitary gland to suppress the release of prolactin. Some evidence suggests that chasteberry is effective for this purpose. For example, a double-blind trial of 104 women compared placebo with two forms of chasteberry (liquid and tablet) for at least three menstrual cycles. The results showed statistically significant and comparable improvements in the treated groups compared with placebo.

Another double-blind, placebo-controlled study, enrolling 178 women, evaluated chasteberry for PMS in general. The results over three menstrual cycles indicated that chasteberry reduced breast tenderness and other PMS symptoms. Benefits were also seen in two other double-blind trials enrolling more than 250 women.

Ginkgo biloba. Although the herb *Ginkgo biloba* is primarily used to enhance memory and mental function, it may also be helpful for breast tenderness. A double-blind, placebo-controlled study evaluated 143 women eighteen to forty-five years of age, with PMS symptoms, and followed them for two menstrual cycles. Each woman received either the ginkgo extract (80 milligrams twice daily) or placebo on day sixteen of the first cycle. Treatment was continued until day five of the next cycle and resumed again on day sixteen of that cycle. Compared with placebo, ginkgo significantly relieved major symptoms of PMS, especially breast pain.

OTHER PROPOSED NATURAL TREATMENTS

Evening primrose oil contains relatively high concentrations of the essential omega-6 fatty acid named gamma-linolenic acid (GLA). On the theory that essential fatty acid imbalances play a role in cyclic mastalgia, evening primrose oil became a popular treatment for this condition. However, despite numerous positive anecdotes, there are considerable doubts regarding whether it is actually effective. The main supporting evidence for GLA comes from three small double-blind studies.

All of these trials, however, had significant limitations in study design and reporting. A large (555-participant) and well-designed study failed to find GLA, with or without antioxidants, any more effective than placebo. The placebo by itself, however, was found to be quite effective, possibly explaining why so many doctors and patients believe that evening primrose oil is helpful. Another well-designed study found that evening primrose oil, by itself or with fish oil, is not more effective than placebo for cyclic breast pain. Other studies found evening primrose oil ineffective for established breast cysts.

Fish oil taken alone has failed to prove effective for cyclic breast pain. According to one small double-blind trial, the substance diindolylmethane might be helpful for cyclic mastalgia.

A small and poorly reported double-blind, placebo-controlled trial provides weak evidence that red clover isoflavones might reduce symptoms of cyclic mastalgia. Another small study suggests possible benefit with soy protein. Weak evidence suggests the supplement iodine may also be helpful for cyclic mastalgia.

Like chasteberry, the herb bugleweed appears to reduce prolactin levels and, for this reason, has also been tried for the treatment of cyclic mastalgia. However, this herb affects the thyroid gland, so it is not recommended.

Many conventional and alternative practitioners suggest avoiding caffeine. However, despite the popularity of this intervention, there is no consistent evidence that caffeine causes breast pain.

EBSCO CAM Review Board

FURTHER READING

Blommers, J., et al. "Evening Primrose Oil and Fish Oil for Severe Chronic Mastalgia." *American Journal of Obstetrics and Gynecology* 187 (2002): 1389-1394.

Goyal, A., and R. E. Mansel. "A Randomized Multicenter Study of Gamolenic Acid (Efamast) with and Without Antioxidant Vitamins and Minerals in the Management of Mastalgia." *Breast Journal* 11 (2005): 41-47.

Horner, N. K., and J. W. Lampe. "Potential Mechanisms of Diet Therapy for Fibrocystic Breast Conditions Show Inadequate Evidence of Effectiveness." *Journal of the American Dietetic Association* 100 (2000): 1368-1380.

Ingram, D. M., et al. "A Double-Blind Randomized Controlled Trial of Isoflavones in the Treatment of Cyclical Mastalgia." *The Breast* 11 (2002): 170-174.

Kollias, J., et al. "Effect of Evening Primrose Oil on Clinically Diagnosed Fibroadenomas. *The Breast* 9 (2000): 35-36.

McFadyen, I. J., et al. "A Randomized Double Blind-Cross Over Trial of Soya Protein for the Treatment of Cyclical Breast Pain." *The Breast* 9 (2000): 271-276.

Schellenberg, R. "Treatment for the Premenstrual Syndrome with Agnus Castus Fruit Extract." *British Medical Journal* 322 (2001): 134-137.

Zeligs, M. A., et al. "Managing Cyclical Mastalgia with Absorbable Diindolylmethane." *Journal of the American Dietetic Association* 8 (2005): 10-20.

See also: Chasteberry; Ginkgo.

Bromelain

CATEGORY: Herbs and supplements
PRINCIPAL PROPOSED USES: Athletic injuries, digestive problems, phlebitis, sinusitis, surgery
OTHER PROPOSED USES: Arthritis, chronic venous in-

sufficiency, easy bruising, gout, hemorrhoids, dysmenorrhea, ulcerative colitis

OVERVIEW

Bromelain is not actually a single substance, but rather a collection of protein-digesting enzymes (also called proteolytic enzymes) found in pineapple juice and in the stem of pineapple plants. It is primarily produced in Japan, Hawaii, and Taiwan, and much of the original research was performed in the first two of those locations. Subsequently, European researchers developed an interest, and by 1995, bromelain had become the thirteenth most common individual herbal product sold in Germany.

THERAPEUTIC DOSAGES

Recommended dosages of bromelain vary with the form used. Because of the wide variation, one should follow the label's instructions.

THERAPEUTIC USES

Bromelain (often in combination with other proteolytic enzymes) is used in Europe to aid in recovery from surgery and athletic injuries, as well as to treat sinusitis and phlebitis. Other proposed uses of bromelain include chronic venous insufficiency (closely related to varicose veins), hemorrhoids, other diseases of the veins, bruising, rheumatoid arthritis, gout, ulcerative colitis, and dysmenorrhea (menstrual pain). However, there is no real evidence that bromelain is effective for these conditions. One study failed to find bromelain effective for osteoarthritis.

Bromelain is definitely useful as a digestive enzyme. Unlike most digestive enzymes, bromelain is active in both the acid environment of the stomach and the alkaline environment of the small intestine. This may make it particularly effective as an oral digestive aid for those who do not digest food properly.

Bromelain may also increase the absorption of various drugs, particularly antibiotics such as amoxicillin and tetracycline. This could offer both risks and benefits. Bromelain is widely available in grocery stores as a meat tenderizer.

SCIENTIFIC EVIDENCE

While most large enzymes are broken down in the digestive tract, those found in bromelain appear to be absorbed whole to a certain extent. This finding makes it reasonable to suppose that bromelain can actually produce systemic (whole-body) effects. Once in the blood, bromelain appears to reduce inflammation, "thin" the blood, and affect the immune system. These influences may be responsible for some of bromelain's therapeutic effects.

Injury and surgery. The evidence for bromelain as a treatment for injuries and surgeries is mixed. A double-blind, placebo-controlled study evaluated 160 women who received episiotomies (surgical cuts in the perineum) during childbirth. Participants given 40 milligram (mg) of bromelain four times daily for three days, beginning four hours after delivery, showed a statistically significant decrease in edema, inflammation, and pain. Ninety percent of persons taking bromelain demonstrated excellent or good responses, compared with 44 percent in the placebo group. However, another double-blind study of 158 women who received episiotomies failed to find significant benefit.

In a double-blind controlled trial, ninety-five patients undergoing treatment for cataracts were given 40 mg of bromelain or a placebo (along with other treatments) four times daily for two days prior to surgery and five days post-operatively. Overall, less inflammation was noted in the bromelain-treated group compared with the placebo group.

Benefits were also seen in double-blind, placebo-controlled studies of dental, nasal, or foot surgery. However, a study of 154 people undergoing facial plastic surgery found no benefit.

A somewhat informal controlled study of 146 boxers suggested that bromelain helps bruises to heal more quickly. Another study–this one without any type of control group–found that bromelain reduced swelling, pain at rest, and tenderness among 59 patients with blunt trauma injuries, including bruising.

People who engage in intense exercise to which they are not accustomed may experience a set of symptoms called delayed onset muscle soreness (DOMS), consisting of pain, reduced flexibility, and weakness of the muscles involved. Bromelain has been proposed for this condition, but a small double-blind, placebo-controlled study failed to find it effective.

Sinusitis. In a double-blind trial, forty-eight patients with moderately severe to severe sinusitis received bromelain or a placebo for six days. All patients were placed on standard therapy for sinusitis, which included antihistamines, analgesics, and antibiotics. Upon completion of the study, inflammation was reduced in 83 percent of those taking bromelain compared with 52 percent of the placebo group. Breathing difficulty was relieved in 78 percent of the bromelain group and 68 percent of the placebo group. Overall, good to excellent results were observed in 87 percent of patients treated with bromelain compared with 68 percent on placebo. Benefits were also seen in two other studies enrolling a total of more than one hundred individuals with sinusitis.

SAFETY ISSUES

Bromelain appears to be essentially nontoxic, and it seldom causes side effects other than occasional mild gastrointestinal distress or allergic reactions. However, because bromelain "thins" the blood to some extent, it should not be combined with drugs such as warfarin (Coumadin) without a doctor's supervision.

According to one small animal study, bromelain might interact with sedative medications, increasing their effect. As noted above, it might also increase blood levels of various antibiotics, which could present risks in some cases. In addition, one trial suggests that doses of bromelain eight times higher than standard recommendations might increase heart rate (but not blood pressure). Safety in young children, pregnant or nursing women, and those with liver or kidney disease has not been established.

IMPORTANT INTERACTIONS

Bromelain might amplify the effect of medications that thin the blood, such as warfarin (Coumadin) or heparin, sedative drugs such as benzodiazepines, or antibiotics.

EBSCO CAM Review Board

FURTHER READING

Brakebusch, M., et al. "Bromelain Is an Accelerator of Phagocytosis, Respiratory Burst and Killing of *Candida albicans* by Human Granulocytes and Monocytes." *European Journal of Medical Research* 6 (2001): 193-200.

Brien, S., et al. "Bromelain as an Adjunctive Treatment for Moderate-to-Severe Osteoarthritis of the Knee." *QJM: An International Journal of Medicine* 99 (2006): 841-850.

Stone, M. B., et al. "Preliminary Comparison of Bromelain and Ibuprofen for Delayed Onset Muscle Soreness Management." *Clinical Journal of Sports Medicine* 12 (2002): 373-378.

See also: Herbal medicine; Sports and fitness support: Enhancing recovery; Venous insufficiency: Homeopathic remedies.

Bromocriptine

CATEGORY: Drug interactions
DEFINITION: An herb sometimes used to treat conditions in which there is too much prolactin, a hormone, in the body.
INTERACTION: Chasteberry
TRADE NAME: Parlodel

CHASTEBERRY

Effect: Theoretical Interference with Drug Action

The herb chasteberry inhibits prolactin secretion and might have unpredictable effects if combined with bromocriptine.

EBSCO CAM Review Board

FURTHER READING

Jarry, H., et al. "In Vitro Prolactin but Not Lh and Fsh Release Is Inhibited by Compounds in Extracts of *Agnus-castus*: Direct Evidence for a Dopaminergic Principle by the Dopamine Receptor Assay." *Experimental and Clinical Endocrinology* 102 (1994): 448-454.

Milewicz, A., et al. "*Vitex agnus-castus* Extract in the Treatment of Luteal Phase Defects Due to Latent Hyperprolactinemia." *Arzneimittel-Forschung* 43, no. 7 (1993): 752-756.

See also: Chasteberry; Food and Drug Administration; Supplements: Introduction.

Bronchitis

CATEGORY: Condition
RELATED TERMS: Acute bronchitis, chest cold, chronic bronchitis
DEFINITION: Treatment of inflammation of the major air passageways in the lungs.
PRINCIPAL PROPOSED NATURAL TREATMENTS: Essential oil monoterpenes (oral), *Pelargonium sidoides*

OTHER PROPOSED TREATMENTS: All treatments used for colds or asthma, combination product containing horseradish and nasturtium, combination product containing thyme and primrose root extract, elecampane, essential oils (inhaled), horehound, licorice, marshmallow, milk avoidance, mullein, slippery elm, vitamin C, yerba santa

INTRODUCTION

The term "bronchitis" refers to inflammation of the major air passageways in the lungs, the bronchi. There are two principal types of bronchitis: acute bronchitis and chronic bronchitis. The latter is closely related to emphysema. Acute bronchitis, the subject of this article, is a condition that frequently develops during the course of a common cold. Symptoms may include a cough (dry or productive), the sensation of heaviness in the chest, and difficulty breathing.

It has become clear that, in many cases, symptoms of bronchitis represent temporary asthma brought on by a respiratory infection. Anti-asthma drugs are now commonly a major component of treatment. Antibiotics may be used too.

PRINCIPAL PROPOSED TREATMENTS

Essential oil monoterpenes. Aromatic essential oils, such as eucalyptus oil and peppermint oil (menthol), have a long history of use as inhalation treatments for respiratory infections. The supporting evidence for such treatments is quite weak. Considerably better evidence supports the use of certain essential oils when taken by mouth.

One combination of essential oils has been extensively evaluated as a treatment for respiratory problems. This mixture, called essential oil monoterpenes, consists of cineole from eucalyptus, d-limonene from citrus fruit, and alpha-pinene from pine. Numerous double-blind, placebo-controlled trials, many of substantial size, indicate that essential oil monoterpenes can aid recovery from sinusitis, bronchitis, and other respiratory conditions.

One large study evaluated the effectiveness of essential oil monoterpenes for acute bronchitis. In this two-week, double-blind, placebo-controlled trial of 676 people with acute bronchitis, participants received either placebo, essential oil monoterpenes, or one of two antibiotics. The results indicate that the essential oil mixture was significantly more effective than placebo and at least as effective as antibiotic therapy.

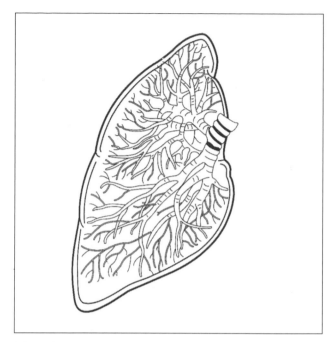

Normal bronchioles.

Pelargonium sidoides. Alcohol extract made from the herb *Pelargonium sidoides* has become popular in Germany as a treatment for various respiratory problems. In one double-blind, placebo-controlled study, 468 adults with recent onset of acute bronchitis were given either placebo or a standard alcohol extract of *P. sidoides* three times daily for a week. The results showed a significantly greater improvement in symptoms in the treatment group compared with the placebo group. On average, participants who received the real treatment were able to return to work two days earlier than those given placebo.

Benefits were also seen in two other studies that enrolled about 350 people. When researchers pooled the results of four well-designed, placebo-controlled trials, they found that a standardized extract of *Pelargonium* performed significantly better than placebo at reducing the symptoms of bronchitis by the seventh day of treatment.

OTHER PROPOSED TREATMENTS

A large (361-person) double-blind, placebo-controlled study found evidence that the use of a standardized combination of thyme and primrose root extract enhanced recovery from acute bronchitis. Symptoms improved rapidly in both groups, but improvement was faster and the response rates were higher for the thyme-primrose combination compared with placebo.

One double-blind, placebo-controlled study found that the use of 200 milligrams (mg) per day of vitamin C enhanced recovery among fifty-seven elderly persons who had been hospitalized for respiratory conditions.

Inhaled essential oils have a long, traditional use for respiratory infections. However, while there is some preliminary scientific support for such treatments, that evidence is still far too weak to rely upon. Another study provides weak evidence that a standardized combination of horseradish and nasturtium might be helpful for the treatment of bronchitis in children.

Numerous herbs have a reputation for helping bronchitis. These include elecampane, horehound, licorice, marshmallow, mullein, slippery elm, and yerba santa.

It is widely believed by many proponents of alternative medicine that cow's milk and related dairy products increase mucus in the lungs and sinuses and should, therefore, be avoided by people with bronchitis problems. However, there has not been sufficient scientific investigation into this belief to either confirm or deny it.

Because acute bronchitis tends to develop during the course of a common cold, all of the natural treatments used to prevent or treat colds are worth considering.

EBSCO CAM Review Board

FURTHER READING

Agbabiaka, T. B., R. Guo, and E. Ernst. "*Pelargonium sidoides* for Acute Bronchitis." *Phytomedicine* 15, no. 5 (2008): 378-385.

Chuchalin, A. G., B. Berman, and W. Lehmacher. "Treatment of Acute Bronchitis in Adults with a *Pelargonium sidoides* Preparation (EPs 7630)." *Explore* 1 (2006): 437-445.

Cohen, B. M., and W. E. Dressler. "Acute Aromatics Inhalation Modifies the Airways: Effects of the Common Cold." *Respiration* 43 (1982): 285-293.

Hunt, C., et al. "The Clinical Effects of Vitamin C Supplementation in Elderly Hospitalised Patients with Acute Respiratory Infections." *International Journal for Vitamin and Nutrition Research* 64 (1994): 212-219.

Matthys, H., and M. Heger. "Treatment of Acute Bronchitis with a Liquid Herbal Drug Preparation from *Pelargonium sidoides* (EPs 7630)." *Current Medical Research and Opinion* 23 (2007): 323-331.

Matthys, H., et al. "Efficacy and Safety of an Extract of *Pelargonium sidoides* (EPs 7630) in Adults with Acute Bronchitis." *Phytomedicine* 10, suppl. 4 (2003): 7-17.

West, John B. *Pulmonary Pathophysiology: The Essentials.* 7th ed. Philadelphia: Wolters Kluwer/Lippincott Williams & Wilkins, 2008.

See also: Colds and flu; Common cold: Homeopathic remedies; Essential oil monoterpenes; Horseradish; *Pelargonium sidoides.*

Bruises

CATEGORY: Condition
RELATED TERMS: Contusions, ecchymoses, hematomas
DEFINITION: Treatment of blood-containing tissue caused by damage to blood vessels from injury or surgery.
PRINCIPAL PROPOSED NATURAL TREATMENTS: Bilberry, citrus bioflavonoids, escin (topical), oligomeric proanthocyanidins, trypsin and chymotrypsin, vitamin C
OTHER PROPOSED NATURAL TREATMENTS: *Arnica* (topical), bromelain, comfrey (topical), sweet clover (topical)

INTRODUCTION

Bruising and bleeding both occur because of damage to blood vessels. When a vein, artery, or capillary is torn or cut, blood flows out into the vessel's surroundings; if the escaped blood is contained within the tissues directly under the skin, a bruise forms.

While all people bruise from time to time, some people bruise particularly easily. A number of factors, besides being accident-prone, can make this occur. One factor contributing to easy bruising is thinning skin, caused by aging or by medications such as corticosteroids. Easy bruising can also be caused by fragile blood vessel walls. Finally, difficulties with blood clotting, including problems with platelets or clotting factors, can also increase bruising. For this reason, strong blood-thinning drugs such as heparin and warfarin (Coumadin) can lead to excessive bruising. If a person

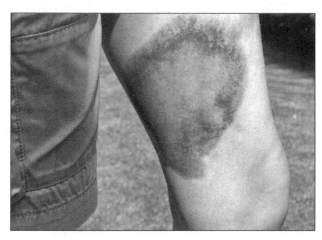

A very severe bruise on a teenager's leg. (©Dambuster/ Dreamstime.com)

is taking these or other anticoagulant drugs and notices increased bruising, he or she should consult a doctor.

Aspirin or natural remedies, such as policosanol, ginkgo, garlic, and high-dose vitamin E, may also thin the blood, possibly raising the risk of bruising and other bleeding problems. Combining two blood-thinning substances could multiply these effects.

Rarely, severe bruising from minor or unnoticed injuries can be a sign of leukemia or another serious health problem. Especially if this is a new development, one should discuss symptoms with a doctor. However, in most cases, there is no identifiable medical cause for easy bruising, and no conventional treatment. Furthermore, once a person has a bruise, no conventional therapy exists to help speed its resolution.

PRINCIPAL PROPOSED NATURAL TREATMENTS

A number of natural substances might be helpful for easy bruising, including citrus bioflavonoids, the related substances oligomeric proanthocyanidins (OPCs) and bilberry, and vitamin C. In addition, if one is already bruised, it might help to take a combination of two proteolytic enzymes, trypsin and chymotrypsin, or a topical preparation of escin (an extract of horse chestnut).

Citrus bioflavonoids and related substances. Bioflavonoids (or flavonoids) are plant substances that bring color to many fruits and vegetables. Citrus fruits are a rich source of bioflavonoids, including diosmin, hesperidin, rutin, and naringen; studies have found these bioflavonoids may help decrease bruising. Two types of natural compounds related to bioflavonoids (OPCs and anthocyanosides) have also shown promise for decreasing the tendency to bruise.

For example, a double-blind, placebo-controlled study of ninety-six people with fragile capillaries found that a combination of the bioflavonoids diosmin and hesperidin decreased the tendency to bruise. Participants took two tablets daily of these bioflavonoids or placebo for six weeks, while researchers used a suction cup to measure their capillaries' tendency to rupture and also looked for spontaneous bruising and other symptoms of fragile capillaries. Those persons who received bioflavonoids had significantly greater improvements in both capillary strength and symptoms, compared to those taking placebo.

Two rather poorly designed studies from the 1960s found benefits with a combination of vitamin C and citrus bioflavonoids for decreasing bruising in collegiate athletes. In a single-blind study of twenty-seven wrestlers, 71 percent of those taking placebo were injured, with bruises making up more than one-half their injuries; in contrast, only 38 percent of those taking the supplement were injured, none of whom sustained bruises. In a follow-up double-blind study of forty football players, the treated group received fewer severe bruises than the group taking placebo.

Test tube studies have found that OPCs protect collagen, partly by inhibiting an enzyme that breaks it down. One rather poorly designed double-blind study of thirty-seven people, most of whom had fragile capillaries, found that OPCs were more effective than placebo in decreasing capillary fragility; however, the authors of this study left many questions unanswered in their report, making it difficult to determine how seriously to take their results.

Anthocyanosides, which are present in high concentrations in bilberry, may also strengthen capillaries through their effects on collagen. Some European physicians believe that these vessel-stabilizing properties make bilberry useful as a treatment for easy bruising, but the evidence is only suggestive.

Vitamin C. Vitamin C is essential for healthy collagen; severe vitamin C deficiency, called scurvy, can lead to easy bruising. Scurvy is extremely rare in Western countries today, but marginal vitamin C deficiency is not rare, and it might lead to increased risk of bruising.

A two-month double-blind study of ninety-four elderly people with marginal vitamin C deficiency found that vitamin C supplements decreased their tendency to bruise. A person whose diet is low in fresh fruits and vegetables may wish to supplement it with vitamin C. In the foregoing study, bruising in elderly people decreased significantly with 1 gram (g) of oral vitamin C given daily for two months.

Trypsin and chymotrypsin. Trypsin and chymotrypsin, naturally produced in the body to help digest protein, are often called proteolytic enzymes. (Bromelain is a proteolytic enzyme from a plant source.) It is theorized that trypsin and chymotrypsin reduce swelling by breaking down protein fibers that trap fluids in the tissues after an injury, thereby restoring normal circulation in the area. Three small double-blind studies involving about eighty athletes found that treatment with proteolytic enzymes significantly speeded healing of bruises and other mild athletic injuries compared with placebo.

Escin. An extract of horse chestnut called escin may also help with bruising. Horse chestnut has been used to treat varicose veins and other problems involving blood vessels and swelling. One double-blind study of seventy people found that about 10 g of 2 percent escin gel, applied externally to bruises in a single dose five minutes after they were induced, reduced bruise tenderness.

OTHER PROPOSED NATURAL TREATMENTS

Bromelain. Like trypsin and chymotrypsin, bromelain is thought to decrease bruising by breaking down proteins that trap fluids in the tissues after an injury, and it is sometimes used in Europe to speed recovery from injuries. However, studies of better quality are needed before bromelain can be said to be effective.

In one controlled study, seventy-four boxers with bruises on their faces and upper bodies were given bromelain until all signs of bruising had disappeared; another seventy-two boxers were given placebo. Fifty-eight of the group taking bromelain had lost all signs of bruising within only four days, compared to ten days taking placebo. This study was apparently not double-blind, meaning that some of its results may have come from the power of suggestion. Another study (this one without any type of control group) found that bromelain reduced swelling, pain at rest,

and tenderness among fifty-nine persons with blunt injuries, including bruising.

Other herbs used. The herbs comfrey, *Arnica*, and sweet clover are widely used externally on bruises and other minor injuries, but despite this traditional use, there is no real scientific evidence that they work. There are various safety concerns involved in using comfrey, *Arnica*, and sweet clover internally. For the treatment of bruising, they are used as topical ointments and salves.

EBSCO CAM Review Board

FURTHER READING

Dinehart, S. M., and L. Henry. "Dietary Supplements: Altered Coagulation and Effects on Bruising." *Dermatologic Surgery* 31, part 2 (2005): 819-826.

MacKay, D., and A. L. Miller. "Nutritional Support for Wound Healing." *Alternative Medicine Review* 8 (2003): 359-377.

Schorah, C. J., et al. "The Effect of Vitamin C Supplements on Body Weight, Serum Proteins, and General Health of an Elderly Population." *American Journal of Clinical Nutrition* 34 (1981): 871-876.

See also: Bilberry; Bromelain; Citrus bioflavonoids; Horse chestnut; Injuries, minor; Oligomeric proanthocyanidins; Proteolytic enzymes; Vitamin C.

Bruises: Homeopathic remedies

CATEGORY: Homeopathy
DEFINITION: The use of highly diluted remedies to treat damage to blood vessels from injury or surgery. The bleeding leads to the development of blood-containing tissue.
Studied homeopathic remedy: *Arnica*

INTRODUCTION

A bruise is the visible evidence of bleeding under the skin. Seldom more than a cosmetic nuisance, it goes through a well-defined series of changes, beginning with a dark purple and red coloration and gradually fading to a greenish yellow color before disappearing. Some people are particularly prone to bruises, developing them after injuries too minor to affect most people.

Scientific Evaluations of Homeopathic Remedies

Homeopathic *Arnica* is so widely believed to be an effective treatment for bruises and other minor traumas that it is found in the medicine cabinets of millions of people, especially in Europe. However, there is no consistent scientific evidence that it is effective.

For example, two preliminary clinical trials were performed to test whether homeopathic *Arnica montana* can reduce the size or discomfort of a bruise caused by injury. The first study tested 10m (quintamillesimal-scale) potency *Arnica* (equivalent to a dilution of one part in 1,020,000); the second used a 30c (centesimal) dilution. About twenty-five persons were enrolled in the two trials.

In these unpleasant-sounding experiments, the participants allowed themselves to be bruised on the inside of their forearms by a 2.3-pound (1,041-gram) weight, which fell from about 1.5 feet (44 centimeters) above the arm. Participants were given either *Arnica* or placebo before the experiment and then were bruised on one arm. Subsequently, they were given a second dose of whatever they had just received and were then followed for three to four days. The goal was to see whether the bruises treated by *Arnica* got better faster than those treated by placebo. Researchers found a hint of benefit in the first study but none in the second study. The numbers of participants in each study were too small to allow for the results to have much statistical meaning.

Another study of people undergoing treatment for varicose veins, along with a study of people undergoing hand surgery, also failed to find benefit in using *Arnica* to reduce bruising. In a double-blind trial of 130 people undergoing treatment for varicose veins, researchers found no benefit with homeopathic *Arnica* at 5x (decimal-scale) potency, compared with placebo. A more recent study, involving face-lift surgery, found equivocal benefits at best.

Finally, researchers have attempted to discover whether homeopathic *Arnica* 10x has any effect on the ability of the blood to clot, as measured by laboratory tests. In a double-blind study of eighteen healthy male volunteers, *Arnica* was indistinguishable from placebo regarding blood coagulation.

Traditional Homeopathic Treatments

Homeopathic practitioners traditionally give *Arnica* to treat traumatic injuries. The classical homeopathic symptom picture for *Arnica* includes the presence of black-and-blue spots, a bruised feeling, and difficulty in finding a comfortable position. It is not difficult to recognize this as a description of minor injury.

EBSCO CAM Review Board

Further Reading

Ramelet, A. A., et al. "Homoeopathic *Arnica* in Postoperative Haematomas." *Dermatology* 201 (2000): 347-348.

Seeley, B. M., et al. "Effect of Homeopathic *Arnica montana* on Bruising in Face-Lifts." *Archives of Facial Plastic Surgery* 8 (2006): 54-59.

Stevinson, C., et al. "Homeopathic *Arnica* for Prevention of Pain and Bruising." *Journal of the Royal Society of Medicine* 96 (2003): 60-65.

See also: Injuries, minor; Pain management; Surgery Support.

Buchu

Category: Herbs and supplements
Related terms: *Agathosma betulina*, *A. crenulata*, *Barosma betulina*
Definition: Natural plant product used as a dietary supplement for specific health benefits.
Principal proposed use: Urinary tract infections and inflammation

Overview

Buchu has a long tradition of use for the treatment of bladder and urinary tract problems, especially urinary tract infections. In South Africa, buchu and other plants similar to it are additionally used for stomach aches, joint pain, and colds and flu. The leaves are the part used medicinally.

Uses and Applications

Many herbalists use buchu as a part of herbal combinations designed for kidney and bladder problems. Buchu is said to have a diuretic effect, meaning that it increases the flow of urine. However, there is no meaningful scientific documentation of this or any other medicinal effect of buchu.

Buchu contains various bioflavonoids, including

diosmin, rutin, and quercetin. Its essential oil contains a variety of aromatic substances, including limonene and menthone, along with the known liver toxin pulegone. While it is commonly said that the essential oil of buchu has antimicrobial effects, the only published study on the subject failed to find activity in this regard. This study did, however, find possible antispasmodic actions, which could potentially reduce the pain of bladder infections.

DOSAGE

Buchu is typically taken with meals at a dose of 1 to 2 grams of dried leaf three times daily. However, because of the toxicity of one of the constituents of buchu, its use is not recommend.

SAFETY ISSUES

Because buchu contains the known liver toxin pulegone, the herb should be used only with great caution, if at all. Buchu also frequently causes stomach upset. It definitely should not be used by young children, pregnant or nursing women, or people with liver or kidney disease.

In addition, if buchu does in fact have diuretic effects as claimed, people taking the medication lithium should use buchu only under the supervision of a physician, as dehydration can be a danger with this medication.

EBSCO CAM Review Board

FURTHER READING

El-Shafae, A. M., and M. M. el-Domiaty. "Improved LC Methods for the Determination of Diosmin and/ or Hesperidin in Plant Extracts and Pharmaceutical Formulations." *Journal of Pharmaceutical and Biomedical Analysis* 26 (2001): 539-545.

Lis-Balchin, M., et al. "Buchu (*Agathosma betulina* and *A. crenulata, Rutaceae*) Essential Oils: Their Pharmacological Action on Guinea-Pig Ileum and Antimicrobial Activity on Microorganisms." *Journal of Pharmacy and Pharmacology* 53 (2001): 579-582.

Moola, A., and A. M. Viljoen. "'Buchu': *Agathosma betulina* and *Agathosma crenulata* (*Rutaceae*)." *Journal of Ethnopharmacology* 119 (2008): 413-419.

Van Wyk, B. E. "A Broad Review of Commercially Important Southern African Medicinal Plants." *Journal of Ethnopharmacology* 119 (2008): 342-355.

See also: Bladder infection; Kidney stones.

Bugleweed

CATEGORY: Herbs and supplements
RELATED TERM: *Lycopus virginicus*
DEFINITION: Natural plant product used to treat specific health conditions.
PRINCIPAL PROPOSED USES: None
OTHER PROPOSED USES: Cyclic mastalgia (cyclic breast pain), hyperthyroidism

OVERVIEW

Bugleweed (*Lycopus virginicus*), from the mint family, is a native of North America. It is closely related to the European herb called gypsywort or gypsyweed (*L. europaeus*). For medicinal purposes, these two plants are often used interchangeably. The leaves of bugleweed are long and thin and grow in pairs from the stem. Small whitish flowers grow around the stem at the base of each pair of leaves. The juice of bugleweed can be used as a fabric dye, and it was reportedly used by gypsies to darken their skin, which may be the origin of the common names applied to the European species of *Lycopus.*

Bugleweed also has a long-standing reputation as a medicinal plant. Herbalists have traditionally used bugleweed as a sedative, to treat mild heart conditions, and to reduce fever and mucus production in influenza and colds. More recently, bugleweed has been suggested as a treatment for hyperthyroidism and mastodynia (breast pain).

THERAPEUTIC DOSAGES

The dosage of bugleweed should be adjusted by measuring thyroid hormone levels.

THERAPEUTIC USES

Several very preliminary studies suggest that bugleweed may be helpful for treating mild hyperthyroidism. Hyperthyroidism is a condition in which the thyroid gland releases excessive amounts of thyroid hormone. Symptoms include weight loss, weakness, heart palpitations, and anxiety. Test tube and animal studies suggest that bugleweed may reduce thyroid hormone by decreasing levels of thyroid-stimulating hormone (TSH) and by impairing thyroid hormone synthesis. In addition, bugleweed may block the action of thyroid-stimulating antibodies found in Grave's disease.

Self-treatment of hyperthyroidism can be dangerous.

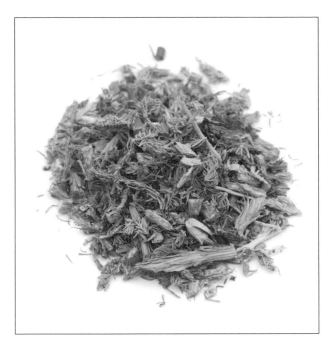

Herbalists have traditionally used bugleweed as a sedative, to treat mild heart conditions, and to reduce fever and mucus production in influenza and colds. (Geoff Kidd/Photo Researchers, Inc.)

Physician supervision is necessary to determine why the thyroid is overactive to design a specific treatment plan.

Bugleweed may also reduce levels of the hormone prolactin, which is primarily responsible for the production of breast milk. Elevated levels of prolactin may also cause breast pain in women; based on this finding, bugleweed has been recommended as a treatment for cyclic mastalgia (breast tenderness that comes and goes with the menstrual cycle). However, because of its effects on thyroid hormone, it is not recommend for this purpose.

SAFETY ISSUES

The safety of bugleweed has not been established. Long-term or high-dose use of the herb may cause an enlarged thyroid. Bugleweed should not be used by individuals with hypothyroidism (low thyroid hormone) or an enlarged thyroid gland. Pregnant or nursing women should also avoid bugleweed because of potential effects on their children as well as on breast milk production.

Bugleweed should not be combined with thyroid medications. It may also interfere with diagnostic procedures that rely on radioactive isotopes to evaluate the thyroid.

IMPORTANT INTERACTIONS

Bugleweed should not be used by those taking thyroid medications, and those undergoing tests of their thyroid function should not use it except on a physician's advice.

EBSCO CAM Review Board

FURTHER READING

Brinker, F. "Inhibition of Endocrine Function by Botanical Agents *I. boraginaceae* and *labiatae*." *Journal of Naturopathic Medicine* 1 (1990): 10-18.

See also: Breast pain, cyclic; Herbal medicine; Hyperthyroidism.

Burdock

CATEGORY: Herbs and supplements
RELATED TERMS: *Arctium lappa*, gobo
DEFINITION: Natural plant product used as a dietary supplement for specific health benefits.
PRINCIPAL PROPOSED USES: Acne, eczema, psoriasis
OTHER PROPOSED USES: Cancer, rheumatoid arthritis

OVERVIEW

The common burdock, that well-known source of annoying burrs matted in the fur of dogs, is also a medicinal herb of considerable reputation. Called *gobo* in Japan, burdock root is said to be a food that provides deep strengthening to the immune system. In ancient China and India, herbalists used it in the treatment of respiratory infections, abscesses, and joint pain. European physicians of the Middle Ages and later used it to treat cancerous tumors, skin conditions, sexually transmitted diseases, and bladder and kidney problems.

Burdock was a primary ingredient in the famous (or infamous) Hoxsey cancer treatment. Harry Hoxsey was a former coal miner who parlayed a traditional family remedy for cancer into the largest privately owned cancer treatment center in the world, with branches around the United States. (The company was shut down in the 1950s by the U.S. Food

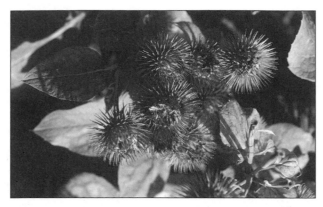

Burdock is widely recommended for the relief of dry, scaly skin conditions such as eczema and psoriasis. (Philippe Garo/ Photo Researchers, Inc.)

and Drug Administration. Hoxsey himself subsequently died of cancer.) Other herbs in Hoxsey's formula included red clover, poke, prickly ash, bloodroot, and barberry. Burdock is also found in the common herbal cancer remedy *Essiac.* Despite this historical enthusiasm, there is no significant evidence that burdock is an effective treatment for cancer or any other illness.

USES AND APPLICATIONS

Burdock is widely recommended for the relief of dry, scaly skin conditions such as eczema and psoriasis. It is also used for treating acne. It can be taken orally and applied directly to the skin. Burdock is sometimes recommended for rheumatoid arthritis. However, there is no real scientific evidence for any of these uses.

DOSAGE

A typical dosage of burdock is 1 to 2 grams of powdered dry root three times per day.

SAFETY ISSUES

As a food commonly eaten in Japan (it is often found in sukiyaki), burdock root is believed to be safe. However, in 1978, the *Journal of the American Medical Association* caused a brief scare by publishing a report of burdock poisoning. Subsequent investigation showed that the herbal product involved was actually contaminated with the poisonous chemical atropine from an unknown source. The safety of burdock use in young children, pregnant or nursing women, and those with severe liver or kidney disease is not established.

IMPORTANT INTERACTIONS

Persons taking insulin or oral medications to reduce blood sugar should note that burdock may possibly increase their effect.

EBSCO CAM Review Board

FURTHER READING

Bryson, P. D., et al. "Burdock Root Tea Poisoning: Case Report Involving a Commercial Preparation." *Journal of the American Medical Association* 239 (1978): 2157.

Chan, Y. S., et al. "A Review of the Pharmacological Effects of *Arctium lappa* (Burdock)." *Inflammopharmacology* (October 28, 2010).

Ferracane, R., et al. "Metabolic Profile of the Bioactive Compounds of Burdock (*Arctium lappa*) Seeds, Roots, and Leaves." *Journal of Pharmaceutical and Biomedical Analysis* 51 (2010): 399-404.

Lou, Z., et al. "Antioxidant Activity and Chemical Composition of the Fractions from Burdock Leaves." *Journal of Food Science* 75 (2010): C413-C419.

See also: Acne; Antioxidants; Eczema; Psoriasis.

Burning mouth syndrome

CATEGORY: Condition
DEFINITION: Treatment of chronic pain of the tongue and mouth.
PRINCIPAL PROPOSED TREATMENT: Lipoic acid
OTHER PROPOSED TREATMENTS: St. John's wort, treatments for yeast hypersensitivity, vitamin B_1, vitamin B_2, vitamin B_6, zinc

INTRODUCTION

Burning mouth syndrome (BMS) is a poorly understood condition in which a person experiences ongoing moderate to severe pain in the tongue or mouth, or both. Although the cause of BMS remains unclear, some patterns have become clear to researchers. The pain is generally worse in the late afternoon and early evening but disappears at night. Most often, more than one part of the mouth is involved. Common areas of burning pain include the tongue, the hard palate (the front part of the roof of the mouth), and the lower lip. Many people recover spontaneously within six or seven years. Dry mouth and altered taste sensations often, but not always, accompany the pain.

BMS is thought to fall in the general category of neuropathic pain, meaning that it probably results from altered nerve function, possibly in the nerves carrying taste sensation. The use of drugs in the angiotensin I-converting enzyme (ACE) inhibitor family has been implicated in some cases of BMS, but the reason for this apparent connection remains unclear.

Conventional treatment for BMS consists of drugs used to treat neuropathic pain in general, including anticonvulsants, sedatives in the benzodiazepine family, and tricyclic antidepressants. There is inadequate research to determine the precise efficacy of these treatments.

Principal Proposed Treatments

The supplement lipoic acid has shown promise for the treatment of diabetic neuropathy, another form of neuropathic pain. Lipoic acid has also been studied for burning mouth syndrome with mixed results.

In a double-blind trial, sixty people with burning mouth syndrome received either lipoic acid (200 milligrams three times daily) or placebo for a period of months. Researchers reported that almost all persons receiving lipoic acid showed significant improvement, while none of those taking placebo improved; relative benefits endured at twelve-month follow-up. The lack of benefit seen in the placebo group is difficult to believe, and it raises concerns about the study's reliability. Subsequently, two double-blind trials involving fifty-two and thirty-nine persons, respectively, failed to find benefit for lipoic acid and noted a large placebo response.

Other Proposed Treatments

The yeast *Candida albicans* can infect the mouth, causing a condition called thrush. Thrush may cause symptoms similar to BMS. Some alternative practitioners believe that excessive *Candida*, or hypersensitivity to it, is the cause of many illnesses. For this reason, they recommend using antifungals to treat BMS. However, no direct evidence supports this approach, and it appears that people with BMS are no more likely to have measurable detectible *Candida* in the mouth than are people without BMS.

Inconsistent evidence suggests that people with BMS might have deficiencies in various nutrients, such as vitamins B_1, B_2, and B_6, and zinc. However, no evidence exists to show that supplementation with these nutrients will have any effect on BMS symptoms.

Also, a placebo-controlled trial involving thirty-nine persons failed to show any significant benefit for twelve weeks of treatment with *Hypericum perforatum* extract (St. John's wort).

Herbs and Supplements to Avoid

Numerous herbs and supplements may interact adversely with drugs used to treat burning mouth syndrome, so one should be cautious when considering the use of herbs and supplements.

EBSCO CAM Review Board

Further Reading

Carbone, M., et al. "Lack of Efficacy of Alpha-Lipoic Acid in Burning Mouth Syndrome." *European Journal of Pain* 13 (May, 2009): 492-496.

Femiano, F., and C. Scully. "Burning Mouth Syndrome (BMS): Double Blind Controlled Study of Alpha-Lipoic Acid (Thioctic Acid) Therapy." *Journal of Oral Pathology and Medicine* 31 (2002): 267-269.

Lopez-Jornet, P., F. Camacho-Alonso, and S. Leon-Espinosa. "Efficacy of Alpha Lipoic Acid in Burning Mouth Syndrome." *Journal of Oral Rehabilitation* 36 (2008): 52-57.

Sardella, A., et al. "*Hypericum perforatum* Extract in Burning Mouth Syndrome." *Journal of Oral Pathology and Medicine* 37 (2008): 395-401.

Ship, J. A., et al. "Burning Mouth Syndrome." *Journal of the American Dental Association* 126 (1995): 842-853.

See also: Canker sores; Leukoplakia; Lipoic acid; Periodontal disease; Tongue diagnosis.

Burns, minor

Category: Condition

Related terms: First-degree burn, scald, superficial burn

Definition: Treatment of relatively minor burns to the top layer of skin.

Principal proposed natural treatments: None

Other proposed natural treatments: Aloe vera, arginine, beta-carotene, *Calendula*, chamomile, comfrey, copper, dehydroepiandrosterone, goldenseal, gotu kola, honey, ornithine alpha-ketoglutarate, potato peel, selenium, vitamin C, vitamin E, zinc

INTRODUCTION

Burns can be caused by heat, electricity, chemicals, and sun exposure. Symptoms can vary in severity from minor pain to life-threatening infection. First-degree burns are the mildest type, damaging only the top layer of skin. The skin gets red, painful, and tender. Though the skin may swell, no blisters form and the area turns white when touched.

Second-degree burns cause damage to deeper layers of the skin. The skin looks much like a first-degree burn except that blisters form at the surface. The blisters may be red or whitish and are filled with a clear fluid. Third-degree burns are the worst type of burn, extending through all layers of the skin and causing nerve damage. Because of this nerve damage, third-degree burns generally are not painful and have no feeling when touched (an ominous sign). The skin may be white, blackened, or bright red. Blisters may also be present.

Only first-degree burns should be self-treated. More severe burns require a doctor's supervision to prevent infection and scarring. Third-degree burns and extensive second-degree burns can cause permanent injury or death.

The best treatment for minor burns is to cool the burn as quickly as possible by immersing the area in cold water. One should keep the burned area clean until it heals.

PROPOSED NATURAL TREATMENTS

Although there are no well-established natural treatments for minor burns, several preliminary studies suggest a few options for reducing pain and speeding healing. A series of studies done in India found that a combination of raw honey and gauze was significantly better than conventional types of bandages for superficial burns treated at a hospital. The burns covered with honey healed faster and with less frequent infection than the burns covered with other types of bandages. Other studies of varying quality have also found evidence of benefit.

Boiled potato peel has also been used successfully in developing countries as a replacement for more expensive conventional bandages. Preliminary studies suggest that the herb gotu kola may speed healing of burns and reduce scarring.

Aloe vera is often recommended as a treatment for minor burns; however, no evidence exists to support

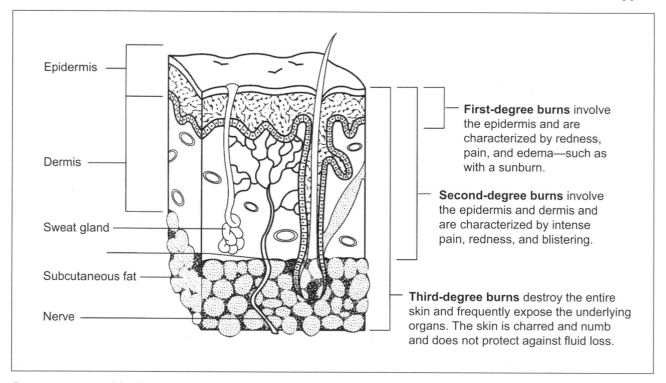

Epidermis

Dermis

Sweat gland

Subcutaneous fat

Nerve

First-degree burns involve the epidermis and are characterized by redness, pain, and edema—such as with a sunburn.

Second-degree burns involve the epidermis and dermis and are characterized by intense pain, redness, and blistering.

Third-degree burns destroy the entire skin and frequently expose the underlying organs. The skin is charred and numb and does not protect against fluid loss.

Burns are measured by the layer(s) of skin affected.

this claim; some studies have found it ineffective. Other popular topical burn treatments include calendula, chamomile, goldenseal, and comfrey.

Oral or topical vitamin C, vitamin E, and beta-carotene, alone or in combination, might be helpful for preventing sunburn. However, the evidence is preliminary and contradictory.

There is some evidence that hospitalized persons with severe burns may benefit from nutritional support with certain supplements, including ornithine alpha-ketoglutarate, arginine, zinc, copper, selenium, and dehydroepiandrosterone.

EBSCO CAM Review Board

FURTHER READING

Donati, L., et al. "Nutritional and Clinical Efficacy of Ornithine Alpha-Ketoglutarate in Severe Burn Patients." *Clinical Nutrition* 18 (1999): 307-311.

Jull, A. B., A. Rodgers, and N. Walker. "Honey as a Topical Treatment for Wounds." *Cochrane Database of Systematic Reviews* (2008): CD005083. Available through *EBSCO DynaMed Systematic Literature Surveillance* at http://www.ebscohost.com/dynamed.

Keswani, M. H., and A. R. Patil. "The Boiled Potato Peel as a Burn Wound Dressing." *Burns, Including Thermal Injury* 11 (1985): 220-224.

Lee, J., et al. "Carotenoid Supplementation Reduces Erythema in Human Skin After Simulated Solar Radiation Exposure." *Proceedings of the Society for Experimental Biology and Medicine* 223 (2000): 170-174.

Maenthaisong R., et al. "The Efficacy of Aloe Vera Used for Burn Wound Healing." *Burns* 33 (2007): 713-718.

Molan, P. C. "Potential of Honey in the Treatment of Wounds and Burns." *American Journal of Clinical Dermatology* 2 (2001): 13-19.

Stahl, W., et al. "Carotenoids and Carotenoids Plus Vitamin E Protect Against Ultraviolet Light-Induced Erythema in Humans." *American Journal of Clinical Nutrition* 71 (2000): 795-798.

Traikovich, S. S. "Use of Topical Ascorbic Acid and Its Effects on Photodamaged Skin Topography." *Archives of Otolaryngology–Head Neck Surgery* 125 (1999): 1091-1098.

See also: Aloe; Burns, minor: Homeopathic remedies; Honey; Injuries, minor; Photosensitivity; Sunburn; Wounds, minor.

Burns, minor: Homeopathic remedies

CATEGORY: Homeopathy
DEFINITION: The use of highly diluted remedies to treat minor burns.
STUDIED HOMEOPATHIC REMEDIES: *Calendula, Cantharis*

SCIENTIFIC EVALUATIONS OF HOMEOPATHIC REMEDIES

One small, double-blind, placebo-controlled study examined the classical remedy *Cantharis*. This trial enrolled thirty-four people who had sustained a minor burn within six hours of admission to the study. The researchers gave the participants acetaminophen (non-aspirin painkiller) and then either one chewable tablet of *Cantharis* 200c (centesimals) or a placebo tablet. On an hourly basis for the next five hours, participants recorded their levels of pain.

The results of the study were not promising. No significant difference was found between the pain levels of the treatment group and the pain levels of the control group.

TRADITIONAL HOMEOPATHIC TREATMENTS

Classical homeopathy offers some homeopathic treatments for minor burns. These therapies are chosen based on various specific details of the person seeking treatment. According to classical homeopathy, lesions that would be described as raw, irritable, and inflamed can be treated with *Calendula*. This remedy can be taken orally or as part of a homeopathically prepared topical lotion or ointment. Persons who are feeling intense and restless from extreme burning pain might also fit the symptom picture for *Cantharis*.

EBSCO CAM Review Board

FURTHER READING

Chandran, P. K., and R. Kuttan. "Effect of *Calendula officinalis* Flower Extract on Acute Phase Proteins, Antioxidant Defense Mechanism, and Granuloma Formation During Thermal Burns." *Journal of Clinical Biochemistry and Nutrition* 43 (2008): 58-64.

"Final report on the Safety Assessment of *Calendula officinalis* Extract and *Calendula officinalis*." *International Journal of Toxicology* 20, suppl. 2 (2001): 13-20.

Leaman, A. M., and D. Gorman. "*Cantharis* in the

Early Treatment of Minor Burns." *Archives of Emergency Medicine* 6 (1989): 259-261.

See also: Burns, minor; Calendula; Homeopathy; Wounds, minor.

Bursitis

CATEGORY: Condition
DEFINITION: Treatment of inflammation of the fluid-filled sacs between tissues and bones.
PRINCIPAL PROPOSED NATURAL TREATMENTS: None
OTHER PROPOSED NATURAL TREATMENTS: Boswellia, devil's claw, evening primrose oil, fish oil, movement therapies (such as Pilates and Feldenkrais), proteolytic enzymes, Tai Chi, white willow, yoga

INTRODUCTION

The muscles and bones of the body work together like a smoothly oiled machine. Some of the "oil" is provided by fluid-filled sacs called bursae. Bursae are strategically located in areas where muscles, ligaments, and tendons might otherwise rub against bones. The smooth surface of a bursa allows tissues to move across each other without friction.

Bursae, however, can become inflamed, leading to a condition called bursitis. One of the main causes of bursitis is repetitive motion. For example, custodians who often use a vacuum cleaner may develop bursitis in the elbow. Excessive pressure, such as that caused by prolonged kneeling, can also injure a bursa. More rarely, gout, arthritis, and certain infections can cause bursitis.

Bursitis occurs most commonly in the hip, knee, elbow, or heel. Symptoms include tenderness, swelling, and pain with motion.

Conventional treatment involves resting the affected area and using anti-inflammatory drugs. If an attack of bursitis does not respond to this treatment, drainage of the bursa and injection of corticosteroids may be used.

Various practical steps can help prevent bursitis. Using knee pads can protect the bursa of the knee from pressure injury. Exercises that strengthen the muscle around a joint are thought to reduce stress on the bursae in the area. Finally, it is important to break up repetitive movements with alternative movement patterns and periods of rest.

OTHER PROPOSED NATURAL TREATMENTS

There are no natural treatments for bursitis that have meaningful scientific support. The herb white willow has effects similar to those of aspirin, and on this basis it might be expected to offer some benefit in bursitis. However, white willow has not been directly studied for that purpose.

Other treatments sometimes recommended for bursitis, but that also lack reliable supporting evidence, include boswellia, fish oil, evening primrose oil, proteolytic enzymes, and devil's claw.

Yoga increases flexibility and might help the symptoms of bursitis by stretching tendons and ligaments and, therefore, releasing tension in the area around the bursa. Movement therapies, such as Pilates and Feldenkrais, involve deliberate retraining of movement and could therefore alter the repetitive movements that can cause bursitis. Tai Chi might also lead to improved movement habits.

EBSCO CAM Review Board

FURTHER READING

Chrubasik, S., et al. "Treatment of Low Back Pain Exacerbations with Willow Bark Extract." *American Journal of Medicine* 109 (2000): 9-14.

Iannotti, J. P., and Y. W. Kwon. "Management of Persistent Shoulder Pain: A Treatment Algorithm." *American Journal of Orthopedics* 34, suppl. 12 (2005): 16-23.

Lewis, J. S., and F. M. Sandford. "Rotator Cuff Tendinopathy: Is There a Role for Polyunsaturated Fatty Acids and Antioxidants?" *Journal of Hand Therapy* 22 (2009): 49-55.

See also: Back pain; Bone and joint health; Chiropractic; Exercise; Injuries, minor; Manipulative and body-based practices; Neck pain; Nonsteroidal anti-inflammatory drugs (NSAIDs); Osteoarthritis; Osteopathic manipulation; Pain management; Soft tissue pain; Tendonitis.

Butcher's broom

CATEGORY: Herbs and supplements
RELATED TERM: *Ruscus aculeatus*
DEFINITION: Natural plant product used to treat specific health conditions.

PRINCIPAL PROPOSED USE: Chronic venous insufficiency

OTHER PROPOSED USES: Hemorrhoids, surgery support (lymphedema following breast cancer surgery)

OVERVIEW

So named because its branches were a traditional source of broom straw used by butchers, the Mediterranean evergreen bush known as butcher's broom has a long history of use in the treatment of urinary conditions. More recently, it has been studied as a treatment for vein-related conditions.

THERAPEUTIC DOSAGES

A typical dose of butcher's broom is 36.0 to 37.5 milligrams (mg) twice daily of a methanol extract concentrated at a level of 15-20:1. This should supply about 7 to 11 mg of ruscogenin (also called ruscogenine) daily. For hemorrhoids, butcher's broom is sometimes applied as an ointment or in the form of a suppository.

THERAPEUTIC USES

Butcher's broom has been approved by Germany's Commission E as supportive therapy for chronic venous insufficiency. Venous insufficiency, a condition closely related to varicose veins, involves pain, swelling and fatigue in the calves. Commission E also recommends butcher's broom for the treatment of hemorrhoids.

This recommendation was in place before any meaningful studies had been performed evaluating butcher's broom for either of these purposes. However, several studies performed subsequently now provide preliminary supporting evidence for its use in chronic venous insufficiency.

No substantial studies have evaluated butcher's broom for hemorrhoids, but because hemorrhoids are similar to varicose veins, it is reasonable to suppose that butcher's broom might be helpful. Various treatments used for venous insufficiency have also shown promise for treating arm swelling (lymphedema) following surgery for breast cancer. One study suggests that butcher's broom may be helpful for this condition as well.

SCIENTIFIC EVIDENCE

Venous insufficiency. A well-designed and -reported double-blind trial evaluated the effectiveness of a

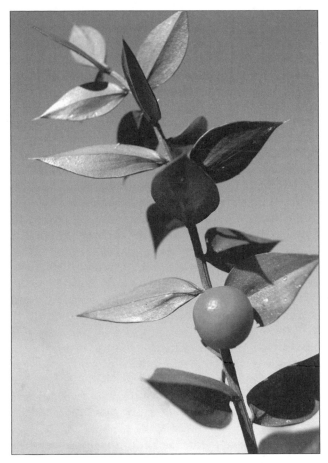

Butcher's broom plant with its red fruit. (©Maljalen/Dreamstime.com.)

standardized butcher's broom extract in 166 women with chronic venous insufficiency. For a period of twelve weeks, participants received either a placebo or butcher's broom (one tablet twice daily containing 36.0 to 37.5 mg of a methanol dry extract concentrated at 15-20:1). The results showed that leg swelling (the primary measurement used) decreased significantly in the butcher's broom group compared with the placebo group. Similar results were seen in a two-week, double-blind, placebo-controlled trial with 148 participants.

Another two-week double-blind, placebo-controlled trial with 141 participants used a combination of butcher's broom extract and the bioflavonoid trimethylhesperidin chalcone and found benefits. Marginal benefits were seen in a much smaller study using this combination.

Lymphedema. In a double-blind study, fifty-seven women with lymphedema received either a placebo or butcher's broom combined with the modified citrus bioflavonoid trimethylhesperidin chalcone. The results indicated that use of the combination therapy resulted in significantly less swelling.

SAFETY ISSUES

In clinical trials, use of butcher's broom has not been associated with any serious adverse effects. However, comprehensive safety studies have not been reported. Maximum safe doses in young children, pregnant or nursing women, and those with liver or kidney disease have not been established.

EBSCO CAM Review Board

FURTHER READING

Lucker, P., et al. "Efficacy and Safety of Ruscus Extract Compared to Placebo in Patients Suffering from Chronic Venous Insufficiency." *Phytomedicine* 7 (2000): 155.

Vanscheidt, W., et al. "Efficacy and Safety of a Butcher's Broom Preparation (*Ruscus aculeatus* L. Extract) Compared to Placebo in Patients Suffering from Chronic Venous Insufficiency." *Arzneimittel-Forschung/Drug Research* 52, no. 4 (2002): 243-250.

See also: Herbal medicine; Venous insufficiency: Homeopathic remedies.

Butterbur

CATEGORY: Herbs and supplements
RELATED TERMS: Blatterdock, bog rhubarb, bogshorns butter-dock, butterly dock, capdockin, flapperdock, langwort, *Petasites hybridus*, umbrella leaves
DEFINITION: Natural plant product used to treat specific health conditions.
PRINCIPAL PROPOSED USES: Allergies, migraine headaches (prevention)
OTHER PROPOSED USES: Asthma, musculoskeletal pain, ulcer protection

OVERVIEW

Butterbur can be found growing along rivers, ditches, and marshy areas in northern Asia, Europe, and parts of North America. It sends up stalks of

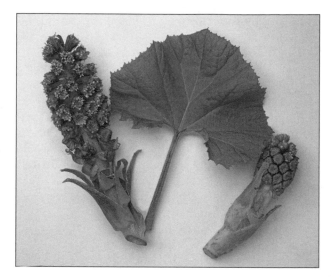

Flowers and leaf of the butterbur plant. (Neil Fletcher/ Getty Images)

reddish flowers very early in spring, before producing very large heart-shaped leaves with a furry gray underside. Once the leaves appear, butterbur somewhat resembles rhubarb; one of its common names is bog rhubarb. It is also sometimes referred to as "umbrella leaves" because of the size of its foliage. Other more or less descriptive common names abound, including blatterdock, bogshorns, butter-dock, butterly dock, capdockin, flapperdock, and langwort.

Butterbur is often described as possessing an unpleasant smell, but being malodorous has not protected it from harvesting by humans. The plant has a long history of use as an antispasmodic, thought to be effective for such conditions as stomach cramps, whooping cough, and asthma.

Externally, butterbur has been applied as a poultice over wounds or skin ulcerations.

THERAPEUTIC DOSAGES

The usual dosage of butterbur is 50 to 75 milligrams (mg) twice daily of a standardized extract that has been processed to remove potentially dangerous chemicals called pyrrolizidine alkaloids. Use of any butterbur product that contains pyrrolizidine alkaloids is not recommended.

THERAPEUTIC USES

A special toxin-free butterbur extract has been investigated for the treatment of a variety of illnesses.

Two double-blind trials suggest that this butterbur extract may be useful for preventing migraine headaches. In addition, meaningful evidence indicates that this extract is helpful for hay fever.

There is some evidence that butterbur has anti-inflammatory and antispasmodic effects, and on this basis it has been proposed as a treatment for a variety of musculoskeletal pain conditions; however, meaningful clinical trials have not been reported. Butterbur has also undergone highly preliminary investigation for treatment of asthma and for protecting the stomach lining from injury, thereby helping to prevent ulcers. Preliminary evidence suggests that butterbur is not likely to be particularly effective for allergic skin diseases, such as eczema.

SCIENTIFIC EVIDENCE

Migraines. Two double-blind, placebo-controlled studies suggest that butterbur extract may be helpful for preventing migraines, although the optimum dosage is not clear. Butterbur extract was tested as a migraine preventive in a double-blind, placebo-controlled study involving sixty men and women who experienced at least three migraines per month. After four weeks without any conventional medications, participants were randomly assigned to take either 50 mg of butterbur extract or a placebo twice daily for three months.

The results were positive: both the number of migraine attacks and the total number of days of migraine pain were significantly reduced in the treatment group compared with the placebo group. Three of four persons taking butterbur reported improvement, compared with only one of four persons in the placebo group. No significant side effects were noted.

In another double-blind, placebo-controlled study performed by different researchers, 202 people with migraine headaches received either 50 mg twice daily of butterbur extract, 75 mg twice daily, or a placebo. Over the three months of the study, the frequency of migraine attacks gradually decreased in all three groups. However, the group receiving the higher dose of butterbur extract showed significantly greater improvement than those in the placebo group. The lower dose of butterbur failed to prove significantly more effective than a placebo.

Based on these two studies, it does appear that butterbur extract is helpful for preventing migraines, and

that 75 mg twice daily is more effective than 50 mg twice daily. However, further research is necessary to establish this with certainty.

Hay fever (allergic rhinitis). Butterbur appears to affect the immune system in ways that suggest it should be helpful for hay fever (technically, "seasonal allergic rhinitis"). On this basis, it has been tested as an allergy treatment, with positive results in substantial studies.

In a two-week double-blind, placebo-controlled study of 186 people with intermittent allergic rhinitis, use of butterbur at a dose of three standardized tablets daily, or one tablet daily, reduced allergy symptoms compared with a placebo. Significantly greater benefits were seen in the higher-dose group. Such "dose dependency" is generally taken as a confirming sign that a treatment really works.

In another double-blind study, 330 people were given either butterbur extract (one tablet three times daily), the antihistamine fexofenadine (Allegra), or a placebo. The results showed that butterbur and fexofenadine were equally effective, and both were more effective than a placebo.

A previous two-week double-blind study of 125 individuals with hay fever compared a standardized butterbur extract against the antihistamine drug certizine. According to ratings by both doctors and patients, the two treatments proved about equally effective. This study did not use a placebo group.

It is not clear how butterbur might work. Unlike standard antihistamines, it does not appear to reduce reactions on allergy skin tests.

SAFETY ISSUES

In studies and postmarketing surveillance involving adults and children, burping and other mild gastrointestinal complaints have been the main side effect of butterbur extract. Butterbur contains liver-toxic and possibly carcinogenic components called pyrrolizidine alkaloids. It is possible to remove these compounds from butterbur products. In Germany, the maximum allowable content of pyrrolizidine alkaloids in butterbur products has been set at 1 microgram per daily recommended dose.

Butterbur should not be used by pregnant or nursing women, young children, or people with severe kidney or liver disease until further safety testing has been performed.

EBSCO CAM Review Board

FURTHER READING

Gray, R. D., et al. "Effects of Butterbur Treatment in Intermittent Allergic Rhinitis." *Annals of Allergy, Asthma, and Immunology* 93 (2004): 56-60.

Jackson, C. M., D. K. Lee, and B. J. Lipworth. "The Effects of Butterbur on the Histamine and Allergen Cutaneous Response." *Annals of Allergy, Asthma, and Immunology* 92 (2004): 250-254.

Lee, D. K., et al. "A Placebo-Controlled Evaluation of Butterbur and Fexofenadine on Objective and Subjective Outcomes in Perennial Allergic Rhinitis." *Clinical and Experimental Allergy* 34 (2004): 646-649.

Lipton, R. B., et al. "*Petasites hybridus* Root (Butterbur) Is an Effective Preventive Treatment for Migraine." *Neurology* 63 (2004): 2240-2244.

Schapowal, A. "Butterbur Ze339 for the Treatment of Intermittent Allergic Rhinitis: Dose-Dependent Efficacy in a Prospective, Randomized, Double-Blind, Placebo-Controlled Study." *Archives of Otolaryngology–Head and Neck Surgery* 130 (2004): 1381-1386.

Schapowal, A. "Randomised Controlled Trial of Butterbur and Cetirizine for Treating Seasonal Allergic Rhinitis." *British Medica Journal* 324 (2002): 144-146.

Thomet, O. A., and H. U. Simon. "Petasins in the Treatment of Allergic Diseases." *International Archives of Allergy and Immunology* 129 (2002): 108-112.

See also: Allergies; Herbal medicines.

C

Calcium

CATEGORY: Herbs and supplements

RELATED TERMS: Bonemeal, calcium aspartate, calcium carbonate, calcium chelate, calcium citrate, calcium citrate malate, calcium gluconate, calcium lactate, calcium orotate, dolomite, oyster shell calcium, tricalcium phosphate

DEFINITION: Natural substance essential for health and used as a dietary supplement for specific health benefits.

PRINCIPAL PROPOSED USES: Osteoporosis, premenstrual syndrome

OTHER PROPOSED USES: Attention deficit disorder, colon polyps and cancer prevention, dysmenorrhea, high cholesterol, hypertension, migraine headaches, periodontal disease, preeclampsia, weight loss

OVERVIEW

Calcium is the most abundant mineral in the body, making up nearly 2 percent of total body weight. More than 99 percent of the calcium in the body is found in bones, but the other 1 percent is perhaps just as important for good health. Many enzymes depend on calcium to work properly, as do the nerves, heart, and blood-clotting mechanisms.

To build bone, a person needs to have enough calcium in his or her diet. However, even with the availability of calcium-fortified orange juice and with the best efforts of the dairy industry, most Americans are calcium deficient. Calcium supplements are a simple way to make sure one is getting enough of this important mineral.

One of the most important uses of calcium is to help prevent and treat osteoporosis, the progressive loss of bone mass to which menopausal women are especially vulnerable. Calcium works best when combined with vitamin D. Other meaningful evidence suggests that calcium may have an additional use: reducing symptoms of premenstrual syndrome (PMS).

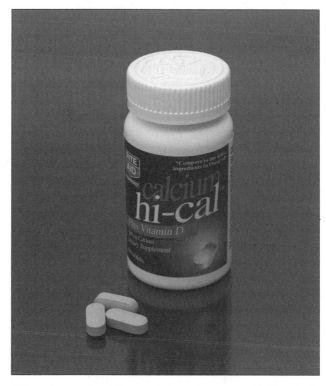

Many forms of calcium supplements are available on the market, each with its own advantages and disadvantages. (GIPhotoStock/Photo Researchers, Inc.)

REQUIREMENTS AND SOURCES

Although there are some variations between recommendations issued by different groups, the official U.S. and Canadian recommendations for daily intake of calcium (in milligrams) are as follows: infants to six months of age (210) and seven to twelve months of age (270); children one to three years of age (500) and four to eight years of age (800); children nine to eighteen years of age (1,300); adults age nineteen to fifty years (1,000), age fifty-one years and older (1,200); and pregnant and nursing girls (1,300) and women (1,000).

To absorb calcium, the body also needs an adequate level of vitamin D. Various medications may impair calcium absorption or metabolism, either directly or through effects on vitamin D. Implicated medications include corticosteroids, heparin, isoniazid, and anticonvulsants. People who use these medications may benefit by taking extra calcium and vitamin D. Calcium carbonate might interfere with the effects of anticonvulsant drugs, so it should not be taken at the same time of day.

Milk, cheese, and other dairy products are excellent sources of calcium. Other good sources include orange juice or soy milk fortified with calcium, fish (such as sardines) canned with its bones, dark green vegetables, nuts and seeds, and calcium-processed tofu. Many forms of calcium supplements are available on the market, each with its own advantages and disadvantages.

Naturally derived forms of calcium. Naturally derived forms of calcium come from bone, shells, or the earth: bonemeal, oyster shell, and dolomite, respectively. Animals concentrate calcium in their shells, and calcium is found in minerals in the earth. These forms of calcium are economical, and a person can get as much as 500 to 600 mg in one tablet. However, there are concerns that the natural forms of calcium supplements may contain significant amounts of lead. The level of contamination has decreased in recent years, but it still may present a health risk. Calcium supplements rarely list the lead content of their sources. The lead concentration should always be less than two parts per million.

Refined calcium carbonate. Refined calcium carbonate is the most common commercial calcium supplement, and it is also used as a common antacid. Calcium carbonate is one of the least expensive forms of calcium, but it can cause constipation and bloating, and it may not be well absorbed by people with reduced levels of stomach acid. Taking it with meals improves absorption because stomach acid is released to digest the food.

Chelated calcium. Chelated calcium is calcium bound to an organic acid (citrate, citrate malate, lactate, gluconate, aspartate, or orotate). The chelated forms of calcium offer some significant advantages and disadvantages compared with calcium carbonate.

Certain forms of chelated calcium (calcium citrate and calcium citrate malate) are widely thought to be significantly better absorbed and more effective for

osteoporosis treatment than calcium carbonate. However, while some studies support this belief, others do not. The discrepancy may come from the particular calcium carbonate products used; some calcium carbonate formulations may dissolve better than others. One study found that calcium citrate malate in orange juice is markedly better absorbed than tricalcium phosphate/calcium lactate in orange juice.

A form of calcium called active absorbable algal calcium has also been promoted as superior to calcium carbonate. The study upon which claims of benefit are founded actually used quite questionable statistical methods (technically, post-hoc subgroup analysis).

Chelated calcium is much more expensive and bulkier than calcium carbonate. In other words, a person would have to take larger pills, and more of them, to get enough calcium. It is not uncommon to need to take five or six large capsules daily to supply the necessary amount, a quantity some people may find troublesome.

THERAPEUTIC DOSAGES

Unlike some supplements, calcium is not taken at extra high doses for special therapeutic benefit. Rather, for all its uses, it should be taken in the recommended amounts, along with the recommended level of vitamin D.

Calcium absorption studies have found evidence that the body cannot absorb more than 500 mg of calcium at one time. Therefore, it is most efficient to take one's total daily calcium in two or more doses.

It is not possible to put all the calcium one needs in a single multivitamin-multimineral tablet, so this is one supplement that should be taken on its own. Furthermore, if taken at the same time, calcium may interfere with the absorption of chromium and manganese. This means that it is best to take the multivitamin-multimineral pill at a different time than the calcium supplement.

Although the calcium in some antacids or supplements may alter the absorption of magnesium, this effect apparently has no significant influence on overall magnesium status. Calcium may also interfere with iron absorption, but the effect may be too slight to cause a problem. Some studies show that calcium may decrease zinc absorption when the two are taken together as supplements; however, studies have found that in the presence of meals, zinc levels may

Calcium for Preventing Colon Cancer

Colorectal adenomas are precancerous polyps that occur in the lower digestive tract. Evidence indicates that the use of calcium supplements can help prevent colon polyps and also reduce colon cancer risk.

A 2007 article in the *Journal of the National Cancer Institute* adds weight to this hypothesis. A total of 930 people with a history of having a colon polyp were given either placebo or calcium carbonate (3 grams daily) for four years. At the end of the four-year trial period, people given calcium showed a significantly lower rate of polyp recurrence compared with those given placebo. Treatment was then stopped, but researchers continued to follow the participants. Remarkably, the protective effect of calcium was maintained for as long as five years after the end of the active part of the study. Even those persons who did not continue to take calcium supplements remained relatively less likely to develop polyps simply on the basis of having taken it.

There are two caveats, however. First, this dose of calcium supplementation is very high and should not be undertaken without a doctor's supervision. Second, there is weak but still potentially worrisome evidence that, when taken by men, calcium supplements may raise the risk of cancer of the prostate.

Steven Bratman, M.D.

be unaffected by increases of either dietary or supplemental calcium. Finally, the use of prebiotics known as inulin fructans may improve calcium absorption.

THERAPEUTIC USES

According to most studies, the use of calcium (especially in the form of calcium citrate) with vitamin D may modestly slow the bone loss that leads to osteoporosis. A rather surprising potential use of calcium came to light when a large, well-designed study found that calcium is an effective treatment for PMS. Calcium supplementation reduced all major symptoms, including headache, food cravings, moodiness, and fluid retention. It is remotely possible that there may be a connection between these two uses of calcium: Weak evidence hints that PMS might be an early sign of future osteoporosis. One small but carefully conducted study suggests that getting enough calcium may help control symptoms of menstrual pain too.

Some observational and intervention studies have found evidence that calcium supplementation may reduce the risk of colon cancer. Risk reduction might continue for years after calcium supplements are stopped. However, calcium supplements might increase risk of prostate cancer in men. For menopausal women, the

use of calcium supplements, especially with vitamin D added, may reduce cancer risk in general.

Persons who are deficient in calcium may be at greater risk of developing high blood pressure. Among persons who already have hypertension, increased intake of calcium might slightly decrease blood pressure, according to some studies. Weak evidence hints that the use of calcium by pregnant women might reduce the risk of hypertension in their children. Calcium supplementation has also been tried as a treatment to prevent preeclampsia in pregnant women. While the evidence from studies is conflicting, calcium supplementation might offer at least a minimal benefit.

The drug metformin, used for diabetes, interferes with the absorption of vitamin B_{12}. Calcium supplements may reverse this, allowing the B_{12} to be absorbed normally. Also, calcium supplements might slightly improve the cholesterol profile.

Rapid weight loss in overweight postmenopausal women appears to slightly accelerate bone loss. For this reason, it may make sense to take calcium and vitamin D supplements when deliberately losing weight. It has been additionally suggested that calcium supplements, or high-calcium diets, may directly enhance weight loss, but the evidence is more negative than positive.

Finally, calcium is also sometimes recommended for attention deficit disorder, migraine headaches, and periodontal disease, but there is no meaningful evidence that it is effective for these conditions. It is important to note that despite the benefits of calcium supplementation for certain conditions, a large placebo-controlled trial involving more than 36,000 postmenopausal women found that daily supplements of 1,000 mg of calcium carbonate combined with 400 international units (IU) of vitamin D(3) for an average of seven years did not significantly reduce death rates from all causes.

SCIENTIFIC EVIDENCE

Osteoporosis. A number of double-blind, placebo-controlled studies indicate that calcium supplements (especially as calcium citrate and taken with vitamin D) are slightly helpful in preventing and slowing bone loss in postmenopausal women. Contrary to some reports, milk does appear to be a useful source of calcium for this purpose. However, the effect of calcium supplementation in any form is relatively mild and may not be strong enough to reduce the rate of osteoporotic fractures. The use of calcium and vitamin D must be continual. Any improvements in bone density rapidly disappear once the supplements are stopped. A large study of more than three thousand postmenopausal women age sixty-five to seventy-one years found that three years of daily supplementation with calcium and vitamin D was not associated with a significant reduction in the incidence of fractures. Calcium carbonate may not be effective.

One study found benefits for elderly men using a calcium- and vitamin D-fortified milk product. Calcium and vitamin D supplementation may help bones heal that have become fractured because of bone thinning. Also, calcium supplements may do a better job of strengthening bones when people have relatively high protein intake.

Heavy exercise leads to a loss of calcium through sweat, and the body does not compensate for this by reducing calcium loss in the urine. The result can be a net calcium loss great enough so that it presents health concerns for menopausal women, already at risk for osteoporosis. One study found that the use of an inexpensive calcium supplement (calcium carbonate), taken at a dose of 400 mg twice daily, is sufficient to offset this loss.

Calcium supplementation could, in theory, be useful for young girls as a way to build a supply of calcium for the future to prevent later osteoporosis. However, the benefits seen in studies have been modest to nonexistent, and this approach may only produce results when exercise is also increased.

Evidence suggests that the use of calcium with vitamin D can help protect against the bone loss caused by corticosteroid drugs, such as prednisone. A review of five studies covering 274 participants reported that calcium and vitamin D supplementation significantly prevented bone loss in corticosteroid-treated persons. For example, in a two-year, double-blind, placebo-controlled study that followed sixty-five persons with rheumatoid arthritis taking low-dose corticosteroids, daily supplementation with 1,000 mg of calcium and 500 IU of vitamin D reversed steroid-induced bone loss, causing a net bone gain. Also, one study found that in calcium-deficient pregnant women, calcium supplements can improve the bones of their unborn children.

There is some evidence that essential fatty acids may enhance the effectiveness of calcium. In one study, sixty-five postmenopausal women were given calcium with either placebo or a combination of omega-6 fatty acids (from evening primrose oil) and omega-3 fatty acids (from fish oil) for eighteen months. At the end of the study period, the group receiving essential fatty acids had higher bone density and fewer fractures than the placebo group. However, a twelve-month, double-blind trial of forty-two postmenopausal women found no benefit. The explanation for the discrepancy may lie in the differences between the women studied. The first study involved women living in nursing homes, while the second studied healthier women living on their own. The latter group of women may have been better nourished and may have been receiving enough essential fatty acids in their diet.

Premenstrual syndrome. According to a large and well-designed study published in 1998 in the *American Journal of Obstetrics and Gynecology*, calcium supplements act as a simple and effective treatment for a variety of PMS symptoms. In a double-blind, placebo-controlled study of 497 women, 1,200 mg daily of calcium as calcium carbonate reduced PMS symptoms by one-half through three menstrual cycles. These symptoms included mood swings, headaches, food cravings, and bloating. These results corroborate earlier, smaller studies.

High cholesterol. In a twelve-month study of 223 postmenopausal women, use of calcium citrate at a dose of 1 gram (g) daily improved the ratio of HDL (good) cholesterol levels to LDL (bad) cholesterol levels. The extent of this improvement was statistically significant (compared with the placebo group) but not very large in practical terms. Similarly modest benefits were seen in a smaller, double-blind, placebo-controlled study. A third double-blind, placebo-controlled study failed to find any statistically significant effects.

Colon cancer. Evidence from observational studies showed that a high calcium intake is associated with a reduced incidence of colon cancer, but not all studies have found this association. Some evidence from intervention trials supports these findings.

A four-year, double-blind, placebo-controlled study

followed 832 persons with a history of colon polyps. Participants received either 3 g daily of calcium carbonate or placebo. The calcium group experienced 24 percent fewer polyps overall than the placebo group. Because colon polyps are the precursor of most colon cancer, this finding strongly suggests benefit. Combining the results for two trials, involving a total of 1,346 participants also with a history of polyps, researchers found that 1,200 or 2,000 mg of daily elemental calcium led to a significant reduction in polyp recurrence compared with placebo in a three-to-four-year period. Another large study found that calcium carbonate at a dose of 1,200 mg daily may have a more pronounced effect on dangerous polyps than on benign ones.

A gigantic (36,282-participant) and long-term (average of seven years) study of postmenopausal women failed to find that calcium carbonate supplements at a dose of 1,000 mg daily had any effect on the incidence of colon cancer. Given these conflicting results, if calcium supplementation does have an effect on colon cancer risk, it is probably small.

Hypertension. A large randomized, placebo-controlled trial of more than 36,000 postmenopausal women found daily supplementation with 1,000 mg of calcium plus 400 IU of vitamin D did not reduce or prevent hypertension during seven years of follow-up. These results are possibly limited by calcium use unrelated to the study.

SAFETY ISSUES

In general, it is safe to take up to 2,500 mg of calcium daily, although this is more than a person needs. Excessive intake of calcium can cause numerous side effects, including dangerous or painful deposits of calcium within the body. For persons with cancer, hyperparathyroidism, or sarcoidosis, calcium should be taken only under a physician's supervision.

Some evidence hints that the use of calcium supplements might slightly increase kidney stone risk. However, increased intake of calcium from food does not seem to have this effect and could even help prevent stones. One study found that if calcium supplements are taken with food, there is no increased risk. Calcium citrate supplements may be particularly safe regarding kidney stones because the citrate portion of this supplement is used to treat kidney stones.

There is preliminary evidence that calcium supplementation in healthy, postmenopausal women may slightly increase the risk of cardiovascular events, such as myocardial infarction. However, it remains far from clear whether this possible risk outweighs the benefits of calcium supplementation in this population.

Large observational studies have found that, in men, higher intakes of calcium are associated with an increased risk of prostate cancer. This seems to be the case whether the calcium comes from milk or from calcium supplements.

Calcium supplements combined with high doses of vitamin D might interfere with some of the effects of drugs in the calcium channel blocker family. It is very important that one consult a physician before trying this combination.

Concerns have been raised that the aluminum in some antacids may be harmful. There is some evidence that calcium citrate supplements might increase the absorption of aluminum; for this reason, one probably should not take calcium citrate at the same time of day as aluminum-containing antacids. Other options are to use different forms of calcium or to avoid antacids containing aluminum.

When taken over the long term, thiazide diuretics tend to increase levels of calcium in the body by decreasing the amount excreted by the body. It is not likely that this will cause a problem. Nonetheless, persons using thiazide diuretics should consult with a physician on the proper doses of calcium and vitamin D.

Finally, calcium may interfere with the absorption of antibiotics in the tetracycline and fluoroquinolone families and with thyroid hormone. Persons taking any of these drugs should take calcium supplements a minimum of two hours before or after the medication dose.

IMPORTANT INTERACTIONS

Persons may need more calcium if also taking corticosteroids, heparin, or isoniazid. Persons taking aluminum hydroxide should take it and calcium citrate a minimum of two hours apart to avoid increasing aluminum absorption.

Persons may need more calcium if they are also taking any of the following anticonvulsants: phenytoin (Dilantin), carbamazepine, phenobarbital, or primidone. It may be advisable to take the dose of anticonvulsant and the calcium supplement a minimum of two hours apart because each substance interferes with the other's absorption.

For persons taking antibiotics in the tetracycline or

fluoroquinolone (cipro, floxin, noroxin) families or taking thyroid hormone, the calcium supplement should be taken a minimum of two hours before or after the dose of medication, because calcium interferes with absorption (and vice versa). Also, one should not take extra calcium except on the advice of a physician if also taking thiazide diuretics. Finally, one should not take calcium with high-dose vitamin D except on the advice of a physician if also taking calcium channel blockers.

Persons may need extra calcium if also taking iron, manganese, zinc, or chromium. Ideally, one should take calcium at a different time of day from these other minerals because it may interfere with their absorption.

Finally, it may be advisable to wait two hours after taking calcium supplements to eat soy (or vice versa). A constituent of soy called phytic acid can interfere with the absorption of calcium.

EBSCO CAM Review Board

FURTHER READING

Caan, B., et al. "Calcium Plus Vitamin D Supplementation and the Risk of Postmenopausal Weight Gain." *Archives of Internal Medicine* 167 (2007): 893-902.

Dodiuk-Gad, R. P., et al. "Sustained Effect of Short-Term Calcium Supplementation on Bone Mass in Adolescent Girls with Low Calcium Intake." *American Journal of Clinical Nutrition* 81 (2005): 168-174.

LaCroix, A. Z., et al. "Calcium plus Vitamin D Supplementation and Mortality in Postmenopausal Women: The Women's Health Initiative Calcium-Vitamin D Randomized Controlled Trial." *Journals of Gerontology: Series A–Biological Sciences and Medical Sciences* 64 (2009): 559-567.

Lappe, J. M., et al. "Vitamin D and Calcium Supplementation Reduces Cancer Risk." *American Journal of Clinical Nutrition* 85 (2007): 1586-1591.

Margolis, K. L., et al. "Effect of Calcium and Vitamin D Supplementation on Blood Pressure." *Hypertension* 52 (2008): 847-855.

Martin, B. R., et al. "Exercise and Calcium Supplementation: Effects on Calcium Homeostasis in Sportswomen." *Medicine and Science in Sports and Exercise* 39 (2007): 1481-1486.

Matkovic, V., et al. "Calcium Supplementation and Bone Mineral Density in Females from Childhood to Young Adulthood." *American Journal of Clinical Nutrition* 81 (2005): 175-188.

Reid, I. R., and M. J. Bolland. "Calcium Supplementation and Vascular Disease." *Climacteric* 11 (2008): 280-286.

Wagner, G., et al. "Effects of Various Forms of Calcium on Body Weight and Bone Turnover Markers in Women Participating in a Weight Loss Program." *Journal of the American College of Nutrition* 26 (2007): 456-461.

Winzenberg, T., et al. "Calcium Supplements in Healthy Children Do Not Affect Weight Gain, Height, or Body Composition." *Obesity* 15 (2007): 1789-1798.

Zemel, M. B., et al. "Effects of Calcium and Dairy on Body Composition and Weight Loss in African-American Adults." *Obesity Research* 13 (2005): 1218-1225.

See also: Bone and joint health; Menopause; Osteoporosis; Premenstrual syndrome (PMS)

Calcium channel blockers

CATEGORY: Drug interactions

DEFINITION: Medications used to treat hypertension, angina, heart arrhythmia, and other heart-related conditions.

INTERACTIONS: Calcium, *Ginkgo biloba*, naringen (a citrus bioflavonoid), vitamin D

DRUGS IN THIS FAMILY: Amlodipine (Norvasc), bepridil hydrochloride (Vascor), diltiazem (Cardizem, Cardizem CD, Cardizem SR, Dilacor XR, Tiamate, Tiazac), felodipine (Plendil), isradipine (DynaCirc, DynaCirc CR), nicardipine hydrochloride (Cardene, Cardene SR), nifedipine (Procardia, Procardia XL, Adalat, Adalat CC), nimodipine (Nimotop), nisoldipine (Sular), verapamil (Calan, Calan SR, Covera-HS, Isoptin, Isoptin SR, Verelan)

CALCIUM AND VITAMIN D

Effect: Possible Decreased Action of Drug

Taking calcium and vitamin D supplements might interfere with some of the effects of calcium channel blockers.

GINKGO BILOBA

Effect: Possible Decreased Action of Drug

According to a study in rats, ginkgo extract may cause the body to metabolize some calcium channel blockers more rapidly, thereby decreasing their effects.

NARINGEN (CITRUS BIOFLAVONOID)

Effect: May Necessitate Reduction in Drug Dosage

Some evidence suggests that the bioflavonoid naringen may interact with medications in the calcium channel blocker family, increasing blood levels of the drug. This may necessitate a reduction in drug dosage.

EBSCO CAM Review Board

FURTHER READING

Guadagnino, V., et al. "Treatment of Severe Left Ventricular Dysfunction with Calcium Chloride in Patients Receiving Verapamil." *Journal of Clinical Pharmacology* 27 (1987): 407-409.

Kuhn, M., and D. L. Schriger. "Low-Dose Calcium Pretreatment to Prevent Verapamil-Induced Hypotension." *American Heart Journal* 124 (1992): 231-232.

Luscher, T. F., et al. "Calcium Gluconate in Severe Verapamil Intoxication." *New England Journal of Medicine* 330 (1994): 718-720.

Margolis, K. L., et al. "Effect of Calcium and Vitamin D Supplementation on Blood Pressure." *Hypertension* 52 (2008): 847-855.

See also: Angina; Arrhythmia; Calcium; Citrus bioflavonoids; Food and Drug Administration; Ginkgo; Herbal medicine; Hypertension; Supplements: Introduction; Vitamin D.

Calendula

CATEGORY: Herbs and supplements

DEFINITION: Natural plant product used to treat specific health conditions.

PRINCIPAL PROPOSED USES: Canker sores, eczema, hemorrhoids, minor burns, minor wounds, varicose veins

OVERVIEW

Calendula, well known as one of the ornamental marigolds, blooms month after month from early spring to first frost. Because *calend* means "month" in Latin, the plant's lengthy flowering season is believed to have given calendula its name. The herb has been used to heal wounds and treat inflamed skin since ancient times.

An active ingredient that might be responsible for calendula's traditional medicinal properties has not been discovered. One theory suggests that volatile oils in the plant act synergistically with other constituents called xanthophylls.

THERAPEUTIC DOSAGES

Calendula cream is generally applied two or three times daily to the affected area. For oral use as a mouthwash, pour boiling water over 1 to 2 teaspoons of calendula flowers and allow to steep for ten to fifteen minutes.

THERAPEUTIC USES

Experiments on rats and other animals suggest that calendula cream exerts wound-healing and anti-inflammatory effects, but double-blind, placebo-controlled studies have not yet been reported. The best study on calendula so far was a controlled trial comparing calendula to the standard treatment trolamine for the prevention of skin irritation caused by radiation therapy. The researchers used trolamine for comparison not because it has been proven effective but more as a kind of acceptable placebo (trolamine is not thought to do much, even though it is widely used). The study found calendula more effective than trolamine. However, because this was not a double-blind study, the results mean little; mere expectation of benefit is likely to cause patients and experimenters to perceive benefit.

Creams made with calendula flower are a nearly ubiquitous item in the German medicine chest, used for everything from children's scrapes to eczema, burns, and poorly healing wounds. These same German products are widely available in the United States as well.

Calendula cream is also used to soothe hemorrhoids and varicose veins, and the tea reportedly reduces the discomfort of canker sores. However, as yet there is no scientific evidence for any of these uses.

SAFETY ISSUES

Calendula is generally regarded as safe. Neither calendula cream nor calendula taken internally has been associated with any adverse effects other than occasional allergic reactions, and animal studies have found no significant toxic effects. However, the same studies found that in high doses, calendula acts like a sedative and also reduces blood pressure. For this reason, it might not be safe to combine calendula with sedative or blood pressure medications.

IMPORTANT INTERACTIONS

In person taking sedative drugs, calendula might increase the sedative effect. Also, internal use of calendula might amplify the blood pressure-lowering effect of medications to reduce blood pressure.

EBSCO CAM Review Board

FURTHER READING

Pommier, P., et al. "Phase III Randomized Trial of *Calendula officinalis* Compared with Trolamine for the Prevention of Acute Dermatitis During Irradiation for Breast Cancer." *Journal of Clinical Oncology* 22 (2004): 1447-1453.

See also: Herbal medicines; Wounds, minor.

CAM on PubMed

CATEGORY: Organizations and legislation
DEFINITION: A U.S.-government-sponsored research and informational database listing scientific journal citations focused on complementary and alternative medicine.
DATE: Founded 2001

INTRODUCTION

The National Center for Complementary and Alternative Medicine (NCCAM) and the National Library of Medicine (NLM), under the auspices of the National Institutes of Health (NIH), joined efforts to create CAM on PubMed, a Web-based resource with a tailored search engine for locating article citations exclusively related to complementary and alternative medicine (CAM). PubMed defines "complementary medicine" as a type of medicine not considered part of routine medical practice but that may be used in addition to conventional treatments; it defines "alternative medicine" as those therapies that are used in place of conventional therapies.

CAM on PubMed was created for a number of reasons. First, it was developed because of the growing popularity of CAM among health consumers. Studies consistently demonstrated that between 38 and 42 percent of Americans had used a minimum of one form of CAM. Second, researchers found that many patients and practitioners believe that CAM has no scientific research or evidence behind it. In fact, the amount of science-based citations on PubMed relating to CAM topics increased by 33 percent from 1988 to 1998. With CAM on PubMed, persons seeking information are assured that the information they find comes from a peer-reviewed journal.

Third, medical professionals and patients did not have a centralized location to search the available and reliable scientific publications on CAM topics. While many European and Asian nations, where CAM is well known and accepted, had already established databases, these databases often were not accessible to persons outside their respective countries of origin. CAM on PubMed, in helping to raise general public awareness about CAM practices, also has helped to increase the likelihood that CAM therapies will become part of routine medical treatment and research.

Although PubMed was created in 1950, the CAM subset was not introduced until 2001. CAM on PubMed contains citations from 1966 through the present. The amount of publications listed on PubMed expands on a daily basis and now exceeds 16 million entries from more than 4,800 medical and life science journals. Approximately 13 percent of the biomedical journals focus on CAM practices. When CAM on PubMed was originally created, 220,000 CAM-related citations were available for searching. In 2011, NCCAM estimated that this number had increased to more than 462,000 citations.

PERFORMING SEARCHES

The CAM on PubMed database is a free Web-based resource open to CAM practitioners, conventional health-care providers, medical researchers, and any other persons interested in the subject. The database does not require user registration. Searches can be made by topic of interest or keyword, such as "acupuncture" or "meditation"; by author; by article title; or by journal title. A literature search provides, at minimum, the journal title and citation information, but an abstract summary of the scientific findings and conclusions is available in approximately 60 percent of cases. PubMed also allows direct connection to the full journal article when the journal is available through open access, meaning the content is free for all users. Certain articles, however, require subscriptions to view the entire paper. Although the site is in English, it lists international scientific publications; many abstracts of these articles have been translated into English.

Specific keyword searches remain a challenge. Many CAM therapies can be described in multiple ways. It is recommended that researchers first perform broad searches and then more specific searches as articles are identified. Research on database reliability and validity has found that when searches are performed comparing CAM on PubMed with other CAM databases, different results will appear because of these limitations. Therefore, several databases might be used together to maximize citation results for users.

Janet Ober Berman, M.S., CGC

FURTHER READING

Boehm, Katja, et al. "An Overview of Forty-five Published Database Resources for Complementary and Alternative Medicine." *Health Information and Libraries Journal* 27, no. 2 (2010): 93-105.

Cogo, E., et al. "Searching for Controlled Trials of Complementary and Alternative Medicine: A Comparison of Fifteen Databases." *Evidence-Based Complementary and Alternative Medicine* (May, 2009): 1-9.

Saxton, Jane, and David Owen. "Developing Optimal Search Strategies for Finding Information on Herbs and Other Medicinal Plants in Medline." *Journal of Alternative and Complementary Medicine* 11, no. 4 (2005): 725-731.

See also: Double-blind, placebo-controlled studies; The Internet and CAM; National Center for Complementary and Alternative Medicine; Regulation of CAM.

Cancer chemotherapy support: Homeopathic remedies

CATEGORY: Homeopathy

DEFINITION: The use of highly diluted remedies to treat side effects from chemotherapy.

STUDIED HOMEOPATHIC REMEDIES: *Arsenicum album*; homeopathic mouthwash containing *Arnica montana, Calendula officinalis, Hamamelis virginiana, Achillea millefolium, Atropa belladonna, Aconitum napellum, Hepar sulfuris, Symphytum, Mercurius solubilis, Bellis perennis, Chamomilla, Echinacea angustifolia, E. purpurea,* and *Hypericum; M. solubilis;* sulphur

INTRODUCTION

While chemotherapy for cancer can be lifesaving, it frequently produces serious side effects. Many of the side effects occur because chemotherapy is designed to attack rapidly dividing cells. These rapidly dividing cells include not only cancer cells but also normal cells in the digestive tract and elsewhere. Symptoms may include nausea, vomiting, and mouth sores. Hair loss and anemia may also occur, again because of chemotherapy's effects on healthy cells that undergo rapid division as part of their normal life cycle. Mouth sores, one complication of chemotherapy, is one side effect that has been studied for its treatment with homeopathic remedies.

SCIENTIFIC EVALUATIONS OF HOMEOPATHIC REMEDIES

In a double-blind trial, thirty children with mouth sores caused by cancer chemotherapy were given either homeopathic or placebo mouthwash, five times daily for a minimum of fourteen days. The results showed that the use of the homeopathic treatment significantly reduced symptoms compared with placebo. The mouthwash used in this trial contained the following ingredients:

Arnica montana, Calendula officinalis, Hamamelis virginiana, Achillea millefolium, Atropa belladonna, Aconitum napellum, Hepar sulfuris, Symphytum, Mercurius solubilis, Bellis perennis, Chamomilla, Echinacea angustifolia, E. purpurea, and *Hypericum.*

TRADITIONAL HOMEOPATHIC TREATMENTS

According to the principles of classical homeopathy, there are many possible homeopathic treatments for cancer chemotherapy support. These therapies are chosen based on various specific details of the person seeking treatment. The traditional symptom picture of homeopathic *Arsenicum album* includes painful mouth sores relieved by warm or hot drinks in a person who feels fatigued and anxious.

Mercurius solubilis may be used when the symptom

picture includes a tongue that is swollen and coated, bleeding gums, and mouth sores that feel worse at night.

Homeopathic sulphur could be indicated for red, inflamed mouth sores that are aggravated by hot drinks. Swollen gums, a bitter taste in the mouth, and dark red lips also can be treated with this remedy.

EBSCO CAM Review Board

FURTHER READING

Guethlin, C., et al. "Characteristics of Cancer Patients Using Homeopathy Compared with Those in Conventional Care." *Annals of Oncology* 21 (2010): 1094-1099.

Kassab, S., et al. "Homeopathic Medicines for Adverse Effects of Cancer Treatments." *Cochrane Database of Systematic Reviews* (2009): CD004845. Available through EBSCO DynaMed Systematic Literature Surveillance at http://www.ebscohost.com/dynamed.

Marian, F., et al. "Patient Satisfaction and Side Effects in Primary Care: An Observational Study Comparing Homeopathy and Conventional Medicine." *BMC Complementary and Alternative Medicine* 8 (2008): 52.

Oberbaum, M., et al. "A Randomized, Controlled Clinical Trial of the Homeopathic Medication Traumeel S in the Treatment of Chemotherapy-Induced Stomatitis in Children Undergoing Stem Cell Transplantation." *Cancer* 92 (2001): 684-690.

See also: Cancer treatment support.

Cancer risk reduction

CATEGORY: Condition
DEFINITION: Prevention and treatment of all cancers.
PRINCIPAL PROPOSED NATURAL TREATMENTS: Folate, garlic, green tea, isoflavones, selenium, soy, tomatoes (lycopene), vitamin C, vitamin E
OTHER PROPOSED NATURAL TREATMENTS: Active hexose correlated compound, beta-carotene, betulin, black tea, blue-green algae, boron, bromelain, calcium, cartilage, catechins (from green tea), citrus bioflavonoids, conjugated linoleic acid, *Cordyceps, Coriolus versicolor*, diindolylmethane, ellagic acid, fiber, fish oil, flaxseed (lignans), flavonoid, genistein, ginseng, glycine, grapes (resveratrol), grass pollen, indole-3-carbinol, inositol hexaphos-

phate (phytic acid), isoflavones, kelp, licorice, ligustrum, melatonin, methyl sulfonyl methane, milk thistle, N-acetylcysteine, nettle, oligomeric proanthocyanidins, papaw tree bark, probiotics, quercetin, rosemary, schisandra, shiitake, sulforaphane, turmeric, vitamin D

INTRODUCTION

Cancer is the second major cause of death (next to heart disease) in the United States. It claims the lives of more than one-half million Americans each year out of the nearly 1.4 million who get the disease. The probability of getting cancer increases with age. Two-thirds of all cases are in people older than age sixty-five.

Cancer is believed to begin with a mutation in a single cell. However, a cell does not become cancerous overnight. Several mutations in a row are necessary to create all the characteristic features of cancer. Ordinarily, cells have a self-destruct mechanism that causes them to die when their deoxyribonucleic acid (DNA) is damaged. However, in developing cancer cells, something interferes with the self-destruct sequence. It may be that the cancer-causing mutations themselves turn off the countdown.

The DNA alterations that create a cancer cell give it a certain independence from the ordinary rules of cell behavior. Normal cells are highly influenced by nearby cells, with the result that they "get along" well with their neighbors. For example, the growth of a healthy cell is ruled by special growth factors given off by surrounding tissues. However, cancer cells either grow without such growth factors or simply make their own. Many types of cancer cells can also trigger the growth of new blood vessels to feed them.

The rate of cancerous mutations is increased by exposure to carcinogenic substances. Cigarette smoke is a powerful carcinogen. Many carcinogens exist in the diet too, even in fruits and vegetables.

PRINCIPAL PROPOSED NATURAL TREATMENTS

It is rather difficult to prove that taking a certain supplement will reduce the chance of developing cancer. One really needs enormous, long-term, double-blind, placebo-controlled studies in which some people are given the studied supplement while others are given placebo. However, relatively few studies of this type have been performed.

For most supplements, the evidence that they help

prevent cancer comes from observational studies, which are much less reliable. Observational studies have found that people who happen to take in high levels of certain vitamins in their diets develop a lower incidence of specific cancers. However, in such studies it is difficult to rule out other factors that may play a role. For example, persons who take vitamins may also exercise more or take better care of themselves in other ways. Such confounding factors make the results of observational studies less reliable.

Although this may sound like a theoretical issue, it has very practical consequences. For example, based primarily on observational studies, hormone replacement therapy (HRT) was promoted as a heart-protective treatment for postmenopausal women. However, when placebo-controlled studies were performed, HRT proved to increase the risk of heart disease.

It is now thought that the apparent benefits of HRT arose because women who used it often belonged to a higher socioeconomic class than those who did not use it. (For a variety of reasons, some of which are obscure, higher income is associated with improved health.) Only a few supplements have any evidence from double-blind trials to support their potential usefulness for cancer prevention, and even that evidence is weak. For all other supplements, supporting evidence is limited to observational studies and to preliminary evidence from animal and test-tube studies.

Vitamin E. The results of observational trials have been mixed, but on balance, they suggest that high intake of vitamin E is associated with reduced risk of many forms of cancer, including stomach, mouth, colon, throat, laryngeal, lung, liver, and prostate cancer. However, the results of observational studies are unreliable as guidelines to treatment. The results of double-blind, placebo-controlled studies are far more persuasive in drawing conclusions about cause and effect. On balance, these studies failed to find vitamin E helpful for the prevention of cancer.

The one positive note came in a double-blind study of 29,133 smokers. Those who were given 50 milligrams (mg) of synthetic vitamin E (dl-alpha-tocopherol) daily for five to eight years showed a 32 percent reduction in the incidence of prostate cancer and a 41 percent drop in prostate cancer deaths. Surprisingly, results were seen soon after the beginning of supplementation. This was unexpected because prostate cancer develops slowly. A cancer that shows up in

a man's prostate today actually started to develop many years ago. That vitamin E almost immediately lowered the incidence of prostate cancer suggests that it may somehow block one of the last steps in the development of detectable prostate cancer.

Nonetheless, the negative results regarding most other types of cancer have made scientists hesitant to place too much hope in these findings. Some researchers believe that better results will be seen with a form of vitamin E called gamma-tocopherol rather than the alpha-tocopherol used in the foregoing trials. Others suggest that vitamin E might be more helpful for cancer prevention in low-risk people.

Selenium. It has long been known that severe selenium deficiency increases the risk of cancer. One double-blind study found some evidence that selenium supplements might help prevent cancer even in the absence of severe deficiency. The study was designed to detect selenium's effects on skin cancer. It followed 1,312 persons, one-half of whom were given 200 micrograms (mcg) of selenium daily. People participating in the study were not deficient in selenium. The participants were treated for an average of 2.8 years and were followed for about six years. Although no significant effect on skin cancer was found, the researchers were startled when the results showed that people taking selenium had a 50 percent reduction in overall cancer deaths and significant decreases in cancer of the lung (40 percent), colon (50 percent), and prostate (66 percent). The findings were so remarkable that the researchers felt obliged to break the blind and allow all the participants to take selenium.

Subsequent reevaluation of the results, including additional data from follow-up, indicated that lung cancer and colon cancer benefits were seen only in participants with somewhat low levels of selenium in the blood to begin with. While this evidence is promising, it has one major flaw: The laws of statistics indicate that when researchers start to deviate from the question their research was designed to answer, the results may not be trustworthy. As an illustration of this, yet another after-the-fact statistical analysis of the data hints that selenium supplements might actually increase the risk of certain forms of skin cancer. This, however, may not be a real concern either, as all such statistical manipulation is suspect.

One study published in 2007 evaluated whether selenium supplements could help prevent skin cancer

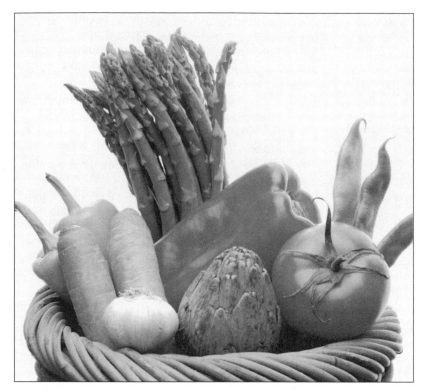

Vegetables are an important part of a cancer-prevention diet.(PhotoDisc)

in transplant patients. People who have undergone organ transplants are at particularly high risk of skin cancer linked to the human papilloma virus (HPV). In this double-blind study, 184 organ transplant recipients were given either placebo or selenium at a dose of 200 mg daily. The results over two years failed to show benefit: Both the placebo group and the selenium group developed precancerous and cancerous lesions at the same rate. Further research will be necessary before it is known whether selenium supplements actually help prevent cancer.

Mixed antioxidants. A large, double-blind, placebo-controlled study evaluated the potential overall cancer-preventive benefits of a low-dose combination antioxidant supplement providing 120 mg of ascorbic acid, 30 mg of vitamin E, 6 mg of beta-carotene, 100 mcg of selenium, and 20 mg of zinc taken daily for about 7.5 years. The results as a whole failed to show benefit. However, analysis by gender showed a significant reduction in cancer incidence in men but not in women. It is not clear whether these results are meaningful. The researchers involved in this study concluded the

following: Low-dose antioxidant supplementation may be helpful in healthy people, without cancer risk, who are deficient in antioxidant nutrition. High doses of antioxidants may be harmful for people who are at higher risk for cancer and may already be in the initial phases of cancer development. Finally, antioxidants in high or low doses are probably not helpful in healthy people with good nutrition.

Another large study failed to find mixed antioxidants helpful for preventing stomach cancer in particular. In a meta-analysis (a detailed mathematical review) of twenty high-quality randomized trials (involving 211,818 participants), researchers concluded that neither beta-carotene, vitamin A, vitamin C, vitamin E, or selenium effectively lowered the risk of gastrointestinal cancers. If anything, they may have slightly increased the risk of death from these cancers.

Beta-carotene. The story of beta-carotene and cancer is full of contradictions. It starts in the early 1980s, when the cumulative results of many studies suggested that people who eat a lot of fruits and vegetables are significantly less likely to get cancer. A close look at the data pointed to carotenes as the active ingredients in fruits and vegetables. It appeared that a high intake of dietary carotene might significantly reduce the risk of cancers of the lung, bladder, breast, esophagus, and stomach.

However, once again, observational studies cannot prove cause and effect. When researchers gave beta-carotene to study participants, the results have been impressively negative.

Beta-carotene's reported benefits came under question in 1994 with the results of the Alpha-Tocopherol, Beta-Carotene study. These results showed that beta-carotene supplements did not prevent lung cancer but actually increased the risk of getting it by 18 percent. This trial followed 29,133 male smokers in Finland who took supplements of about 50 international units (IU) of vitamin E (alpha-tocopherol), 20 mg of beta-carotene (more than ten times the amount necessary to provide the daily requirement of vitamin

A), both, or placebo daily for five to eight years. (In contrast, vitamin E was found to reduce the risk of cancer, especially prostate cancer.)

In January, 1996, researchers monitoring the Beta-carotene and Retinol Efficacy Trial (CARET) confirmed the earlier negative news with more of their own: The beta-carotene group had 46 percent more cases of lung cancer deaths. This study involved smokers, former smokers, and workers exposed to asbestos. Alarmed, the National Cancer Institute ended the $42 million CARET trial twenty-one months before it was scheduled to end.

At about the same time, the twelve-year Physicians' Health Study of 22,000 male physicians was finding that 50 mg of beta-carotene (about twenty-five times the amount necessary to provide the daily requirement of vitamin A) taken every other day had no effect–good or bad–on the risk of cancer or heart disease. In this study, 11 percent of the participants were smokers and 39 percent were former smokers.

Similarly, another study of beta-carotene supplements failed to find any effect on the risk of cancer in women. In a final indictment of beta-carotene's safety and effectiveness, researchers, who combined the results of twelve recent placebo-controlled trials investigating the association between antioxidant supplementation and cancer, found that beta-carotene use was associated with an increased incidence of cancer among smokers. However, the story does not end there. In yet another careful analysis of four randomized trials involving 109,394 smokers and former smokers, researchers found that smokers who consumed between 20 and 30 mg of beta-carotene were at significantly greater risk of developing lung cancer. There was no such risk among former smokers.

One possible explanation for these discrepancies is that beta-carotene alone is not effective. Fruits and vegetables contain many carotenoids (carotene-like substances) that may be more important for preventing cancer than beta-carotene. One researcher suggested that taking beta-carotene supplements actually depletes the body of other beneficial carotenoids. It is also possible that intake of carotenes as such is unrelated to cancer and that some unrelated factor common to persons with a high carotene diet is the cause of the benefits seen in observational trials.

Tomatoes (lycopene). Lycopene, a carotenoid like beta-carotene, is found in high levels in tomatoes and pink grapefruit. Lycopene appears to exhibit about twice the antioxidant activity of beta-carotene and may be more helpful for preventing cancer.

In one observational study, elderly Americans consuming a diet high in tomatoes showed a 50 percent reduced incidence of cancer. Men and women who ate at least seven servings of tomatoes weekly developed less stomach and colorectal cancers compared to those who ate only two servings weekly.

In another study, 47,894 men were followed for four years in an observational study looking for influences on prostate cancer. Their diets were evaluated on the basis of how often they ate fruits, vegetables, and foods containing fruits and vegetables. High levels of tomatoes, tomato sauce, and pizza in the diet were strongly connected to reduced incidence of prostate cancer. After an evaluation of known nutritional factors in these foods compared to other foods, lycopene appeared to be the common denominator. Additional impetus has been given to this idea by the discovery of lycopene in reasonably high levels in the human prostate, evidence from test-tube studies that lycopene might slow DNA synthesis in prostate cells, and evidence that men with higher lycopene levels in the blood have a lower risk of prostate cancer. Similarly weak evidence suggests that foods containing lycopene might help prevent other forms of cancer, including lung, colon, and breast cancer. A few poorly designed intervention trials have also been performed, and these suggest that lycopene or a standardized tomato extract containing lycopene might be helpful for the prevention or treatment of prostate or breast cancer.

Vitamin C. Several observational studies have found a strong association between high dietary vitamin C intake and a reduced incidence of stomach cancer. It has been proposed that vitamin C may prevent the formation of carcinogenic substances known as N-nitroso compounds in the stomach.

Observational studies have also linked higher vitamin C in the diet with reduced risk of cancers of the colon, esophagus, larynx, bladder, cervix, rectum, breast, and perhaps lung. However, dietary vitamin C intake does not appear to be associated with reduced rate of prostate cancer.

One study found that vitamin C supplementation at 500 mg or more daily was associated with a lower incidence of bladder cancer. However, another study found no association. Similarly, in another observational study, 500 mg or more of vitamin C daily for six years was not associated with reduced incidence of breast cancer. Another study found similar results.

Green tea. Both green tea and black tea come from the plant *Camellia sinensis*, which has been cultivated in China for centuries. The key difference between the two is in preparation. For black tea, the leaves are allowed to oxidize, a process believed to lessen the potency of the presumed active ingredients in green tea, catechin polyphenols. Green tea is made by lightly steaming the freshly cut leaf, a process that prevents oxidation and possibly preserves more of the therapeutic effects.

Laboratory and animal studies suggest that tea consumption protects against cancers of the stomach, lung, esophagus, duodenum, pancreas, liver, breast, and colon. A 1994 study of skin cancer in mice found that both black and green teas, even decaffeinated versions, inhibited skin cancer in mice exposed to ultraviolet light and other carcinogens. After thirty-one weeks, mice given the teas brewed at the same concentration humans drink had 72 to 93 percent fewer skin tumors than mice that were given only water.

However, results from observational studies in humans have not been so clear-cut; some have found evidence of a protective effect, and others have not. One study followed 8,552 Japanese adults for nine years. Women who drank more than ten cups of green tea daily had a delay in the onset of cancer and also a 43 percent lower total rate of cancer occurrence. Men had a 32 percent lower cancer incidence, but this finding was not statistically significant.

A study in Shanghai, China, found that those who drank green tea had significantly less risk of developing cancers of the rectum and pancreas than those who did not. No significant association with colon cancer incidence was found. A total of 3,818 residents age thirty to seventy-four years were included in the population study. For men, those who drank the most tea had a 28 percent lower incidence of rectal cancer and a 37 percent lower incidence of pancreatic cancer compared to those who did not drink tea regularly. For women, the respective differences in cancer frequency were even greater: 43 percent and 47 percent.

Another study in Shanghai found similar associations for stomach cancer. Green tea drinkers were 29 percent less likely to get stomach cancer than nondrinkers, with those drinking the most tea having the least risk. The risk of stomach cancer did not depend on the person's age at which he or she started drinking green tea. Researchers suggested that green tea may disrupt the cancer process at both the intermediate and the late stages.

Green tea may exert an estrogen-blocking effect that is helpful in preventing breast and uterine cancer, and another study suggests that it might prevent the development of tumors by blocking the growth of new blood vessels. In a review of nine studies (none of which were clinical trials) involving more than 5,600 persons, researchers found weak evidence for reduction in breast cancer recurrence among people who consumed more than three cups of green tea every day, but they failed to find reliable evidence for a reduction in the incidence of breast cancer.

However, in an observational study of 26,311 Japanese persons, researchers saw no reduction in stomach cancer rates. Lack of benefit was also seen in a study conducted in Hawaii. Also, combining the results of thirteen observational studies, researchers found conflicting evidence for green tea's effect on the risk of stomach cancer. However, in a small Japanese randomized trial, persons who supplemented their regular diet with an extra 1.5 grams of green tea extract per day for one year lowered their risk of recurrent colorectal polyps compared to those who took no supplement. In a review of multiple studies, including forty-three observational studies, four randomized trials and one meta-analysis (a mathematical summation of the results from several studies), researchers concluded that there was inconsistent evidence supporting green tea's effectiveness for cancer prevention.

The main catechin polyphenol found in green tea is epigallocatechin gallate (EGCG). Preliminary experimental studies suggest that EGCG may help prevent skin cancer if it is applied directly to the skin.

Soy. In many animal studies, soybeans, soy protein, or other soy extracts decreased cancer risk, and observational studies in people have found suggestive associations between higher soy consumption and lower incidence of hormone-related cancers such as prostate, breast, and uterine cancer. Soybeans provide estrogen-like compounds known as isoflavones, especially genistein and daidzein. These substances bind to the same sites in the body as estrogen, occupying these sites and keeping natural estrogen away. Estrogen stimulates certain forms of cancer, but soy isoflavones exert a milder estrogen-like effect that may not stimulate cancer as much as natural estrogen.

This could help protect against cancer. Soy may additionally reduce levels of the body's own estrogen, which would also have a protective effect.

However, not all evidence on soy and cancer is positive. Because the isoflavones work somewhat like estrogen, there are theoretical concerns that they may not be safe for women who have already had breast cancer. Studies in animals have found suggestive evidence that under certain circumstances soy isoflavones might stimulate breast cancer cells. Furthermore, evidence from two preliminary studies in humans found changes suggesting that soy might slightly increase breast cancer risk. Other studies in women have found reassuring results; nonetheless, women who have had breast cancer, or are at high risk for it, should consult a physician before taking any isoflavone product.

Men have very low levels of circulating estrogen, so the net effect of increased soy consumption might be to increase estrogen-like activity in the body. Because real estrogen is used as a treatment to suppress prostate cancer, it has been hypothesized that the mild estrogen-like activity of isoflavones has a similar effect. There are also indications that isoflavones might decrease testosterone levels and alter ratios of certain forms of estrogen, both of which would be expected to provide benefit. Thus, there are several possible ways in which isoflavones might be useful for preventing or treating prostate cancer. Whether or not they actually help has been tested in a few preliminary trials.

For example, in one double-blind study, men with early prostate cancer were given either isoflavones or placebo, and their PSA levels were monitored. (PSA is a marker for prostate cancer, with higher values generally showing an increased number of cancer cells.) The results did show that the use of isoflavones (60 mg daily) slightly reduces PSA levels. Whether this meant that soy actually slowed the progression of the cancer or simply lowered PSA directly is not clear from this study alone. However, another study of apparently healthy men (not known to have prostate cancer) found that soy isoflavones at a dose of 83 mg per day did not alter PSA levels. Taken together, these two studies provide some direct evidence that soy isoflavones may be helpful for treating or preventing prostate cancer, but the case, nonetheless, remains highly preliminary.

A special highly concentrated extract of soy, Bowman-Birk inhibitor (BBI), has also shown promise for helping to prevent various types of cancer. There exists weak evidence that besides the isoflavone found in soy, flavonoids (found, for example, in beans, onions, apples, and tea) may reduce the recurrence of colorectal polyps, common precancerous lesions found in the colon and rectum.

Folate. Observational studies have suggested that folate deficiency may predispose persons toward developing cancer of the cervix, colon, lung, breast, pancreas, and mouth. Other observational studies have suggested that folate supplements may help prevent colon cancer, especially when they are taken for many years or by people with ulcerative colitis. However, observational studies are notoriously unreliable; large double-blind, placebo-controlled studies are needed to prove a treatment effective.

One such study performed on folate for cancer prevention among 1,000 people over a five-year period found folate ineffective for preventing early colon cancer. Also, in a large controlled trial involving more than 5,400 women, supplements combining folate plus vitamins B_6 and B_{12} taken for seven years did not reduce the risk of a cancer compared with placebo. However, a much smaller study involving ninety-four persons with colon polyps (a precancerous condition) found that folate may reduce the risk of recurrent polyps over a three-year period.

OTHER PROPOSED NATURAL TREATMENTS

Some observational and intervention studies have found evidence that calcium supplementation may reduce the risk of colon cancer. Risk reduction might continue for years after calcium supplements are stopped. In men, however, calcium supplements might increase risk of prostate cancer. For menopausal women, calcium supplementation, especially when taken with vitamin D, appears to reduce overall cancer incidence.

Some studies have connected higher vitamin D levels with a lower incidence of cancer of the breast, colon, pancreas, and prostate, and of melanoma, but overall research has yielded mixed results. In an extremely large study involving more than 36,000 postmenopausal women, supplementing the diet with 1,000 mg of calcium plus 400 IU of vitamin D daily did not lower the risk of breast cancer in a period of seven years. Based on the results of this placebo-controlled study, there does not appear to be a connection between vitamin D and breast cancer risk.

Increasing dietary fiber has long been thought to

help reduce the incidence of colon polyps. However, several late studies found either little evidence of benefit or no evidence. For example, one large study enrolled almost two thousand people with a history of colon polyps and compared the ordinary American diet with a diet high in fiber, fruits, and vegetables and low in saturated fat. In the four years of the study, plus an additional four years of follow-up, this presumably healthier diet failed to reduce polyp recurrence.

Substances known as lignans are found in several foods and may produce anticancer benefits. Lignans are converted in the digestive tract to estrogen-like substances known as enterolactone and enterodiol. Like soy isoflavones, these substances prevent estrogen from attaching to cells and may thereby block its cancer-promoting effects. Lignans are found most abundantly in flaxseed, a high-fiber grain that has been cultivated since ancient Egyptian times. Both flaxseed and flaxseed oil have been recommended for the prevention or treatment of cancer, but the supporting evidence is still extremely preliminary. Contrary to some reports, flaxseed oil contains no lignans. Instead, it contains the alpha-linolenic acid, which is also hypothesized to have cancer-preventive effects.

Evidence from observational studies suggests that garlic taken in the diet as food may help prevent cancer, particularly cancer of the colon and stomach. In one of the best of these studies, the Iowa Women's Study, women who ate significant amounts of garlic were found to be about 30 percent less likely to develop colon cancer. Similar results were seen in other observational studies performed in China, Italy, and the United States. In addition, one preliminary intervention trial also found some evidence that aged garlic may reduce risk of colon cancer.

Resveratrol is a phytochemical found in at least seventy-two different plants, including mulberries and peanuts. Grapes and red wine are particularly rich in resveratrol. This substance has shown anticancer properties in test-tube studies.

One large observational study suggests that higher intake of boron may reduce the risk of prostate cancer. Provocative evidence suggests that a substance called sulforaphane, found in broccoli and related vegetables, may possess anticancer properties. Broccoli sprouts have been touted for cancer prevention on the basis of their high content of sulforaphane. However, this recommendation is still highly speculative. Another constituent of broccoli-family vegetables, in-

dole-3-carbinol, has also shown promise as a cancer-preventive agent; however, there is some evidence that this substance might actually increase the risk of cancer in certain circumstances. Much the same is true of the related substance diindolylmethane.

In one large, randomized-controlled trial, diets rich in fish and omega-3 fatty acids from fish were associated with a significant reduction in the risk of developing colorectal cancer among men in a twenty-two-year period. Another study provides preliminary supporting evidence for the notion that fish oil reduces the risk of prostate cancer. However, on balance, there is still relatively little evidence that the consumption of fish oil reduces the risk of cancer.

Weak evidence hints that N-acetylcysteine treatment may help to prevent colon cancer. Also, several studies have experimented with using very high doses of vitamin A to prevent skin cancer, doses considerably above levels ordinarily considered safe. Some have found possible benefits regarding preventing some forms of skin cancer, while others have not. This approach should not be tried except under physician supervision. Vitamin K has shown some promise for helping to prevent liver cancer in people with chronic viral hepatitis.

Innumerable other herbs and supplements have shown minimal promise in test-tube and animal studies, including but not limited to active hexose correlated compound, *Cordyceps*, *Coriolus versicolor*, ligustrum, quercetin, citrus bioflavonoids, conjugated linoleic acid, *Morina citrifolia* (noni), turmeric, rosemary, betulin (from white birch tree), bromelain, ellagic acid (from grapes, raspberries, strawberries, apples, walnuts, and pecans), ginseng, glycine, grass pollen, inositol hexaphosphate (phytic acid, IP6), kelp, licorice, melatonin, methyl sulfonyl methane, milk thistle, nettle, oligomeric proanthocyanidins, papaw tree bark, probiotics (friendly bacteria), royal jelly, shiitake, schisandra, and blue-green algae.

While it is commonly stated as a fact that high consumption of fruits and vegetables reduces cancer risk, the evidence is limited to inherently unreliable observational studies, and even among these the results are inconsistent. As noted, a large study failed to find that a diet high in fruits and vegetables reduced risk of colon polyps. Similarly, meat consumption, widely stated to increase colon cancer risk, might or might not do so (the evidence is not compelling). Data do not suggest that diets high in sugar or other simple carbohydrates increase colon cancer risk or that reducing fat in the diet reduces colon, uterine, or breast cancer risk. Higher levels of exercise might potentially help reduce the risk of various forms of cancer, especially colon cancer.

EBSCO CAM Review Board

FURTHER READING

Bardia, A., et al. "Efficacy of Antioxidant Supplementation in Reducing Primary Cancer Incidence and Mortality." *Mayo Clinic Proceedings* 83 (2008): 23-34.

Bjelakovic, G., et al. "Systematic Review and Meta-analysis: Primary and Secondary Prevention of Gastrointestinal Cancers with Antioxidant Supplements." *Alimentary Pharmacology and Therapeutics* 28 (2008): 689-703.

Bobe, G., et al. "Dietary Flavonoids and Colorectal Adenoma Recurrence in the Polyp Prevention Trial." *Cancer Epidemiology, Biomarkers, and Prevention* 17 (2008): 1344-1353.

Buring, J. E. "Aspirin Prevents Stroke but Not MI in Women–Vitamin E Has No Effect on CV Disease or Cancer." *Cleveland Clinic Journal of Medicine* 73 (2006): 863-870.

Chlebowski, R. T., et al. "Calcium plus Vitamin D Supplementation and the Risk of Breast Cancer." *Journal of the National Cancer Institute* 100 (2008): 1581-1591.

Hall, M. N., et al. "A Twenty-Two-Year Prospective Study of Fish, N-3 Fatty Acid Intake, and Colorectal Cancer Risk in Men." *Cancer Epidemiology, Biomarkers, and Prevention* 17 (2008): 1136-1143.

Michels, K. B., and W. C. Willett. "The Women's Health Initiative Randomized Controlled Dietary Modification Trial: A Post-mortem." *Breast Cancer Research and Treatment* 114 (2009): 1-6.

Myung, S. K., et al. "Green Tea Consumption and Risk of Stomach Cancer." *International Journal of Cancer* 124 (2009): 670-677.

Ogunleye, A. A., F. Xue, and K. B. Michels. "Green Tea Consumption and Breast Cancer Risk or Recurrence." *Breast Cancer Research and Treatment* 119 (2010): 477-484.

Peters, U., et al. "Vitamin E and Selenium Supplementation and Risk of Prostate Cancer in the Vitamins and Lifestyle (VITAL) Study Cohort." *Cancer Causes and Control* 19 (2008): 75-87.

Prentice, R. L., et al. "Low-Fat Dietary Pattern and Risk of Invasive Breast Cancer: The Women's Health Initiative Randomized Controlled Dietary Modification Trial." *Journal of the American Medical Association* 295 (2006): 629-642.

Tanvetyanon, T., and G. Bepler. "Beta-Carotene in Multivitamins and the Possible Risk of Lung Cancer Among Smokers Versus Former Smokers: A Meta-analysis and Evaluation of National Brands." *Cancer* 113 (2008): 150-157.

Weingarten, M., A. Zalmanovici, and J. Yaphe. "Dietary Calcium Supplementation for Preventing Colorectal Cancer and Adenomatous Polyps." *Cochrane Database of Systematic Reviews* (2008): CD003548. Available through *EBSCO DynaMed Systematic Literature Surveillance* at http://www.ebscohost.com/dynamed.

Wright, M. E., et al. "Supplemental and Dietary Vitamin E Intakes and Risk of Prostate Cancer in a Large Prospective Study." *Cancer Epidemiology, Biomarkers, and Prevention* 16 (2007): 1128-1135.

Zhang, S. M., et al. "Effect of Combined Folic Acid, Vitamin B6, and Vitamin B12 on Cancer Risk in Women." *Journal of the American Medical Association* 300 (2008): 2012-2021.

See also: Beta-carotene; Cancer chemotherapy support: Homeopathic remedies; Cancer treatment support; Folate; Green tea; Lycopene; Selenium; Soy; Vitamin C; Vitamin E.

Cancer treatment support

CATEGORY: Condition

DEFINITION: The use of herbs, supplements, and alternative therapies to complement conventional cancer treatment.

PROPOSED NATURAL TREATMENTS

- *Improving the effectiveness of conventional treatment:* Active hexose correlated compound, *Coriolus versicolor*, docosahexaenoic acid, *Eleutherococcus senticosus*, *Ginkgo biloba*, lycopene, melatonin, mistletoe extract (injected), N-acetylcysteine, *Panax ginseng*, relaxation therapies, shark cartilage, shiitake, social support, vitamin A, vitamin C, vitamin D

- *Reducing the side effects of chemotherapy:* Acetyl-L-carnitine, acupuncture-acupressure, active hexose correlated compound, aromatherapy, beta-carotene, chamomile cream, coenzyme Q_{10}, colostrum, creatine, docosahexaenoic acid, ginger, glutamine, hypnosis, massage, melatonin, milk thistle, N-acetylcysteine, probiotics, relaxation therapy, sea buckthorn, traditional Chinese herbal medicine, vitamin E

- *Reducing the side effects of radiation therapy:* Aloe vera gel, calendula cream, chamomile cream, multivitamin-multimineral supplements, probiotics, proteolytic enzymes, sea buckthorn, zinc
- *Treating lymphedema caused by breast cancer surgery:* Citrus bioflavonoids, oligomeric proanthocyanidins, oxerutins

HERBS AND SUPPLEMENTS TO USE ONLY WITH CAUTION: Alfalfa, androstenedione, beta-carotene, black cohosh, boron, dong quai, estriol, folate, genistein, hops, licorice, *Panax ginseng,* red clover, resveratrol, St. John's wort, soy, vitamin C, vitamin E

INTRODUCTION

Cancer is the second leading cause of death in the United States (after heart disease), and its insidious nature gives it a special terror. Most diseases give warning in the form of escalating symptoms, while others strike suddenly. Cancer follows a different, stealthier path. A person who feels perfectly well may come back from the doctor's office with a diagnosis of potentially fatal cancer and plenty of time to fear what comes next.

Conventional treatments for cancer also have frightening qualities to them, including disfiguring surgery, arduous chemotherapy, and treatment with invisible radiation. In many cases, when cancer is found early enough, conventional treatment can lead to a permanent cure. Often, though, the prognosis is given in statistics (a percentage chance of survival) or, worse, in months remaining to live.

Some alternative therapies for cancer may truly work, even if they have not been proven. Most studies of alternative therapies for cancer have involved adding a natural treatment to a standard cancer regimen; alternatively, they enrolled persons who have already failed to respond to existing methods. These latter circumstances could potentially hide the benefits of an effective natural therapy. If a treatment only worked in the absence of chemotherapy, for example (as some alternative cancer therapy proponents claim about their methods) or could only cure early cases of cancer, these ethical obstacles would prevent researchers from finding out.

The relatively small amount of information that is known from a scientific perspective about alternative treatments for cancer is discussed here, as are natural options that may reduce side effects of standard cancer therapies. Possible interactions between herbs and supplements and drugs are also discussed.

PROPOSED NATURAL TREATMENTS

Various natural supplements have shown some promise for improving the effectiveness of conventional cancer therapy (specifically surgery, chemotherapy, and radiation) or reducing its side effects. In most cases, however, the supporting evidence remains weak, and the most rigorous studies have often failed to find benefit. Persons receiving cancer treatment should not use any herbs or supplements except under the supervision of a physician.

IMPROVING EFFECTIVENESS OF CONVENTIONAL TREATMENT

Numerous natural therapies have been proposed for enhancing the cancer-fighting effects of standard therapies. However, most of the supporting research falls short of the necessary standard for proof: a double-blind, placebo-controlled study.

Shark cartilage. Based on the belief that sharks do not get cancer, shark cartilage has been heavily marketed as a cure for cancer. While this is a myth (sharks do get cancer), shark cartilage has shown some promise. Shark cartilage tends to inhibit the growth of new blood vessels, a process called angiogenesis. Because cancerous tumors must build new blood vessels to feed themselves, this effect might be beneficial.

Shark cartilage also inhibits substances called matrix metalloproteases (MMPs). These little-understood enzymes affect the extracellular matrix, the framework of substances that lie between cells in the body. MMPs are thought to play a role in diseases of the cornea, gums, skin, blood vessels, and joints, and in cancer and illnesses that involve excessive fibrous tissue.

A number of test-tube experiments have found that shark cartilage extracts prevent new blood vessels from forming in chick embryos and other test systems. These findings have led to other test-tube experiments, animal studies, and preliminary human trials to investigate the possible anticancer effects of shark cartilage. The results appeared to suggest that a particular liquid shark cartilage extract might be useful in the treatment of various cancers, including lung, prostate, and breast cancer. However, the two

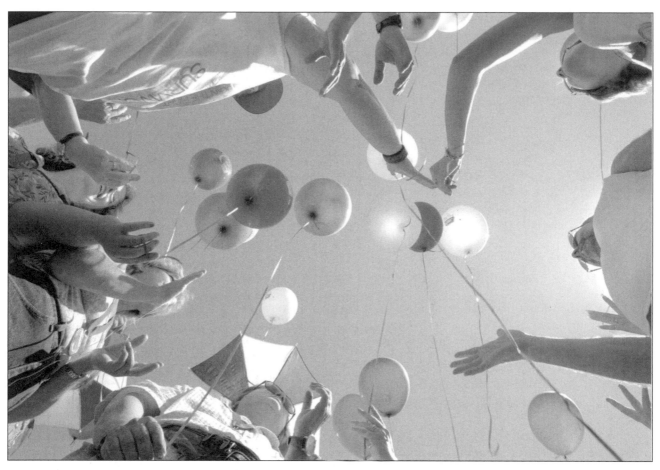

Cancer survivors can find comfort by participating in support groups and events such as the cancer walk. (AP/Wide World Photos)

most recent and best designed of these studies have failed to find benefit.

Social support and other psychological factors. Cancer treatment puts tremendous stress, both physical and emotional, on those who undergo it. Several studies have examined the potential benefits of social support for women with breast cancer. According to most studies, such support improves survival and enhances quality of life. In one well-known study of women with advanced breast cancer, participants who attended a support group twice weekly doubled their survival time compared to study participants who did not attend the group.

It is also commonly said that certain psychological coping styles (for example, fighting spirit versus helpless acceptance) can lead to longer life in people with cancer. However, a review of the evidence found that there is little to no evidence that psychological attitude makes much of a difference. People with cancer should not feel pressured into adopting particular coping styles to improve survival or reduce the risk of recurrence, the study's authors concluded.

Relaxation therapies. One study evaluated guided imagery and relaxation therapy following surgery for colon cancer. The results indicated no more than a short-term, mood-elevating benefit; those receiving the treatment did not recover more quickly.

Another study on relaxation therapy involved 126 hospitalized persons with cancer pain. Researchers found that those who listened to relaxing music for thirty minutes and received pain medication had more relief than the group who received only the medication.

Vitamin C. Cancer treatment is one of the more controversial proposed uses of vitamin C. An early study tested vitamin C in eleven hundred terminally ill persons with cancer. One hundred persons received 10,000 milligrams (mg) daily of vitamin C, while the other one thousand persons (the control group) did not receive vitamin C. Those taking the vitamin C survived more than four times longer on average (210 days) than those in the control group (50 days). A large (1,826 subjects) follow-up study by the same researchers found a nearly doubled survival rate (343 days versus 180 days) in vitamin C-treated persons whose cancers were deemed incurable, compared to people not treated with vitamin C. Benefits were also seen in a similarly designed Japanese study.

However, while these results seem promising and almost miraculous, they show next to nothing because they lacked a placebo group. When proper double-blind, placebo-controlled studies were performed on vitamin C for cancer, they failed to find any benefit. Vitamin C proponents have criticized these trials on various grounds, but the fact remains that there is no reliable positive evidence for vitamin C in cancer.

PC-SPES for prostate cancer. PC-SPES is a formulation of eight natural substances: seven are plants and one is a fungus. The name is derived from the common abbreviation for prostate cancer (PC) and the Latin word *spes*, meaning "hope."

After its commercial launch in 1996, PC-SPES received increasing interest from the general public and prostate cancer researchers. Preliminary evidence suggested that it has significant effects on prostate cancer cells, perhaps because of its estrogen-like action.

However, chemical analysis reported in 2002 showed that PC-SPES is not truly a purely herbal product; samples of the product dating to 1996 have been found to contain a form of pharmaceutical estrogen, diethylstilbestrol (DES), as well as indomethacin (an anti-inflammatory medication in the ibuprofen family) and warfarin (a strong blood thinner). Samples subsequent to 1999 contain less DES; but they also have shown less effectiveness in treating prostate cancer.

There is little doubt that DES is active against prostate cancer, but it presents a variety of risks, including blood clots in the legs. The other two pharmaceutical contaminants might actually reduce the risk of blood clots (which may be why they were covertly added), but present various risks all on their own. For these reasons, PC-SPES use is not recommended.

Other natural treatments. Hundreds of herbs and supplements have been shown in test-tube studies to fight cancer cells. However, it is a long way from a test tube to a human body, and such findings are not meaningful.

Several natural supplements that have received at least preliminary study in humans are discussed here. None of the positive studies cited here reached the level of rigor required to truly show a treatment effective. (Most lacked a control group, for example.) In contrast, several properly designed studies failed to find benefit.

A double-blind study of fifty-three people undergoing cancer treatment found equivocal evidence that treatment with a special form of *Panax ginseng* (modified to contain higher levels of certain constituents) could improve general well-being of people with cancer. Another study investigating the effects of *P. ginseng* on survival of persons being treated for lung cancer showed no additional benefit. One study provides indirect but promising evidence that a mixture of the supplements coenzyme Q_{10} (100 mg daily), riboflavin (10 mg daily), and niacin (50 mg daily) might help reduce the chance of breast cancer metastasis, or recurrence.

According to most of the highly preliminary trials, extracts of the fungus *Coriolus versicolor* may enhance the effectiveness of various forms of standard cancer therapy. *Coriolus* is thought to work by stimulating the immune system. The fungi products active hexose correlated compound and shiitake are also advocated for this purpose.

The supplement docosahexaenoic acid, a constituent of fish oil, has shown promise for enhancing the effects of the cancer chemotherapy drug doxorubicin. The herb *Ginkgo biloba* is thought to increase blood flow. An uncontrolled study evaluated combination therapy with ginkgo extract and the chemotherapy drug 5-FU for the treatment of pancreatic cancer, on the theory that ginkgo might enhance blood flow to the tumor and thereby help 5-FU penetrate better. The results were promising. Scant preliminary evidence suggests that American ginseng may increase the effectiveness of treatment for breast cancer and that Siberian ginseng (properly known as *Eleutherococcus senticosus*) may be useful in the treatment of breast cancer and other forms of cancer.

A small unblinded study using a no-treatment control group found indications that the use of a standardized tomato extract containing the supplement lycopene might slow the growth of prostate cancer. In a small, double-blind, placebo-controlled study, a combination of soy, isoflavones, lycopene, silymarin (from milk thistle), and antioxidants showed some potential benefit for preventing recurrence of prostate cancer after prostate cancer surgery. Another study enrolled men with rising PSA levels (a symptom of worsening cancer) and found that the use of lycopene helped stabilize these levels. Because this study failed to include a placebo control group, its results fail to indicate that lycopene lowers PSA levels and therefore, by inference, slows prostate cancer. However, researchers did compare lycopene alone with lycopene plus isoflavones and found that the combined treatment seemed to be less effective, as if the isoflavones somehow antagonized the effects of lycopene.

Preliminary studies, including unblinded-controlled trials, suggest that the hormone melatonin may enhance the effectiveness of standard therapy for breast cancer, prostate cancer, brain glioblastomas, non-small-cell lung cancer, and other forms of cancer. However, no double-blind studies have been reported. Melatonin may also help decrease cancer chemotherapy side effects.

Mistletoe extract (Iscador) taken by injection has been evaluated as a cancer treatment in a number of studies, including double-blind, placebo-controlled trials. In general, though, these studies failed to attain adequate levels of scientific rigor or clinical relevance. The best studies found benefit; more rigorous studies found no improvement in survival time, survival rate, or quality of life. A review of forty-one studies found mistletoe use was associated with improved survival in persons with cancer. An analysis of these studies limited to randomized trials showed no effect. The safety of mistletoe is not established, and one report suggests that it can damage the liver.

An uncontrolled study found that the use of a special spleen extract (spleen peptide preparation) somewhat reduced side effects of chemotherapy for head and neck cancer. In a double-blind, placebo-controlled trial, neither vitamin A nor N-acetylcysteine proved helpful for enhancing survival in head and neck cancer or lung cancer. Vitamin D may decrease bone pain and increase muscle strength in men with prostate cancer.

Traditional Chinese medicine has been evaluated in a number of studies in persons being treated for cancer. In one such study, acupuncture has shown some promise for reducing the sense of fatigue that commonly occurs in cancer. Similarly, medical qigong (two ninety-minute sessions weekly) was associated with improved quality of life, fatigue, and mood disturbance in another study. A review of fifteen mostly poor-quality trials involving 862 persons receiving chemotherapy for non-small-cell lung cancer suggested that Chinese herbal medicine might improve quality of life. A 2010 review of seven studies, however, found insufficient evidence to conclude whether or not Tai Chi improves quality of life or psychological or physical outcomes in persons with breast cancer. One study tested whether a diet very high in vegetables, fruit, and fiber, and low in fat could enhance survival or reduce recurrence rates in women diagnosed with breast cancer; no benefits were seen.

Reducing Side Effects of Chemotherapy

Various herbs and supplements have shown promise for reducing the side effects of chemotherapy. Many chemotherapy drugs work by interfering with rapidly dividing cells. Cancer cells, however, are not the only cells that divide rapidly. The intestinal tract constantly rebuilds its lining, and chemotherapy may interfere with that process. The result is gastrointestinal side effects, such as mouth sores, nausea, loss of appetite, and diarrhea. Several herbs and supplements have shown promise for alleviating these conditions, although none have been definitively proven effective.

Diarrhea and other gastrointestinal side effects. A well-designed, double-blind, placebo-controlled trial of seventy participants undergoing cancer chemotherapy with the drug 5-FU evaluated the potential benefits of the supplement glutamine for reducing chemotherapy-induced diarrhea. The results suggest that the use of glutamine at a dose of 18 grams daily may reduce intestinal damage and diminish symptoms of diarrhea. These promising findings indicate a need for larger trials to accurately determine the extent of benefit.

A double-blind, placebo-controlled study of 150 people undergoing chemotherapy with 5-FU found some evidence that a probiotic (friendly bacterium) called *Lactobacillus rhamnosus* can reduce the diarrhea that is a common complication of this treatment. Another, more unusual probiotic, a special, nonpathogenic form of *Escherichia coli*, has also shown promise. Preliminary evidence hints that the supplement active hexose correlated compound and colostrum might help reduce chemotherapy-induced gastrointestinal side effects. In one study, the use of the supplement creatine failed to help maintain muscle mass in people undergoing chemotherapy for colon cancer.

Mouth sores. In an uncontrolled study, the use of the herb chamomile as a mouthwash appeared to help prevent mouth sores in people undergoing various forms of chemotherapy. However, uncontrolled studies prove nothing. A rigorous, double-blind, placebo-controlled trial of 164 people did not find chamomile mouthwash effective for treating the mouth sores caused by the chemotherapy drug 5-FU. Beta-carotene and vitamin E have also shown some promise for preventing mouth sores (caused by various forms of cancer treatment) in preliminary studies, but rigorous studies of adequate size have not been reported.

Nausea. A preliminary trial hints that ginger may reduce nausea caused by the chemotherapy drug 8-MOP. However, another study failed to find ginger helpful for nausea in people using the drug cisplatin. In a third trial, ginger did not add to the effectiveness of standard medications to treat chemotherapy-induced nausea and vomiting.

Massage has shown some benefit for reducing nausea caused by chemotherapy. Psychological methods such as hypnosis and relaxation therapy have also shown promise for nausea. One study found that the use of aromatherapy massage (combined massage therapy and the use of fragrant essential oils) reduced symptoms of anxiety or depression (or both) in people undergoing treatment for cancer, at least for the short-term. However, the authors of a review of ten massage therapy studies were unable to draw firm conclusions about its benefits for a wide range of symptoms in persons undergoing treatment for cancer. Studies of acupressure or acupuncture for reducing nausea in people undergoing chemotherapy have reached contradictory results, though on balance, there may be some benefit.

A double-blind study performed in Hong Kong evaluated the potential benefits in cancer chemotherapy of personalized herbal formulas designed according to the principles of traditional Chinese herbal medicine. In this study, 120 people undergoing chemotherapy for early-stage breast or colon cancer were given either a personalized formula or placebo. Researchers evaluated numerous possible effects of the treatment but found benefits in only one: reduction of nausea. Even this single result is less meaningful than it may seem; it is statistically questionable to use a multiplicity of outcome measures.

Other side effects of chemotherapy. In highly preliminary trials, the supplement N-acetylcysteine has shown promise for reducing various side effects of the drug ifosfamide. An animal study suggests that a constituent of fish oil called docosahexaenoic acid might decrease side effects caused by the drug irenotecan. The hormone melatonin has shown some promise for reducing the side effects of various chemotherapy drugs.

In preliminary studies, various antioxidants have shown promise for preventing heart damage and other side effects of the drug doxorubicin. One animal study hints that the herb milk thistle might protect against kidney damage caused by the drug cisplatin. In addition, there is some evidence that acetyl-L-carnitine, glutamine, and vitamin E supplementation might each reduce peripheral neuropathy (painful damage to nerves outside the spinal column) symptoms in persons receiving cisplatin or paclitaxel.

Sea buckthorn berry has been advocated for reducing side effects of chemotherapy, but the evidence that it works is far too preliminary to be relied upon. A review of thirty-three studies supports the view that antioxidants in general (with the exception of vitamin A) may reduce the toxic effects of chemotherapy. However, because of inconsistencies among these studies, it is unclear what antioxidants are best for this purpose.

REDUCING SIDE EFFECTS OF RADIATION THERAPY

Although the symptoms are generally less intense than with chemotherapy, radiation therapy can also cause problems, such as diarrhea, skin damage, and fatigue. Certain supplements and alternative therapies may offer benefit.

Two double-blind, placebo-controlled studies enrolling a total of almost seven hundred people undergoing radiation therapy found that the use of probiotics significantly improved diarrhea. However, of eighty-five women receiving pelvic radiation for cervical or uterine cancer, those who consumed a probiotic-enriched yogurt had no less diarrhea than those who took a placebo drink.

An unblinded-controlled study of seventy-five people receiving radiation therapy for various forms of cancer found some evidence that soap enriched with aloe vera gel can help protect the skin from radiation damage. However, researchers had to use questionable statistical methods to find evidence of benefit, making the results less than fully reliable. A double-blind, placebo-controlled study that evaluated the effects of aloe gel in 225 women undergoing radiation therapy for breast cancer failed to find benefit. Another study failed to find aloe vera beneficial for reducing side effects of radiation therapy for head and neck cancer.

One study compared cream made from calendula flowers with the standard treatment trolamine for protecting the skin during radiation therapy and found calendula more effective. However, it is not known whether trolamine is beneficial, neutral, or harmful when used for this purpose, and for this reason it is not possible to draw firm conclusions from the study. Cream made from chamomile has also been tried for protecting the skin from damage caused by radiation therapy, but the one controlled trial on the subject failed to find benefit.

One study failed to find oligomeric proanthocyanidins from grape seed helpful for reducing the local side effects of radiation therapy for breast cancer. Radiation treatment in the vicinity of the mouth may cause alterations in taste sensation. In a small, double-blind, placebo-controlled trial, the use of zinc supplements tended to counter this symptom. However, a larger follow-up study failed to find this benefit. Another study did find that the use of zinc could modestly decrease inflammation of the mucous membranes and skin caused by radiation therapy.

Radiation treatment to the pelvic area can cause nausea, vomiting, and fatigue. A double-blind, placebo-controlled trial with fifty-six participants evaluated the potential effectiveness of proteolytic enzymes for reducing these symptoms. No benefits were seen. Another study failed to find proteolytic enzymes helpful for reducing mouth sores or other symptoms that occur during radiation therapy of head and neck cancers.

In a double-blind study of forty people undergoing radiation therapy for breast cancer, the use of a standard multivitamin preparation failed to reduce fatigue compared with placebo. People in the placebo group may have done somewhat better than those given the vitamin.

A large study failed to find aromatherapy more helpful than placebo for reducing psychological distress among people undergoing radiation therapy for cancer. A small randomized trial found that effleurage massage, a common massage technique, had no significant effect on anxiety, depression, or quality of life among twenty-two women undergoing radiation therapy for breast cancer.

As with chemotherapy, sea buckthorn berry has been advocated for reducing side effects of radiation therapy, but again, reliable evidence is lacking. The use of antioxidants during radiation therapy is controversial. One study found that the use of antioxidants decreased radiation therapy side effects but also may have decreased radiation therapy effectiveness. In a small trial, persons who wore acupressure bands for up to seven days following radiation therapy reported less nausea than persons who received only usual care.

TREATING SIDE EFFECTS CAUSED BY BREAST CANCER SURGERY

Many women experience lymphedema (chronic arm swelling caused by damage to the lymph drainage system) following breast cancer surgery. Natural treatments for this condition include oxerutins, citrus bioflavonoids, and oligomeric proanthocyanidins. Another small randomized trial of seventy persons found that acupuncture may decrease dry mouth and pain after removing lymph nodes in the neck for cancer treatment.

Hot flashes after mastectomy. Women who have had breast cancer surgery frequently experience annoying hot flashes. Estrogen treatment is not an option, as it might increase the risk of cancer recurrence.

In a two-month double-blind trial, eighty-five women who had undergone treatment for breast cancer received either the herb black cohosh or placebo. The results were not encouraging: Black cohosh did not reduce overall hot-flash symptoms. Four double-blind, placebo-controlled trials evaluated soy isoflavones as a treatment for hot flashes, but these also failed to find benefit.

A trial involving seventy-two women with breast cancer failed to find real acupuncture significantly more effective than sham acupuncture for treatment of hot flashes. A 2008 review of all existing studies on the subject concluded that the evidence does not support a beneficial effect for acupuncture in women with breast cancer who also have hot flashes. In a small randomized trial, hypnosis appeared to reduce hot flashes and improve mood and sleep among fifty-one breast cancer survivors.

Treating side effects caused by chemotherapy. In a small randomized trial of forty-three persons with breast cancer, six weeks of acupuncture twice weekly reduced joint pain attributed to aromatase-inhibitor therapy.

TREATING WEIGHT LOSS CAUSED BY CANCER OR CANCER TREATMENT

Cancer can cause a condition called tumor-induced weight loss, in which symptoms of starvation occur despite apparently adequate nutrition. The cause is thought to be a particular form of inflammation caused by the cancer. Cancer chemotherapy can also cause weight loss.

CANCER CURES

Numerous herbs, including bloodroot, burdock, cat's claw, flaxseed (based on lignan content), lapacho, maitake, noni, Oregon grape, pokeroot, red clover, and reishi, have been claimed effective for the treatment of cancer. However, there is no reliable evidence to indicate that these herbs actually help, and one, pokeroot, is actively toxic.

Various herbal combinations have also been promoted for the treatment of cancer, including the Hoxsey cancer cure, Essiac, and Jason Winter's cancer-cure tea. Again, however, there is no reliable evidence that they really work. Similarly, various dietary approaches that have been claimed to help treat cancer, such as macrobiotics and raw foods, lack meaningful supporting evidence.

HERBS AND SUPPLEMENTS TO USE ONLY WITH CAUTION

Various herbs and supplements may interact adversely with drugs used to treat cancer. It is strongly recommend that persons under treatment for cancer not use any herb or supplement except under a physician's supervision.

The herb St. John's wort interacts with many medications, including various chemotherapy drugs. The drug methotrexate causes the body to become deficient in folate. For this reason, people who take methotrexate for rheumatoid arthritis, juvenile rheumatoid arthritis, or psoriasis are sometimes advised to take folate supplements. Studies indicate that in those conditions, the use of folate does not impair the action of the drug. However, no studies have established that folate supplements are safe to take with methotrexate when it is used to treat cancer. The citrus bioflavonoid tangeretin may interact with the breast cancer drug tamoxifen. One highly preliminary study found that black cohosh might interfere with the action of the chemotherapy drug cisplatin.

The antioxidant controversy. Heated disagreement exists regarding whether it is safe or appropriate to combine antioxidants (such as vitamin E, vitamin C, and beta-carotene) with standard chemotherapy drugs. The reasoning behind the concern is that some chemotherapy drugs may work in part by creating free radicals that destroy cancer cells, and antioxidants might interfere with this beneficial effect.

There is little reliable evidence, though, that antioxidants interfere with chemotherapy drugs. Additionally, there is growing evidence that antioxidants may not cause harm and, in certain cases, may offer benefits. However, the effects are likely to vary with the specific situation (for example, type and stage of cancer and kind of treatment used), and there is far more research to be done. Therefore, it is strongly recommend that one not take antioxidants (or any other supplements) while undergoing cancer chemotherapy, except on the advice of a physician.

A similar situation exists regarding radiation therapy. One study found that the use of antioxidants decreased radiation therapy side effects but also may have decreased radiation therapy effectiveness. Another study found some evidence that people who both smoked cigarettes and used antioxidants while undergoing radiation therapy for head and neck cancer had increased risk of treatment failure compared to smokers who did not use antioxidants.

After reviewing much of the research on this controversial topic, one group of researchers published an article in the *Journal of the National Cancer Institute*, in which they conclude that antioxidants should be discouraged during either chemotherapy or radiation therapy because of their potential to reduce the effectiveness of these treatments.

Herbs that may increase breast cancer recurrence risk. Women who have had breast cancer are at high risk for a recurrence. The use of estrogen promotes the development of breast cancer, and for this reason it is "off limits." However, certain natural products may present a similar risk. Numerous herbs and supplements have estrogen-like properties, including alfalfa, genistein, hops, licorice, red clover, resveratrol, and soy. Contrary to popular belief, black cohosh is probably not estrogenic.

Other supplements, such as androstenedione and boron, may raise estrogen levels in the body. Finally, although the herbs dong quai and *P. ginseng* do not appear to act in an estrogen-like manner, they may nonetheless stimulate the growth of breast cancer cells. Women who have undergone breast cancer surgery should use these herbs and supplements only under the advice of a physician.

The weak estrogen estriol is sometimes advocated by alternative practitioners as a safer choice than standard estrogen. However, test-tube studies suggest that estriol is just as likely to cause breast cancer as any other form of estrogen.

EBSCO CAM Review Board

Further Reading

Billhult, A., I. Bergbom, and E. Stener-Victorin. "Massage Relieves Nausea in Women with Breast Cancer Who Are Undergoing Chemotherapy." *Journal of Alternative and Complementary Medicine* 13 (2007): 53-58.

Block, K. I., et al. "Impact of Antioxidant Supplementation on Chemotherapeutic Toxicity." *International Journal of Cancer* 123 (2008): 1227-1239.

Crew, K. D., et al. "Randomized, Blinded, Sham-Controlled Trial of Acupuncture for the Management of Aromatase Inhibitor-Associated Joint Symptoms in Women with Early-Stage Breast Cancer." *Journal of Clinical Oncology* 28 (2010): 1154-1160.

Elkins, G., et al. "Randomized Trial of a Hypnosis Intervention for Treatment of Hot Flashes Among Breast Cancer Survivors." *Journal of Clinical Oncology* 26 (2008): 5022-5026.

Horneber, M. A., et al. "Mistletoe Therapy in Oncology." *Cochrane Database of Systematic Reviews* (2008): CD003297. Available through *EBSCO DynaMed Systematic Literature Surveillance* at http://www.ebscohost.com/dynamed.

Huang, S. T., M. Good, and J. A. Zauszniewski. "The Effectiveness of Music in Relieving Pain in Cancer Patients." *International Journal of Nursing Studies* 47 (2010): 1354-1362.

Lee, M. S., T. Y. Choi, and E. Ernst. "Tai Chi for Breast Cancer Patients." *Breast Cancer Research and Treatment* 120 (2010): 309-316.

Oh, B., et al. "Impact of Medical Qigong on Quality of Life, Fatigue, Mood, and Inflammation in Cancer Patients." *Annals of Oncology* 21 (2010): 608-614.

Vaishampayan, U., et al. "Lycopene and Soy Isoflavones in the Treatment of Prostate Cancer." *Nutrition and Cancer* 59 (2007): 1-7.

Wilkinson, S., K. Barnes, and L. Storey. "Massage for Symptom Relief in Patients with Cancer." *Journal of Advanced Nursing* 63 (2008): 430-439.

Wilkinson, S., et al. "Effectiveness of Aromatherapy Massage in the Management of Anxiety and Depression in Patients with Cancer." *Journal of Clinical Oncology* 25 (2007): 532-539.

Zick, S. M., et al. "Phase II Trial of Encapsulated Ginger as a Treatment for Chemotherapy-Induced Nausea and Vomiting." *Supportive Care in Cancer* 17 (2009): 563-572.

See also: Cancer chemotherapy support: Homeopathic remedies; Cancer risk reduction; Doxorubicin; Pain management; Surgery support; Weight loss, undesired.

Candida/yeast hypersensitivity syndrome

Category: Condition

Related terms: Candidiasis hypersensitivity syndrome, chronic candida, yeast syndrome

Definition: Treatment of yeast infections of moist areas of the body.

Principal proposed natural treatments: None

Other proposed natural treatments: Barberry, betaine hydrochloride, caprylic acid, essential oils such as lavender oil, oregano oil, peppermint oil, and tea tree oil, garlic, grapefruit seed extract, lapacho, probiotics, red thyme

Introduction

Candida albicans is a naturally occurring yeast that flourishes in moist areas such as the digestive tract, the vagina, and skin folds. Ordinarily, its population is kept in check by bacteria that live in the same areas. When normal bacteria are disturbed by antibiotics, however, yeast populations can grow to abnormally high levels.

For women, the most common form of excess

Candida is a vaginal yeast infection, as marked by itchiness, redness, burning on urination, and a yeasty odor. *Candida* can also overpopulate in the mouth (as thrush), in the warm moist environment under a diaper (as diaper rash), and in other areas.

Candida usually confines itself to the surface of mucous membranes and does not penetrate deeply into the body. However, in people whose immune systems are severely compromised, such as those persons with acquired immunodeficiency syndrome or leukemia, *Candida* can become a dangerous, invasive organism. The medical name for this rare and dire condition is systemic candidiasis.

Besides this official meaning, "systemic candidiasis" has another meaning that was coined in the world of complementary and alternative medicine (CAM). "Systemic candidiasis," among CAM practitioners, is a loose term connoting a whole syndrome of symptoms related to *Candida* overgrowth. Equivalent terms are "chronic candida," "yeast syndrome," "yeast hypersensitivity syndrome," and simply "candida." Conventional medicine does not recognize these alternative terms as valid.

Yeast syndrome came to public awareness in 1983, when Orion Truss published *The Missing Diagnosis*. This was followed by William Crook's better-known *The Yeast Connection*. These books claim that a person who is chronically colonized by too much *Candida* may develop an allergy-like hypersensitivity to it. The symptoms of this allergy are said to be similar to those of other allergies, including sinus congestion, fatigue, intestinal gas, difficulty concentrating, depression, and muscle aches.

The regimen outlined by Crook consists of two parts: treatments toward diminishing the total body burden of *Candida* and less convincing recommendations that attempt to lessen allergic reactions toward yeast in general. For decreasing the amount of yeast in the body, Crook recommended avoiding certain substances, including antibiotics, corticosteroids, birth control pills, sugar, and most sweet foods. (He argued that dietary sugar "feeds yeast.") He also recommended the use of various supplements and even strong prescription drugs to directly kill yeast or, at minimum, interfere with its growth.

Next, Crook recommended avoiding foods containing yeast of any type, for he believed that those who are allergic to *Candida* will also be allergic to other members of the fungus family. Thus, Crook recommended avoiding fermented foods, such as beer, cheese, breads containing baker's yeast, tomato paste (which has a significant mold content), and even mushrooms.

Some evidence suggests that persons diagnosed with this condition do not in fact have excessive growth of *Candida* in the digestive tract. Nonetheless, one study suggests that antifungal treatment might provide some benefits, perhaps through effects on other yeasts. This four-week, double-blind, placebo-controlled study of 116 persons with symptoms believed to be characteristic of the yeast syndrome evaluated the effects of treatment with the antifungal drug nystatin. The results showed that treatment with nystatin modestly improved overall symptoms compared with placebo. In addition, some participants voluntarily undertook a sugar-free and yeast-free diet and reported even better results; how much of this latter effect was from the power of suggestion cannot be determined. A previous study of forty-two women failed to find benefit with nystatin, but the study design was somewhat convoluted.

PROPOSED NATURAL TREATMENTS

Many treatments can reduce the amount of yeast in the body, but it is not possible to eliminate *C. albicans* permanently. No matter how successful a treatment may be, as soon as it is stopped, *Candida* will return. (It is a natural inhabitant of the body.) However, it is known from other conditions, such as vaginal yeast infections, that sufficient intake of probiotics, or friendly bacteria, can help keep yeast regrowth within reasonable bounds. It is probably best to use a mixture of organisms, including acidophilus, bulgaricus, and bifidus.

Other agents that may reduce the amount of yeast in the body (especially the digestive tract) include caprylic acid, grapefruit seed extract, betaine hydrochloride, barberry, red thyme, pau d'arco (also called lapacho), and garlic. Various essential oils have also been proposed for this purpose, including peppermint oil, oregano oil, lavender oil, and tea tree oil. However, the scientific foundation for the use of any of these treatments in *Candida* infections is weak, and some may be toxic if taken to excess or for prolonged periods.

EBSCO CAM Review Board

FURTHER READING

Dismukes, W. E., et al. "A Randomized, Double-Blind Trial of Nystatin Therapy for the Candidiasis Hypersensitivity Syndrome." *New England Journal of Medicine* 323 (1990): 1717-1723.

National Candida Center. http://www.nationalcandida-center.com.

Quick Access Patient Information on Conditions, Herbs, and Supplements. New York: Thieme, 2000.

Santelmann, H., et al. "Effectiveness of Nystatin in Polysymptomatic Patients: A Randomized, Double-Blind Trial with Nystatin Versus Placebo in General Practice." *Family Practice* 18 (2001): 258-265.

See also: Probiotics; Vaginal infection; Women's health.

Candling

CATEGORY: Therapies and techniques

RELATED TERM: Coning

DEFINITION: The use of a hollow lighted candle to treat specific health conditions of the ear.

PRINCIPAL PROPOSED USE: Ear cleansing

OTHER PROPOSED USES: Meniere's disease, otitis media, sinus pressure and pain, tinnitus

OVERVIEW

The origins of candling are uncertain, but this ancient practice possibly started in Asia, Egypt, or the pre-Columbian Americas. Practitioners of candling (also called coning) use special candles made of linen or cotton soaked in wax or paraffin that are placed in the ear.

MECHANISM OF ACTION

A lit candle, hollow and about 10 inches long, is placed in the ear to create a low-level vacuum that sucks wax and other debris from the ear canal.

USES AND APPLICATIONS

Many claims are made about the effects of candling. Proponents believe that candling can treat ear-wax build-up and can cure the following conditions: tinnitus, otitis media, sinus pressure and pain, and Meniere's disease.

SCIENTIFIC EVIDENCE

There is no scientific evidence to support the claims that candling works. In addition, no plausible reasoning exists for how candling might work. Furthermore, each of the conditions that candling is claimed to cure occurs on the inner side of the eardrum and is, therefore, out of reach of candles. For other conditions closer to the site of candling, such as swimmer's ear or temporomandibular disorder, no evidence exists to show that candling is helpful. Many other health benefits associated with candling are vague or scientifically meaningless. Some examples are "strengthen the brain," "purify the mind," "stabilize emotions," "clear the eyes," "purify the blood," and "release blocked energy."

Using candling to treat ear wax build-up also has been criticized. According to one group of researchers, the negative pressure needed to pull sticky wax from the ear canal would have to be so powerful that it would rupture the eardrum during the process. After actually measuring the pressure during candling, the researchers found that no negative pressure was created. In any case, there are much safer and easier ways to remove wax.

SAFETY ISSUES

Many doctors have concerns about the safety of ear candling. Twenty-one of 122 ear, nose, and throat specialists who took part in a survey had seen patients who were harmed by ear candling. Of these patients, thirteen had external burns, seven had ear canal obstruction from candle wax, and one had a ruptured eardrum.

The U.S. Food and Drug Administration (FDA) considers the ear candle an unregulated medical device and has taken action to prevent the sale and distribution of ear candles in the United States. The FDA also has warned consumers about the risk of serious injury from candling. Despite these actions, ear candles are still widely available at health food stores and online.

According to the American Academy of Otolaryngology, earwax is healthy in normal amounts and serves to coat the skin of the ear canal, where it acts as a temporary water repellent. The absence of earwax may result in dry, itchy ears.

Amy Scholten, M.P.H.;
reviewed by Brian Randall, M.D.

FURTHER READING

American Academy of Otolaryngology–Head and Neck Surgery. http://www.entnet.org.

Canadian Society of Otolaryngology. http://www.csohns.com.

Seely, D. R., S. M. Quigley, and A. W. Langman. "Ear Candles: Efficacy and Safety." *Laryngoscope* 106 (1996): 1226-1229.

U.S. Food and Drug Administration. "Ear Candles: Risk of Serious Injuries." Available at http://www.fda.gov.

See also: Cupping; Ear infections; Hearing loss; Home health; Hydrotherapy; Swimmer's ear.

Candytuft

CATEGORY: Herbs and supplements
RELATED TERMS: Clown's mustard, *Iberis amara*
DEFINITION: Natural plant product used to treat specific health conditions.
PRINCIPAL PROPOSED USE: Dyspepsia (in herbal combinations)
OTHER PROPOSED USES: Gastrointestinal side effects caused by medications, irritable bowel syndrome

OVERVIEW

Candytuft, also known as clown's mustard, is a white flowering plant found originally in Spain. It is a member of the Brassicaceae family, making it a relative of cabbage and broccoli. Traditionally, it was used in the treatment of arthritis, gout, enlarged heart, and asthma. The seeds, stems, roots, and leaves have all been used medicinally.

THERAPEUTIC DOSAGES

A typical dosage of the tested candytuft preparation is twenty drops three times daily.

THERAPEUTIC USES

Candytuft is widely used in Germany for treatment of dyspepsia. This term indicates chronic digestive distress that occurs in the absence of any identifiable cause, such as an ulcer. Symptoms include stomach discomfort, gas, bloating, belching, appetite loss, and nausea.

Several studies, enrolling a total of more than six hundred participants, have found benefits for dyspepsia with use of a proprietary herbal combination therapy containing candytuft as the primary ingredient. Besides dyspepsia, candytuft combinations have shown potential for decreasing the gastrointestinal side effects caused by a variety of medications and for reducing lower digestive tract symptoms of irritable bowel syndrome.

The product tested in these studies has undergone change over time. The original version included, along with candytuft, matricaria flower (chamomile), peppermint leaves, caraway, licorice root, and lemon balm. Subsequently, an augmented preparation was tested that utilized, in addition to the above, a mixture of angelica root, celandine, and milk thistle. This second preparation later became the one used by the manufacturer in lieu of the original.

SCIENTIFIC EVIDENCE

An eight-week double-blind study of 315 people with functional dyspepsia tested the newer candytuft product and found it significantly more effective than a placebo. This was a high-quality study with adequate design and reporting, and its results provide a strong indication that the treatment actually works.

An earlier double-blind, placebo-controlled trial of 120 people with dyspepsia evaluated the original candytuft combination. The design of this study was excessively complicated, but in essence it found that four weeks of treatment with the product was more effective than a placebo in reducing dyspepsia symptoms.

In another double-blind study, this one enrolling sixty people with dyspepsia, use of either the original or the newer candytuft herbal combination proved more effective than a placebo. Benefits with the original mixture were also seen in two other double-blind, placebo-controlled studies enrolling a total of about two hundred people. In addition, a double-blind, comparative study found that both candytuft combinations and the standard drug cisapride were equally effective.

SAFETY ISSUES

In controlled clinical trials, use of the tested candytuft preparation has not resulted in any significant side effects. The studied preparation is manufactured in Germany under conditions that are more closely regulated than herbal manufacturing in the United

Candytuft and Dyspepsia

"Dyspepsia" is a catchall term that includes a variety of digestive problems such as stomach discomfort, gas, bloating, belching, appetite loss, and nausea. Although many serious medical conditions can cause similar symptoms, the term "dyspepsia" is used in those cases when no other identifiable medical cause can be determined.

Because dyspepsia has, by definition, no known medical cause, there is no apparent way to develop medical treatments to address it. Many people with dyspepsia simply experiment with medications or with alterations to their diet. However, substantial double-blind, placebo-controlled studies suggest that a proprietary herbal combination may provide benefit. Sold under the trade name Iberogast, this preparation consists primarily of candytuft, along with chamomile, peppermint leaves, caraway, licorice root, lemon balm, angelica root, celandine, and milk thistle.

A double-blind study published in 2007 enrolled 315 people with dyspepsia. Researchers evaluated the severity of the condition through the use of a standardized questionnaire, the Gastrointestinal Symptom Score (GIS) scale. Participants received either placebo or Iberogast at a dose of twenty drops three times daily. In the eight-week study period, participants given Iberogast showed significantly greater improvement in GIS scores than those given placebo.

Several earlier double-blind studies, enrolling a total of about three hundred people, also had shown benefit. However, many of these studies used an earlier type of Iberogast that lacked some of the herbs used in the product used today.

Steven Bratman, M.D.

States. Formulations made outside Germany might present unrecognized safety risks. Even with the tested product, comprehensive safety studies have not been performed. Safety for pregnant or nursing women, young children, and individuals with severe liver or kidney disease has not been established.

EBSCO CAM Review Board

FURTHER READING

Gundermann, K. J., E. Godehardt, and M. Ulbrich. "Efficacy of a Herbal Preparation in Patients with Functional Dyspepsia." *Advances in Therapy* 20 (2003): 43-49.

Madisch, A., et al. "A Plant Extract and Its Modified Preparation in Functional Dyspepsia." *Zeitschrift fur Gastroenterologie* 39 (2001): 511-517.

_____. "Treatment of Functional Dyspepsia with a Herbal Preparation." *Digestion* 69, no. 1 (2004): 45-52.

Melzer, J., et al. "*Iberis amara* L. and Iberogast: Results of a Systematic Review Concerning Functional Dyspepsia." *Journal of Herbal Pharmacotherapy* 4 (2005): 51-59.

Rosch, W., B. Vinson, and I. Sassin. "A Randomized Clinical Trial Comparing the Efficacy of a Herbal Preparation STW 5 with the Prokinetic Drug Cisapride in Patients with Dysmotility Type of Functional Dyspepesia." *Zeitschrift fur Gastroenterologie* 40 (2002): 401-408.

Von Arnim, U., et al. "STW 5, a Phytopharmacon for Patients with Functional Dyspepsia." *American Journal of Gastroenterology* 102 (2007): 1268-1275.

See also: Caraway; Dyspepsia; Herbal medicine; Lemon balm; Licorice; Peppermint.

Canker sores

CATEGORY: Condition
RELATED TERM: Aphthous stomatitis
DEFINITION: Treatment of mouth ulcers or sores.
PRINCIPAL PROPOSED NATURAL TREATMENTS: None
OTHER PROPOSED NATURAL TREATMENTS: Acidophilus, calendula, caraway, deglycyrrhizinated licorice, lactic acid, oak bark, *Rhizophora mangle* (red mangrove), slippery elm, vitamin B$_1$, witch hazel

INTRODUCTION

Canker sores are small ulcers in the mouth caused by an assortment of viruses. A susceptibility to canker sores tends to run in families. No successful conventional treatment is available.

PROPOSED NATURAL TREATMENTS

A preliminary study suggests that a chemically altered form of the herb licorice known as deglycyrrhizinated licorice may be useful for speeding the resolution of canker sores. In a second, better-designed trial employing a dissolving adhesive patch with glycyrrhiza root extract, researchers noted an improvement in ulcer size and pain compared with the use of a placebo patch.

A product containing vitamins and minerals and the herbs paprika, rosemary, peppermint, milfoil, hawthorn, and pumpkin seed has been used in Scandinavia for many years as a treatment for various mouth-related conditions. A small six-month study reported that the use of this product could reduce frequency of canker sores. However, two subsequent studies failed to find any meaningful benefit. One small double-blind study found benefits with an extract of the bark of the red mangrove tree, *Rhizophora mangle*.

A study performed in Iraq reported benefits through the use of a mouthwash containing 5 percent lactic acid. Other herbs and supplements sometimes recommended for canker sores but lacking supporting evidence include caraway, oak bark, witch hazel, acidophilus, calendula, slippery elm, and vitamin B_1. Another study failed to find that alpha-linolenic acid from perilla oil reduced the incidence of canker sores.

EBSCO CAM Review Board

FURTHER READING

Brateli, J., et al. "The Effect of LongoVital on Recurrent Aphthous Stomatitis in a Controlled Clinical Trial." *Oral Health and Preventive Dentistry* 3 (2005): 3-8.

De Armas, E., et al. "Efficacy of *Rhizophora mangle* Aqueous Bark Extract (RMABE) in the Treatment of Aphthous Ulcers." *Current Medical Research and Opinion* 21 (2005): 1711-1715.

Hamazaki, K., et al. "Effects of Cooking Plant Oils on Recurrent Aphthous Stomatitis." *Nutrition* 22 (2006): 534-538.

Kolseth, I., et al. "Norwegian LongoVital and Recurrent Aphthous Ulceration." *Oral Diseases* 11 (2005): 374-378.

Martin, M. D., et al. "A Controlled Trial of a Dissolving Oral Patch Concerning Glycyrrhiza (Licorice) Herbal Extract for the Treatment of Aphthous Ulcers." *General Dentistry* 56 (2008): 206-210.

Sharquie, K. E., et al. "Lactic Acid 5 Percent Mouthwash Is an Effective Mode of Therapy in Treatment of Recurrent Aphthous Ulcerations." *Dermatology Online Journal* 12 (2006): 2.

See also: Burning mouth syndrome; Herpes; Leukoplakia; Witch hazel.

Caraway

CATEGORY: Herbs and supplements
RELATED TERM: *Carum carvi*
DEFINITION: Natural plant product used to treat specific health conditions.
PRINCIPAL PROPOSED USES: Dyspepsia (nonspecific indigestion), intestinal gas
OTHER PROPOSED USES: Irritable bowel syndrome, canker sores, periodontal disease

OVERVIEW

Caraway has a long history of use as a "carminative," an herb said to relieve gas pain. Mentions of caraway for digestive problems can be found in Egyptian records, and the herb has been used in Europe for this purpose since at least the Middle Ages. The seeds, in the form of their essential oil, are the part of the plant used medicinally.

THERAPEUTIC DOSAGES

A typical dose of caraway is 0.05 to 0.2 milliliters of the essential oil taken three times daily.

THERAPEUTIC USES

Only double-blind, placebo-controlled studies can prove a treatment effective, and thus far such studies have not been performed on caraway alone. However, a few double-blind studies have been reported on combination products containing caraway oil for the treatment of dyspepsia (nonspecific stomach distress).

For example, a double-blind, placebo-controlled study of thirty-nine people found that an enteric-coated peppermint oil and caraway oil combination taken three times daily by mouth for four weeks significantly reduced dyspepsia pain compared with a placebo. Of the treatment group, 63.2 percent of participants were painfree after four weeks, compared with 25 percent of the placebo group. In other double-blind, placebo-controlled studies, a combination of caraway, bitter candytuft, feverfew, peppermint leaves, licorice root, and lemon balm also proved effective for dyspepsia.

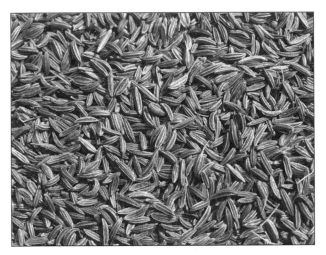

Caraway seeds, or their essential oil, are used medicinally. (©Petr Pokorny/Dreamstime.com)

Double-blind comparative studies have also been reported. One such study of 118 people found that the combination of peppermint and caraway oil was about as effective as the standard drug cisapride (a drug used for dyspepsia that is no longer available). After four weeks, the herbal combination reduced dyspepsia pain by 69.7 percent, whereas the conventional treatment reduced pain by 70.2 percent. Finally, a preparation of peppermint, caraway, fennel, and wormwood oil was compared with the drug metoclopramide in a double-blind study enrolling 60 people. After seven days, 43.3 percent of the treatment group was painfree, compared with 13.3 percent of the metoclopramide group.

Far weaker evidence hints that caraway extracts may have anticancer, antibacterial, and antidiabetic actions. However, the evidence for these potential benefits is far too weak to rely on.

Caraway oil is said to be helpful for irritable bowel syndrome. Teas made from caraway are recommend for periodontal disease and canker sores. However, there is no meaningful supporting evidence for any of these uses.

SAFETY ISSUES

Caraway is generally regarded as safe when used in recommended doses. However, essential oils can be toxic to very young children, and excessive doses could be dangerous for adults as well. Maximum safe dosages in young children, pregnant or nursing women, and people with severe liver or kidney disease have not been established.

EBSCO CAM Review Board

FURTHER READING

Gundermann, K. J., E. Godehardt, and M. Ulbrich. "Efficacy of a Herbal Preparation in Patients with Functional Dyspepsia." *Advances in Therapy* 20 (2003): 43-49.

Iacobellis, N. S., et al. "Antibacterial Activity of *Cuminum cyminum* L. and *Carum carvi* L. Essential Oils." *Journal of Agricultural and Food Chemistry* 53 (2005): 57-61.

Madisch, A., et al. "Treatment of Functional Dyspepsia with a Herbal Preparation." *Digestion* 69, no. 1 (2004): 45-52.

Singh, G., et al. "Studies on Essential Oils: Part 10–Antibacterial Activity of Volatile Oils of Some Spices." *Phytotherapy Research* 16 (2002): 680-682.

See also: Candytuft; Dyspepsia; Feverfew; Herbal medicine; Lemon balm; Licorice; Peppermint.

Carbamazepine

CATEGORY: Drug interactions

DEFINITION: An anticonvulsant agent used primarily to prevent seizures in conditions such as epilepsy.

INTERACTIONS: Biotin, calcium, carnitine, dong quai, folate, ginkgo, glutamine, grapefruit juice, hops, ipriflavone, kava, nicotinamide, passionflower, St. John's wort, valerian, vitamin D, vitamin K

TRADE NAMES: Atretol, Carbatrol, Epitol, Tegretol, Tegretol XR

DRUGS IN THIS FAMILY: Phenobarbital, phenytoin, primidone, valproic acid

GINKGO

Effect: Possible Harmful Interaction

The herb ginkgo (*Ginkgo biloba*) has been used to treat Alzheimer's disease and ordinary age-related memory loss, among many other conditions. This interaction involves potential contaminants in ginkgo, not ginkgo itself.

A recent study found that a natural nerve toxin present in the seeds of *Ginkgo biloba* made its way into standardized ginkgo extracts prepared from the

Drug Reactions

Medicines are helpful, most of the time. They reduce aches and pains, fight infections, and control problems such as seizures, high blood pressure, and diabetes. However, medicines can also cause unwanted physical reactions.

For example, interactions between a drug such as the anticonvulsant agent carbamazepine and the herbal supplement *Ginkgo biloba* can change the actions of one or both substances. The products might not work, or they could cause side effects, some of which can be serious. Persons starting a new prescription or over-the-counter medication should be sure to understand the proper way to take that medication and to know what other medications, dietary supplements, and foods to avoid.

leaves. This toxin has been associated with convulsions and death in laboratory animals.

The detected amounts of this toxic substance are considered harmless. However, given the lack of satisfactory standardization of herbal formulations in the United States, it is possible that some batches of product might contain greater amounts of the toxin depending on the season of harvest. In light of these findings, taking a ginkgo product that happened to contain significant levels of the nerve toxin might theoretically prevent an anticonvulsant from working as well as expected.

GLUTAMINE
Effect: Possible Harmful Interaction

The amino acid glutamine is converted to glutamate in the body. Glutamate is thought to act as a neurotransmitter (chemical that enables nerve transmission). Because anticonvulsants work (at least in part) by blocking glutamate pathways in the brain, high dosages of the amino acid glutamine might theoretically diminish an anticonvulsant's effect and increase the risk of seizures.

GRAPEFRUIT JUICE
Effect: Possible Harmful Interaction

Grapefruit juice slows the body's normal breakdown of several drugs, including the anticonvulsant carbamazepine, allowing it to build up to potentially dangerous levels in the blood. A recent study indicates this effect can last for three days or more following the last glass of juice. Because of this risk, if one uses carbamazepine, the safest approach is to avoid grapefruit juice altogether.

IPRIFLAVONE
Effect: Possible Harmful Interaction

Ipriflavone, a synthetic isoflavone that slows bone breakdown, is used to treat osteoporosis. Test-tube studies indicate that ipriflavone might increase blood levels of the anticonvulsants carbamazepine and phenytoin when they are taken therapeutically. Ipriflavone was found to inhibit a liver enzyme involved in the body's normal breakdown of these drugs, thus allowing them to build up in the blood. Higher drug levels increase the risk of adverse effects.

Because anticonvulsants are known to contribute to the development of osteoporosis, a concern is that the use of ipriflavone for this drug-induced osteoporosis could result in higher blood levels of the drugs with potentially serious consequences. Persons taking either of these drugs should use ipriflavone only under medical supervision.

HOPS, KAVA, PASSIONFLOWER, VALERIAN
Effect: Possible Harmful Interaction

The herb kava (*Piper methysticum*) has a sedative effect and is used for anxiety and insomnia. Combining kava with anticonvulsants, which possess similar depressant effects, could result in "add-on" or excessive physical depression, sedation, and impairment. In one case report, a fifty-four-year-old man was hospitalized for lethargy and disorientation, side effects attributed to his having taken the combination of kava and the anti-anxiety agent alprazolam (Xanax) for three days.

Other herbs having a sedative effect that might cause problems when combined with anticonvulsants include ashwagandha (*Withania somnifera*), calendula (*Calendula officinalis*), catnip (*Nepeta cataria*), hops (*Humulus lupulus*), lady's slipper (*Cypripedium* species), lemon balm (*Melissa officinalis*), passionflower (*Passiflora incarnata*), sassafras (*Sassafras officinale*), skullcap (*Scutellaria lateriflora*), valerian (*Valeriana officinalis*), and yerba mansa (*Anemopsis californica*). Because of the potentially serious consequences, one should avoid combining these herbs with anticonvulsants or other drugs that also have sedative or depressant effects, unless advised by a physician.

NICOTINAMIDE

Effect: Possible Harmful Interaction

Nicotinamide (also called niacinamide) is a compound produced by the body's breakdown of niacin (vitamin B$_3$). It is a supplemental form that does not possess the flushing side effect or the cholesterol-lowering ability of niacin. Nicotinamide appears to increase blood levels of carbamazepine and primidone, possibly requiring a reduction in drug dosage to prevent toxic effects.

Carbamazepine blood levels increased in two children with epilepsy after they were given nicotinamide, but the fact that the children were on several anticonvulsant drugs clouds the issue somewhat. Similarly, nicotinamide given to three children on primidone therapy increased blood levels of primidone. It is thought that nicotinamide may interfere with the body's normal breakdown of these anticonvulsant agents, allowing them to build up in the blood.

DONG QUAI, ST. JOHN'S WORT

Effect: Possible Harmful Interaction

St. John's wort (*Hypericum perforatum*) is primarily used to treat mild to moderate depression. The herb dong quai (*Angelica sinensis*) is often recommended for menstrual disorders such as dysmenorrhea, premenstrual syndrome (PMS), and irregular menstruation.

The anticonvulsant agents carbamazepine, phenobarbital, and valproic acid have been reported to cause increased sensitivity to the sun, amplifying the risk of sunburn or skin rash. Because St. John's wort and dong quai may also cause this problem, taking them during treatment with these drugs might add to this risk.

It may be a good idea to use sunscreen or wear protective clothing during sun exposure if one takes one of these herbs while using these anticonvulsants.

BIOTIN

Effect: Supplementation Possibly Helpful, but Take at a Different Time of Day

Anticonvulsants may deplete biotin, an essential water-soluble B vitamin, possibly by competing with it for absorption in the intestine. It is not clear, however, whether this effect is great enough to be harmful.

Blood levels of biotin were found to be substantially lower in 404 people with epilepsy on long-term treatment with anticonvulsants compared with 112

untreated people with epilepsy. The effect occurred with phenytoin, carbamazepine, phenobarbital, and primidone. Valproic acid appears to affect biotin to a lesser extent than other anticonvulsants. A test-tube study suggested that anticonvulsants might lower biotin levels by interfering with the way biotin is transported in the intestine.

Biotin supplementation may be beneficial if one is on long-term anticonvulsant therapy. To avoid a potential interaction, one should take the supplement two to three hours apart from the drug. It has been suggested that the action of anticonvulsant drugs may be at least partly related to their effect of reducing biotin levels. For this reason, it may be desirable to take enough biotin to prevent a deficiency, but not an excessive amount.

FOLATE

Effect: Supplementation Possibly Helpful

Folate (also known as folic acid) is a B vitamin that plays an important role in many vital aspects of health. Carbamazepine appears to lower blood levels of folate by speeding up its normal breakdown by the body and also by decreasing its absorption. Other antiseizure drugs can also reduce levels of folate in the body.

Low folate can lead to anemia and reduced white blood cell count, and folate supplements have been shown to help prevent these complications of carbamazepine treatment.

Adequate folate intake is also necessary to prevent neural tube birth defects, such as spina bifida and anencephaly. Because anticonvulsant drugs deplete folate, babies born to women taking anticonvulsants are at increased risk for such birth defects. Anticonvulsants may also play a more direct role in the development of birth defects.

The low serum folate caused by anticonvulsants can raise homocysteine levels, a condition hypothesized to increase the risk of heart disease. However, the case for taking extra folate during anticonvulsant therapy is not as simple as it might seem. It is possible that folate supplementation itself might impair the effectiveness of anticonvulsant drugs, and physician supervision is necessary.

CALCIUM

Effect: Supplementation Probably Helpful, but Take at a Different Time of Day

Anticonvulsant drugs may impair calcium absorption

and, in this way, increase the risk of osteoporosis and other bone disorders. Calcium absorption was compared in twelve people on anticonvulsant therapy (all taking phenytoin and some also taking carbamazepine, phenobarbital, and/or primidone) and twelve people who received no treatment. Calcium absorption was found to be 27 percent lower in the treated participants.

An observational study found low calcium blood levels in 48 percent of 109 people taking anticonvulsants. Other findings in this study suggested that anticonvulsants might also reduce calcium levels by directly interfering with parathyroid hormone, a substance that helps keep calcium levels in proper balance. A low blood level of calcium can itself trigger seizures, and this might reduce the effectiveness of anticonvulsants.

Calcium supplementation may be beneficial for people taking anticonvulsant drugs. However, some studies indicate that antacids containing calcium carbonate may interfere with the absorption of phenytoin and perhaps other anticonvulsants. For this reason, one should take calcium supplements and anticonvulsant drugs several hours apart if possible.

CARNITINE

Effect: Supplementation Possibly Helpful

Carnitine is an amino acid that has been used for heart conditions, Alzheimer's disease, and intermittent claudication. Intermittent claudication is a possible complication of atherosclerosis, in which impaired blood circulation causes severe pain in calf muscles during walking or exercising.

Long-term therapy with anticonvulsant agents, particularly valproic acid, is associated with low levels of carnitine. However, it is not clear whether the anticonvulsants cause the carnitine deficiency or whether it occurs for other reasons. It has been hypothesized that low carnitine levels may contribute to valproic acid's damaging effects on the liver. The risk of this liver damage increases in children younger than twenty-four months, and carnitine supplementation may be protective. However, in one double-blind crossover study, carnitine supplementation produced no real improvement in well-being as assessed by parents of children receiving either valproic acid or carbamazepine.

L-carnitine supplementation may be advisable in certain cases, such as in infants and young children (especially those younger than two years) who have

neurologic disorders and are receiving valproic acid and multiple anticonvulsants.

VITAMIN D

Effect: Supplementation Possibly Helpful

Anticonvulsant drugs may interfere with the activity of vitamin D. As proper handling of calcium by the body depends on vitamin D, this may be another way that these drugs increase the risk of osteoporosis and related bone disorders.

Anticonvulsants appear to speed up the body's normal breakdown of vitamin D, decreasing the amount of the vitamin in the blood. A survey of forty-eight people taking both phenytoin and phenobarbital found significantly lower levels of calcium and vitamin D in many of them compared with thirty-eight untreated persons. Similar but lesser changes were seen in thirteen people taking phenytoin or phenobarbital alone. This effect may be apparent only after several weeks of treatment.

Another study found decreased blood levels of one form of vitamin D but normal levels of another. Because there are multiple forms of vitamin D circulating in the blood, the body might be able to adjust in some cases to keep vitamin D in balance, at least for a time, despite the influence of anticonvulsants.

Adequate sunlight exposure may help overcome the effects of anticonvulsants on vitamin D by stimulating the skin to manufacture the vitamin. Of 450 people on anticonvulsants residing in a Florida facility, none was found to have low blood levels of vitamin D or evidence of bone disease. This suggests that environments providing regular sun exposure may be protective. Persons regularly taking anticonvulsants, especially those taking combination therapy and those with limited exposure to sunlight, may benefit from vitamin D supplementation.

VITAMIN K

Effect: Supplementation Possibly Helpful for Pregnant Women

Phenytoin, carbamazepine, phenobarbital, and primidone speed up the normal breakdown of vitamin K into inactive byproducts, thus depriving the body of active vitamin K. This can lead to bone problems, such as osteoporosis. In addition, use of these anticonvulsants can lead to a vitamin K deficiency in babies born to mothers taking the drugs, resulting in bleeding disorders or facial bone abnormalities in the newborns. Mothers who take these anticonvulsants may need vitamin K supplementation during pregnancy to prevent these conditions in their newborns.

EBSCO CAM Review Board

Further Reading

Asadi-Pooya, A. A., and E. Ghetmiri. "Folic Acid Supplementation Reduces the Development Abnormalities in Children Receiving Carbamazepine." *Epilepsy and Behavior* 8 (2006): 228-231.

De Vivo, D. C., et al. "L-carnitine Supplementation in Childhood Epilepsy." *Epilepsia* 39 (1998): 1216-1225.

Kishi, T., et al. "Mechanism for Reduction of Serum Folate by Antiepileptic Drugs During Prolonged Therapy." *Journal of the Neurological Sciences* 145 (1997): 109-112.

Lewis, D. P., et al. "Drug and Environmental Factors Associated with Adverse Pregnancy Outcomes: Part 1–Antiepileptic Drugs, Contraceptives, Smoking, and Folate." *Annals of Pharmacotherapy* 32 (1998): 802-817.

Ono, H., et al. "Plasma Total Homocysteine Concentrations in Epileptic Patients Taking Anticonvulsants." *Metabolism* 46 (1997): 959-962.

Takanaga, H., et al. "Relationship Between Time After Intake of Grapefruit Juice and the Effect on Pharmacokinetics and Pharmacodynamics of Nisoldipine in Healthy Subjects." *Clinical Pharmacology and Therapeutics* 67 (2000): 201-214.

See also: Biotin; Calcium; Carnitine; Dong quai; Food and Drug Administration; Folate; Ginkgo; Glutamine; Hops; Ipriflavone; Kava; Nicotinamide; Passionflower; St. John's wort; Supplements: Introduction; Valerian; Vitamin D; Vitamin K.

Cardiomyopathy

Category: Condition

Related terms: Arrhythmogenic right ventricular cardiomyopathy, dilated cardiomyopathy, hypertrophic cardiomyopathy, idiopathic dilated cardiomyopathy, idiopathic hypertrophic cardiomyopathy, idiopathic restrictive cardiomyopathy, restrictive cardiomyopathy

Definition: Treatment of the diseased muscle tissue of the heart.

Principal proposed natural treatments: None
Other proposed natural treatments: Carnitine, coenzyme Q_{10}

Introduction

Cardiomyopathy is a little-understood condition in which the muscle tissue of the heart becomes diseased. There are several distinct forms of cardiomyopathy that may or may not be similar in origin. Medical treatment consists mainly of medications that attempt to compensate for the increasing failure of the heart to function properly. A heart transplant may ultimately be necessary.

Proposed Natural Treatments

Coenzyme Q_{10}. Preliminary evidence suggests that the naturally occurring substance coenzyme Q_{10} (CoQ_{10}) might offer benefit in some forms of cardiomyopathy. In a six-year trial, 143 people with moderately severe cardiomyopathy were given CoQ_{10} daily in addition to standard medical care. The results showed a significant improvement in cardiac function (technically, ejection fraction) in 84 percent of the study participants. Most of them improved by several stages on a scale that measures the severity of heart failure (technically, as classified by the New York Heart Association). Furthermore, a comparison with persons on conventional therapy alone appeared to show a reduction in mortality.

This study was an open trial, meaning that participants knew that they were being treated, and such studies are not fully reliable. There have been a few double-blind, placebo-controlled trials of CoQ_{10} in cardiomyopathy too. One such trial followed eighty people with various forms of cardiomyopathy for three years. Of those treated with CoQ_{10}, 89 percent improved significantly, but when the treatment was stopped, their heart function deteriorated. No benefit was seen in another double-blind study, but it was a smaller and shorter trial and enrolled only people who had one particular type of cardiomyopathy (idiopathic dilated cardiomyopathy).

Carnitine. A small amount of evidence indicates that the vitamin-like supplement carnitine may be useful in cardiomyopathy.

Herbs and Supplements to Use Only with Caution

Various herbs and supplements may interact

adversely with drugs used to treat cardiomyopathy, so one should be cautious when considering the use of herbs and supplements.

EBSCO CAM Review Board

FURTHER READING

Langsjoen, H., et al. "Usefulness of Coenzyme Q10 in Clinical Cardiology." *Molecular Aspects of Medicine* 15, suppl. (1994): S165-S175.

Nodari, S., et al. "The Role of N-3 PUFAs in Preventing the Arrhythmic Risk in Patients with Idiopathic Dilated Cardiomyopathy." *Cardiovascular Drugs and Therapy* 23 (2008): 5-15.

Pepine, C. J. "The Therapeutic Potential of Carnitine in Cardiovascular Disorders." *Clinical Therapeutics* 13 (1991): 2-21.

Winter, S., et al. "The Role of L-carnitine in Pediatric Cardiomyopathy." *Journal of Child Neurology* 10, suppl. 2 (1995): S45-S51.

See also: Angina; Arrhythmia; Atherosclerosis and heart disease prevention; Carnitine; Coenzyme Q_{10}; Congestive heart failure; Heart attack.

Carnitine

CATEGORY: Herbs and supplements

RELATED TERMS: Acetyl-L-carnitine, L-acetyl-carnitine, L-carnitine, propionyl-L-carnitine

DEFINITION: Natural substance promoted as a dietary supplement for specific health benefits.

PRINCIPAL PROPOSED USES: Angina, chronic obstructive pulmonary disease, congestive heart failure, diabetic peripheral neuropathy, heart attack, hyperthyroidism, intermittent claudication, male infertility, male sexual dysfunction, Peyronie's disease

OTHER PROPOSED USES: Alzheimer's disease, attention deficit disorder, celiac disease, chronic fatigue syndrome, depression, diabetes, diabetic cardiac autonomic neuropathy, enhancing mental function in the elderly, fibromyalgia, high cholesterol, human immunodeficiency virus infection, hyperactivity in fragile X syndrome, liver cirrhosis, sports performance, weight loss

OVERVIEW

Carnitine is a substance used by the body to turn fat into energy. It is not normally considered an essential nutrient because the body can manufacture all it needs. However, supplemental carnitine could in theory improve the ability of certain tissues to produce energy. This has led to the use of carnitine for various muscle diseases and heart conditions.

REQUIREMENTS AND SOURCES

There is no dietary requirement for carnitine. However, some people have a genetic defect that hinders the body's ability to make carnitine. In addition, diseases of the liver, kidneys, or brain may inhibit carnitine production. Certain medications, especially the antiseizure drugs valproic acid (Depakene) and phenytoin (Dilantin), may reduce carnitine levels; however, whether taking extra carnitine would be helpful has not been determined. Heart muscle tissue, because of its high energy requirements, is particularly vulnerable to carnitine deficiency.

The principal dietary sources of carnitine are meat and dairy products. To obtain therapeutic dosages, however, a supplement is necessary.

THERAPEUTIC DOSAGES

Typical adult dosages for the diseases described here range from 500 to 1,000 milligrams (mg) three times daily. For children, one study used 50 mg per kilogram twice daily, up to a maximum of 4 grams daily.

Carnitine is taken in three forms: L-carnitine (for heart and other conditions), propionyl-L-carnitine (for heart conditions), and acetyl-L-carnitine (for Alzheimer's disease). The dosage is the same for all three forms.

THERAPEUTIC USES

Carnitine is primarily used for heart-related conditions. Some evidence suggests that it can be used along with conventional treatment for angina to improve symptoms and reduce medication needs. When combined with conventional therapy, it may or may not help prevent medical complications or sudden cardiac death in the months following a heart attack.

Lesser evidence suggests that it may be helpful for a condition called intermittent claudication (pain in the legs after walking due to narrowing of the arteries) and for congestive heart failure. In addition, a few studies suggest that carnitine may be useful for cardiomyopathy.

Carnitine may also be helpful for improving

Carnitine for Athletic Performance

Some athletes take carnitine to improve their performance. However, more than twenty years of research finds no consistent evidence that carnitine supplements can improve exercise or physical performance in healthy persons—at doses ranging from 2 to 6 grams per day, administered for one to twenty-eight days. (The total body content of carnitine is about 20 grams in a man weighing 155 pounds, almost all of it in the skeletal muscle.) For example, carnitine supplements do not appear to increase the body's use of oxygen or improve metabolic status when exercising. Furthermore, carnitine supplements do not necessarily increase the amount of carnitine in muscle. Excess carnitine is excreted in the urine.

exercise tolerance in people with chronic obstructive pulmonary disease (COPD), also known as emphysema. One should not attempt to self-treat any of the foregoing serious medical conditions or use carnitine as a substitute for standard drugs.

Growing, if not entirely consistent, evidence suggests that L-carnitine or acetyl-L-carnitine, or their combination, may be helpful for improving sperm function and thereby provide benefits in male infertility. Two studies found evidence that carnitine is helpful for Peyronie's disease, a condition affecting the penis.

Carnitine has also shown promise for improving mental and physical fatigue in the elderly. Some studies have found evidence that one particular form of carnitine, acetyl-L-carnitine, might be helpful in Alzheimer's disease, but the two most recent and largest studies found no benefit. One review evaluated published and unpublished double-blind, placebo-controlled trials and concluded that acetyl-L-carnitine may only be helpful for very mild Alzheimer's disease.

In preliminary trials, acetyl-L-carnitine has shown some promise for the treatment of depression or dysthymia (a milder condition related to depression). Some evidence suggests that carnitine may be useful for improving blood sugar control in people with type 2 diabetes. Better evidence suggests benefit with acetyl-L-carnitine for a major complication of diabetes, diabetic peripheral neuropathy (injury to nerves of the extremities caused by diabetes). Acetyl-L-carnitine might help prevent diabetic cardiac autonomic neu-

ropathy (injury to the nerves of the heart caused by diabetes). However, one study found that carnitine supplements had an adverse effect on triglyceride levels in people with diabetes.

Much weaker evidence suggests possible benefits for neuropathy caused by the chemotherapy drugs cisplatin and paclitaxel. Weak evidence hints that carnitine might help reduce liver and heart toxicity caused by the chemotherapy drug adriamycin.

Some evidence suggests that carnitine may be able to improve cholesterol profile. One small study demonstrated a beneficial effect of L-carnitine on anemia and high cholesterol in persons on hemodialysis for chronic renal failure.

A genetic condition called fragile X syndrome can cause behavioral disturbances such as hyperactivity, along with intellectual disability, autism, and alterations in appearance. A preliminary study of seventeen boys found that acetyl-L-carnitine might help to reduce hyperactive behavior associated with this condition. Evidence for the effectiveness of L-carnitine in attention deficit disorder (ADD) has been mixed.

Celiac disease is an autoimmune disease affecting the digestive tract. Fatigue is a common symptom of the disease. One small double-blind trial found evidence that the use of L-carnitine at a dose of 2 g daily might help alleviate this symptom.

Weak evidence hints that carnitine may help people with degeneration of the cerebellum (the structure of the brain responsible for voluntary muscular movement). One small study suggests carnitine may be helpful for reducing symptoms of chronic fatigue syndrome. Another study suggests that carnitine may be of value for treating hyperthyroidism and for severe liver disease. A substantial study marred by poor design (specifically, far too many primary endpoints) found equivocal evidence that L-carnitine, taken at dose of 500 mg three times daily, might be more effective than placebo for the treatment of fibromyalgia.

Other weak evidence suggests that carnitine may be helpful for decreasing the muscle toxicity of AZT (a drug used to treat HIV infection). Other weak evidence hints that the acetyl-L-carnitine might reduce nerve-related side effects caused by HIV drugs in general.

One study failed to find carnitine effective for promoting weight loss, although another found that carnitine might lead to improvements in body composition (fat-muscle ratio). Carnitine is widely touted as a physical performance enhancer, but there is no real evidence that it is effective, and some research indicates that it is not.

Little to no evidence supports other claimed benefits, such as treating irregular heartbeat, Down syndrome, muscular dystrophy, and alcoholic fatty liver disease. However, in a randomized trial involving twenty-five persons with liver cirrhosis and early brain dysfunction (hepatic encephalopathy) associated with severe forms of this condition, carnitine appeared to significantly improve the function of both the liver and the brain after three months of treatment.

SCIENTIFIC EVIDENCE

Angina. Carnitine might be a good addition to standard therapy for angina. In one controlled study, two hundred persons with angina (the exercise-induced variety) either took 2 g daily of L-carnitine or were left untreated. All the study participants continued to take their usual medication for angina. Those taking carnitine showed improvement in several measures of heart function, including a significantly greater ability to exercise without chest pain. They were also able to reduce the dosages of some of their heart medications (under medical supervision) as their symptoms decreased.

The results of this study cannot be fully trusted because researchers did not use a double-blind protocol. Another trial with a double-blind, placebo-controlled design tested L-carnitine in fifty-two people with angina and found evidence of benefit.

In addition, several small studies (some of them double-blind) tested propionyl-L-carnitine for the treatment of angina and also found evidence of benefit.

Intermittent claudication. People with advanced hardening of the arteries, or atherosclerosis, often have difficulty walking because of a lack of blood flow to the legs, a condition called intermittent claudication. Pain may develop after walking less than half a block. Although carnitine does not increase blood flow, it appears to improve the muscle's ability to function under difficult circumstances.

A twelve-month, double-blind, placebo-controlled trial of 485 persons with intermittent claudication evaluated the potential benefits of propionyl-L-carnitine. Participants with relatively severe disease showed a 44 percent improvement in walking distance, com-

pared with placebo. However, no improvement was seen in those persons with mild disease. Another double-blind study followed 245 people and also found benefit.

Similar results have been seen in most other studies of L-carnitine or propionyl-L-carnitine. Propionyl-L-carnitine may be more effective for intermittent claudication than plain carnitine.

Congestive heart failure. Several small studies have found that carnitine, often in the form of propionyl-L-carnitine, can improve symptoms of congestive heart failure. In one trial, benefits were maintained for sixty days after treatment with carnitine was stopped.

After a heart attack. L-carnitine has shown inconsistent promise for use after a heart attack. A double-blind, placebo-controlled study followed 101 people for one month after those persons had experienced a heart attack. The study found that the use of L-carnitine, in addition to standard care, reduced the size of the infarct (dead heart tissue).

In the months following a severe heart attack, the left ventricle of the heart often enlarges, and the pumping action of the heart becomes less efficient. Some evidence suggests that L-carnitine can help prevent heart enlargement but that it does not improve heart function. In a twelve-month, double-blind, placebo-controlled study of 472 persons who had just had a heart attack, the use of carnitine at a dose of 6 g per day significantly decreased the rate of heart enlargement. However, heart function was not significantly altered.

A three-month, double-blind, placebo-controlled study of sixty persons who had just had a heart attack also failed to find improvements in heart function. (Heart enlargement was not studied.)

Results consistent with the foregoing studies were seen in a six-month double blind, placebo-controlled study of 2,330 people who had just had a heart attack. Carnitine failed to produce significant reductions in mortality or heart failure (serious decline in heart function) over the six-month period. However, the study did find reductions in early death. (For statistical reasons, the meaningfulness of this last finding is questionable. Reduction in early death was a secondary endpoint rather than a primary one.) Carnitine is used with conventional treatment, not as a substitute for it.

Diabetic neuropathy. High levels of blood sugar can damage the nerves leading to the extremities, causing pain and numbness. This condition is called diabetic peripheral neuropathy. Nerve damage may also develop in the heart, a condition called cardiac autonomic neuropathy. Acetyl-L-carnitine has shown considerable promise for diabetic peripheral neuropathy and some promise for cardiac autonomic neuropathy.

Two fifty-two-week, double-blind, placebo-controlled studies, involving a total of 1,257 people with diabetic peripheral neuropathy, evaluated the potential benefits of acetyl-L-carnitine taken at 500 or 1,000 mg daily. The results showed that the use of acetyl-L-carnitine, especially at the higher dose, improved sensory perception and decreased pain levels. In addition, the supplement appeared to promote nerve fiber regeneration. A small study found some potential benefits for cardiac autonomic neuropathy.

Male sexual function. Carnitine has shown promise for improving male sexual function. One double-blind, placebo-controlled study of 120 men compared a combination of propionyl-L-carnitine (2 g per day) and acetyl-L-carnitine (2 g per day) with testosterone for the treatment of male aging symptoms (sexual dysfunction, depression, and fatigue). The results indicated that both testosterone and carnitine improved erectile function, mood, and fatigue, compared with placebo. However, no improvements were seen in the placebo group. This is an unusual occurrence in studies of erectile dysfunction, so it casts some doubt on the study results.

A double-blind study of forty men evaluated propionyl-L-carnitine (2 g per day) in diabetic men with erectile dysfunction who had not responded well to Viagra. The results indicated that carnitine significantly enhanced the effectiveness of Viagra. In another double-blind study, a combination of the propionyl and acetyl forms of carnitine enhanced the effectiveness of Viagra in men who suffered from erectile dysfunction caused by prostate surgery.

Male infertility. Growing evidence suggests that L-carnitine or acetyl-L-carnitine, or their combination, may be helpful for improving sperm quality and function, thereby benefiting male infertility. For example, in one double-blind, placebo-controlled study of sixty men, the use of combined L-carnitine (2 g per day) and acetyl-L-carnitine (also at 2 g per day) significantly improved sperm quality.

Chronic obstructive pulmonary disease (COPD). Evidence from three double-blind, placebo-controlled studies enrolling a total of forty-nine people suggests that L-carnitine can improve exercise tolerance in COPD, presumably by improving muscular efficiency in the lungs and other muscles.

Alzheimer's disease. Numerous double-blind or single-blind studies involving a total of more than fourteen hundred people have evaluated the potential benefits of acetyl-L-carnitine in the treatment of Alzheimer's disease and other forms of dementia. However, while early studies found evidence of modest benefit, two large and well-designed studies failed to find acetyl-L-carnitine effective.

The first of these studies was a double-blind, placebo-controlled trial that enrolled 431 participants for one year. Overall, acetyl-L-carnitine proved no better than placebo. However, because a close look at the data indicated that the supplement might help people who develop Alzheimer's disease at an unusually young age, researchers performed a follow-up trial. This one-year, double-blind, placebo-controlled trial evaluated acetyl-L-carnitine in 229 persons with early onset Alzheimer's. No benefits were seen here either. One review of the literature concluded that acetyl-L-carnitine may be helpful for mild cases of Alzheimer's disease, but not for more severe cases.

Mild depression. A double-blind study of sixty elderly persons with dysthymia (a mild form of depression) found that treatment with 3 g of carnitine daily for two months significantly improved symptoms, compared with placebo. Positive results were seen in two other studies too, one of depression and one of dysthymia.

Hyperthyroidism. Enlargement of the thyroid (goiter) can be due to many causes, including cancer and iodine deficiency. In some cases, thyroid enlargement occurs without any known cause, resulting in benign goiter.

Treatment of benign goiter generally consists of taking thyroid hormone pills. This causes the thyroid gland to become less active, and the goiter shrinks. However, undesirable effects may result. Symptoms of hyperthyroidism (too much thyroid hormone) can develop, including heart palpitations, nervousness, weight loss, and bone breakdown.

A double-blind, placebo-controlled trial found evidence that the use of L-carnitine could alleviate many of these symptoms. This six-month study evaluated the effects of L-carnitine in fifty women who were taking thyroid hormone for benign goiter. The results showed that a dose of 2 or 4 g of carnitine daily protected participants' bones and reduced other symptoms of hyperthyroidism.

Carnitine is thought to affect thyroid hormone by blocking its action in cells. This suggests a potential concern—carnitine might be harmful for people who have low or borderline thyroid levels to begin with. This possibility has not been well explored.

Peyronie's disease. Peyronie's disease is an inflammatory condition of the penis that develops in stages. In the first stage, penile pain occurs with erection; next, the penis becomes curved; finally, erectile dysfunction may occur. Many medications have been tried for Peyronie's disease, with some success. One such drug is tamoxifen, which is better known as a treatment to prevent breast cancer recurrence. A three-month, double-blind study compared the effectiveness of acetyl-L-carnitine to the drug tamoxifen in forty-eight men with Peyronie's disease. Acetyl-L-carnitine (at a dose of 1 g daily) reduced penile curvature, while tamoxifen did not; in addition, the supplement reduced pain and slowed disease progression to a greater extent than tamoxifen.

SAFETY ISSUES

L-carnitine in its three forms appears to be quite safe. However, persons with low or borderline-low thyroid levels should avoid carnitine because it might impair the action of thyroid hormone. Persons on dialysis should not receive this (or any other supplement) without a physician's supervision. The maximum safe dosages for young children, pregnant or nursing women, and those with severe liver or kidney disease have not been established.

IMPORTANT INTERACTIONS

Persons taking antiseizure medications, particularly valproic acid (Depakote, Depakene) but also phenytoin (Dilantin), may need extra carnitine. Persons taking thyroid medication should not take carnitine except under a physician's supervision.

EBSCO CAM Review Board

FURTHER READING

Arnold, L. E., et al. "Acetyl-L-Carnitine (ALC) in Attention-Deficit/Hyperactivity Disorder." *Journal of Child and Adolescent Psychopharmacology* (2007): 791-802.

Cavallini, G., et al. "Carnitine Versus Androgen Administration in the Treatment of Sexual Dysfunction, Depressed Mood, and Fatigue Associated with Male Aging." *Urology* 63 (2004): 641-646.

Gentile, V., et al. "Preliminary Observations on the Use of Propionyl-L-Carnitine in Combination with Sildenafil in Patients with Erectile Dysfunction and Diabetes." *Current Medical Research and Opinion* 20 (2004): 1377-1384.

Maestri, A., et al. "A Pilot Study on the Effect of Acetyl-L-Carnitine in Paclitaxel- and Cisplatin-Induced Peripheral Neuropathy." *Tumori* (2005): 135-138.

Malaguarnera, M., L. Cammalleri, et al. "L-Carnitine Treatment Reduces Severity of Physical and Mental Fatigue and Increases Cognitive Functions in Centenarians." *American Journal of Clinical Nutrition* 86 (2007): 1738-1744.

Malaguarnera, M., M. P. Gargante, et al. "Acetyl-L-Carnitine Treatment in Minimal Hepatic Encephalopathy." *Digestive Diseases and Sciences* 53 (2008): 3018-3025.

Rossini, M., et al. "Double-Blind, Multicenter Trial Comparing Acetyl-L-Carnitine with Placebo in the Treatment of Fibromyalgia Patients." *Clinical and Experimental Rheumatology* 25 (2007): 182-188.

Sima, A. A., et al. "Acetyl-L-Carnitine Improves Pain, Nerve Regeneration, and Vibratory Perception in Patients with Chronic Diabetic Neuropathy." *Diabetes Care* 28 (2004): 89-94.

Smith, W., et al. "Effect of Glycine Propionyl-L-Carnitine on Aerobic and Anaerobic Exercise Performance." *International Journal of Sport Nutrition and Exercise Metabolism* 18 (2008): 19-36.

Youle, M., and M. Osio. "A Double-Blind, Parallel-Group, Placebo-Controlled, Multicentre Study of Acetyl-L-Carnitine in the Symptomatic Treatment of Antiretroviral Toxic Neuropathy in Patients with HIV-1 Infection." *HIV Medicine* 8 (2007): 241-250.

See also: Alzheimer's disease and non-Alzheimer's dementia; Angina; Chronic fatigue syndrome; Chronic obstructive pulmonary disease; Congestive heart failure; Diabetes, complications of; Elder health; Fatigue; Fibromyalgia: Homeopathic remedies; Heart attack; Hyperthyroidism; Infertility, male; Intermittent claudication; Men's health; Peyronie's disease; Sexual dysfunction in men.

Carnosine

CATEGORY: Herbs and supplements

DEFINITION: Natural substance of the human body used as a supplement to treat specific health conditions.

PRINCIPAL PROPOSED USE: Antiaging nutrient

OTHER PROPOSED USES: Alzheimer's disease and related conditions, autism, cataracts, sports and fitness support: enhancing performance

OVERVIEW

Carnosine (L-carnosine), not to be confused with L-carnitine, is a substance manufactured in the human body, made by combining the amino acids alanine and histidine. The highest levels of carnosine are found in the brain and nervous system, the lens of the eye, and skeletal muscle tissue. Its exact function in the body is not known.

REQUIREMENTS AND SOURCES

The body manufactures carnosine from common dietary proteins, and for this reason, there is no daily requirement of this substance.

THERAPEUTIC DOSAGES

Among advocates of carnosine, there is a controversy regarding whether the proper dose is 50 to 150 milligrams (mg) per day or nearer to 1,000 mg daily. However, until carnosine has actually been shown to have any medical benefits, this argument cannot be settled.

SCIENTIFIC EVIDENCE

Like numerous other substances, carnosine has antioxidant properties, meaning that it neutralizes dangerous, naturally occurring substances called free radicals. Free radicals are thought to play a role in many illnesses. On this basis, many antioxidant substances have been studied for potential health-promoting properties. Some Web sites claim that carnosine acts as an antioxidant in a unique way, fighting the "second wave" effects that follow attacks by free radicals. However, there is no meaningful evidence to support this theory or the hypothesis that such an effect, if it truly exists, would provide any health benefits.

Antiaging. Carnosine is widely marketed as an antiaging nutrient. There are numerous studies that hint carnosine might help slow various aspects of aging. The quality of these studies, though, is too low to provide any reliable evidence for benefit.

Autism. There is some very preliminary evidence that carnosine may be helpful for children with autistic spectrum disorders. In a double-blind, placebo-controlled trial, thirty-one children with autism were given either carnosine (400 mg twice daily) or a placebo for a period of eight weeks. The children given carnosine showed significant improvements compared with those given a placebo.

Brain disorders. Carnosine has been studied in Parkinson's disease. In a small controlled trial, adding carnosine to the diet of people being treated for Parkinson's disease improved their symptoms. There is also weak evidence that carnosine may be helpful for Alzheimer's disease and other forms of dementia. Carnosine can be found in the olfactory tissue, which is responsible for the sense of smell. Because of this, some researchers have suggested that carnosine should be administered through the nose (rather than by mouth), especially considering that people with Alzheimer's disease often have problems with their ability to detect odors. This use for carnosine and this method of administering it are in need of further study.

Sports performance. It has been suggested that taking supplements of the amino acid alanine can raise carnosine levels in muscle and, in turn, enhance sports performance. In one small trial, twenty-six men were randomized to receive 6,400 mg daily of carnosine or a placebo over the course of ten weeks. The men then went through an exercise training program, and their physical fitness was assessed after a ten-week period. Researchers, though, did not find any significant differences between the two groups.

Other conditions. Other weak evidence hints that oral carnosine might be helpful for cataracts, wound healing, conditions of the digestive tract, and various forms of heart disease, such as atherosclerosis (hardening of the arteries). For example, one study found that carnosine may interfere with the development of low density lipoproteins (LDL, or bad cholesterol).

SAFETY ISSUES

The use of carnosine has not been associated with any significant side effects. However, the body deploys a range of enzymes, called carnosinases, to break down carnosine. There may be a reason for the presence of these enzymes, and overcoming them by providing large amounts of supplemental carnosine could conceivably cause harm in some as-yet unrecognized way. Maximum safe doses in young children, pregnant or nursing women, and people with severe liver or kidney disease have not been established.

EBSCO CAM Review Board

FURTHER READING

Argirova, M., and O. Argirova. "Inhibition of Ascorbic Acid-Induced Modifications in Lens Proteins by Peptides." *Journal of Peptide Science* 9 (2003): 170-176.

Babizhayev, M. A., et al. "Efficacy of N-acetylcarnosine in the Treatment of Cataracts." *Drugs in R&D* 3 (2002): 87-103.

Chez, M. G., et al. "Double-Blind, Placebo-Controlled Study of L-carnosine Supplementation in Children with Autistic Spectrum Disorders." *Journal of Child Neurology* 17 (2002): 833-837.

Hipkiss, A. R., et al. "Reaction of Carnosine with Aged Proteins: Another Protective Process?" *Annals of the New York Academy of Sciences* 959 (2002): 285-294.

Shao, L., Q. H. Li, and Z. Tan. "L-carnosine Reduces Telomere Damage and Shortening Rate in Cultured Normal Fibroblasts." *Biochemical and Biophysical Research Communications* 324 (2004): 931-936.

Wang, A. M., et al. "Use of Carnosine as a Natural Anti-senescence Drug for Human Beings." *Biochemistry* (Moscow) 65 (2000): 869-871.

Yuneva, A. O., et al. "Effect of Carnosine on *Drosophila melanogaster* Lifespan." *Bulletin of Experimental Biology and Medicine* 133 (2002): 559-161.

See also: Aging; Herbal medicine; Sports and fitness support: Enhancing performance.

Carob

CATEGORY: Functional foods

RELATED TERM: Locust bean gum

DEFINITION: Natural product promoted as a dietary supplement for specific health benefits.

PRINCIPAL PROPOSED USES: Diarrhea, high cholesterol

OTHER PROPOSED USE: Esophageal reflux in infants

OVERVIEW

Carob is a warm-climate tree that grows up to fifty feet in height. Its long, reddish pods contain seeds

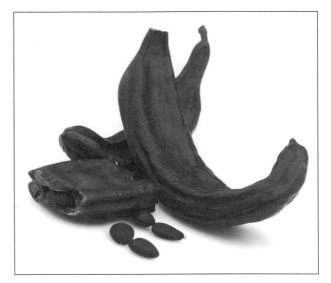

Carob pods and seeds. (©Margo555/Dreamstime.com)

used as medicine and food. The seed consists of three different parts: the outer husk, the nutritive endosperm (analogous to the white edible portion of the coconut), and the inner seed, or germ. The endosperm is converted to locust bean gum, a thickening agent used in numerous prepared foods. The entire pod, when dried and ground, is called carob powder. Carob powder is used both as a chocolate-like flavoring and as a medicinal substance for the treatment of diarrhea.

USES AND APPLICATIONS

Carob is rich in insoluble fiber. Like other sources of fiber, carob has shown some promise for improving cholesterol profile. In a small (fifty-eight-participant), double-blind, placebo-controlled study, the use of carob powder at a dose of 15 grams daily significantly reduced levels of LDL (bad) cholesterol compared with placebo.

Carob also contains tannins, astringent substances found in many plants. Foods rich in tannins are often recommended for the treatment of diarrhea. A double-blind clinical trial of forty-one infants with diarrhea found that carob powder (at a dose of 1 gram per kilogram of body weight per day) significantly speeded resolution of diarrhea compared with placebo.

The portion of carob that is made into locust bean gum contains soluble fiber in the galactomannan family. Like other forms of soluble fiber, it has shown potential (though not proven) benefit for enhancing weight loss and controlling blood sugar levels.

Some infants have a tendency to regurgitate after eating. A small, double-blind, placebo-controlled study found that the use of locust bean gum as a thickening agent significantly reduced the amount and frequency of regurgitation.

DOSAGE

A typical dose of carob powder for the treatment of diarrhea or high cholesterol in adults is 15 to 20 grams daily. The dose is reduced proportionately by weight for treating diarrhea in children. Like other fiber sources, carob should be taken with plenty of water. Severe diarrhea in infants and children requires professional medical care.

SAFETY ISSUES

Carob powder and locust bean gum, as widely consumed foods, are believed to have a high degree of safety. Locust bean gum has been extensively evaluated and found noncarcinogenic and nontoxic. There are no known risks for pregnant or nursing women.

EBSCO CAM Review Board

FURTHER READING

Brennan, C. S. "Dietary Fibre, Glycaemic Response, and Diabetes." *Molecular Nutrition and Food Research* 49 (2005): 560-570.

Wenzl, T. G., et al. "Effects of Thickened Feeding on Gastroesophageal Reflux in Infants: A Placebo-Controlled Crossover Study Using Intraluminal Impedance." *Pediatrics* 111 (2003): 355-359.

Zunft, H. J., et al. "Carob Pulp Preparation Rich in Insoluble Fibre Lowers Total and LDL Cholesterol in Hypercholesterolemic Patients." *European Journal of Nutrition* 42 (2003): 235-242.

See also: Chocolate; Cholesterol, high; Diarrhea; Functional foods: Introduction; Gastroesophageal reflux disease.

Carotenoids

CATEGORY: Functional foods
DEFINITION: Natural substance promoted as a dietary supplement for specific health benefits.

OVERVIEW

Carotenoids are red, orange, and yellow pigments found in fruits and vegetables. About six hundred carotenoids have been identified, and all of them have antioxidant properties. Some carotenoids can be converted in the body to vitamin A, and these are called provitamin A carotenoids. The best-known carotenoids include beta-carotene, lutein, lycopene, astaxanthin, and zeaxanthin.

The results of some observational studies suggest that a diet high in these carotenoids can reduce the risk of developing various illnesses, including cardiovascular disease, age-related vision loss, and various types of cancer. These findings led to large-scale studies of synthetic beta-carotene for preventing cancer (especially lung cancer), heart disease, cataracts, strokes, and macular degeneration. The results showed, at best, no benefit and, at worst, a possible increase in disease risk.

Many proponents of alternative medicine considered this outcome paradoxical and attempted to explain the outcome in various ways, such as beta-carotene alone may not be as useful as mixed carotenoids (and other healthful substances) found in fruits and vegetables, and synthetic beta-carotene may be less effective than natural beta-carotene. Also, the participants in these studies were inappropriate for the trials (generally, they were smokers).

However, while any of these explanations may be correct, it is also quite possible that carotenoids simply do not provide any of the healthful effects attributed to them. Observational studies are notoriously unreliable for proving a treatment effective. Such studies only find associations between events, rather than cause and effect. It is quite possible, for example, that people who tend to eat more fruits and vegetables may be healthier in various other ways than those who do not, and that these other factors account for the apparent improvements.

Consider the history of medical beliefs about hormone replacement therapy (HRT) for menopausal women. Observational studies had found evidence that women who used HRT had less heart disease, and on this basis millions of women were prescribed HRT. However, when proper double-blind studies were done, the results indicated that HRT actually caused heart disease.

Similarly, nothing more reliable than observational studies underlies the widespread belief that lycopene can prevent prostate cancer and that lutein can do the same for cataracts. One double-blind study does hint that mixed carotenoid supplementation is beneficial for people with human immunodeficiency virus infection, but the results were statistically weak. Thus, while it is a good idea to eat fruits and vegetables, it is not clear that taking concentrated extracts of various substances found in fruits and vegetables provides any health benefits.

EBSCO CAM Review Board

FURTHER READING

Age-Related Eye Disease Study Research Group. "A Randomized, Placebo-Controlled Clinical Trial of High-Dose Supplementation with Vitamins C and E and Beta Carotene for Age-Related Cataract and Vision Loss." *Archives of Ophthalmology* 119 (2001): 1439-1452.

Austin, J., et al. "A Community Randomized Controlled Clinical Trial of Mixed Carotenoids and Micronutrient Supplementation of Patients with Acquired Immunodeficiency Syndrome." *European Journal of Clinical Nutrition* 60 (2006): 1266-1276.

Epstein, K. R. "The Role of Carotenoids on the Risk of Lung Cancer." *Seminars in Oncology* 30 (2003): 86-93.

Hak, A. E., et al. "Plasma Carotenoids and Tocopherols and Risk of Myocardial Infarction in a Low-Risk Population of US Male Physicians." *Circulation* 108 (2003): 802-807.

Peterson, C. E., et al. "Combined Antioxidant Carotenoids and the Risk of Persistent Human Papillomavirus Infection." *Nutrition and Cancer* 62 (2010): 728-733.

See also: Beta-carotene; Functional foods: Introduction; Lutein; Lycopene.

Carpal tunnel syndrome

CATEGORY: Condition

DEFINITION: Treatment of the compression of the median nerve of the wrist.

PRINCIPAL PROPOSED NATURAL TREATMENTS: None

OTHER PROPOSED NATURAL TREATMENTS: *Arnica*, bromelain, laser therapy, magnet therapy, proteolytic enzymes, vitamin B_6, vitamin B_{12}, yoga

INTRODUCTION

Carpal tunnel syndrome (CTS) is a common and often disabling condition most often associated with data entry and general computer use, but it can affect anyone who performs repetitive hand motions. CTS occurs in women more often than men and is a relatively common temporary complication of pregnancy (because of fluid retention). It also occurs frequently among people with rheumatoid arthritis or diabetes.

CTS is caused by compression of the median nerve. On its way to the hand, the median nerve passes through an opening in the wrist called the carpal tunnel. Constant, repetitive hand motion may aggravate the ligaments and tendons encased in the tunnel, causing them to swell. As the tunnel walls close in, they compress the median nerve. This causes tingling and numbness in the thumb, index finger, middle finger, and half of the ring finger. The discomfort of CTS often wakes people during the night and eventually makes it difficult to grasp small objects.

Most instances of CTS are job-related. Paying attention to proper ergonomics is essential for preventing CTS. This might involve repositioning a computer keyboard or taking breaks more often. Conventional medical treatment for more stubborn CTS cases is variable in its success. Splinting the affected hand, especially at night, may help reduce symptoms. Nonsteroidal anti-inflammatory medications, such as ibuprofen or naproxen, may help slightly. Surgery is considered the ultimate treatment, but corticosteroid injections may be equally or slightly more effective. In some cases, a person with work-related CTS may have no choice but to change vocation.

PROPOSED NATURAL TREATMENTS

There are no natural treatments for carpal tunnel syndrome that have any meaningful supporting evidence. Those that have been scientifically evaluated to any extent include vitamin B_6, yoga, and magnet therapy.

Vitamin B_6. Late in the twentieth century, researchers noted that people with CTS seemed to be deficient in vitamin B_6. This led to widespread use of vitamin B_6 as a CTS remedy. However, a more recent study found no association between CTS and vitamin B_6 deficiency. In any case, even if vitamin B_6 deficiency were common in CTS, that by itself would not prove that taking vitamin B_6 supplements can reduce symptoms.

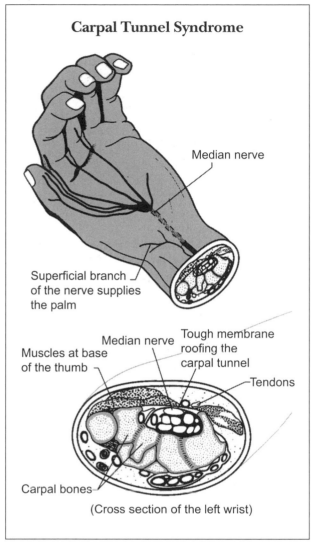

Carpal Tunnel Syndrome

Median nerve

Superficial branch of the nerve supplies the palm

Muscles at base of the thumb

Median nerve

Tough membrane roofing the carpal tunnel

Tendons

Carpal bones

(Cross section of the left wrist)

Repetitive wrist motion such as typing may put excessive pressure on the median nerve and cause numbness and tingling in the hands, a condition known as carpal tunnel syndrome. If rest, wrist splints, and painkillers do not alleviate the problem, surgery may be needed to relieve the pressure.

A few studies have investigated the effectiveness of vitamin B$_6$ for CTS. Most were poorly designed and involved few people. The two (albeit small) randomized, double-blind, placebo-controlled studies that do exist found no evidence that vitamin B$_6$ effectively treats CTS. The first study, which enrolled only fifteen people, found no significant difference after ten weeks among those taking vitamin B$_6$, placebo, or nothing. The second study, involving thirty-two people, did find

some benefits, but these were fairly minor. There was no improvement in nighttime pain, numbness, or tingling, or in objective measurements of median nerve function. Some benefit, however, was seen in the relatively less important symptoms of finger swelling and discomfort after repetitive motion.

Because vitamin B$_6$ has not been proven effective and may be harmful in high doses, it is not recommend for treating carpal tunnel syndrome.

Yoga. Hatha yoga, a system of stretching and balancing exercises, has been tried for CTS. In one study, forty-two persons with CTS were randomly assigned to receive either yoga instruction or a wrist splint for eight weeks. The results indicated that yoga was more effective than the wrist splint.

However, this study has a serious flaw: Participants in the control group were simply offered the wrist splint and given the choice of using it or not. It would have been preferable for them to have received an option such as fake laser acupuncture or, even better, phony yoga postures. Experience from numerous studies shows that when people believe they are receiving an effective treatment, they report improvement, regardless of the nature of the treatment.

Magnet therapy. In the one reported double-blind, placebo-controlled study of magnet therapy for CTS, thirty people with CTS received treatment with either a real or a fake static magnet. Dramatic, long-lasting benefits were seen with the magnet treatment. However, identical dramatic and long-lasting benefits were seen with placebo treatment too. This study underscores the need for a placebo group in studies; had there not been one in this trial, magnet therapy would have shown itself quite effective for CTS. In two more small, randomized trials, researchers again found that there were no differences between the treatment and the placebo groups. Both groups experienced an improvement in symptoms.

Other treatments. Bromelain and other proteolytic enzymes are sometimes recommended for the treatment of CTS, but there is no evidence that they are effective. In a double-blind, placebo-controlled study of thirty-seven people undergoing surgery for CTS, an ointment made from the herb *Arnica* (combined with homeopathic *Arnica* tablets) proved slightly more effective than placebo for relieving pain after surgery.

People who have a stroke that renders one hand paralyzed may develop CTS from overuse of the remaining functional hand. One poorly designed study found preliminary evidence that mecobalamin, a form of vitamin B_{12}, might provide some benefit. Another study failed to find low-level laser therapy helpful for CTS.

EBSCO CAM Review Board

FURTHER READING

Carter, R., C. B. Aspy, and J. Mold. "The Effectiveness of Magnet Therapy for Treatment of Wrist Pain Attributed to Carpal Tunnel Syndrome." *Journal of Family Practice* 51 (2002): 38-40.

Colbert, A. P., et al. "Static Magnetic Field Therapy for Carpal Tunnel Syndrome." *Archives of Physical Medicine and Rehabilitation* 91 (2010): 1098-1104.

Hui, A. C., et al. "A Randomized Controlled Trial of Surgery vs. Steroid Injection for Carpal Tunnel Syndrome." *Neurology* 64 (2005): 2074-2078.

Irvine, J., et al. "Double-Blind Randomized Controlled Trial of Low-Level Laser Therapy in Carpal Tunnel Syndrome." *Muscle and Nerve* 30 (2004): 182-187.

Jeffrey, S., and J. Belcher. "Use of *Arnica* to Relieve Pain After Carpal-Tunnel Release Surgery." *Alternative Therapies in Health and Medicine* 8 (2002): 66-68.

Ly-Pen, D., et al. "Surgical Decompression Versus Local Steroid Injection in Carpal Tunnel Syndrome." *Arthritis and Rheumatism* 52 (2005): 612-619.

See also: Bone and joint health; Bursitis; Fibromyalgia: Homeopathic remedies; Magnet therapy; Nonsteroidal anti-inflammatory drugs (NSAIDs); Osteoarthritis; Pain management; Rheumatoid arthritis; Tendonitis; Vitamin B_6; Yoga.

Cartilage

CATEGORY: Herbs and supplements

RELATED TERMS: Bovine cartilage, shark cartilage

DEFINITION: Natural substance of the body of humans and other animals used as a supplement to treat specific health conditions.

PRINCIPAL PROPOSED USES: None

OTHER PROPOSED USES: Cancer treatment, minor wounds, osteoarthritis, psoriasis

OVERVIEW

Cartilage is a tough connective tissue found in many parts of the body. Human ears and nose are made from cartilage, and so is the gliding surface in human joints.

One constituent of cartilage, chondroitin, is widely used in Europe to treat osteoarthritis. Cartilage itself has also been proposed as a treatment for osteoarthritis.

The most commonly used forms of cartilage come from cows (bovine cartilage) and sharks. Provocative evidence had suggested that shark cartilage might have some value in the treatment of cancer. However, properly designed studies have so far failed to find benefit.

REQUIREMENTS AND SOURCES

The preferred source of cartilage is a health-food store or pharmacy, where the supplements can be purchased in pill or powdered form.

THERAPEUTIC DOSAGES

Various doses of cartilage have been used in different studies, ranging from 2.5 milligrams to 60 grams daily.

THERAPEUTIC USES

Based on the belief that sharks do not get cancer, shark cartilage has been heavily marketed as a cure for cancer. Although this justification is a myth (sharks do get cancer), shark cartilage has, in fact, shown some promise for cancer treatment. Shark cartilage (like other forms of cartilage) contains substances that tend to inhibit angiogenesis (the growth of new blood vessels). Because cancers must build new blood vessels to feed themselves, this effect might be beneficial. Double-blind, placebo-controlled studies on special formulations of shark cartilage for the treatment of cancer are now under way. It has also been suggested that the anti-angiogenic properties of shark cartilage may make it helpful for psoriasis, but this hypothesis has not yet undergone proper study.

Shark cartilage also inhibits substances called matrix metalloproteases (MMPs). These little-understood enzymes affect the "extracellular matrix," the framework of substances that lie between cells in the body. MMPs are thought to play a role in diseases of the cornea, gums, skin, blood vessels, and joints, as well as cancer and illnesses that involve excessive fibrous tissue. On this basis, shark cartilage has been proposed for a wide variety of medical conditions, from cataracts to scleroderma; however, there are no meaningful studies as yet that can tell us whether it offers any benefit.

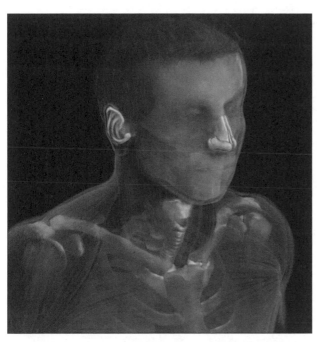

An illustration of areas containing cartilage on the human body. (Anatomical Travelogue/Photo Researchers, Inc.)

Cartilage in general has been proposed as a treatment for the common "wear and tear" type of arthritis known as osteoarthritis. The idea behind this is straightforward: Because osteoarthritis is a disease of the joints and because cartilage is one of the elements that make up the joints, adding cartilage to the diet might help. This idea sounds a bit too simplistic to be believable, but it is the same principle behind the use of glucosamine and chondroitin (specific substances found in the joints) for osteoarthritis. Since well-designed studies have found those treatments effective, perhaps cartilage itself will ultimately be proven to work. However, such studies of cartilage have not yet been performed.

Finally, highly preliminary studies hint that cartilage may help heal minor wounds.

SCIENTIFIC EVIDENCE

A number of test-tube experiments have found that shark cartilage extracts prevent new blood vessels from forming in chick embryos and other test systems. As mentioned, this effect could conceivably mean that shark cartilage might fight cancer. These findings have led to other test-tube experiments, animal studies, and preliminary human trials to investi-

gate the possible anticancer effects of shark cartilage. The results suggest that a particular liquid shark cartilage extract might be useful in the treatment of various cancers, including lung, prostate, and breast cancer. However, not all studies have been positive.

In any case, only double-blind, placebo-controlled trials can provide conclusive data. The only reported studies of this type on shark cartilage for cancer failed to find benefit.

SAFETY ISSUES

Because cartilage is just common, ordinary gristle, it is presumably safe to consume. However, for reasons that are not clear, there is a report of an individual who developed liver inflammation after taking shark cartilage supplements. He recovered fully when the supplements were discontinued.

EBSCO CAM Review Board

FURTHER READING

Loprinzi, C., et al. "Evaluation of Shark Cartilage in Patients with Advanced Cancer." *Cancer* 104, no. 1 (2005): 176-182.

Riviere, M., et al. "AE-941 (Neovastat), an Inhibitor of Angiogenesis: Phase I/II Cancer Clinical Trial Results." *Cancer Investigation* 17 (1999): 16-17.

Wojtowicz-Praga, S. "Clinical Potential of Matrix Metalloprotease Inhibitors." *Drugs in R&D* (New Zealand) 1 (1999): 117-129.

See also: Chondroitin; Glucosamine; Herbal medicine; osteoarthritis.

Cataracts

CATEGORY: Condition

DEFINITION: Treatment of the decline of vision caused by an opaque buildup of damaged proteins in the lens of the eye.

PRINCIPAL PROPOSED NATURAL TREATMENTS: Antioxidants, beta-carotene, lutein, lycopene, vitamin C, vitamin E

OTHER PROPOSED NATURAL TREATMENTS: Bilberry, carnosine, ginkgo, lipoic acid, oligomeric proanthocyanidins, selenium, taurine, turmeric, vitamin B$_2$ (riboflavin), vitamin B$_3$ (niacin), whey protein, zinc

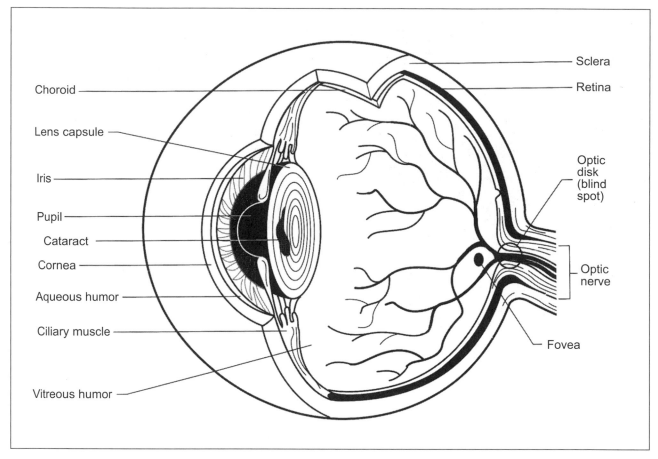

Cataracts are dark regions in the eye lens that lead gradually to obscured vision and blindness.

INTRODUCTION

Cataracts, an opaque buildup of damaged proteins in the lens of the eye, are the leading cause of visual decline in persons older than age sixty-five years. Most people in this age group have at minimum the beginnings of cataract formation. Many factors contribute to the development of cataracts, but damage by free radicals is believed to play a major role.

Cataracts can be removed surgically. Although this has become a relatively quick, safe, easy, and painless surgery, it does not result in completely normal vision.

PRINCIPAL PROPOSED NATURAL TREATMENTS

Antioxidants. Numerous observational studies suggest that high intake of antioxidants, such as vitamin C, vitamin E, and carotenoids (beta-carotene, lutein, astaxanthin, and lycopene), are associated with a re-duced incidence of cataracts. However, this by itself does not prove that the use of antioxidant supplements can prevent cataracts. Only double-blind, placebo-controlled studies can do that. The results of several large studies of this type were not encouraging.

In an enormous, double-blind, placebo-controlled trial involving almost forty thousand female health-care professionals, the use of natural vitamin E at a dose of 600 milligrams (mg) every other day for ten years failed to have any effect on cataract development. Another placebo-controlled trial studied the effects of antioxidant supplements in 4,629 older persons. Participants received either placebo or an antioxidant supplement containing 500 mg of vitamin C, 400 international units (IU) of vitamin E, and 15 mg of beta-carotene. The results over more than six years showed no effect on the risk of development of cataracts or on the rate at which existing cataracts progressed to greater severity. Finally, a five-year double-blind, placebo-controlled study of 798 people in Southern India failed to find benefit with supplemental antioxidants, despite dietary antioxidant deficiency being common among the people studied.

In addition, a previous double-blind, placebo-controlled study examining the use of beta-carotene or vitamin E alone in male smokers failed to find the supplements effective. On a more positive note, though, one large study found that beta-carotene supplements helped prevent cataracts in the subgroup of study participants who smoked. However, no benefits were seen in the group as a whole. In any case, people who smoke are generally not advised to take extra beta-carotene.

In another long-term study involving more than one thousand older adults, taking multivitamin-multimineral supplements led to a significant decrease in the development of cataracts compared with placebo over a nine-year period. However, these favorable results were tempered by an inexplicable increase in the number of a subtype of cataracts (posterior subcapsular) occurring among those taking the multivitamin-multimineral supplements. A small two-year study found some evidence that lutein may improve visual function in people who already have cataracts.

OTHER PROPOSED NATURAL TREATMENTS

Herbs high in antioxidant flavonoids are frequently suggested for preventing cataracts. These herbs include bilberry, ginkgo, oligomeric proanthocyanidins, and turmeric. For various theoretical reasons, the supplements carnosine, lipoic acid, niacin (vitamin B_3), riboflavin (vitamin B_2), selenium, taurine, whey protein, and zinc have also been proposed. However, there is little evidence that any of these treatments help.

EBSCO CAM Review Board

FURTHER READING

Chasan-Taber, L., et al. "A Prospective Study of Carotenoid and Vitamin A Intakes and Risk of Cataract Extraction in U.S. Women." *American Journal of Clinical Nutrition* 70 (1999): 509-516.

Christen, W. G., et al. "Vitamin E and Age-Related Cataract in a Randomized Trial of Women." *Ophthalmology* 115 (200): 822-829.

Christen, W. G, J. E. Manson, et al. "A Randomized Trial of Beta Carotene and Age-Related Cataract in U.S. Physicians." *Archives of Ophthalmology* 121 (2003): 372-378.

Olmedilla, B., et al. "Lutein, but Not Alpha-Tocopherol, Supplementation Improves Visual Function in Patients with Age-Related Cataracts." *Nutrition* 19 (2003): 21-24.

See also: Aging; Antioxidants; Beta-carotene; Conjunctivitis; Glaucoma; Lutein; Lycopene; Macular degeneration; Retinitis pigmentosa; Uveitis; Vitamin C; Vitamin E.

Catnip

CATEGORY: Herbs and supplements
RELATED TERM: *Nepeta cataria*
DEFINITION: Natural plant product used to treat specific health conditions.
PRINCIPAL PROPOSED USES: None
OTHER PROPOSED USES: Indigestion (especially when caused by stress), insomnia

OVERVIEW

Although catnip has a stimulating effect on virtually all felines, in humans it is traditionally used as a sleep aid. It has also been used for digestive and menstrual problems, as a uterine stimulant in childbirth, and as a symptomatic treatment for colds. Publications from the late 1960s suggested that the plant, when smoked, produced a psychedelic high not unlike marijuana, but it was later discovered that the researchers had, in fact, mixed up the two plants.

THERAPEUTIC DOSAGES

Catnip tea is most commonly made by mixing 1 to 2 teaspoons (1 to 2 grams) of the dried herb, or half that amount of the liquid extract, per cup of water (240 milliliters) and can be consumed up to three times a day.

THERAPEUTIC USES

Catnip is primarily used by today's herbalists as a treatment for insomnia, as well as for mild stomach upset, especially when caused by stress. One ingredient of catnip, trans-cis-nepetalactone, is the active ingredient so far as cats are concerned. Most (but not all) cats respond to this substance with a complex reaction called the "catnip response" that can go on for about an hour.

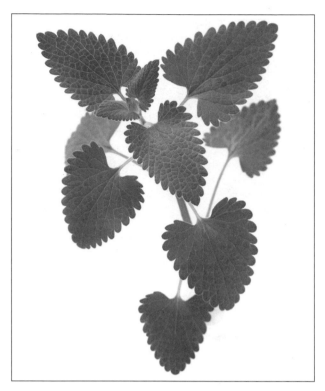

Leaves from the catnip plant. (©Ppy2010ha/Dreamstime. com)

Nepetalactone is similar to a class of substances called valepotriates, found in the sedative herb valerian. This has attracted some attention, as valerian also is used for insomnia and stomach discomfort. However, as valepotriates are no longer considered to be the active ingredients in valerian, it is not clear that this relationship has any significance.

There is no real evidence that catnip produces any effect in humans. Tests conducted on chicks and rats have produced conflicting results, although high doses of essential oil of catnip have increased sleeping times in the latter.

SAFETY ISSUES

Although comprehensive safety studies have not been performed, catnip tea is generally regarded as safe. However, because of its traditional use as a uterine stimulant, pregnant women should probably avoid catnip. Safety for young children or individuals with severe liver or kidney disease has not been established.

EBSCO CAM Review Board

FURTHER READING

McGuffin, M., ed. *American Herbal Products Association's Botanical Safety Handbook.* Boca Raton, Fla.: CRC Press; 1997.

See also: Herbal medicine; Insomnia; Valerian.

Cat's claw

CATEGORY: Herbs and supplements
RELATED TERMS: *Uncaria guianensis, U. tomentosa*
DEFINITION: Natural plant product used to treat specific health conditions.
PRINCIPAL PROPOSED USES: Acquired immunodeficiency syndrome, feline leukemia virus, genital and oral herpes, osteoarthritis, rheumatoid arthritis, shingles
OTHER PROPOSED USES: Allergies, ulcers

OVERVIEW

Cat's claw is an herb popular among the indigenous peoples of Peru, where it is used to treat cancer, diabetes, ulcers, arthritis, and infections and to assist in recovery from childbirth. It is also used as a contraceptive. There are two primary species of cat's claw used medicinally: *Uncaria tomentosa* and *U. guianensis.*

THERAPEUTIC DOSAGES

Numerous widely varying forms of cat's claw are available commercially. The optimum dosage of each type is not known. In addition, the precise differences in action between the two species of cat's claw, *U. tomentosa* and *U. guianensis*, as well as the pentacyclic and tetracyclic forms of *U. tomentosa* are not known.

THERAPEUTIC USES

Cat's claw is most often marketed as a treatment for viral diseases, such as herpes, shingles, acquired immunodeficiency syndrome, and feline leukemia virus. However, the evidence for these uses is extremely preliminary.

The most meaningful study yet performed on cat's claw suggests that the *U. guianensis* species might be helpful for an entirely different condition: osteoarthritis. In addition, one double-blind trial indicates that a certain type of *U. tomentosa* may be modestly helpful for people with rheumatoid arthritis. Cat's claw has also been proposed as a treatment for allergies and stomach ulcers, but there is no meaningful evidence as yet that it is effective for these conditions.

Scientific Evidence

Osteoarthritis. A four-week double-blind, placebo-controlled trial evaluated the potential benefits of cat's claw (*U. guianensis* species) for the treatment of osteoarthritis. A total of forty-five individuals with osteoarthritis were enrolled. Of these, thirty were treated with cat's claw extract, and fifteen were given placebo. Individuals in the treatment group showed reduced pain with activity compared with those in the placebo group. However, no comparative improvements were seen in knee pain at rest or at night, nor in knee circumference.

This pilot trial suggests that the *U. guianensis* species of cat's claw may be a useful treatment for osteoarthritis. Another study compared the effectiveness of a proprietary combination of cat's claw with glucosamine sulfate, a widely used dietary supplement for osteoarthritis. Researchers reported the results as positive, but because there was no placebo group, the overall effectiveness of this cat's claw combination product cannot be determined. More research will be necessary to verify this potential use of the herb.

Rheumatoid arthritis. In a double-blind, placebo-controlled trial of forty individuals undergoing conventional treatment for rheumatoid arthritis, use of an extract made from *U. tomentosa* modestly improved symptoms in individuals with rheumatoid arthritis compared with a placebo. The researchers conducting this trial made use of recent information indicating that there are two different subtypes of *U. tomentosa*, identifiable based on the chemicals found in them. For this trial, they used the form containing pentacyclic oxindole alkaloids, as opposed to tetracyclic oxindole alkaloids.

Safety Issues

In general, use of cat's claw has not been associated with adverse effects more serious than occasional digestive upset or allergic reactions. However, full safety studies have not been completed, and there has been one report of kidney failure apparently triggered by cat's claw.

Safety in young children, in pregnant or nursing women, and in those with severe liver or kidney disease has not yet been established. Some evidence suggests that cat's claw might interact with various medications by affecting their metabolism in the liver, but the extent of this effect has not been fully determined.

EBSCO CAM Review Board

Further Reading

Budzinski, J. W., et al. "An In Vitro Evaluation of Human Cytochrome P450 3A4 Inhibition by Selected Commercial Herbal Extracts and Tinctures." *Phytomedicine* 7 (2000): 273-282.

Mehta, K., et al. "Comparison of Glucosamine Sulfate and a Polyherbal Supplement for the Relief of Osteoarthritis of the Knee." *BMC Complementary and Alternative Medicine* 7 (October 31, 2007): 34.

Mur, E., et al. "Randomized Double Blind Trial of an Extract from the Pentacyclic Alkaloid-Chemotype of *Uncaria tomentosa* for the Treatment of Rheumatoid Arthritis." *Journal of Rheumatology* 29 (2002): 678-681.

Piscoya, J., et al. "Efficacy and Safety of Freeze-Dried Cat's Claw in Osteoarthritis of the Knee: Mechanisms of Action of the Species *Uncaria guianensis.*" *Inflammatory Research* 50 (2001): 442-448.

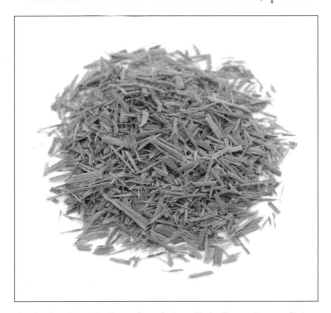

Cat's claw is an herb used traditionally in Peruvian medicine. (Geoff Kidd/Photo Researchers, Inc.)

See also: Glucosamine; Herbal medicine; Osteoarthritis; Rheumatoid arthritis.

Cavity prevention

CATEGORY: Condition
RELATED TERMS: Caries prevention, dental caries, tooth decay
DEFINITION: Prevention and treatment of the dissolving of the enamel of teeth.
PRINCIPAL PROPOSED NATURAL TREATMENT: Xylitol
OTHER PROPOSED NATURAL TREATMENTS: Black tea, calcium, chitosan, cranberry, hops, myrrh, probiotics, propolis, sanguinaria, sorbitol

INTRODUCTION

Cavities, technically called dental caries, are caused by the bacterium *Streptococcus mutans*. This bacterium lives in the mouth and thrives on sugar and other carbohydrates. In the presence of carbohydrates, *S. mutans* produces acids that dissolve the enamel of teeth, causing cavities.

Strong evidence indicates that fluoride toothpastes help prevent cavities. These toothpastes are so widely used that water fluoridation is probably of little to no value except in poorer, less developed countries where the use of fluoride toothpastes is not so common and widespread.

Fluoride rinses may offer some additional benefit. However, there is little to no scientific support for the use of the much more expensive, professionally applied fluoride varnishes.

PRINCIPAL PROPOSED NATURAL TREATMENTS

Double-blind studies enrolling almost four thousand people, mostly children, have found that the natural sugar xylitol can prevent cavities. These trials used xylitol-sweetened gum, candies, or toothpaste. The best evidence regards xylitol gum. One study suggested that the candy "gummy bears" may be an effective alternative method of administering xylitol to children. Xylitol is thought to prevent cavities by inhibiting the growth of *S. mutans*.

In one of the largest of these trials, researchers tested gum sweetened with various concentrations of xylitol or sorbitol (or both) with gum sweetened with sucrose and a control group receiving no gum. This forty-month trial was completed by 861 children. Gum containing 100 percent xylitol reduced the incidence of cavities the most. However, all of the xylitol and sorbitol gum groups showed significant reductions in cavities compared to the control group. In

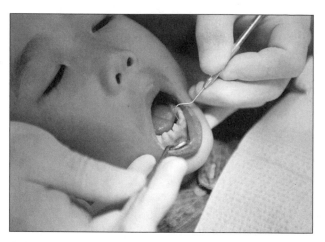

A dentist checks a child's teeth. Proper dental care is important for both deciduous and permanent teeth. (PhotoDisc)

contrast, the children receiving sucrose-sweetened gum had a slight increase in cavities compared to the control group.

A double-blind, placebo-controlled study of 1,677 children compared a standard fluoride toothpaste with a similar toothpaste that also contained 10 percent xylitol. Over the three-year study period, children given the xylitol-enriched toothpaste developed significantly fewer cavities than those in the fluoride-only group. Studies in adults and children have shown similar results for xylitol gum and candy. Another series of studies suggests that children acquire cavity-causing bacteria from their mothers and that regular use of xylitol by a mother of a newborn child may provide long-lasting protection to the child.

OTHER PROPOSED NATURAL TREATMENTS

Another sugar substitute called sorbitol may work as well as xylitol for the prevention of cavities in children. However, xylitol appears to work better than sorbitol for preventing cavities in adults.

Friendly bacteria (probiotics) have been proposed for the prevention of cavities, on the belief that they can fight harmful cavity-causing bacteria. The best evidence regards a probiotic product called *Lactobacillus GG* (LGG). In a double-blind, placebo-controlled trial, 594 children age one to six years were given either normal milk or milk with LGG. After the seven-month trial, the results showed significantly fewer cavities in the children receiving LGG.

One preliminary study found suggestive evidence

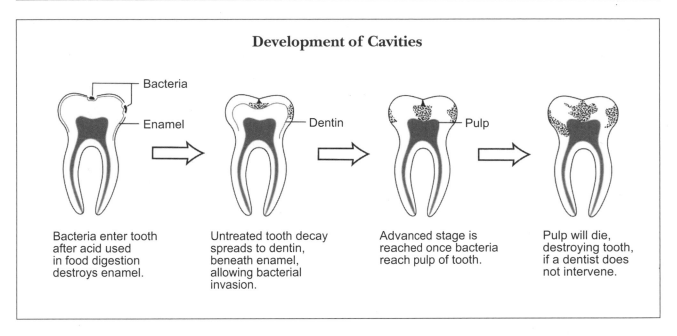

Development of Cavities

Bacteria enter tooth after acid used in food digestion destroys enamel.

Untreated tooth decay spreads to dentin, beneath enamel, allowing bacterial invasion.

Advanced stage is reached once bacteria reach pulp of tooth.

Pulp will die, destroying tooth, if a dentist does not intervene.

that the use of a toothpaste containing the herb sanguinaria (bloodroot) plus fluoride is more effective for cavity prevention than fluoride alone. Weak evidence hints at benefits with chewing gum that contains chitosan. Cranberry juice has also shown some promise, as has a special extract of hops called hop bracts polyphenols.

One study failed to find benefit through the use of calcium-rich chewing gum. Other natural treatments that have been proposed for preventing cavities, but that lack any meaningful scientific support, include black tea, myrrh, and propolis.

EBSCO CAM Review Board

FURTHER READING

Ly, K. A., et al. "Xylitol Gummy Bears Snacks." *BMC Oral Health* 8 (2008): 20.

Marinho, V. C., J. P. Higgins, and S. Logan et al. "Fluoride Mouthrinses for Preventing Dental Caries in Children and Adolescents." *Cochrane Database of Systematic Reviews* (2003): CD002284. Available through *EBSCO DynaMed Systematic Literature Surveillance* at http://www.ebscohost.com/dynamed.

Marinho, V. C., J. P. Higgins, and A. Sheiham et al. "Fluoride Toothpastes for Preventing Dental Caries in Children and Adolescents." *Cochrane Database of Systematic Reviews* (2003): CD002278. Available through *EBSCO DynaMed Systematic Literature Surveillance* at http://www.ebscohost.com/dynamed.

Nase, L., et al. "Effect of Long-Term Consumption of a Probiotic Bacterium, *Lactobacillus rhamnosus* GG, in Milk on Dental Caries and Caries Risk in Children." *Caries Research* 35 (2001): 412-420.

Nikawa, H., et al. "*Lactobacillus reuteri* in Bovine Milk Fermented Decreases the Oral Carriage of Mutans Streptococci." *International Journal of Food Microbiology* 95 (2004): 219-223.

Pizzo, G., et al. "Community Water Fluoridation and Caries Prevention." *Clinical Oral Investigations* 11 (2007): 189-193.

Schirrmeister, J. F., et al. "Effects of Various Forms of Calcium Added to Chewing Gum on Initial Enamel Carious Lesions In Situ." *Caries Research* 41 (2007): 108-114.

Soderling, E., et al. "Influence of Maternal Xylitol Consumption on Acquisition of Mutans Streptococci by Infants." *Journal of Dental Research* 79 (2000): 882-887.

See also: Canker sores; Fluoride; Xylitol.

Cayenne

CATEGORY: Herbs and supplements
RELATED TERMS: *Capsicum annuum, C. frutescens*
DEFINITION: Natural plant product used to treat specific health conditions.

PRINCIPAL PROPOSED USES:
- *Topical:* Osteoarthritis, peripheral neuropathy, post-herpetic neuralgia
- *Oral:* Dyspepsia

OTHER PROPOSED USES:
- *Topical:* Back pain, cluster headaches, fibromyalgia, nerve pain following surgery, psoriasis
- *Oral:* Protecting the stomach from ulcers caused by anti-inflammatory drugs

OVERVIEW

Cayenne and related peppers have a long history of use as digestive aids in many parts of the world, but the herb's recent popularity has come through conventional medicine. The capsicum family includes red peppers, bell peppers, pimento, and paprika, but the most famous medicinal member of this family is the common cayenne pepper.

REQUIREMENTS AND SOURCES

Many people think that hot peppers cause inflammation of tissues and that this is the source of the classic hot pepper sensation. However, hot peppers do not actually have any damaging effect; they merely simulate the sensations produced by damage. (Herbs such as garlic, ginger, horseradish, and mustard actually can cause tissue damage.)

THERAPEUTIC DOSAGES

Capsaicin creams are approved over-the-counter drugs and should be used as directed. If the burning sensation that occurs with initial use is too severe, using weaker forms of the cream at first may be advisable. For treatment of dyspepsia, cayenne may be taken at a dosage of 0.5 to 1.0 grams (g) three times daily (prior to meals).

THERAPEUTIC USES

All hot peppers contain a substance called capsaicin. When applied to tissues, capsaicin causes release of a chemical called substance P. Substance P is ordinarily released when tissues are damaged; it is part of the system the body uses to detect injury. When hot peppers artificially elicit the release of substance P, they trick the nervous system into thinking that an injury has occurred. The result: a sensation of burning pain.

When capsaicin is applied regularly to a part of the body, substance P becomes depleted in that location.

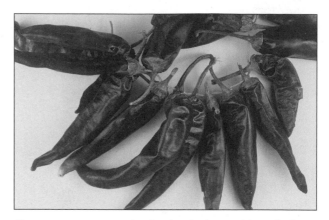

Cayenne peppers contain the chemical capsaicin, which has various medicinal uses. (Astrid and Hanns-Frieder Michler/Photo Researchers, Inc.)

This is why individuals who consume a lot of hot peppers gradually build up a tolerance.

It is also the basis for a number of medical uses of capsaicin. When levels of substance P are reduced in an area, all pain in that area is somewhat reduced. Because of this effect, capsaicin cream is widely used for the treatment of various painful conditions.

Under the brand name Zostrix, a cream containing concentrated capsaicin has been approved by the U.S. Food and Drug Administration for the treatment of post-herpetic neuralgia, the pain that often lingers after an attack of shingles. There is also relatively good evidence that topical capsaicin can modestly decrease the pain of diabetic peripheral neuropathy, other forms of peripheral neuropathy nerve pain following cancer surgery, as well as the pain of arthritis. Capsaicin cream may also be helpful for other forms of pain, including fibromyalgia, back pain, and cluster headaches. However, the benefits seen with capsaicin are seldom dramatic; in many cases, other pain-relieving treatments are used simultaneously. Besides pain-related conditions, some evidence indicates that topical capsaicin may be helpful for psoriasis and possibly other skin conditions as well (especially those that involve itching).

Cayenne can be taken internally as well. It appears that oral use of cayenne might reduce the pain of minor indigestion (dyspepsia). This may seem like an odd use of the herb; intuitively, it seems that hot peppers should be hard on the stomach. However, remember that hot peppers do not actually damage tissues; they merely produce sensations similar to those caused by actual damage. Apparently, by depleting substance P in the stomach, they reduce sensations of discomfort. In fact, some evidence suggests that oral use of cayenne or capsaicin can actually protect the stomach against ulcers caused by anti-inflammatory drugs. However, contrary to some reports, cayenne does not appear to be able to kill *Helicobacter pylori*, the stomach bacterium implicated as a major cause of ulcers. In addition, it appears that, contrary to long-standing belief, hot peppers do not cause increased pain in people with hemorrhoids.

SCIENTIFIC EVIDENCE

Oral uses of cayenne. In a double-blind, placebo-controlled study, thirty individuals with dyspepsia were given either 2.5 g daily of red pepper powder (divided up and taken prior to meals) or a placebo for five weeks. By the third week of treatment, individuals taking red pepper were experiencing significant improvements in pain, bloating, and nausea compared with a placebo, and these relative improvements lasted through the end of the study. A placebo-controlled, crossover study failed to find benefit, but it only enrolled eleven participants, far too few to have much chance of identifying a treatment effect.

Topical uses of cayenne. All double-blind studies of topical capsaicin (or cayenne) suffer from one drawback: It is not really possible to hide the burning sensation that occurs during initial use of the treatment. For this reason, such studies probably are not truly double-blind. It has been suggested that instead of an inactive placebo, researchers should use some other substance (such as camphor) that causes at least mild burning. However, such treatments might also have therapeutic benefits; they have a long history of use for pain as well. Because of these complications, the evidence for topical treatments cited here is less meaningful than it might at first appear.

Capsaicin cream is well established as a modestly helpful pain-relieving treatment for post-herpetic neuropathy (the pain that lingers after an attack of shingles), peripheral neuropathy (nerve pain that occurs most commonly as a complication of diabetes, but may occur with human immunodeficiency virus infection and other conditions), pain after surgery for cancer or hernia repair, and osteoarthritis.

Weaker evidence supports the use of topical capsaicin for fibromyalgia. Capsaicin instilled into the nose may be helpful for cluster headache.

Actual cayenne rather than capsaicin has been tested for pain as well. A three-week double-blind trial of 154 individuals with back pain found that cayenne applied topically as a "plaster" improved pain to a greater extent than a placebo.

A double-blind, placebo-controlled trial of nearly two hundred individuals found that use of topical capsaicin can improve itching as well as overall severity of psoriasis. Benefits were also seen in a smaller double-blind study of topical capsaicin for psoriasis. Topical capsaicin is thought to be helpful for various itchy skin conditions, such as prurigo nodularis, but double-blind studies are lacking.

Intranasal uses of cayenne. One study of 208 patients with idiopathic rhinitis found that using a capsicum nasal spray three times daily for three days (4 micrograms per puff) may reduce symptom frequency.

SAFETY ISSUES

Capsaicin creams commonly cause an unpleasant burning sensation when they are first applied; this sensation disappears over subsequent days as treatment is continued. As a commonly used food, cayenne is generally recognized as safe. Contrary to some reports, cayenne does not appear to aggravate stomach ulcers.

IMPORTANT INTERACTIONS

Cayenne might increase the amount of absorption of the asthma drug theophylline, possibly leading to toxic levels. However, cayenne might protect the stomach from damage caused by nonsteroidal anti-inflammatory drugs.

EBSCO CAM Review Board

FURTHER READING

Alper, B. S., and P. R. Lewis. "Treatment of Postherpetic Neuralgia: A Systematic Review of the Literature." *Journal of Family Practice* 51 (2002): 121-128.

Bortolotti, M., et al. "The Treatment of Functional Dyspepsia with Red Pepper." *Alimentary Pharmacology and Therapeutics* 16 (2002): 1075-1082.

Frerick, H., et al. "Topical Treatment of Chronic Low Back Pain with a Capsicum Plaster." *Pain* 106 (2003): 59-64.

Jensen, P. G., and J. R. Larson. "Management of Painful Diabetic Neuropathy." *Drugs and Aging* 18 (2001): 737-749.

McCleane, G. "Topical Application of Doxepin

Hydrochloride, Capsaicin, and a Combination of Both Produces Analgesia in Chronic Human Neuropathic Pain." *British Journal of Clinical Pharmacology* 49 (2000): 574-579.

Rodriguez-Stanley, S., et al. "The Effects of Capsaicin on Reflux, Gastric Emptying, and Dyspepsia." *Alimentary Pharmacology and Therapeutics* 14 (2000): 129-134.

Stander, S., T. Luger, and D. Metze. "Treatment of Prurigo Nodularis with Topical Capsaicin." *Journal of the American Academy of Dermatology* 44 (2001): 471-478.

Todd, C. "Meeting the Therapeutic Challenge of the Patient with Osteoarthritis." *Journal of the American Pharmaceutical Association* 42 (2002): 74-82.

See also: Dyspepsia; Gastrointestinal health; Herbal medicine; Osteoarthritis; Pain management.

Cephalosporins

CATEGORY: Drug interactions
DEFINITION: Class of antibiotics that work similarly to penicillin but have been chemically modified to have a broader spectrum of effect.
INTERACTION: Vitamin K
DRUGS IN THIS FAMILY: Cefadroxil (Duricef), cephalexin (Cefanex, Keflex, Keftab, Biocef), cephradine (Velosef), cefaclor (Ceclor, Ceclor CD), cefprozil (Cefzil), cefuroxime (Ceftin), loracarbef (Lorabid), cefdinir (Omnicef), cefixime (Suprax), cefpodoxime proxetil (Vantin), ceftibuten (Cedax)

VITAMIN K
Effect: Supplementation Possibly Helpful

Like all other antibiotics, cephalosporins might interfere with vitamin K levels by killing vitamin K-producing bacteria in the intestines. In addition, antibiotics in the cephalosporin family may also interfere with the way vitamin K works. For this reason, taking extra vitamin K may be a good idea when using cephalosporins over the long term.

EBSCO CAM Review Board

FURTHER READING
Shils, M., et al., eds. *Modern Nutrition in Health and Disease.* 9th ed. Baltimore: Williams and Wilkins, 1999.

See also: Antibiotics, general; Food and Drug Administration; Supplements: Introduction; Vitamin K; Vitamins and minerals.

Cervical dysplasia

CATEGORY: Condition
RELATED TERMS: Abnormal pap smear, abnormal pap test
DEFINITION: Treatment of the precancerous stages of cervical cancer.
PRINCIPAL PROPOSED NATURAL TREATMENTS: None
OTHER PROPOSED NATURAL TREATMENTS: Black cohosh, blessed thistle, dehydroepiandrosterone, diindolylmethane, emmenagogue herb, false unicorn, folate, indole-3-carbinol, motherwort, multivitamin-multimineral supplement, selenium, squaw vine, true unicorn

INTRODUCTION
Few cancers can be identified so far ahead of the danger point as cancer of the cervix. A decade or more before invasive cancer develops, the cells lining the surface of the cervix begin to show changes visible under a microscope–in plenty of time for definitive treatment. For this reason, a regular, properly performed and interpreted Pap test is one of medicine's most effective preventive methods.

The stages of progression from a healthy cervix to one that is cancerous begin with what is called mild dysplasia: precancerous alterations in structure and activity. Prolonged infection with human papilloma virus (HPV) is thought to be the primary cause of these changes. Subsequently, altered cells spread from the surface of the cervix down toward the underlying tissue. In the early stages, cancerous changes may disappear on their own, but once these cells fully penetrate the lining, progression to true cancer usually occurs within five to ten years.

Medical treatment consists of watchful waiting for spontaneous regression during the early stages of dysplasia and, if no regression occurs, more aggressive removal of the cervical lining by laser, freezing, or other techniques. These options are usually successful; however, they are invasive and frequently uncomfortable. The vaccine for preventing HPV infection is expected to also markedly reduce cervical cancer risk.

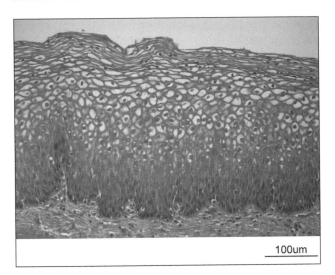

Microscopy of cervical dysplasia cells. (J. L. Carson/Getty Images)

PROPOSED NATURAL TREATMENTS

It has been claimed that certain natural herbs and supplements can improve the odds of early stages of dysplasia returning to normal cells. If a woman's physician suggests watchful waiting and a repeat examination, it should be safe to try some of these methods during the waiting period. There is, however, no reliable scientific evidence that these treatments are effective, and in all circumstances, close medical supervision is necessary to verify good results or to identify failure. Alternative treatment is definitely not advisable for advanced cervical dysplasia.

Folate deficiency is thought to increase the ease with which cervical cancer can develop. However, taking extra folate does not appear to reverse cervical dysplasia once it has occurred. Indole-3-carbinol (I3C) is a substance found in vegetables of the broccoli family. One small, double-blind, placebo-controlled trial found evidence that I3C at a dose of 200 or 400 milligrams (mg) per day can improve the chances of cervical dysplasia returning to normal by itself. The related substance diindolylmethane might also help.

Observational studies have found that women with cervical dysplasia tend to show a high frequency of general nutritional deficiencies, as high as 67 percent in one survey. Particular vitamin deficiencies most closely associated with cervical dysplasia include beta-carotene, vitamin C, vitamin B_6, selenium, and folate.

However, observational studies are notoriously unreliable; it is quite possible, for example, that people who do not eat healthily also have other risk factors for cervical dysplasia. Only double-blind, placebo-controlled studies can actually show a treatment effective, and these have not been promising. For example, a double-blind placebo-controlled study of 141 women found that neither vitamin C nor beta-carotene supplements taken daily in doses of 500 mg and 30 mg, respectively, could reverse cervical dysplasia. Negative results were also seen in studies that investigated beta-carotene by itself.

Some practitioners of herbal medicine feel that a class of herbs known as emmenagogues can be helpful in cervical dysplasia. These include squaw vine, motherwort, true unicorn, false unicorn, black cohosh, and blessed thistle. However, there is no meaningful scientific evidence to indicate that any of these herbs are effective for cervical dysplasia. Vaginal use of the hormone dehydroepiandrosterone has also been suggested for the treatment early cervical dysplasia, but no controlled studies have been reported.

EBSCO CAM Review Board

FURTHER READING

Bell, M. C., et al. Placebo-Controlled Trial of Indole-3-Carbinol in the Treatment of CIN." *Gynecological Oncology* 78 (2000): 123-129.

Keefe, K. A., et al. "A Randomized, Double Blind, Phase III Trial Using Oral Beta-Carotene Supplementation for Women with High-Grade Cervical Intraepithelial Neoplasia." *Cancer Epidemiology, Biomarkers, and Prevention* 10 (2001): 1029-1035.

Mackerras, D., et al. "Randomized Double-Blind Trial of Beta-Carotene and Vitamin C in Women with Minor Cervical Abnormalities." *British Journal of Cancer* 79 (1999): 1448-1453.

Suh-Burgmann, E., et al. "Long-Term Administration of Intravaginal Dehydroepiandrosterone on Regression of Low-Grade Cervical Dysplasia." *Gynecologic and Obstetric Investigation* 55 (2003): 25-31.

Zoorob, J. R. "CAM and Women's Health: Selected Topics." *Primary Care* 37, no. 2 (2010): 367-387.

See also: Amenorrhea; Beta-carotene; Cancer risk reduction; Cancer treatment support; Dysmenorrhea; Folate; Indole-3-carbinol; Vaginal infection; Women's health.

Cetylated fatty acids

CATEGORY: Herbs and supplements
PRINCIPAL PROPOSED USE: Osteoarthritis
OTHER PROPOSED USE: Psoriasis

OVERVIEW

In 2004, a special mixture of fats called cetylated fatty acids began to be widely marketed as a treatment for osteoarthritis. Although the claims associated with this product appear to exceed what has actually been proven, it is fair to say that cetylated fatty acids have shown definite promise in preliminary trials.

REQUIREMENTS AND SOURCES

There is no dietary requirement for cetylated fatty acids.

THERAPEUTIC DOSAGES

Cetylated fatty acids are used both orally and as a topical cream. A typical oral dose of cetylated fatty acids is 1,000 to 2,000 milligrams daily. Cetylated fatty acid creams are applied two to four times daily to the affected area.

THERAPEUTIC USES

Three double-blind, placebo-controlled studies have found cetylated fatty acids helpful for osteoarthritis. Two involved a topical product, and one used an oral formulation.

In one study using a cream, forty people with osteoarthritis of the knee applied either cetylated fatty acids or a placebo to the affected joint. The results over thirty days showed greater improvements in range of motion and functional ability among people using the real cream than among those using the placebo cream. In another thirty-day study, also enrolling forty people with knee arthritis, use of cetylated fatty acid cream improved postural stability, presumably because of decreased pain levels.

In addition, a sixty-eight-day double-blind, placebo-controlled study of sixty-four people with knee arthritis tested an oral cetylated fatty acid supplement (the supplement also contained lesser amounts of lecithin and fish oil.) Participants in the treatment group experienced improvements in swelling, mobility, and pain level compared with those in the placebo group. Inexplicably, the study report does not discuss whether side effects occurred.

Although this is a promising body of research, it is far from definitive. Current advertising claims for cetylated fatty acids go far beyond the existing evidence. For example, a number of Web sites claim that cetylated fatty acids are more effective than glucosamine or chondroitin. However, no comparison studies have been performed upon which such a claim could be rationally based.

It is not known how cetylated fatty acids might help osteoarthritis. Proponents cite the known benefits of fish oil for rheumatoid arthritis, but since the fatty acids in fish oil are rather different from those in cetylated fatty acids, and the origin of rheumatoid arthritis is quite unlike that of osteoarthritis, there is little relevance to these observations. Proponents also make multiple specific claims, including that cetylated fatty acids reduce inflammation, protect cartilage from damage, lubricate cell membranes, and increase fluid in joints. However, none of these explanations have more than speculative scientific support. If cetylated fatty acids do help osteoarthritis, their mechanism is not known. Cetylated fatty acid creams have also been proposed for treatment of psoriasis.

SAFETY ISSUES

Cetylated fatty acids appear to have a low level of toxicity, according to safety studies conducted by the primary manufacturer. However, maximum safe doses in young children, pregnant or nursing women, and people with severe liver or kidney disease have not been established.

EBSCO CAM Review Board

FURTHER READING

Hesslink, R. Jr., et al. "Cetylated Fatty Acids Improve Knee Function in Patients with Osteoarthritis." *Journal of Rheumatology* 29 (2002): 1708-1712.

Kraemer, W. J., et al. "Effects of Treatment with a Cetylated Fatty Acid Topical Cream on Static Postural Stability and Plantar Pressure Distribution in Patients with Knee Osteoarthritis." *Journal of Strength and Conditioning Research* 19 (2005): 115-121.

See also: Chondroitin; Fish oil; Glucosamine; Herbal medicine; Osteoarthritis.

Chamomile

CATEGORY: Herbs and supplements
RELATED TERMS: *Chamaemelum nobile, Matricaria recutita*
DEFINITION: Natural plant product used to treat specific health conditions.
PRINCIPAL PROPOSED USES: Skin inflammation (eczema, skin inflammation caused by radiation therapy)
OTHER PROPOSED USES: Digestive upset, mouth sores caused by chemotherapy, tension, and stress

OVERVIEW

Two distinct plants known as chamomile are used interchangeably: German and Roman chamomile. Although distantly related botanically, they both look like miniature daisies and are traditionally thought to possess similar medicinal benefits.

More than one million cups of chamomile tea are drunk daily, testifying, at least, to its good taste. Chamomile was used by early Egyptian physicians for fevers, and by ancient Greeks, Romans, and Indians for headaches and disorders of the kidneys, liver, and bladder.

The modern use of chamomile dates back to 1921, when a German firm introduced a topical form. This cream became a popular treatment for a wide variety of skin disorders, including eczema, bedsores, skin inflammation caused by radiation therapy, and contact dermatitis (from poison ivy).

THERAPEUTIC DOSAGES

Chamomile cream is applied to the affected area one to four times daily. Chamomile tea can be made by pouring boiling water over 2 to 3 heaping teaspoons of flowers and steeping for ten minutes. Chamomile tinctures and pills should be taken according to the directions on the label. Alcoholic tincture may be the most potent form for internal use.

THERAPEUTIC USES

Germany's Commission E authorizes the use of topical chamomile preparations for a variety of diseases of the skin and mouth. Chamomile tea is also said to reduce mild tension and stress and to aid indigestion.

SCIENTIFIC EVIDENCE

There is no reliable evidence that chamomile is effective for the treatment of any health condition.

Skin diseases. A controlled study of 161 individuals found chamomile cream just as effective as 0.25

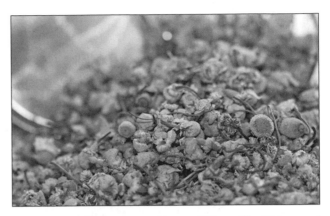

Dried chamomile flowers used in tea. (©Jennifer Pitiquen/ Dreamstime.com)

percent hydrocortisone cream for the treatment of eczema. However, this study did not use a placebo group and does not appear to have been double-blind. For this reason, the results are not reliable.

A study of seventy-two individuals with eczema found somewhat odd results. In this trial, chamomile was not significantly more effective than placebo, but both were better than 0.5 percent hydrocortisone cream. It is difficult to interpret what these paradoxical results actually mean, but they certainly cannot be taken as proof that chamomile cream is effective.

In a double-blind study, chamomile cream proved less effective for reducing inflammation of the skin than hydrocortisone cream or witch hazel cream. Finally, in a single-blind trial, fifty women receiving radiation therapy for breast cancer were treated with either chamomile or placebo. Chamomile failed to prove superior to a placebo for preventing skin inflammation caused by the radiation therapy.

Mouth sores. A double-blind, placebo-controlled trial of 164 individuals did not find chamomile mouthwash effective for treating the mouth sores caused by chemotherapy with the drug 5-FU.

SAFETY ISSUES

Chamomile is listed on the U.S. Food and Drug Administrations's generally recognized as safe (GRAS) list. Reports that chamomile can cause severe reactions in people allergic to ragweed have received significant media attention. However, when all the evidence is examined, it does not appear that chamomile is actually more allergenic than any other plant. The cause of these reports may be products contaminated with "dog chamomile," a highly allergenic and bad-tasting plant of similar appearance.

Chamomile also contains naturally occurring coumarin compounds that might act as blood thinners under certain circumstances. There is one case report in which it appears that the use of chamomile combined with the anticoagulant warfarin led to excessive blood thinning, resulting in internal bleeding. Some evidence suggests that chamomile might interact with other medications as well through effects on drug metabolism, but the extent of this effect has not been fully determined.

Safety in young children, pregnant or nursing women, and those with liver or kidney disease has not been established, although there have not been any credible reports of toxicity caused by this common beverage tea.

IMPORTANT INTERACTIONS

Chamomile may increase the effect of blood-thinning medications such as warfarin (Coumadin), heparin, clopidogrel (Plavix), ticlopidine (Ticlid), or pentoxifylline (Trental), potentially causing problems.

EBSCO CAM Review Board

FURTHER READING

Budzinski, J. W., et al. "An In Vitro Evaluation of Human Cytochrome P450 3A4 Inhibition by Selected Commercial Herbal Extracts and Tinctures." *Phytomedicine* 7 (2000): 273-282.

Patzelt-Wenczler, R., and E. Ponce-Poschl. "Proof of Efficacy of KamillosanW Cream in Atopic Eczema." *European Journal of Medical Research* 5 (2000): 171-175.

Segal, R., and L. Pilote. "Warfarin Interaction with *Matricaria chamomilla.*" *Canadian Medical Association Journal* 174 (2006): 1281-1282.

See also: Dyspepsia; Herbal medicine.

Chaparral

CATEGORY: Herbs and supplements
RELATED TERMS: Creosote bush, *Larrea tridentate*
DEFINITION: Natural plant product used to treat specific health conditions.
PRINCIPAL PROPOSED USES: None

OVERVIEW

Chaparral is a tough plant with a long history of medicinal use by the indigenous peoples of North America. Traditionally, it was taken internally to treat joint pain and to eliminate worms. Chaparral tea was applied externally to painful joints and minor wounds and also used as a mouthwash and hair rinse. When European herbalists encountered chaparral, they initially used it to treat colds, flu, and intestinal infections. Later, based on a number of unsubstantiated cases, chaparral gained a reputation as a miracle cancer cure. There are a number of reports in which it appears that internal use of chaparral has caused serious liver injury.

THERAPEUTIC DOSAGES

The internal use of chaparral is not recommended. For external use, chaparral may be prepared as a tea or allowed to diffuse its contents into oil over several days or weeks. The resulting preparation is then applied in the form of a wet or oil-soaked cloth.

THERAPEUTIC USES

There are no scientifically established medicinal uses of chaparral, and reports of liver injury have made it substantially less popular in recent years. The presumed active ingredient in chaparral is the antioxidant compound nordihydroguaiaretic acid (NDGA). NDGA is used as a preservative in packaged and processed foods. Some evidence from animal and test-tube studies hints that NGDA, or synthetic chemicals related to it, might have anticancer effects. However, the same can be said of thousands of substances. So far, NGDA and its analogues have not shown themselves promising enough to warrant human trials.

Other proposed actions of chaparral and its constituents lack more than the most minimal of scientific evidence. These include anti-inflammatory, antimicrobial, and liver-protective effects.

SAFETY ISSUES

Considerable confusion exists regarding the safety of chaparral. Chaparral itself does not appear to be toxic even when given to animals in very high doses. In particular, it does not appear to contain any liver toxins. Nonetheless, there have been recurrent reports of severe liver or kidney injury associated with use of the herb. While in some of these cases cause and effect was poorly established, in others the connection seems clear.

Almost all reports involved chaparral tablets or extracts rather than the more traditional tea; however, the significance of this distinction is not clear. It is quite likely, though not proven, that the liver or kidney toxicity is an "idiosyncratic reaction," something in the nature of a rare allergy. However, until this situation is cleared up, internal use of chaparral should be regarded as presenting unknown risks. Because chaparral has no established benefits, it is probably best to avoid it.

EBSCO CAM Review Board

FURTHER READING

Chen, J. H., et al. "A Novel Lipoxygenase Inhibitor Nordy Attenuates Malignant Human Glioma Cell Responses to Chemotactic and Growth Stimulating Factors." *Journal of Neuro-Oncology* 84, no. 3 (2007): 223-231.

Kauma, H., et al. "Toxic Acute Hepatitis and Hepatic Fibrosis After Consumption of Chaparral Tablets." *Scandinavian Journal of Gastroenterology* 39 (2004): 1168-1171.

Meyer, G. E., et al. "Nordihydroguaiaretic Acid Inhibits Insulin-like Growth Factor Signaling, Growth, and Survival in Human Neuroblastoma Cells." *Journal of Cellular Biochemistry* 102, no. 6 (2007): 1529-1549.

Ping, Y. F., et al. "The Anti-cancer Compound Nordy Inhibits CXCR4-Mediated Production of IL-8 and VEGF by Malignant Human Glioma Cells." *Journal of Neuro-Oncology* 84, no. 1 (2007): 21-29.

Zavodovskaya, M., et al. "Nordihydroguaiaretic Acid (NDGA), an Inhibitor of the HER2 and IGF-1 Receptor Tyrosine Kinases, Blocks the Growth of HER2-Overexpressing Human Breast Cancer Cells." *Journal of Cellular Biochemistry* 103, no. 2 (2008): 624-635.

See also: Herbal medicine.

Charaka

CATEGORY: Biography
ALSO KNOWN AS: Cakara
IDENTIFICATION: Indian physician and a principal practitioner of Ayurvedic medicine
BORN: 300 B.C.E.; India
DIED: Unknown

OVERVIEW

Charaka, an Indian physician also considered the founder of Indian medicine and of anatomy, was a primary contributor to the ancient Indian practice of Ayurveda, a set a healing practices involving medicine and lifestyle. This alternative medicine system is grounded in metaphysics and involves the intentional balance of three "energies," which are often referred to as wind, bile, and phlegm, to sustain a healthy lifestyle. Ayurveda is a fairly integrative technique that involves exercise, diet, yoga, and meditation.

According to translations of Charaka's writings, Charaka thought that neither health nor disease was predetermined, and that intentionally making certain lifestyle choices could prolong a person's life. In line with Ayurveda, his philosophies were rooted in the idea that prevention of disease was primary. In one of his books, Charaka indicated that his medical philosophy was based on the principle that a physician who treats a patient blindly (without considering the patient's various life details) will fail to effectively treat the person's disease. Instead, he thought that a physician should consider all factors associated with the person, including his or her environment, and then customize treatment accordingly. Moreover, Charaka recognized the importance of preventive medicine and thought more emphasis should be placed on this aspect of human health, rather than on curing already present ailments.

Charaka is believed to be the first doctor to discuss the concepts of metabolism and immunities—but in premature terms. According to translations of one of his books, he speculated that the human body functions because it contains certain energies that are produced when the *dhatus* (blood, flesh, and marrow) interact with the food that a person ingests. Related to metabolism, he indicated that even if different persons eat the same amount of food, their bodies respond to the food differently, which serves to explain the broad spectrum of human body size and shape. Regarding immunity, he believed that illness was caused by a person having imbalanced energies. He administered various natural preparations to overcome health issues, in addition to prescribing other interventions, including amendment of a person's diet and exercise regimen.

Charaka spent much time investigating anatomy. In particular, he theorized about the number of bones in the human body and about the makeup of various bodily organs. Although his ideas on such issues were, by modern standards, flawed, the ideas were ahead of their time and inspired many physicians and academics thereafter.

Charaka also is credited with understanding some basic genetic principles that are now taken for granted, such as that some defects in newborns are caused not by obvious health defects or disorders in the parents, but instead by problems in the fertilized egg of the mother or in the sperm of the father.

Brandy Weidow, M.S.

FURTHER READING

Gerson, Scott. *Ayurveda: The Ancient Healing Art.* 2d ed. Colfax, Wash.: Cougar Graphics, 2001.

Ninivaggi, Frank John. *Ayurveda: A Comprehensive Guide to Traditional Indian Medicine for the West.* Westport, Conn.: Praeger, 2008.

See also: Ayurveda; Chopra, Deepak; Diet-based therapies; Traditional healing; Whole medicine; Yoga.

Chasteberry

CATEGORY: Herbs and supplements
RELATED TERMS: *Agnus-castus, vitex*
DEFINITION: Natural plant product used to treat specific health conditions.
PRINCIPAL PROPOSED USES: Cyclic breast discomfort (often associated with premenstrual syndrome, or PMS), other PMS symptoms
OTHER PROPOSED USES: Amenorrhea, female infertility, irregular menstruation, menopausal symptoms

OVERVIEW

Chasteberry is frequently called by its Latin name *vitex* or, alternatively, *agnus-castus*. A shrub in the Verbena family, chasteberry is commonly found on riverbanks and nearby foothills in central Asia and around the Mediterranean Sea. After its violet flowers have bloomed, a dark brown, peppercorn-size fruit with a pleasant odor reminiscent of peppermint develops. This fruit is used medicinally.

As the name implies, for centuries chasteberry was thought to counter sexual desire. A drink prepared from the plant's seeds was used by the Romans to diminish libido, and in ancient Greece, young women

celebrating the festival of Demeter wore chasteberry blossoms to show that they were remaining chaste in honor of the goddess. Monks in the Middle Ages used the fruit for similar purposes, yielding the common name "monk's pepper."

THERAPEUTIC DOSAGES

The typical dose of dry chasteberry extract is 20 milligrams taken one to three times daily. Chasteberry is also sold as a liquid extract to be taken at a dosage of 40 drops each morning. However, extracts that require lower or higher dosing are also available.

THERAPEUTIC USES

The modern use of chasteberry dates to the 1950s, when the German pharmaceutical firm Madaus first produced a standardized extract. This herb has become a standard European treatment for cyclic breast tenderness, a condition related to premenstrual syndrome (PMS) that is sometimes called cyclic mastitis, cyclic mastalgia, mastodynia, or fibrocystic breast disease. Chasteberry also appears to be useful for general PMS symptoms.

Chasteberry is believed to work by suppressing the release of prolactin from the pituitary gland. Prolactin is a hormone that naturally rises during pregnancy to stimulate milk production. Inappropriately increased production of prolactin may be a factor in cyclic breast tenderness, as well as other symptoms of PMS.

Elevated prolactin levels can also cause a woman's period to become irregular and even stop. For this reason, chasteberry is sometimes tried when

---

Chasteberry: Side Effects and Cautions

Chasteberry has not been associated with serious side effects. However, it can cause gastrointestinal problems, acne-like rashes, and dizziness.

Chasteberry may affect certain hormone levels. Women who are pregnant, who are taking birth control pills, or who have a hormone-sensitive condition (such as breast cancer) should not use chasteberry.

Because chasteberry may affect the dopamine system in the brain, people taking dopamine-related medications, such as certain antipsychotic drugs and Parkinson's disease medications, should avoid using chasteberry.

menstruation is irregular or stops altogether (amenorrhea). Persons should not attempt to self-treat significant menstrual irregularities without a full medical evaluation. Serious medical conditions could result.

High prolactin levels can also cause infertility in women. For this reason, chasteberry is sometimes tried as a fertility drug; however, the two double-blind studies performed to evaluate this possible use failed to return statistically significant results. Finally, chasteberry is sometimes used for menopausal symptoms, but there is as yet no evidence that it is effective, either alone or in combination with other herbs.

SCIENTIFIC EVIDENCE

There is a growing body of scientific research supporting the use of chasteberry.

Cyclic mastalgia. A double-blind, placebo-controlled trial of ninety-seven women with symptoms of cyclic mastalgia found that treatment with chasteberry extract significantly reduced pain intensity by the end of one menstrual cycle. The reduction continued to increase throughout the second menstrual cycle, and at the end of both the first and the second cycle, women in the treated group were doing better than those receiving a placebo.

However, in the third cycle, the benefits of chasteberry treatment reached a plateau, while the placebo group continued to improve. At the end of the third cycle, those receiving chasteberry were still doing better, but the difference was no longer statistically significant.

Another double-blind trial of 104 women compared a placebo against two forms of chasteberry (liquid and tablet) for at least three menstrual cycles. The results showed statistically significant and comparable improvements in the treated groups, compared with a placebo.

Benefits were also seen in a double-blind trial that enrolled 160 women with cyclic breast pain. The women were given either chasteberry, a drug related to progesterone, or a placebo, and were followed for at least four menstrual cycles. Although there were many dropouts, the results again suggest that chasteberry is superior to a placebo.

Premenstrual syndrome (PMS). A double-blind, placebo-controlled study of 178 women found that treatment with chasteberry over three menstrual cycles significantly reduced general PMS symptoms. The dose used was one tablet three times daily of a dry

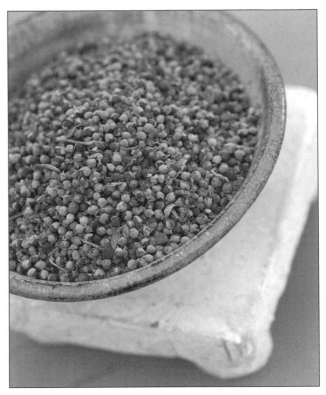

Chasteberry appears to be useful for general premenstrual syndrome (PMS) symptoms (©Antaratma Images/Dreamstime.com)

chasteberry extract. Women in the treatment group experienced significant improvements in symptoms, including irritability, depression, headache, and breast tenderness. In a similar study, 217 women with moderate to severe PMS were randomized to receive chasteberry extract or placebo. After three menstrual cycles, the women in the treatment group reported fewer symptoms. A smaller trial involving 67 women also reported on the effectiveness of chasteberry for PMS. Chasteberry in combination with St. John's wort was also studied for PMS symptoms during late menopause with favorable results in at least one small trial.

There is also some conflicting evidence, though. A double-blind trial compared chasteberry to vitamin B_6 (pyridoxine) instead of a placebo. The two treatments proved equally effective. However, because vitamin B_6 itself has not been shown effective for PMS, these results mean little.

Two other studies are often cited in support of chasteberry as a treatment for PMS. These were rather informal reports of a total of about three thousand women with PMS given chasteberry by their physicians. The physicians rated chasteberry as effective about 90 percent of the time, but in the absence of a control group, these reports are not very meaningful.

Irregular menstruation. One double-blind trial followed fifty-two women with a form of irregular menstruation known as luteal phase defect. This condition is believed to be related to excessive prolactin release. After three months, the women who took chasteberry showed significant improvements.

SAFETY ISSUES

There have not been any detailed studies of the safety of chasteberry. However, its widespread use in Germany has not led to any reports of significant adverse effects, other than a single case of excessive ovarian stimulation possibly caused by chasteberry.

Because it lowers prolactin levels, chasteberry is not an appropriate treatment for pregnant or nursing women. Safety in young children or those with severe liver or kidney disease has not been established.

There are no known drug interactions associated with chasteberry. However, it is quite conceivable that the herb could interfere with hormones or medications that affect the pituitary gland. Chasteberry may interfere with the action of hormones or drugs that affect the pituitary.

EBSCO CAM Review Board

FURTHER READING

Halaska, M., et al. "Treatment of Cyclical Mastalgia with a Solution Containing a *Vitex agnus castus* Extract." *Breast* 8 (1999): 175-181.

He, Z., et al. "Treatment for Premenstrual Syndrome with *Vitex agnus castus*: A Prospective, Randomized, Multi-center Placebo Controlled Study in China." *Maturitas* 63, no. 1 (2009): 99-103.

Ma, L., et al. "Evaluating Therapeutic Effect in Symptoms of Moderate-to-Severe Premenstrual Syndrome with *Vitex agnus castus* (BNO 1095) in Chinese Women." *Australian and New Zealand Journal of Obstetrics and Gynaecology* 50, no. 2 (2010): 189-193.

Schellenberg, R. "Treatment for the Premenstrual Syndrome with *Agnus castus* Fruit Extract." *British Medical Journal* 322 (2001): 134-137.

Van Die, M. D., et al. "Effects of a Combination of *Hypericum perforatum* and *Vitex agnus-castus* on PMS-like Symptoms in Late-Perimenopausal Women: Findings from a Subpopulation Analysis." *Journal of Alternative and Complementary Medicine* 15, no. 9 (2009): 1045-1048.

See also: Breast pain, cyclic; Dysmenorrhea; Herbal medicine; Infertility, female; Menopausal symptoms; Premenstrual syndrome (PMS); Women's health.

Chelation therapy

CATEGORY: Therapies and techniques
RELATED TERM: Ethylenediaminetetraacetic acid chelation
DEFINITION: Therapy for heart disease using ethylenediaminetetraacetic acid, a synthetic substance that removes calcium and heavy metals from the body.

OVERVIEW

When medical researchers first investigated the phenomenon known as hardening of the arteries (closely related to atherosclerosis), they discovered that the damaged, brittle vessels found in people with heart disease were lined with calcium deposits. This finding inspired the notion that calcium deposits were the cause of the problem.

Some early researchers investigated the possible therapeutic effect of removing such deposits. However, subsequent research indicated that the calcium deposits of atherosclerosis were a symptom rather than a cause, and mainstream interest turned elsewhere. Certain physicians nonetheless maintained an interest in removing calcium; thus, chelation therapy was born.

Chelation therapy for heart disease consists of intravenous infusions of a chemical called ethylenediaminetetraacetic acid (EDTA). This synthetic substance is used in conventional medicine to remove heavy metals, such as lead, from the body, but it also has an effect on calcium, which is why it came into use in chelation therapy.

Proponents claim that EDTA chelation is an effective alternative to heart surgery and that it also offers many other health benefits. To support these claims, proponents cite numerous anecdotes of cures apparently brought about by its use. However, anecdotes cannot possibly prove a treatment effective. Only double-blind, placebo-controlled trials can do so, and such studies have failed to find chelation therapy effective.

In 2000, a highly respected researcher reviewed the literature on chelation therapy and concluded that

> The most striking finding is the almost total lack of convincing evidence for efficacy. . . . Only 2 controlled clinical trials were located. They provide no evidence that chelation therapy is efficacious beyond a powerful placebo effect. . . . Given the potential of chelation therapy to cause severe adverse effects, this treatment should now be considered obsolete.

Subsequent to this review, a well-designed study compared chelation therapy to placebo in eighty-four people with coronary artery disease. People receiving EDTA chelation showed improvement; however, those receiving placebo also improved, and did so to the same extent. This finding is a reminder of why double-blind, placebo-controlled studies are necessary to establish the effectiveness of a treatment. If researchers had performed this study without a placebo group, they might have concluded that EDTA chelation really works. Instead, the fact that the same level of benefits was seen in the fake-treatment group indicates that chelation therapy does not work.

Another double-blind study evaluated the potential benefits of chelation therapy when added to conventional therapy in the treatment of people with coronary artery disease. Researchers were looking for improvements in the ability of a blood vessel in the arm (the brachial artery) to dilate, but they did not find any. However, this study had several limitations in its design, making its results less meaningful than they might have been.

Safety Issues

EDTA chelation not only appears to be ineffective; it also may present some safety risks. This treatment is generally given in a series of ten to thirty sessions. If the practitioner fails to take proper precautions, severe adverse consequences, such as kidney damage, may result. While it appears to be the case that properly performed chelation therapy is unlikely to cause harm, there is no justification for using such an invasive method in the absence of evidence that it will help.

EBSCO CAM Review Board

Further Reading

Anderson, T. J., et al. "Effect of Chelation Therapy on Endothelial Function in Patients with Coronary Artery Disease." *Journal of the American College of Cardiology* 41 (2003): 420-425.

Ernst, E. "Chelation Therapy for Coronary Heart Disease: An Overview of All Clinical Investigations." *American Heart Journal* 140 (2000): 4-5.

Knudtson, M. L., et al. "Chelation Therapy for Ischemic Heart Disease." *Journal of the American Medical Association* 287 (2002): 481-486.

See also: Atherosclerosis and heart disease prevention; Congestive heart failure; Heart attack; Hypertension.

Cherries

Category: Functional foods
Related terms: Cherry juice, *Prunus avium*
Definition: A food consumed for specific health benefits.
Principal proposed uses: None
Other proposed uses: Antioxidant, gout, pain relief, sports and fitness

Overview

Cherries and cherry juice have a long history of use in food and cooking all over the world. Mention of cherries can be found in the literature of the ancient Chinese, Greeks, and South Asians.

Medicinally, cherries have been used for a variety of pain-related conditions, including arthritis, gout, back pain, and tendon injuries. It is often said that tart cherries have more medicinal value than sweet cherries.

Uses and Applications

Tart cherries contain relatively high levels of substances known as anthocyanins, which are also found in bilberry, cranberry, and other foods. Anthocyanins are antioxidants, and most health claims for cherries are based on this fact. However, the case that antioxidants provide health benefits has become weaker rather than stronger, and therefore, merely finding antioxidant content in cherries is inadequate to show benefit. Only double-blind, placebo-controlled studies can actually provide evidence of efficacy, and

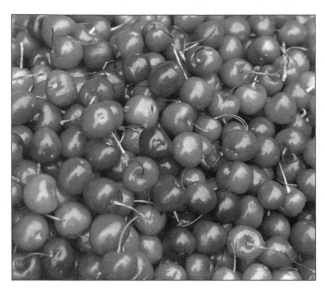

Medicinally, cherries have been used for a number of pain-related conditions. (©Lieska/Dreamstime.com)

for cherries, only one small study of this type has been reported.

In this study, fourteen male athletes were given either tart cherry juice (12 ounces) or placebo twice daily before performing intensive arm exercises. The results of this trial indicated that the use of cherry juice reduced pain and strength loss caused by the excessive exercise. Based on this, it has been suggested that cherry juice might be helpful for athletes in training by enhancing recovery from heavy exercise, because of its antioxidant actions. However, this was a very small study, and more research would be necessary to actually document benefit. Other antioxidants have failed to prove helpful for this purpose.

Cherries are also claimed to be helpful for gout, based primarily on a single study performed in the 1950s. However, this study was far too poorly designed to prove anything, because it did not utilize a placebo group. A much later study did find some evidence that cherry consumption might lower levels of urate in the blood. Because high levels of urate are associated with gout, this finding does provide some suggestive evidence that cherries might be helpful. However, this study was small, preliminary, and somewhat poorly designed. Furthermore, it does not directly show benefit: Many substances reduce urate levels but do not help gout, and many cases of gout are

not associated with elevated urate. One animal study hints that the anthocyanins in tart cherries may have general pain-relieving and anti-inflammatory properties.

DOSAGE

For use in reducing pain after intensive exercise, a dose of 12 ounces of cherry juice twice daily has been tested in the small study noted. A typical dosage recommendation for gout is one-half pound of whole cherries daily.

SAFETY ISSUES

As a widely consumed food, cherries are presumed to have a high level of safety. However, maximum safe doses in pregnant or nursing women, young children, and people with severe liver or kidney disease have not been determined.

EBSCO CAM Review Board

FURTHER READING

Connolly, D. A., et al. "Efficacy of a Tart Cherry Juice Blend in Preventing the Symptoms of Muscle Damage." *British Journal of Sports Medicine* 40 (2006): 679-683.

Ferretti, G., et al. "Cherry Antioxidants: From Farm to Table." *Molecules* 15 (2010): 6993-7005.

Jacob, R. A., et al. "Consumption of Cherries Lowers Plasma Urate in Healthy Women." *Journal of Nutrition* 133 (2003): 1826-1829.

See also: Antioxidant; Functional foods: Introduction; Gout; Sports and fitness support: Enhancing performance.

Childbirth support: Homeopathic remedies

CATEGORY: Homeopathy

DEFINITION: The use of highly diluted remedies to alleviate unpleasant and painful symptoms of labor and childbirth.

STUDIED HOMEOPATHIC REMEDIES: *Arnica montana*; *Caulophyllum*; belladonna; *Cimicifuga*; homeopathic remedy containing *Arnica, Caulophyllum, Actea racemosa, Pulsatilla,* and *Gelsemium*

INTRODUCTION

Medical advances have made childbirth safer, but it remains a painful and difficult experience for most women. Homeopathy has shown some promise for alleviating the challenges of giving birth.

SCIENTIFIC EVALUATIONS OF HOMEOPATHIC REMEDIES

A double-blind, placebo-controlled trial involving ninety-three pregnant women evaluated the effectiveness of a combination remedy consisting of *Arnica, Caulophyllum, Actea racemosa, Pulsatilla,* and *Gelsemium,* each at a potency of 5c (centesimals). For the women receiving treatment, the duration of labor was decreased by an average of about 3.5 hours compared with placebo. Furthermore, only 11.3 percent of women given the homeopathic remedy experienced difficult labor, versus 40 percent in the placebo group. However, a double-blind pilot study of 161 women that evaluated the effectiveness of *Arnica montana* D6 alone versus placebo failed to find benefit.

TRADITIONAL HOMEOPATHIC TREATMENTS

Classical homeopathy offers many possible homeopathic treatments for childbirth support. These therapies are chosen based on various specific characteristics of the woman seeking treatment.

Homeopathic *Caulophyllum* is a common homeopathic remedy in childbirth. Although *Caulophyllum* is made from the toxic herb blue cohosh, it is safe when given at homeopathic potencies. The symptom picture of this remedy includes a history of irregular menstruation and previous difficult deliveries, including sharp needle-like pains occurring during labor; trembling; nervousness; and a sense of uterine weakness.

Belladonna is traditionally used for women in labor exhibiting delirious agitation, confusion, flushing, and fever. The classic symptom picture of *Cimicifuga* includes painful spasms that travel a long distance, deep sighs, and gloominess expressed by statements that labor will be impossible to complete.

EBSCO CAM Review Board

FURTHER READING

Gregg, D. "Like Cures Like: Homeopathy for Labor and Birth." *Midwifery Today with International Midwife* 95 (2010): 13-16, 64.

Hofmeyr, G. J., V. Piccioni, and P. Blauhof. "Postpartum Homoeopathic *Arnica montana:* A Potency-Finding Pilot Study." *British Journal of Clinical Practice* 44 (1990): 619-621.

Smith, C. A. "Homoeopathy for Induction of Labour." *Cochrane Database of Systematic Reviews* (2003): CD003399. Available through EBSCO DynaMed Systematic Literature Surveillance at http://www.ebscohost.com/dynamed.

Steen, M., and J. Calvert. "Homeopathy for Childbirth: Remedies and Research." *RCM Midwives* 9 (2006): 438-440.

See also: Breast-feeding support; Homeopathy; Women's health.

Childbirth techniques

CATEGORY: Therapies and techniques
RELATED TERMS: Birth assistant, doula, water-birthing
DEFINITION: Alternative and complementary techniques and methods to aid in labor and childbirth.

OVERVIEW

With the growing openness of medical staff to complementary and alternative therapies, now often called integrative medicine, mothers-to-be are investigating and choosing new options for delivering their babies. So many parents elect nontraditional paths that "what used to be alternative is now the norm," says Loma Ellis, nursing manager for California's Alameda Hospital Birthing Center. As a result, parents now have more birthing choices than ever before.

BIRTH ASSISTANCE

A birth assistant, or doula, is a professional person hired privately by parents to attend their child's birth. A doula serves as a support and coach for the laboring woman. The doula does not replace the role of the pregnant woman's partner and is not a member of the health care team. The doula is present solely to attend the laboring woman. Usually highly trained in childbirth, a doula can serve as a stand-in when a pregnant woman's partner is not available. However, many parents hire doulas even if a partner is present.

"The doula is a safety net," says Sandi Miller, owner of Before Birth and Beyond in San Jose, California. "Whatever happens, whether it's a cesarean or whatever, the parents know what's going on and the doula is watching out for them."

Studies show that doulas, whose services start at $100 on average for a doula-in-training and can go as high as $1,000 or more, have positive medical effects on both mother and newborn. A study published in the *British Medical Journal* suggests that the employment of doulas results in fewer cesareans and shorter labors and in a lower admission rate to neonatal intensive care for infants. A review found that continuous support by a doula reduces anxiety, shortens labor, decreases the need for cesarean deliveries and other forms of assisted birth, and reduces rates of postpartum depression.

WATER-BIRTHING

Water can smooth away aches and drain off tension. Women who labor or deliver (or both) their babies in a birthing pool report less pain and greater relaxation. According to the Israeli medical journal *Harefuah*, water-birthing women are more relaxed and comfortable; water immersion may also speed the dilation of the cervix, leading to a shorter labor. The following benefits also may be passed to the infant:

Less fetal discomfort. Barbara Harper, director of Oregon-based Waterbirth International and the author of *Gentle Birth Choices* (2005), says that when the laboring woman is relaxed, the unborn child spends less time in the birth canal and undergoes minimal discomfort.

Less trauma. Proponents of water births also believe the method is less traumatic for newborns. "Babies seem to be very relaxed. They open their eyes and focus on people," says Beah Haber of the Birth Home in Pleasanton, California, who has attended hundreds of water births. However, there is no scientific evidence to document this claim.

Smoother transition. The easier transition is partly a response to the relaxed state of the laboring woman and partly because of the insulating effects of water, according to Harper. "The baby has hearing even in utero, but it's muffled and muted . . . the same way it is underwater," she says. Underwater, the newborn is protected from harsh lights, sounds, and even touch and thus is more relaxed and comfortable. Again, however, scientific evidence is lacking.

Despite the rising interest in water-birthing, the American Congress of Obstetricians and Gynecologists (ACOG) has not endorsed this practice. ACOG

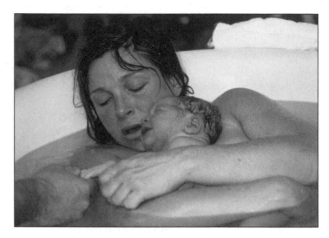

Mother holding her newborn in a birthing pool. (Eddie Lawrence/Photo Researchers, Inc.)

warns that not enough information exists, specifically concerning rates of infection, to recommend warm-water immersion as a safe and appropriate birthing alternative. There are concerns, for example, that a baby can develop an infection if he or she begins breathing while underwater and inhales the soiled birthing water.

Marion McCartney, certified nurse midwife and director of professional services for the American College of Nurse Midwives, says, however, that "most research has found that healthy babies do not gasp upon delivery, rather they do not take a breath until they are removed from the water and reach the air."

Although these studies have been quite small, evidence from larger studies involving almost two thousand women suggests that water birth does not increase rate of infection, and it may reduce the duration of labor and the need for pain control. Nonetheless, ACOG maintains that water-birthing should be performed only under the strictest measures of infection control. All experts agree that water-birthing should be considered for healthy women and healthy fetuses only.

LABOR PAIN

Many nonpharmaceutical options are available to manage the pain and discomfort of labor. These options include relaxation and alternative remedies, such as herbs, acupressure, and acupuncture.

Relaxation techniques. The first step to pain management is relaxation. The tenser one is, the higher the sensation of pain. Relaxation starts with the environment. Even in the hospital, one can dim the lights, play soft music, light candles, or use aromatherapy to create a safe feeling. Lavender and sage are especially soothing scents. Other relaxation techniques include massage, showers, and baths.

The mind is one of the most effective pain-fighting tools available. Hypnotism, visualization, and imagery are all methods for pain relief, and there is some scientific support for their use.

Alternative remedies. Acupressure and acupuncture have been studied as natural treatments for reducing labor pain. Each of these methods may offer some benefits, but more research is needed.

Although red raspberry is an herb traditionally used during pregnancy and labor, a double-blind, placebo-controlled trial evaluating the effects of red raspberry in 192 pregnant women failed to find benefit. The herb blue cohosh is sometimes recommended by midwives, but it is a toxic herb and should not be used.

Lain Chroust Ehmann; reviewed by Ganson Purcell, Jr., M.D., FACOG, FACPE

FURTHER READING

Bodner, K., et al. "Effects of Water Birth on Maternal and Neonatal Outcomes." *Wiener klinische Wochenschrift* 114 (2003): 391-395.

Fehervary, P., et al. "Water Birth: Microbiological Colonisation of the Newborn, Neonatal, and Maternal Infection Rate in Comparison to Conventional Bed Deliveries." *Archives of Gynecology and Obstetrics* 270 (2004): 6-9.

Hjelmstedt, A., et al. "Acupressure to Reduce Labor Pain." *Acta Obstetricia et Gynecologica Scandinavica* 89, no. 11 (2010): 1453-1459.

Lieberman, A. B., et al., eds. *Easing Labor Pain: The Complete Guide to a More Comfortable and Rewarding Birth.* Boston: Harvard Common Press, 1992.

Nesheim, B. I., et al. "Acupuncture During Labor Can Reduce the Use of Meperidine." *Clinical Journal of Pain* 19 (2003): 187-191.

Ramnero, A., et al. "Acupuncture Treatment During Labour." *BJOG: An International Journal of Obstetrics and Gynaecology* 109 (2002): 637-644.

Scott, K. D., et al. "The Obstetrical and Postpartum Benefits of Continuous Support During Childbirth." *Journal of Women's Health and Gender-Based Medicine* 8 (2000): 1257-1264.

Simpson, M., et al. "Raspberry Leaf in Pregnancy: Its Safety and Efficacy in Labor." *Journal of Midwifery and Women's Health* 46 (2001): 51-59.

Skilnand, E, et al. "Acupuncture in the Management of Pain in Labor." *Acta Obstetricia et Gynecologica Scandinavica* 81 (2002): 943-948.

Thoeni, A., et al. "Review of Sixteen Hundred Water Births: Does Water Birth Increase the Risk of Neonatal Infection?" *Journal of Maternal-Fetal and Neonatal Medicine* 17 (2005): 357-361.

See also: Acupressure; Acupuncture; Balneotherapy; Childbirth support: Homeopathic remedies; Children's health; Hydrotherapy; Pain management; Pregnancy support; Women's health.

Children's health

CATEGORY: Issues and overviews
RELATED TERM: Integrative pediatrics
DEFINITION: Complementary and alternative medicines and therapies that are focused on infants, toddlers, and young children.

OVERVIEW

Children's health issues can range from mild to severe. For milder, common conditions, many parents turn to complementary and alternative medicine (CAM) to relieve their child's symptoms. The 2007 National Health Interview Survey (NHIS) found that 12 percent of children in the United States had used some form of alternative medicine. The use is greater among children whose parents used CAM and whose parents had higher education levels, had multiple health conditions, and were white. The use of CAM was also greater among families who delayed conventional care because of cost.

While it is thought that CAM will spare the child from harsh conventional medications and treatments, caution is warranted. Many alternative treatments are not tested and regulated for safety in children. In addition, some treatments, such as restrictive diets, may be difficult for children to adhere to. Also, some parents may think that one can give children extra natural medicine without causing harm, but even natural substances in the wrong doses can be toxic.

While additional research needs to be done, evidence regarding CAM has increased for certain

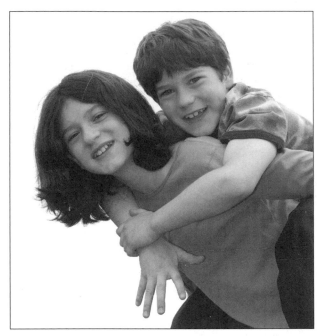

The 2007 National Health Interview Survey (NHIS) found that 12 percent of children in the United States had used some form of alternative medicine. (©Elena Elisseeva/ Dreamstime.com)

therapies. Many of these studies, however, were based on the testing of adults, not of children or adolescents. With a pediatrician's guidance, conventional and alternative medicine can be used together safely.

The most commonly used natural therapies among children in the United States, in descending order, are herbal products, chiropractic/osteopathic care, deep breathing, yoga, homeopathic treatment, traditional healing, massage, meditation, diet-based therapies, and progressive relaxation. Children are most often using CAM for back and neck pain, head and chest colds, anxiety and stress, musculoskeletal conditions, attention deficit disorder (ADD), and insomnia.

The National Center for Complementary and Alternative Medicine, part of the National Institutes of Health, places CAM into four major categories: biologically based (supplementing the diet with nutrients, herbs, particular foods, and extracts), manipulative and body-based (using touch and manipulation, such as chiropractic and massage), mind/body (connecting the mind to the body and spirit in practices such as yoga and meditation), and energy therapies

(aiming to restore balance to the body's energy with therapies such as qigong). Other whole, ancient, medical systems include traditional Chinese medicine, Ayurveda, homeopathic medicine, and naturopathic medicine.

COMMON HEALTH ISSUES

There are a number of health issues that predominate during childhood, including infant colic and ear infections. CAM is one place to begin to address these issues. Other good starting points for optimum health during these growth years are proper nutrition, adequate rest, and good coping skills.

Alternative therapies for colic. Infant colic (excessive fussiness, crying, and discomfort for more than three hours at a time and for a minimum of three days per week) is a condition experienced by many parents and their newborns between about four and five months of age. There is supporting evidence that fennel oil improves symptoms and is effective in reducing crying time for infants with colic. Also used for indigestion, fennel is a carminative. That is, it helps the body expel gas. Herbal combinations such as fennel, chamomile, vervain, licorice, and balm mint have also been shown to help relieve colic.

Alternative therapies for ear infections. Xylitol is a sweetener and natural sugar found in plums, strawberries, and raspberries. It inhibits the growth of certain types of bacterial strains, such as *Streptococcus mutans* and related species, and of *Haemophilus influenzae.* Chewing gum with xylitol and ingesting xylitol sweetener five times per day can help to prevent middle ear infections. Lower doses, however, are not effective. Some homeopathic ear drops provide symptom relief in children with mild to moderate pain too.

HERBAL AND NUTRITION THERAPIES

The NHIS reported the most common natural health products being used by children. These products include echinacea, fish oil/omega 3, combination herbal pills, and flaxseed oil/pills.

Echinacea is commonly used by children, teenagers, and adults for colds and flu. Double-blind, placebo-controlled studies enrolling more than one thousand people found that various forms and species of echinacea can reduce the symptoms and duration of a common cold, in adults. It is thought that echinacea works by temporarily stimulating, strengthening, and nourishing the immune system. There is

Common Health Conditions of Children

Allergies
Asthma
Attention deficit disorder
Autism
Bed-wetting
Bumps, bruises, and other injuries
Canker sores
Colic
Diarrhea

Ear infection
Eczema
Fever
Headaches
Hives
Insect bites
Irritable bowel syndrome
Strep throat
Warts

limited scientific evidence, however, to support these claims. Although echinacea might stimulate the immune system temporarily, there is no evidence of long-term effectiveness.

As with all herbal medicines, the precise species and part or parts of the plant being used are key. There are three main species of echinacea: *E. purpurea, E. angustifolia,* and *E. pallida.* The flowers, leaves, and stems of *E. purpurea,* when used together, provide the best supporting evidence for benefits in treating colds and influenza. The root of *E. purpurea* has not been shown to be effective, while the root of *E. pallida* may be the active, and effective, part of that species.

Echinacea may be beneficial in reducing symptoms or halting a cold once it has started. However, echinacea does not appear to prevent colds. It may not be effective in children and adolescents and has not been studied in these populations. As with all herbal supplements, the actual dosing, potency, and quality of the over-the-counter product are not regulated or guaranteed.

Omega-3 is the second most commonly used natural supplement in children. It has been broadly studied for its impact on heart health and on arthritis, asthma, cancer prevention, depression, and many more diseases. Many children's natural vitamin products include fish oil or some form of omega-3. Supportive evidence for its benefits to heart health led the U.S. Food and Drug Administration (FDA) to allow the following statement on products containing fish oil: "Supportive but not conclusive research shows that consumption of EPA and DHA omega-3 fatty acids may reduce the risk of coronary heart disease."

Omega-3 is also approved by the FDA as an aid in lowering levels of bad cholesterol. Evidence for ome-ga-3's benefits has been mounting. One randomized control trial even showed that women who took fish oil supplements during the third trimester of pregnancy helped to reduce the risk of asthma in their children for up to sixteen years. There is, however, no daily requirement or omega-3 standard recommended dose for children.

Parents should use caution before giving children herbs or supplements, because most of these alternative products have not been tested on children. Herbalists may suggest taking one-quarter the adult dose. Many common herbs, such as ephedra, kava kava, lavender, monkshood, wormwood, deadly nightshade, foxglove, desert herb, star anise, lobelia, and mistletoe, as well as Ayurvedic herbal remedies, have been shown to be toxic to the cardiac and central nervous systems. Parents should discuss with their family doctor any plans to use alternative medications or other products for their children, especially because these medications could alter the effectiveness of traditional medication or could otherwise threaten the child's health.

MIND/BODY THERAPIES

The power of the mind to heal and bring about well-being has been demonstrated in self-reported quality-of-life measures. Strong evidence in the form of randomized controlled trials is lacking, in part because of the difficulty in devising placebo therapies and because of funding obstacles. Many practices, such as yoga, meditation, and Tai Chi may help children reduce symptoms and bring about a sense of relaxation.

Even young children are under a great deal of stress. Family and economic issues, the daily stresses of homework, chores, and being involved in every activity, can affect children deeply. Deep breathing and yoga are two of the more common mind/body therapies used by children, according to a national survey. Yoga emphasizes a healthy spine for a healthy body and incorporates deep-breathing exercises. Different poses and movements involving twisting and balancing are believed to stimulate the nerves along the spine and promote circulation and the flow of energy. Many professional athletes practice some form of yoga for increased flexibility, and yoga is often incorporated into cross-training exercise routines. Yoga practitioners claim that yoga can help children develop a good body- and self-image, self-control, flexibility, and body awareness. Children with ADD may also benefit from yoga poses, which can help instill a sense of calm and centeredness. Simple deep-breathing is a good coping strategy for children who feel overwhelmed or stressed.

MANIPULATIVE THERAPIES

After herbal products, chiropractic/osteopathic care is the second most commonly used complementary and alternative therapy. Pediatric conditions that are often treated by chiropractors and osteopaths include earache, asthma, allergies, colic, bed-wetting, sinus disorders, migraines, and muscle pain.

Chiropractic care is founded on the belief that adjustments to the spinal vertebrae (or other parts of the body) free the nerves from compression and maximize the body's ability to heal itself and feel well. There are several chiropractic techniques, including diversified, activator, and sacrooccipital, to promote adjustments of the body and spine. Imaging studies are common in chiropractic care. In one study, chiropractors reported performing fewer imaging studies on children and charging less for pediatric visits. Chiropractors may also recommend herbal remedies or dietary supplements. There is scant research evidence to support or reject its effectiveness, especially in children.

A 2000 cross-sectional study done in the Boston area showed that 420,000 pediatric chiropractic visits were made in the area in one year, costing approximately $14 million (approximately one-half of the fees were covered by insurance). The study showed that pediatric chiropractic care was often inconsistent with recommended medical guidelines. More research is needed to assess its safety and effectiveness in children.

Similarly, osteopathic care is centered on touch therapy. Osteopaths manipulate muscles and joints by stretching, adding resistance and gentle pressure. It is thought that these movements help diagnose, treat, and prevent injury.

Deanna M. Neff, M.P.H.

FURTHER READING

American Academy of Pediatrics: Provisional Section for Complementary, Holistic, and Integrative Medicine. http://www.aap.org/sections/chim. The complementary, holistic, and integrative medicine section of the American Academy of Pediatrics Web site.

EBSCO Publishing. *Health Library: Children's Health.* Available through http://www.ebscohost.com. An overview of children's health.

Freeman, Lyn. *Mosby's Complementary and Alternative Medicine: A Research-Based Approach.* 3d ed. St. Louis, Mo.: Mosby/Elsevier, 2009. A comprehensive resource on CAM, from a research perspective.

Kemper, K., and P. Gardiner. "Herbal Medicines." In *Nelson Textbook of Pediatrics*, edited by Richard E. Behrman, Robert M. Kliegman, and Hal B. Jenson. 18th ed. Philadelphia: Saunders/Elsevier, 2007. A thorough chapter examining the use of herbal medicines for children and adolescents.

Lee, A., D. Li, and K. Kemper. "Chiropractic Care for Children." *Archives of Pediatric Adolescent Medicine* 154 (2000): 401-407. Focused on the use of chiropractic care in treating children and adolescents.

See also: Adolescent and teenage health; Attention deficit disorder; Autism spectrum disorder; Compulsive overeating; Depression, mild to moderate; Eating disorders; Herbal medicine; Mental health.

Chinese medicine

CATEGORY: Therapies and techniques

RELATED TERMS: Asian medicine, Eastern medicine, traditional Chinese herbal medicine, traditional Chinese medicine

DEFINITION: A complex healing system that reflects the belief that health exists when the body is balanced and its energy is flowing freely.

OVERVIEW

Traditional Chinese medicine (TCM) is one of the most complex and highly developed traditional healing

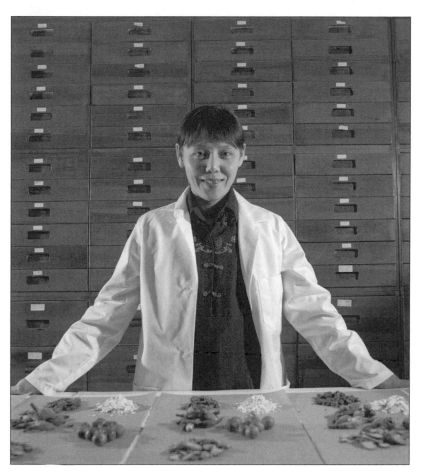

Herbal medicine is a component of Chinese medicine. (Bob Barkany/Getty Images)

forth in the *Inner Classic of Medicine*, or *Nei Jing*, first published in 206 B.C.E. during the Han Dynasty. Chinese herbal medicine, however, developed somewhat later. It received its first rudimentary theoretical foundations in the first or second century C.E., but it was not until the twelfth century that the deeper principles of Chinese medicine were fully applied to herbal treatment.

Chinese medical theories involving diet follow along much the same lines as herbal theory. Essentially, each food is an herb and has its own characteristic effects on the body. (A variation of this system known as macrobiotics has become well known.)

The relative importance of the two fields has waxed and waned over time. Herbology reached a state of high development in the fourteenth and fifteenth centuries; acupuncture then reached what might be called a golden age under the Ming Dynasty in the late sixteenth and early seventeenth centuries. Subsequently, herbal medicine gained in importance; by the time acupuncture came back in vogue in twentieth-century China, it had undergone a major transformation sometimes called the herbalization of acupuncture.

theories in the world, rivaled in its scope only by Ayurveda. TCM comprises several parts: acupuncture, traditional Chinese herbal medicine, dietary interventions, exercise systems such as Tai Chi and qigong, and theories about architecture and interior design known as feng shui. Its principles are essentially Daoist in nature and encompass (in principle) every aspect of human existence.

HISTORY

The principles of Chinese medicine developed within the larger sphere of the Daoist religion. Primitive acupuncture needles dating to around 1000 B.C.E. have been discovered in archaeologic finds of the Shan Dynasty in China. The theoretical framework underlying the practice of acupuncture was first set

The martial arts also developed within the context of Daoism and, therefore, follows principles consistent with Chinese medicine. The healing martial art known as Tai Chi is said to have been invented by the monk Chang San-Feng sometime in the Middle Ages; however, the exact dates (and even the existence of this monk) are disputed.

In China today, various aspects of TCM are used with conventional Western medical treatment. Considerable attempts have been made to subject acupuncture, herbal therapy, and healing martial arts to scientific evaluation; however, most of the published Chinese studies on the subject fall far short of current scientific standards. (For example, they frequently lack a control group.)

In neighboring Japan, a variation of the traditional

Chinese herbal system known as Kampo has become extremely popular, and many Kampo remedies have been approved for medical use by the Japanese health ministry. The scientific basis for these remedies remains inadequate, but several studies of moderately good quality have been reported.

What is traditional Chinese medicine? Traditional Chinese medicine (TCM) is an all-embracing system that, in theory, encompasses all aspects of human existence. Even a basic introduction to its principles far exceeds the scope of this article.

According to the principles of TCM, health exists when the body is balanced and its energy, or qi, is flowing freely. Qi is the life energy that is said to animate the body. The term "balance" refers to the relative factors of yin and yang, the classic Daoist opposing forces of the universe. Yin and yang find their expression in various subsidiary antagonists such as cold versus heat, dampness versus dryness, descending versus ascending, at rest versus active, and full versus empty.

In an ideal state, yin and yang in all their forms are perfectly balanced in every part of the body. However, external or internal factors can upset this balance, which then leads to disease. Chinese medical diagnosis and treatment involve identifying the factors that are out of balance and attempting to bring them back into harmony.

Besides yin and yang, there are five elements or phases that can exist in harmony or disharmony. These are translated into English as wood, metal, water, earth, and fire. Each of these elements has characteristic properties and affects various organs, personality, and overall health in unique ways.

It is important to realize that diagnosis according to TCM differs greatly from Western diagnosis. For example, one patient with a migraine headache might be said to have "dryness in the liver and ascending qi," while another might be diagnosed with "exogenous wind-cold." For this reason, there is no such thing as a TCM remedy for migraines per se; rather, treatment must be individualized to the imbalance determined by traditional theory.

USES AND APPLICATIONS

TCM addresses all possible physical, psychological, and spiritual problems. In the West, TCM is primarily used to treat long-term chronic conditions (such as rheumatoid arthritis and menopausal symptoms) and some acute conditions that are not life-threatening (such as menstrual pain and colds). TCM is also widely used to promote wellness and prevent disease.

SCIENTIFIC EVIDENCE

There is no meaningful scientific evidence that the overarching principles of TCM reflect true insights into health. There is some evidence, however, that certain TCM therapies may be helpful for specific conditions. Nonetheless, even here there are serious problems. Studies of TCM performed in China generally fall far short of modern Western standards of scientific rigor. Furthermore, even studies performed according to the highest standards have some inherent problems because of the nature of the treatments themselves.

SAFETY ISSUES

Acupuncture appears to be a relatively safe form of medicine if practiced appropriately. However, there are serious safety concerns regarding traditional Chinese herbal therapy.

EBSCO CAM Review Board

FURTHER READING

Bauer, R., and K. Chan. "Traditional Chinese Medicine." *Planta Medica* 76 (2010).

Vickers, A., et al. "Do Certain Countries Produce Only Positive Results? A Systematic Review of Controlled Trials." *Controlled Clinical Trials* 19 (1998): 159-166.

Wang, G., et al. "The Quality of Reporting of Randomized Controlled Trials of Traditional Chinese Medicine." *Clinical Therapeutics* 29 (2007): 1456-1467.

See also: Acupuncture; Alternative versus traditional medicine; Ayurveda; Folk medicine; Herbal medicine; Home health; Naturopathy; Qigong; Tai Chi; Traditional Chinese herbal medicine; Traditional healing.

Chinese skullcap

CATEGORY: Herbs and supplements
RELATED TERMS: Baicalein, baicalin, *Scutellaria baicalensis*
DEFINITION: Natural plant product used to treat specific health conditions.

PRINCIPAL PROPOSED USES: None
OTHER PROPOSED USES: Anxiety, cancer treatment, enhancing antibiotic activity, hypertension, liver protection

OVERVIEW

Chinese skullcap (*Scutellaria baicalensis*) is a member of the mint family and has long been used in traditional Chinese herbal medicine. Chinese skullcap has been incorporated in herbal formulas designed to treat such widely varying conditions as cancer, liver disease, allergies, skin conditions, and epilepsy. The root is the part used medicinally. Chinese skullcap is substantially different from American skullcap (*S. lateriflora*).

THERAPEUTIC DOSAGES

The optimum doses, if any, of baicalin, wogonin, and baicalein have not been established. Chinese skullcap is typically taken at a dose of 3 to 9 grams daily as part of an herbal combination.

THERAPEUTIC USES

The root of Chinese skullcap contains the flavonoids baicalin, wogonin, and baicalein, and most studies have involved these substances rather than the whole herb. Highly preliminary evidence suggest that baicalin can enhance the activity of antibiotics against antibiotic-resistant staph bacteria. Other highly preliminary evidence suggests that baicalin, wogonin, and baicalein may have anticancer, anti-inflammatory, liver-protective, antianxiety, and antihypertensive effects. However, for none of these uses does the evidence approach the level necessary to truly establish a treatment as effective. Research involving combination herbal therapies containing Chinese skullcap are discussed in the article on traditional Chinese herbal medicine.

SAFETY ISSUES

Baicalin, wobogin, and baicalein appear to have a low order of toxicity, though comprehensive safety studies have not been performed. There have been case reports of liver injury associated with use of skullcap products, but these may have been caused by adulteration by the herb germander.

One animal study found worrisome evidence that baicalin might markedly reduce the absorption of drug cyclosporine, used to prevent organ transplant rejection. Another study found that baicalin might reduce blood levels of drugs in the statin family, used to improve cholesterol profile. Safety in young children, pregnant or nursing women, or people with severe liver or kidney disease has not been established.

IMPORTANT INTERACTIONS

Those persons taking cyclosporine should not use Chinese skullcap or its constituents. Also, the use of Chinese skullcap may reduce the effectiveness of cholesterol-lowering drugs in the statin family.

EBSCO CAM Review Board

FURTHER READING

Bonham, M., et al. "Characterization of Chemical Constituents in *Scutellaria baicalensis* with Antiandrogenic and Growth-Inhibitory Activities Toward Prostate Carcinoma." *Clinical Cancer Research* 11 (2005): 3905-3914.

Chi, Y. S., et al. "Effects of Wogonin, a Plant Flavone from *Scutellaria radix*, on Skin Inflammation: In Vivo Regulation of Inflammation-Associated Gene Expression." *Biochemical Pharmacology* 66 (2003): 1271-1278.

Liu, J. J., et al. "Baicalein and Baicalin Are Potent Inhibitors of Angiogenesis: Inhibition of Endothelial Cell Proliferation, Migration, and Differentiation." *International Journal of Cancer* 106 (2003): 559-565.

Ong, E. S., et al. "Differential Protein Expression of the Inhibitory Effects of a Standardized Extract from *Scutellariae radix* in Liver Cancer Cell Lines Using Liquid Chromatography and Tandem Mass Spectrometry." *Journal of Agricultural and Food Chemistry* 53 (2005): 8-16.

Wang, J., et al. "Baicalein Induces Apoptosis Through ROS-Mediated Mitochondrial Dysfunction Pathway in HL-60 Cells." *International Journal of Molecular Medicine* 14 (2004): 627-632.

Wozniak, D., et al. "Antimutagenic and Antiradical Properties of Flavones from the Roots of *Scutellaria baicalensis Georgi*." *Die Nahrung* 48 (2004): 9-12.

Yang, Z. C., et al. "The Synergistic Activity of Antibiotics Combined with Eight Traditional Chinese Medicines Against Two Different Strains of *Staphylococcus aureus*." *Colloids and Surfaces: B, Biointerfaces* 41 (2005): 79-81.

See also: Chinese medicine; Herbal medicine.

Chiropractic

CATEGORY: Therapies and techniques

RELATED TERM: Spinal manipulation

DEFINITION: Technique that involves spinal adjustments and, in some cases, the use of vitamins, herbs, and other alternative treatment methods.

PRINCIPAL PROPOSED USES: Back pain, migraine headaches, neck pain, painful conditions of the upper extremities, scoliosis, tension headaches

OTHER PROPOSED USES: Asthma, bed-wetting, dysmenorrhea, high blood pressure, infantile colic, phobias, premenstrual syndrome

OVERVIEW

Chiropractic is one of the most widely used health services. It has gained increasing acceptance as a treatment for back and neck pain, and it is covered by many health insurance plans. Millions of people would report that chiropractic spinal manipulation has brought them relief. Nonetheless, the research record for its effectiveness is inconclusive.

Daniel David Palmer founded chiropractic in 1895, after an experience in which he apparently believed he cured a man's deafness by manipulating his back. Palmer then opened the Palmer School of Chiropractic and began teaching spinal manipulation. This college still exists and has a fully accredited program.

One of Palmer's first students was his son, Bartlett Joshua (B. J.) Palmer. It was B. J. Palmer who truly popularized the technique. Later Willard Carver, an Oklahoma City lawyer, opened a competing school. He believed that chiropractic physicians needed to offer other methods of treatment in addition to spinal manipulation. This opened a schism in the chiropractic world that still exists. Followers of Palmer and his methods focus only on spinal adjustments, an approach called "straight" chiropractic. Those who, like Carver, use various approaches to healing are called "mixers." Mixers may use vitamins, herbs, and any other treatment methods they find useful (and are allowed to practice by law).

Medical treatments in the nineteenth and early twentieth centuries were not based on scientific evidence of effectiveness, and chiropractic treatment was no exception. It became a widespread technique long before there was any real evidence that it worked. Chiropractic schools utilized their profits and resources to further develop programs for training people in chiropractic techniques, not for verifying the theory and practice of chiropractic. However, in the 1970s, proper scientific research into chiropractic began to draw interest. In 1977, the Foundation for Chiropractic Education and Research established a program to train chiropractic researchers. Since then, efforts have been made to fund scientific trials testing the effectiveness of chiropractic techniques and to establish a scientific foundation for the practice.

There are many different chiropractic techniques, some with proprietary names such as the Gonstead and Maitland techniques. In general, most involve rapid (high-velocity) short (low-amplitude) thrusts. Manipulation may be purely manual or mechanically assisted. For example, some chiropractors use what is called an "activator," a small metal tool that applies a force directly to one vertebra.

In addition, some chiropractors use a related therapy called spinal mobilization. This method involves gentle, extended movements (low-velocity, high-amplitude) rather than the "back cracking" of classic chiropractic spinal manipulation.

MECHANISM OF ACTION

Since its origin, chiropractic theory has based itself on subluxations, or vertebrae that have shifted position in the spine. These subluxations are said to impede nerve outflow and cause disease in various organs. A chiropractic treatment is supposed to "put back in" these "popped out" vertebrae; for this reason, it is called an "adjustment."

However, no real evidence has ever been presented showing that a given chiropractic treatment alters the position of any vertebrae. In addition, there is as yet no real evidence that impairment of nerve outflow is a major contributor to common illnesses, or that spinal manipulation changes nerve outflow in such a way as to affect organ function.

Later theories suggest that chiropractic manipulation may relieve pain by "loosening" vertebrae that have become relatively immobile rather than by changing their position. In addition, the movements associated with manipulation may alter the response patterns of nerves in the central nervous system, including both the spine and the brain, leading to pain relief.

USES AND APPLICATIONS

Chiropractic spinal manipulation is widely used for the treatment of back pain, neck pain, and headaches, whether acute or chronic. It is also frequently tried for pain in other areas, such as the shoulders, knees, and jaw, and for breech birth positioning of a fetus, infantile colic, frequent colds, and many other conditions.

Some chiropractic physicians promote comprehensive chiropractic care as a means of staying healthy. This approach may include diet, exercise, and supplements, along with regular chiropractic manipulation.

SCIENTIFIC EVIDENCE

Chiropractic spinal manipulation has been evaluated scientifically to determine its efficacy and its costs compared to other forms of health care. However, the evidence is not compelling in either case.

Efficacy. Although there is some evidence that chiropractic spinal manipulation may be helpful for various medical purposes, in general the evidence is not strong. There are several reasons for this, but one is fundamental: Even with the best of intentions, it is difficult to properly ascertain the effectiveness of a hands-on therapy like chiropractic.

Only one form of study can truly prove that a treatment is effective: the double-blind, placebo-controlled trial. However, it is difficult to fit chiropractic into a study design of this type. Because of this, all studies of chiropractic manipulation fall short of optimum design. Many have compared chiropractic treatment with no treatment. However, studies of this type cannot provide reliable evidence about the efficacy of a treatment. If a benefit is seen, there is no way to determine whether it was caused by chiropractic manipulation specifically or by attention generally. (Attention alone will almost always produce some reported benefit.)

More meaningful trials used some sort of unrelated fake treatment for the control group, such as phony laser acupuncture. However, it is less than ideal to use a placebo treatment that is so very different in form from the treatment under study. Better studies compare real chiropractic manipulation with sham forms of manipulation, such as light touch. Studies of this type are a definite step forward. However, it is quite likely that the practitioners unconsciously conveyed more enthusiasm and optimism when performing the real therapy than the fake therapy; this, too, could affect the outcome. It has been suggested that the only way to get around this problem would be to compare the effectiveness of trained practitioners to that of actors trained only enough to provide simulated treatment; however, such studies have not been reported.

Still other studies have simply involved treating people with chiropractic spinal manipulation and seeing whether they improve. These trials are particularly meaningless; it has been proven that both participants and examining physicians will think that they observe improvement in people given a treatment, regardless of whether the treatment does anything on its own.

Finally, other trials have compared chiropractic manipulation to competing therapies, such as massage therapy or conventional physical therapy. However, neither of these therapies has been proven effective. When one compares unproven therapies to each other, the results cannot possibly prove that any of the tested treatments are effective. Given these caveats, the following discussion will focus on what science knows about the effects of chiropractic.

Cost of care. Besides effectiveness, another important consideration is cost of care. There are many aspects to the cost of treatment, including number of visits to the chosen provider, cost of evaluation procedures such as X rays, insurance reimbursement versus patient out-of-pocket expense, and costs for missed work time.

However, it is difficult to develop accurate cost-comparison figures because there are many complicating factors in research on the subject. For example, one approach is to simply identify people with similar injuries who choose one treatment or another and add up the total cost. The results of such a study can be misleading. People with more or less severe back pain might tend to choose different forms of treatment; if those with more severe pain usually chose surgical treatment, this would tend to inflate the comparative costs of conventional care and make chiropractic seem less expensive.

Another potentially complicating factor is that, to a great extent, insurance companies control utilization of treatment. If they are less inclined to authorize chiropractic visits, people who choose chiropractic care might find their care cut off more rapidly than others who choose, say, physical therapy. This too would lead to artificially low costs of chiropractic treatment compared to physical therapy, skewing the results of the study.

These problems could be solved by conducting a

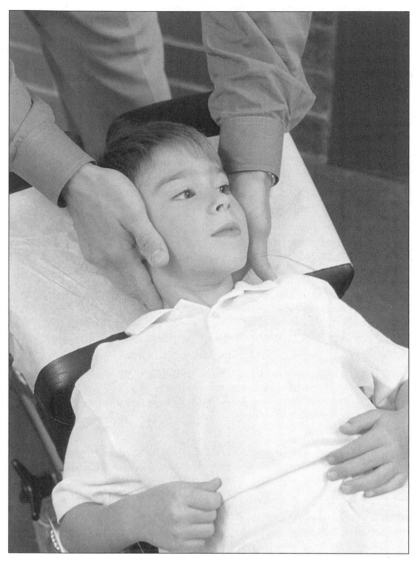

A chiropractor performs a manipulation on the neck of a young patient. (PhotoDisc)

placebo, if not by a great deal. For example, a single-blind controlled study of eighty-four people with low back pain compared manipulation to treatment with a diathermy machine (a physical therapy machine that uses microwaves to create heat beneath the skin) that was not actually functioning. The researchers asked the participants to assess their own pain levels within fifteen minutes of the first treatment then three and seven days after treatment. The only statistically significant difference between the two groups was found with fifteen minutes of the manipulation. (Chiropractic had better results at that point.)

In another single-blind, placebo-controlled study, researchers assigned 209 participants to one of three groups: a high-velocity, low-amplitude (HVLA) spinal manipulation, a sham manipulation, or a back-education program. Although this has been reported as a positive study, most of the differences seen among the groups were not statistically significant. In addition, because almost one-half of the participants dropped out of the study before the end, the results cannot be regarded as meaningful.

Unimpressive results were also seen in a well-designed study of 321 people with back pain comparing chiropractic manipulation, a special form of physical therapy (the Mackenzie method), and the provision of an educational booklet in treating low back pain. All groups improved to about the same extent.

study in which researchers randomly assign participants to certain treatments, with the length of treatment determined entirely by the treating physician. Studies of this type have not been conducted.

Back pain. Chiropractic spinal manipulation is one of the most popular treatments for acute and chronic back pain in the United States, and it may provide modest benefit. However, research evidence has failed to find chiropractic manipulation convincingly more effective than standard medical care.

Chiropractic does seem to be more effective than

Several studies evaluated the effectiveness of chiropractic manipulation combined with a different kind of treatment called mobilization, but they too found little to no benefit. On a positive note, one study of one hundred people with back pain and sciatica symptoms (pain down the leg caused by disc protrusion) found that chiropractic manipulation was significantly more effective at relieving symptoms than was sham chiropractic manipulation.

Several studies have found that chiropractic is at least as helpful as other commonly used therapies for low back pain, such as muscle relaxants, anti-inflammatory medication, soft-tissue massage, conventional medical care, and physical therapy. For example, a large well-designed study found chiropractic manipulation more effective than general medical care and exercise therapy.

Physical therapy, the main conventional therapy for back pain, also lacks consistent supporting evidence. For example, in one large study of people with back pain, a single session of advice proved just as effective as a full course of physical therapy for back pain.

Neck pain. As with back pain, there is no reliable evidence that spinal manipulation works for neck pain. Of the limited number of studies performed, most have failed to find manipulation (with or without mobilization or massage) convincingly more effective than placebo or no treatment. One large study (almost two hundred participants) found that a special exercise program (MedX) was more effective than manipulation. However, a study reported in 2006 found that a single HVLA manipulation of the neck was more effective than a single mobilization procedure in improving range of motion and pain in people with neck pain.

Upper extremity pain. Persons often seek chiropractic care for painful conditions affecting their upper extremities (such as the shoulder, elbow, forearm, wrist, and hand). A recent search and analysis of all published studies examining the effectiveness of chiropractic for these conditions revealed mostly case studies, an unreliable source of evidence. The few uncovered controlled trials were of insufficient quality to draw any reliable conclusions about the effectiveness of chiropractic for painful conditions of the upper extremity.

Tension and cervicogenic headaches. Many people experience headaches caused by muscle tension, neck problems, or a combination of the two. Because these tension headaches and cervicogenic headaches (those caused by neck problems) overlap, they are discussed together here. Chiropractic spinal manipulation has shown some promise for these conditions, but the evidence remains incomplete and somewhat contradictory. In a controlled trial of 150 people, investigators compared spinal manipulation to the drug amitriptyline for the treatment of chronic tension-type headaches. By the end of the six-week treatment period,

participants in both groups had improved similarly. However, four weeks after treatment was stopped, people who had received spinal manipulation showed greater reduction in headache intensity and frequency and over-the-counter medication usage than those who used the medication. The difference in the amount of improvement between the groups was statistically significant.

In another positive trial, fifty-three people with cervicogenic headaches received chiropractic spinal manipulation or laser acupuncture plus massage. Chiropractic manipulation was more effective. However, a similar study of seventy-five people with recurrent tension headaches found no difference between the two groups. Other, smaller studies of spinal manipulation have been reported too, with mixed results.

Finally, in a controlled trial, two hundred people with cervicogenic headaches were randomly assigned to receive one of four therapies: manipulation, a special exercise technique, exercise plus manipulation, or no therapy. Each participant received a minimum of eight to twelve treatments for six weeks. All three treatment approaches produced better results than no treatment, and each had approximately the same effect as the others. However, these results prove little because any treatment whatsoever will generally produce better results than no treatment.

Migraine headaches. There is some evidence that chiropractic manipulation may provide both long-term and short-term benefits for migraine headaches. In a double-blind, placebo-controlled study, 123 participants with migraine headaches were treated for two months with chiropractic manipulations or fake electrical therapy (in which electrodes were placed on the body without electrical current sent between them) as placebo. The study lasted six months: two months pretreatment, two months of treatment, and two months post-treatment. After two months of treatment, those receiving chiropractic manipulation showed statistically significant improvement in headache severity and frequency compared with the control group. Furthermore, these benefits persisted to a two-month follow-up evaluation.

Chiropractic manipulation also produced relatively prolonged benefits in another trial. In this study, 218 people with migraine headaches were divided into three groups: manipulation, medication (amitriptyline), or manipulation plus medication. During the four weeks of treatment, all three groups experienced comparable benefits. During the follow-up four-week period, however, people who had received manipulation alone experienced more benefit than those who had been in the other two groups.

A study of eighty-five people with migraines compared spinal manipulation with two other treatments: mobilization and manipulation performed by someone other than a chiropractor. The results showed no difference among groups.

Chiropractic has been evaluated for many other conditions, including the following, but the results show little evidence of benefit.

Infantile colic. Infantile colic is a common and frustrating problem. Although chiropractic manipulation has been promoted as a treatment for this condition, there is little evidence that it offers specific benefits.

In a single-blind, placebo-controlled trial, eighty-six infants either received three chiropractic treatments or were held for ten minutes by a nurse. While a high percentage of infants improved, there was no significant difference between the two groups. Another trial compared spinal manipulation to the drug dimethicone. While chiropractic proved more effective than the medication, dimethicone itself has never been proven effective for infantile colic, and the study did not use a placebo group. For this reason, the results of this study indicate little about the effectiveness of chiropractic treatment for infantile colic.

Premenstrual syndrome. A small crossover trial of chiropractic for premenstrual symptoms found equivocal results.

Phobias. A small trial compared real and sham activator-style chiropractic treatment in people with phobias and found some evidence of benefit.

Asthma. In two controlled studies comparing spinal manipulation to sham manipulation for the treatment of people with asthma, the results showed equal improvement for participants in the two groups. These results suggest that the benefits were most likely caused by the attention given by the chiropractor and not by the spinal manipulation itself. However, one of these studies has been sharply criticized for using as a sham treatment a chiropractic method perfectly capable of producing a therapeutic effect. This could hide real benefits of the tested form of chiropractic. (If the "placebo" treatment used in a study is actually better than placebo, and the tested treatment does no better than this "placebo," the results would appear to indicate that the tested treatment is no better than placebo and, hence, is ineffective.)

Dysmenorrhea. A single-blind, placebo-controlled study of 138 women complaining of dysmenorrhea (menstrual pain) compared spinal manipulation with sham manipulation for four menstrual cycles and found no differences between the two groups.

High blood pressure. In a study of 148 people with mild high blood pressure, the use of chiropractic spinal manipulation plus dietary changes failed to prove more effective for reducing blood pressure than dietary changes alone.

Bed-wetting. A single-blind, placebo-controlled trial compared real and sham chiropractic (activator technique) in forty-six children with bed-wetting problems but failed to find a statistically significant difference between the groups.

Scoliosis. Weak evidence hints that chiropractic could be somewhat helpful for adolescent idiopathic scoliosis (curvature of the spine that occurs for no clear reason in adolescents).

WHAT TO EXPECT DURING TREATMENT

Depending on the condition, chiropractic treatment is usually conducted two or three times per week for one month or more. Chiropractic is also sometimes used on an as-needed basis or in a once or twice a month maintenance form. For many chiropractors, X rays are essential at the first visit and at some follow-up visits.

Each session involves hands-on manipulation following the methods of whatever manipulation technique the practitioner chooses to use. Sometimes other modalities may be used too, such as massage or hot or cold packs. Chiropractic physicians may also provide general wellness counseling and prescribe or recommend herbs or supplements.

SAFETY ISSUES

Chiropractic manipulation appears to be generally safe and rarely causes serious side effects. However, a temporary increase of symptoms may occur relatively frequently. Other side effects include temporary headache, tiredness, and discomfort radiating from the site of the adjustment.

More serious complications may occur on rare occasions. These are primarily associated with manipulation of the neck. Articles have been published that document almost two hundred cases of more serious complications associated with neck manipulation, including stroke, vertebral fracture, disc herniation, severely increased sensation of nerve pinching, and rupture of the windpipe. More than one-half of these reports involve some form of stroke, often caused by a tear in a major blood vessel at the base of the neck (the vertebral artery).

Although attempts have been made to determine in advance who will experience strokes following chiropractic, these attempts have not been successful. Thus, stroke must be considered an unpredictable, though rare, side effect of chiropractic manipulation of the neck.

To put this in perspective, however, the rate of complications from chiropractic is extremely low. According to one estimate, only one complication per million individual sessions occurs. Among people receiving a course of treatment involving manipulation of the neck, the rate of stroke is perhaps 1 per 100,000 people; the rate of death is 1 per 400,000. By comparison, serious medical complications involving common drugs in the ibuprofen family (nonsteroidal anti-inflammatory drugs, or NSAIDs) are far more common. Among people using them for arthritis, NSAIDs result in hospitalizations at a rate of about 4 in 1,000 people and death at a rate of 4 in 10,000 people. To put it another way, the rate of complications with these common over-the-counter drugs is perhaps one hundred to four hundred times greater than with chiropractic.

Certain health conditions preclude spinal manipulation. These conditions include nerve impingement causing severe nerve damage and significant disease of the spinal bones.

EBSCO CAM Review Board

FURTHER READING

Hoiriis, K. T., et al. "A Randomized Clinical Trial Comparing Chiropractic Adjustments to Muscle Relaxants for Subacute Low Back Pain." *Journal of Manipulative and Physiological Therapeutics* 27 (2004): 388-398.

Hurwitz, E. L., et al. "Frequency and Clinical Predictors of Adverse Reactions to Chiropractic Care in the UCLA Neck Pain Study." *Spine* 30 (2005): 1477-1484.

Jüni, P., et al. "A Randomised Controlled Trial of Spinal Manipulative Therapy in Acute Low Back Pain." *Annals of the Rheumatic Diseases* 68 (2009): 1420-1427.

McHardy, A., et al. "Chiropractic Treatment of Upper Extremity Conditions." *Journal of Manipulative and Physiological Therapeutics* 31 (2008): 146-159.

Martinez-Segura, R., et al. "Immediate Effects on Neck Pain and Active Range of Motion After a Single Cervical High-Velocity Low-Amplitude Manipulation in Subjects Presenting with Mechanical Neck Pain." *Journal of Manipulative and Physiological Therapeutics* 29 (2006): 511-517.

Schmid, A., et al. "Paradigm Shift in Manual Therapy? Evidence for a Central Nervous System Component in the Response to Passive Cervical Joint Mobilisation." *Manual Therapy* 13 (2008): 387-396.

Wilkey, A., et al. "A Comparison Between Chiropractic Management and Pain Clinic Management for Chronic Low-Back Pain in a National Health Service Outpatient Clinic." *Journal of Alternative and Complementary Medicine* 14 (2008): 465-473.

See also: Acupressure; Acupuncture; Alternative versus traditional medicine; Back pain; Bone and joint health; Headaches, tension; Manipulative and body-based therapies; Migraine headaches; Neck pain; Osteopathic manipulation; Pain management; Palmer, Daniel David.

Chitosan

CATEGORY: Herbs and supplements

RELATED TERM: Chitin

DEFINITION: Natural substance used to treat specific health conditions.

PRINCIPAL PROPOSED USES: None

OTHER PROPOSED USES: Antimicrobial, high blood pressure, high cholesterol, kidney failure, preventing cavities, weight loss, wound healing

OVERVIEW

Chitosan is a form of fiber chemically processed from crustacean shells. Like other forms of fiber, such as oat bran, chitosan is not well digested by the human body. As it passes through the digestive tract, it seems to have an ability to bond with ingested fat and carry it out in the stool. For this reason, it has been tried as an agent for lowering cholesterol and reducing weight. However, the results in studies have been more negative than positive. In addition, chitosan has been tried as a treatment for kidney failure and as an aid in wound healing.

REQUIREMENTS AND SOURCES

Chitosan can be extracted from the shells of shrimp, crab, or lobster. It is also found in yeast and some fungi. Another inexpensive source of chitin is squid pens, a by-product of squid processing; these are small, plastic-like, inedible pieces of squid that are removed before the squid is consumed.

THERAPEUTIC DOSAGES

The standard dosage of chitosan is 3 to 6 grams (g) per day, to be taken with food. Chitosan can deplete the body of certain minerals. For this reason, when using chitosan, it may be helpful to take supplemental calcium, vitamin D, selenium, magnesium, and other minerals. Also, according to a preliminary study in rats, taking vitamin C along with chitosan might provide additional benefit in lowering cholesterol.

THERAPEUTIC USES

On the basis of chitosan's supposed ability to bind fat in the intestines, it has been tried as a treatment for high cholesterol. However, the evidence regarding whether it really works is generally more negative than positive. At best, chitosan appears to offer no more than minimal benefit for high cholesterol.

Chitosan has also been proposed as a weight-loss treatment on the same principle. However, despite some mildly positive results, the current balance of evidence suggests chitosan does not in fact significantly aid weight loss.

Weak evidence hints that chitosan may be helpful in kidney failure. When used for this purpose, it is thought to work by binding with toxins in the digestive tract and causing them to be excreted.

Studies in dogs have found that topically applied chitosan can help heal wounds. This effect might be caused by stimulation of new tissue growth; in addition, topical chitosan appears to kill bacteria such as those in the *Streptococcus* species, which may also contribute to wound healing. Chitosan may also have activity against *Candida albicans*, a form of yeast that causes vaginal infections.

Highly preliminary evidence suggests that oral chitosan may inhibit the expected rise in blood pressure after a high-salt meal. Other weak evidence hints that chitosan chewing gum might help prevent cavities. It

has been suggested that chitosan can stimulate the immune system and prevent cancer, but there is no reliable evidence as yet that it offers these benefits.

Animal studies suggest that some forms of chitosan may help to prevent bone loss; however, because chitosan also interferes with mineral absorption, the net effect in humans might actually be to increase bone loss.

SCIENTIFIC EVIDENCE

High cholesterol. An eight-week double-blind, placebo-controlled trial of fifty-one women found that use of chitosan at a dose of 1,200 milligrams (mg) twice daily slightly reduced low density lipoproteins (LDL, or bad cholesterol) compared with a placebo but did not affect total or high density lipoprotein (HDL, or good cholesterol) levels. Another eight-week trial, this one enrolling eighty-four people, also found modest benefits.

However, a four-month double-blind, placebo-controlled trial of 88 individuals found no improvement in cholesterol with 1,000 mg three times daily of a different chitosan product. A seven-month study of 84 men given a placebo or 1,200 mg of chitosan daily also failed to find any benefit. Furthermore, in a ten-month double-blind, placebo-controlled study of 130 men and women, use of a special microcrystalline form of chitosan at a dose of 1,200 mg twice daily again failed to improve cholesterol profile. These contradictory results suggest that if chitosan actually improves cholesterol profile, it does so to only a minimal extent.

Weight loss. Chitosan has been widely advocated as a weight-loss supplement on the basis of its supposed ability to bind fat in the digestive tract. However, despite some positive results, the largest and best-designed trial failed to find benefit. In this six-month double-blind, placebo-controlled study of 250 overweight people, use of chitosan at a dose of 3 g daily failed to enhance weight loss to any meaningful extent, compared with a placebo.

Kidney failure. People with kidney failure experience numerous health problems, including anemia, fatigue, and loss of appetite. In one open study, researchers tested chitosan supplements in eighty people with kidney failure receiving ongoing hemodialysis treatment. Half the participants were given 45 mg tablets for a total of about 1,500 mg of chitosan daily for twelve weeks; the other half were not given a supplement. Those in the treatment group showed a significant decrease in urea and creatinine levels. Further, they had a rise in hemoglobin levels and reported improved overall strength, appetite, and sleep.

SAFETY ISSUES

There is significant evidence that long-term, high-dose chitosan supplementation can result in malabsorption of some crucial vitamins and minerals, including calcium, magnesium, selenium, and vitamins A, D, E, and K. In turn, this appears to lead to a risk of osteoporosis in adults and delayed growth in children. For this reason, adults taking chitosan should also take supplemental vitamins and minerals, making especially sure to get enough vitamin D, calcium, and magnesium. Another possible risk of long-term ingestion of high doses of chitosan is that it could change the intestinal flora and allow the growth of unhealthful bacteria.

Finally, there has been a case report of arsenic poisoning caused by long-term use of chitosan supplements. Shellfish, it appears, can concentrate arsenic in their shells as part of their normal development; this in turn may lead to arsenic-laced chitosan supplements. Pregnant or nursing women and young children should probably avoid chitosan altogether.

EBSCO CAM Review Board

FURTHER READING

Bokura, H., and S. Kobayashi. "Chitosan Decreases Total Cholesterol in Women." *European Journal of Clinical Nutrition* 57 (2003): 721-725.

Guha, S., et al. "Effect of Chitosan on Lipid Levels When Administered Concurrently with Atorvastatin." *Journal of the Indian Medical Association* 103 (2005): 418, 420.

Ho, S. C., et al. "In the Absence of Dietary Surveillance, Chitosan Does Not Reduce Plasma Lipids or Obesity in Hypercholesterolaemic Obese Asian Subjects." *Singapore Medical Journal* 42 (2001): 6-10.

Lehtimaki, T., et al. "Microcrystalline Chitosan Is Ineffective to Decrease Plasma Lipids in Both Apolipoprotein E Epsilon4 Carriers and Non-carriers: A Long-term Placebo-Controlled Trial in Hypercholesterolaemic Volunteers." *Basic and Clinical Pharmacology and Toxicology* 97 (2005): 98-103.

Metso, S., et al. "The Effect of Long-term Microcrystalline Chitosan Therapy on Plasma Lipids and Glucose Concentrations in Subjects with Increased Plasma Total Cholesterol." *European Journal of Clinical Pharmacology* 59, no. 10 (2003): 721-726.

Mhurchu, C. N., et al. "The Effect of the Dietary Supplement, Chitosan, on Body Weight: A Randomised Controlled Trial in 250 Overweight and Obese Adults." *International Journal of Obesity and Related Metabolic Disorders* 28 (2004): 1149-1156.

Schiller, R. N., et al. "A Randomized, Double-Blind, Placebo-Controlled Study Examining the Effects of a Rapidly Soluble Chitosan Dietary Supplement on Weight Loss and Body Composition in Overweight and Mildly Obese Individuals." *Journal of the American Nutraceutical Association* 4 (2001): 42-49.

See also: Herbal medicine.

Chocolate

CATEGORY: Functional foods
RELATED TERMS: Cocoa, *Theobroma cacao*
DEFINITION: A food made from the cocoa bean that is consumed for specific health benefits.
PRINCIPAL PROPOSED USE: Cardiovascular disease prevention
OTHER PROPOSED USES: Aging-skin prevention, chronic fatigue syndrome, cough treatment, high blood pressure, high cholesterol, photosensitivity prevention, sunburn prevention

OVERVIEW

Made from the beans of the cocoa tree, chocolate was first developed as a food in South America, where it was primarily consumed as a bitter beverage. Cocoa was not combined with sugar until the Spaniards brought chocolate back to Europe from the Americas. The Latin name of the cocoa tree is *Theobroma cacao* (*theobroma* means "food of the gods"), and because of this, one of the stimulant substances in chocolate is named theobromine. This caffeine-related substance, however, does not contain the element bromine.

POSSIBLE HEALTH BENEFITS

Chocolate is rich in antioxidants in the flavonol family, substances similar to those found in green tea, red wine, grapes, soy, and other potentially healthful foods. However, this alone is not enough to prove that chocolate provides any health benefits. In gigantic

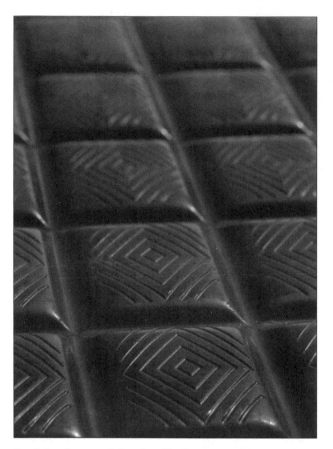

Dark chocolate may help reduce blood pressure. (©Dreamstime. com)

studies of other strong antioxidants, such as vitamin E, none of the hoped-for benefits materialized. Only double-blind, placebo-controlled studies can prove a treatment effective, and for chocolate, few of these studies have been performed.

Nonetheless, some potential benefits have been seen in preliminary trials. A controlled study of twenty males with mild hypertension compared the effects of 100 grams (g) daily of a flavonol-rich dark chocolate compared with a flavonol-free white chocolate. Results appeared to indicate that the dark chocolate produced improvements in blood pressure. A subsequent study of similar design, this one enrolling forty-four people with mild hypertension, found that a much lower dose of dark chocolate (6.3 g daily), also significantly reduced blood pressure levels. Also, a review including several additional studies drew the same conclusion regarding chocolate's modest yet favorable effect on blood pressure.

Chocolate has also shown some promise for improving cholesterol profile. In one study, fifty-seven people with high cholesterol were given either a standard snack bar or a snack bar enriched with cocoa flavonols. In six weeks, the results appeared to indicate that cocoa improved cholesterol levels to a greater extent than placebo. Two other preliminary studies found evidence that the consumption of chocolate can improve levels of HDL (good) cholesterol.

One double-blind study failed to find that flavonol-rich cocoa improved blood vessel health in people with established cardiovascular disease. Besides flavonols, chocolate contains a fat called stearic acid. Although it is a saturated fat, stearic acid is hypothesized to improve cardiovascular health. However, this has not been proven.

Like other antioxidants, the consumption of high-flavonol cocoa might also offer some protection to the skin from ultraviolet damage. This could, in theory, help prevent sunburn, reduce symptoms of photosensitivity, and help prevent age-related skin changes. However, the benefits would be small compared with standard sun block.

An unpublished double-blind study reportedly found that dark chocolate is helpful for chronic fatigue syndrome. The theobromine in cocoa, in addition to being a stimulant, might also have a cough-suppressant effect.

DOSAGE

In studies, the typical daily dose of flavonols from chocolate thought to offer a beneficial effect range widely from 30 to 500 milligrams (mg) per day. The flavonol content of chocolate itself also varies widely. White chocolate contains little to no flavonols, and commercial dark chocolate can contain as much as 500 to 2,000 mg of flavonols per 100 g of chocolate. Special flavonol-enriched forms of chocolate are also available.

SAFETY ISSUES

As a widely consumed food, chocolate is assumed to have a high safety factor. However, because of its caffeine and theobromine content, it would be expected to have potential side effects similar to those of coffee and black tea, namely heartburn, gastritis, insomnia, anxiety, and heart arrhythmia (benign palpitations or more serious disturbances of heart rhythm). All drug interactions that can occur with caffeine would be expected to occur with chocolate. Also, most chocolate products are high in calories and therefore could lead to weight gain.

IMPORTANT INTERACTIONS

Persons taking monoamine oxidase inhibitors should note that the caffeine in chocolate could cause dangerous drug interactions. Stimulant drugs such as ritalin might amplify the stimulant effects of chocolate. Chocolate also might interfere with drugs that prevent heart arrhythmias or with drugs that treat insomnia, heartburn, ulcers, or anxiety.

EBSCO CAM Review Board

FURTHER READING

Baba, S., et al. "Plasma LDL and HDL Cholesterol and Oxidized LDL Concentrations Are Altered in Normo- and Hypercholesterolemic Humans After Intake of Different Levels of Cocoa Powder." *Journal of Nutrition* 137 (2007): 1436-1441.

Heinrich, U., et al. "Long-Term Ingestion of High Flavanol Cocoa Provides Photoprotection Against UV-Induced Erythema and Improves Skin Condition in Women." *Journal of Nutrition* 136 (2006): 1565-1569.

Hooper, L., et al. "Flavonoids, Flavonoid-Rich Foods, and Cardiovascular Risk." *American Journal of Clinical Nutrition* 88 (2008): 38-50.

Ried, K., et al. "Does Chocolate Reduce Blood Pressure?" *BMC Medicine* 8 (2010): 39.

Rusconi, M., and A. Conti. "*Theobroma cacao* L., the Food of the Gods: A Scientific Approach Beyond Myths and Claims." *Pharmacological Research* 61 (2010): 5-13.

Taubert, D., et al. "Effects of Low Habitual Cocoa Intake on Blood Pressure and Bioactive Nitric Oxide." *Journal of the American Medical Association* 298 (2007): 49-60.

See also: Carob; Cholesterol, high; Functional foods: Introduction.

Cholesterol, high

CATEGORY: Condition
RELATED TERMS: Hyperlipidemia, hypercholesterolemia
DEFINITION: Treatment of abnormally high levels of cholesterol in the blood that lead to heart disease and other serious conditions.
PRINCIPAL PROPOSED NATURAL TREATMENTS: Artichoke leaf, fiber, soy, stanols, vitamin B_3 (niacin)
OTHER PROPOSED NATURAL TREATMENTS: *Achillea wilhelmsii*, alfalfa, ashwagandha, berberine (goldenseal), beta-glucan, black cohosh, black tea, broccoli and cabbage, caigua, calcium, carob, chocolate, chitosan, chromium, cinnamon, *Cordyceps*, creatine, curcumin, *Eclipta alba*, fenugreek, flaxseed, flaxseed oil, gamma oryzanol, garlic, genistein, glucomannan, green tea, guggul, He shou wu, honey, L-carnitine, lecithin, lifestyle changes, maitake, mesoglycan, multivitamin-multimineral supplements, nopal, olive oil, pantethine, policosanol, prebiotics, probiotics, red yeast rice, royal jelly, spirulina, tocotrienols

INTRODUCTION

One of the most significant discoveries in preventive medicine is that elevated levels of cholesterol in the blood accelerate atherosclerosis, a condition commonly known as hardening of the arteries. Like high blood pressure, inactivity, smoking, and diabetes, high cholesterol has proven to be one of the most important factors in the development of heart disease, strokes, and peripheral vascular disease (blockage of circulation to the extremities, usually the legs).

Cholesterol does not directly clog arteries like grease clogs pipes. The current theory is that elevated levels of cholesterol irritate the walls of blood vessels and cause them to undergo harmful changes. Because most cholesterol is manufactured by the body itself, dietary sources of cholesterol (such as eggs) are not usually the most important problem. The relative proportion of unsaturated fats (from plants) and saturated fats (mainly from animal products) in the diet is more significant.

When the consequences of elevated cholesterol were first being researched, total cholesterol was the only measurement considered. Today, the overall lipid profile is taken into account. LDL (bad) cholesterol, HDL (good) cholesterol, and triglycerides are the most common measurements related to cholesterol. Lipoprotein A and oxidized LDL cholesterol are also drawing increasing attention.

This change in emphasis has placed doubt on some long-standing recommendations. For example, reducing total fat intake generally decreases total cholesterol. On this basis, medical authorities long ago adopted a policy of recommending low-fat diets. However, when other lipid measurements are taken into account, it is clear that reducing fat intake is not the key. Low-fat diets improve total and LDL cholesterol levels, but they worsen HDL and triglyceride levels. Conversely, low-carbohydrate (carb), high-fat diets tend to raise levels of LDL and total cholesterol, but they reduce triglycerides and raise HDL. Some researchers use these effects as proof that the low-fat diet is healthier, but the current state of knowledge does not indicate whether the changes in lipids produced by low-fat diets are better or worse than the changes produced by low-carb diets. It is possible that a diet low in carbohydrates and high in monounsaturated fats (such as olive oil) offers the best of both worlds, but this has not been conclusively proven. What is clear is that losing weight is extremely important. If one is overweight and loses weight, one's cholesterol profile is almost certain to improve.

Increasing exercise and losing weight may produce adequate improvements in the lipid profile. If such lifestyle changes are not effective, however, there are many highly effective drugs to choose from. Medications in the statin family are most effective, and they have been shown to prevent heart attacks and reduce mortality. Other useful conventional options include ezetimibe (Zetia), fibrate drugs, and various forms of the vitamin niacin.

PRINCIPAL PROPOSED NATURAL TREATMENTS

Several herbs and supplements appear to help lower cholesterol levels. For some (such as stanols-sterols, vitamin B$_3$, fiber, and soy), the evidence is sufficiently strong to have produced mainstream acceptance.

Stanols and sterols. Stanols are substances that occur naturally in various plants. Their cholesterol-lowering effects were first observed in animals in the 1950s. Since then, a substantial amount of research suggests that plant stanols (usually modified into stanol esters) can help to lower cholesterol in persons with normal or mildly to moderately elevated cholesterol levels. Stanols are available in margarine spreads, salad dressings, and dietary supplement tablets. Related substances called plant sterols appear to have equivalent effects. In the following subsection, sterols and stanols and their esters will be referred to somewhat interchangeably.

Plant stanol esters reduce serum cholesterol levels by inhibiting cholesterol absorption. Because they are structurally similar to cholesterol, stanols (and sterols) can displace cholesterol from the "packages" that deliver cholesterol for absorption from the intestines to the bloodstream. The displaced cholesterol is then excreted from the body. This not only interferes with the absorption of cholesterol from food but has the additional (and probably more important) effect of removing cholesterol from substances made in the liver that are recycled through the digestive tract.

Numerous double-blind, placebo-controlled studies, ranging in length from thirty days to twelve months, have found stanol esters and their chemical relatives effective for improving cholesterol profile levels. The combined results suggest that these substances can reduce total cholesterol and LDL (bad) cholesterol by about 10 to 15 percent. However, stanols-sterols do not appear to have any significant effect on HDL (good) cholesterol or triglycerides.

Fish oil has also been shown to have a favorable effect on fats in the blood, in particular triglycerides. A study investigating the possible benefit of combining sterols with fish oil found that together they significantly lowered total cholesterol, LDL cholesterol, and triglycerides, and raised HDL cholesterol in persons with undesirable cholesterol profiles.

Persons taking statin drugs also may benefit from using stanols-sterols. According to one study, persons on statins and who start taking sterol ester margarine will see improvement in their cholesterol level to the same extent as if they had doubled the dose of statin. Stanols or sterols also appear to enhance the effects of cholesterol-lowering diets. Stanols or sterols also appear to be safe and effective in helping to improve cholesterol profile in people with type 2 (adult-onset) diabetes.

Niacin. The common vitamin niacin, also called vitamin B$_3$, is an accepted medical treatment for elevated cholesterol with solid science behind it. Several well-designed, double-blind, placebo-controlled studies have found that niacin reduced LDL cholesterol by approximately 10 percent and triglycerides by 25 percent, and raised HDL cholesterol by 20 to 30 percent. Niacin also lowers levels of lipoprotein A (another risk factor for atherosclerosis) by about 35 percent. Furthermore, long-term use of niacin has been shown to significantly reduce death rates from cardiovascular disease.

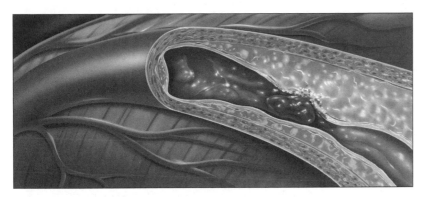

High levels of cholesterol can lead to a blocked coronary artery. (John Bavosi/ Photo Researchers, Inc.)

Niacin appears to be a safe and effective treatment for high cholesterol in people with diabetes too and (contrary to previous reports) does not seem to raise blood sugar levels. Niacin, if taken in sufficient quantities to lower cholesterol, can cause an annoying flushing reaction and occasionally liver inflammation. Close medical supervision is essential when using niacin to lower cholesterol.

Combining high-dose niacin with statin drugs (the most effective medications for high cholesterol) further improves lipid profile by raising HDL cholesterol. There are real concerns, however, that this combination therapy could cause a potentially fatal condition called rhabdomyolysis.

A growing body of evidence, however, suggests that the risk is relatively slight in persons with healthy kidneys. Furthermore, even much lower doses of niacin than the usual dose given to improve cholesterol levels (100 milligrams [mg] versus 1,000 mg or more) may provide a similar benefit. At this dose, the risk of rhabdomyolysis should be decreased. Nonetheless, it is not safe to try this combination except under close physician supervision because rhabdomyolysis can be fatal.

Soluble fiber. Water-soluble fiber supplements (such as psyllium, hydroxymethylcellulose and its relatives, and beta glucan from oats) are thought to lower cholesterol, and the U.S. Food and Drug Administration (FDA) has permitted products containing this form of fiber to carry a "heart-healthy" label. The bulk of the supporting evidence for this theory comes from studies of oats conducted by manufacturers of oat products. A typical dose of oat bran is 5 to 10 grams (g) with each meal and at bedtime; psyllium is taken at 10 g with each meal.

Soy protein. Soy protein appears capable of modestly lowering total cholesterol, LDL cholesterol, and triglycerides by approximately 5 to 15 percent. The FDA has allowed foods containing soy protein to make the heart-healthy claim on the label. One study suggests that substituting as little as 20 g daily of soy protein for animal protein can significantly improve cholesterol levels. Higher doses appear to lead to increased benefit.

Although it was once thought that isoflavones are the active ingredients in soy responsible for improving cholesterol profile, evidence suggests otherwise. Other substances, such as certain soy proteins, may be more important. However, it also has been suggested that soy protein must be kept in its original state to be effective. Ordinary soy protein extracts are somewhat damaged ("denatured"). In a double-blind study of 120 people, a special "preserved" soy protein extract proved more effective for improving cholesterol profile than standard denatured soy protein extracts.

Artichoke leaf. Although primarily used to stimulate gallbladder function, artichoke leaf also may be helpful for high cholesterol. In a double-blind, placebo-controlled study of 143 persons with elevated cholesterol, artichoke leaf extract significantly improved cholesterol readings. Total cholesterol fell by 18.5 percent compared to 8.6 percent in the placebo group; LDL cholesterol fell by 23 percent versus 6 percent; and the LDL to HDL ratio decreased by 20 percent versus 7 percent. In a subsequent study of seventy-five otherwise healthy people with high cholesterol, artichoke leaf extract significantly reduced total cholesterol compared with placebo, but it did not affect LDL, HDL, or triglycerides levels.

Artichoke leaf may work by interfering with cholesterol synthesis. A compound in artichoke called luteolin may play a role in reducing cholesterol.

OTHER PROPOSED NATURAL TREATMENTS

There are several other promising alternative treatments for high cholesterol. Numerous studies enrolling a total of many thousands of persons purported to show that the substance policosanol, made from sugarcane, can markedly improve cholesterol profile. However, the single Cuban research group behind these studies has a financial connection to the product. Not until 2006 did independent research groups begin to report their results on the use of policosanol for hyperlipidemia. Nine such independent studies have been reported, enrolling more than five hundred people, and in not one of these studies has policosanol proved to be more effective than placebo.

Red yeast rice is a traditional Chinese medicinal substance that is made by fermenting a type of yeast called *Monascus purpureus* over rice. It contains cholesterol-lowering chemicals in the statin family, including one identical to the drug lovastatin. Like statin drugs, red yeast rice appears to be effective for improving various aspects of lipid profile, including total cholesterol, LDL cholesterol, and the LDL/HDL ratio. Presumably it also presents the same safety risks as statins, compounded by the uncertainty regarding how much active drug any particular batch of red yeast rice contains.

In a twelve-month study of 223 postmenopausal women, calcium supplements (calcium citrate at a dose of 1 g daily) significantly improved the ratio of HDL cholesterol to LDL cholesterol. This appears to have been primarily caused by a meaningful rise in HDL levels.

Krill are tiny shrimplike crustaceans that flourish in the Antarctic Ocean and provide food for numerous aquatic animals. Krill oil, similar but not identical to fish oil, may improve cholesterol profile. Fish oil may enhance the effectiveness of drugs in the statin family. Eicosapentaenoic acid, another constituent of fish oil, may help prevent severe heart complications in people with high cholesterol who are already taking statins.

One double-blind study found evidence that cinnamon, taken at a dose of 1 to 6 grams daily, improved triglyceride, LDL cholesterol, and total cholesterol, without worsening HDL cholesterol. Inconsistent evidence hints that flaxseed might reduce LDL cholesterol and, overall, slow down atherosclerosis. Flaxseed oil may be helpful too, although evidence is again inconsistent. It may be the generic fiber and not the other specific ingredients in flaxseed that benefit cholesterol levels. Studies of purified lignans (found in flaxseed) have yielded mixed results. Also, a growing body of evidence suggests that increased consumption of nuts such as almonds, walnuts, pecans, and macadamia nuts may improve lipid profile and re-

duce heart disease risk, presumably because of their high monounsaturated fat content.

Olive oil is known to improve cholesterol profile. Until recently, it had been thought that the monounsaturated fats in olive oil are its primary active ingredients. However, some evidence hints that polyphenols in olive oil (particularly, virgin olive oil) also may play a positive role.

Some studies suggest that friendly bacteria (probiotics) might improve cholesterol profile. Prebiotics, substances that enhance the growth of friendly bacteria, have shown inconsistent benefit in studies. One study found that any improvement, if it does occur, is short-lived.

Both black and green teas enriched with either theaflavin or catechins have shown promise for lowering cholesterol. Without such enhancement, both green tea and black tea may be ineffective. Dark chocolate contains substances related to those in black and green tea, and it too has shown some promise for improving cholesterol profile.

Other preliminary double-blind trials suggest potential benefit with the Iranian herb *Achillea wilhelmsii*, the Peruvian herb caigua (*Cyclanterha pedata*), carob fiber, caterpillar fungus (*Cordyceps sinensis*), *Ipomoea batatus* (sweet potato), and a drink containing broccoli and cabbage. Chitosan, a type of insoluble fiber derived from crustacean shells, has been proposed for reducing cholesterol levels. Evidence suggests that if it does offer any benefits, they are minimal at best.

A comprehensive review combining the results of fourteen studies found that glucomannan, a dietary fiber derived from the tubers of *Amorphophallus konjac*, significantly reduced total and LDL cholesterol levels. Weaker, and in some cases inconsistent, evidence suggests potential benefit with alfalfa; berberine (found in goldenseal, honey, Oregon grape, and barberry); beta-hydroxy-beta-methylbutyrate; blue-green algae; conjugated linoleic acid; L-carnitine; the Ayurvedic herb *Eclipta alba* (also known as Bhringraja or Keshraja); grape polyphenols; mesoglycan; and nopal cactus.

Studies on whether the mineral chromium can improve cholesterol levels have returned mixed results. However, this mineral may offer benefit for people taking drugs in the beta-blocker family. These medications, used for high blood pressure and other conditions, sometimes reduce HDL cholesterol levels. Chromium supplements may offset this side effect.

One study provides preliminary evidence that the herb black cohosh may improve lipid profiles in postmenopausal women. Rice bran oil, like other vegetables oils, appears to favorably change lipid profile and to reduce heart disease risk in other ways. Weaker evidence suggests that gamma oryzanol, a substance found in rice bran oil, can also improve lipid profiles.

Substances related to vitamin E called tocotrienols are sometimes promoted as improving cholesterol levels. However, while benefit has been reported in test-tube studies, animal studies, and nonblinded human trials, properly designed studies have failed to find it effective. Other herbs and supplements sometimes recommended for high cholesterol include ashwagandha, fenugreek, He shou wu, maitake, and royal jelly, but there is no evidence that they work.

A number of studies published in the 1980s and 1990s reported that various garlic preparations, including raw garlic, stabilized garlic powder, and aged garlic, can lower cholesterol. However, several more recent and generally better-designed studies have found that if any benefits exist, they are so small as to be of little help in real life.

Although lecithin is commonly believed to reduce cholesterol levels, evidence indicates that it does not work. Similarly, guggul, the sticky gum resin from the mukul myrrh tree, has been widely marketed as a cholesterol-reducing herb. However, while preliminary studies found evidence of benefit, the studies all had significant design flaws; a well-designed study did not find guggul effective.

Vitamin C, cranberry, curcumin (turmeric), and elderberry have failed to prove effective in studies thus far. Also, one study failed to find special fats called medium-chain triacylglycerols more effective for reducing cholesterol than ordinary unsaturated fats.

Herbs and Supplements to Use Only with Caution

One study, in which participants took more than 50 mg of zinc daily, showed that zinc might reduce levels of HDL, or good, cholesterol. Unexpected results in a single trial hint that the sports supplement pyruvate might negate some of the beneficial effects of exercise on HDL levels. In addition, various herbs and supplements may interact adversely with drugs used to treat high cholesterol.

EBSCO CAM Review Board

Further Reading

Allen, R. R., et al. "Daily Consumption of a Dark Chocolate Containing Flavanols and Added Sterol Esters Affects Cardiovascular Risk Factors in a Normotensive Population with Elevated Cholesterol." *Journal of Nutrition* 138 (2008): 725-731.

Baba, S., et al. "Continuous Intake of Polyphenolic Compounds Containing Cocoa Powder Reduces LDL Oxidative Susceptibility and Has Beneficial Effects on Plasma HDL-Cholesterol Concentrations in Humans." *American Journal of Clinical Nutrition* 85 (2007): 709-717.

Berglund, L., et al. "Comparison of Monounsaturated Fat with Carbohydrates as a Replacement for Saturated Fat in Subjects with a High Metabolic Risk Profile: Studies in the Fasting and Postprandial States." *American Journal of Clinical Nutrition* 86 (2007): 1611-1620.

Bloedon, L. T., et al. "Flaxseed and Cardiovascular Risk Factors." *Journal of the American College of Nutrition* 27 (2008): 65-74.

Castro Cabezas, M., et al. "Effects of a Stanol-Enriched Diet on Plasma Cholesterol and Triglycerides in Patients Treated with Statins." *Journal of the American Dietetic Association* 106 (2006): 1564-1569.

Covas, M. I., et al. "The Effect of Polyphenols in Olive Oil on Heart Disease Risk Factors." *Annals of Internal Medicine* 145 (2006): 333-341.

Gardner, C. D., et al. "Effect of Raw Garlic vs Commercial Garlic Supplements on Plasma Lipid Concentrations in Adults with Moderate Hypercholesterolemia." *Archives of Internal Medicine* 167 (2007): 346-353.

Gardner, C. D., et al. "Effect of Two Types of Soy Milk and Dairy Milk on Plasma Lipids in Hypercholesterolemic Adults." *Journal of the American College of Nutrition* 26 (2007): 669-677.

Griel, A. E., et al. "A Macadamia Nut-Rich Diet Reduces Total and LDL-Cholesterol in Mildly Hypercholesterolemic Men and Women." *Journal of Nutrition* 138 (2008): 761-767.

Hughes, S., and S. Samman. "The Effect of Zinc Supplementation in Humans on Plasma Lipids, Antioxidant Status, and Thrombogenesis." *Journal of the American College of Nutrition* 25 (2006): 285-291.

Kelly, S., et al. "Wholegrain Cereals for Coronary Heart Disease." *Cochrane Database of Systematic Reviews* (2007): CD005051. Available through *EBSCO DynaMed Systematic Literature Surveillance* at http://www.ebscohost.com/dynamed.

Lichtenstein, A. H. "Dietary Fat and Cardiovascular Disease Risk: Quantity or Quality?" *Journal of Women's Health* 12 (2003): 109-114.

Mukamal, K. J., et al. "A Six-Month Randomized Pilot Study of Black Tea and Cardiovascular Risk Factors." *American Heart Journal* 154 (2007): 724.

Nagao, T., T. Hase, and I. Tokimitsu. "A Green Tea Extract High in Catechins Reduces Body Fat and Cardiovascular Risks in Humans." *Obesity* 15 (2007): 1473-1483.

Reynolds, K., et al. "A Meta-analysis of the Effect of Soy Protein Supplementation on Serum Lipids." *American Journal of Cardiology* 98 (2006): 633-640.

Tay, J., et al. "Metabolic Effects of Weight Loss on a Very-Low-Carbohydrate Diet Compared with an Isocaloric High-Carbohydrate Diet in Abdominally Obese Subjects." *Journal of the American College of Cardiology* 51 (2008): 59-67.

See also: Artichoke; Heart attack; Hypertension; Policosanol; Red yeast rice; Soy; Stanols and sterols; Strokes; Triglycerides, high; Vitamin B_3.

Chondroitin

CATEGORY: Herbs and supplements
RELATED TERM: Chondroitin sulfate
DEFINITION: Natural substance of the human body used as a supplement to treat specific health conditions.
PRINCIPAL PROPOSED USE: Osteoarthritis
OTHER PROPOSED USES: Atherosclerosis, high cholesterol, sports and fitness support: enhancing recovery

OVERVIEW

Chondroitin sulfate is a naturally occurring substance in the body. It is a major constituent of cartilage, the tough, elastic connective tissue found in the joints.

Based on the evidence of preliminary double-blind studies, chondroitin is widely used as a treatment for osteoarthritis, the typical arthritis that many people suffer as they get older. However, the supporting evidence for this use is weak.

There is some evidence that chondroitin might go beyond treating symptoms and actually protect joints from damage. Current medical treatments for osteoarthritis, such as nonsteroidal anti-inflammatory drugs (NSAIDs), treat the symptoms but do not actually slow the disease's progression, and they may actually make it get worse faster. Chondroitin (along with glucosamine) may take the treatment of osteoarthritis to a new level. However, more research needs to be performed to prove definitively that this possibility is real.

REQUIREMENTS AND SOURCES

Chondroitin is not an essential nutrient. Animal cartilage is the only dietary source of chondroitin. (Animal cartilage in food is called gristle.) Chondroitin comes in pill form and can be purchased from a health-food store or pharmacy.

THERAPEUTIC DOSAGES

The usual dosage of chondroitin is 400 milligrams (mg) taken three times daily, indefinitely. Two studies (mentioned below) used an on-and-off schedule of chondroitin (taking it for three months, going off of it for three months, and then taking it again). Other studies involved taking chondroitin daily. Regardless of how it is taken, the results are thought to take weeks to develop.

In commercial products, chondroitin is often combined with glucosamine. Preliminary information from one animal study suggests that this combination may be superior to treatment by either substance alone.

There are large differences between chondroitin products based on their chemical structure. This can be expected to lead to significant differences in absorption and hence effectiveness. Most likely, chondroitin products with physically smaller molecules (fewer than 16,900 daltons) are better absorbed. In addition, a review conducted in 2003 by a respected testing organization found that some products sold as providing chondroitin actually contained far less chondroitin than stated on the label, or even no chondroitin. It may be advisable to use the exact products that were tested in double-blind trials.

THERAPEUTIC USES

Numerous double-blind studies have found evidence that chondroitin can relieve the symptoms of osteoarthritis and possibly also slow the progression of the disease. However, most of these studies suffer from serious problems in design, statistical analysis, and reporting. When pooled together, the results of the three best studies failed to demonstrate benefit. On balance, the evidence for chondroitin's effectiveness for osteoarthritis is inconsistent and incomplete.

Chondroitin has also been proposed as a treatment for other conditions, such as atherosclerosis, interstitial cystitis, and high cholesterol, but as yet the evidence that the supplement might help is far too weak to rely upon. One small double-blind study evaluated chondroitin for reducing muscle soreness caused by intense exercise but failed to find benefit.

SCIENTIFIC EVIDENCE

For years, experts stated that oral chondroitin could not possibly work because its molecules are so big that it seemed doubtful that they could be absorbed through the digestive tract. However, in 1995, researchers laid this objection to rest when they found evidence that up to 15 percent of chondroitin is absorbed intact.

Reducing symptoms of osteoarthritis. Many but not all double-blind, placebo-controlled studies indicate that chondroitin can relieve symptoms of osteoarthritis. For example, one study enrolled eighty-five people with osteoarthritis of the knee and followed them for six months. Participants received either 400 mg of chondroitin sulfate twice daily or a placebo. At the end of the trial, doctors rated the improvement as good or very good in 69 percent of those taking chondroitin sulfate, but in only 32 percent of those taking a placebo.

Another way of comparing the results is to look at maximum walking speed among participants. Whereas individuals in the chondroitin group were able to improve their walking speed gradually over the course of the trial, walking speed did not improve in the placebo group. Additionally, there were improvements in other measures of osteoarthritis, such as pain level, with benefits seen as early as one month. This suggests that chondroitin was able to stop the arthritis from gradually getting worse.

Good results were seen in a twelve-month double-blind trial that compared chondroitin against placebo in 104 people, a twelve-month trial of 42 people, and a twelve-month study of 120 people. In two of these studies, chondroitin was taken for two separate three-month periods separated by three months of no treatment; in the others, it was taken continuously. No

comparison of these two ways of using chondroitin has been published.

Benefits were also seen in two other double-blind, placebo-controlled trials involving a total of more than 350 individuals. Another double-blind study compared chondroitin to the anti-inflammatory drug diclofenac and found equivalent benefits.

Additional studies combined glucosamine with chondroitin. A six-month double-blind, placebo-controlled study of ninety-three people with knee arthritis found that a combination of glucosamine and chondroitin (along with manganese) was more effective than a placebo. Another double-blind, placebo-controlled study evaluated chondroitin/glucosamine for temporomandibular joint (TMJ) disease but had equivocal results.

However, a very large (1,583 participants) and well-designed study failed to find either chondroitin or glucosamine plus chondroitin more effective than a placebo. When this study is pooled together with the two other best-designed trials, no overall benefit is seen. Yet another study also failed to find benefit with glucosamine plus chondroitin. Finally, in a systematic review including ten randomized trials involving 3,803 patients with osteoarthritis of hip or knee, researchers found that chondroitin alone or with glucosamine did not improve pain. It has been suggested that chondroitin, like glucosamine, may primarily appear effective in studies funded by manufacturers of chondroitin products.

Slowing the progression of osteoarthritis. Osteoarthritis tends to worsen with time. As mentioned earlier, no conventional treatment for osteoarthritis protects joints from progressive damage. Some evidence hints that chondroitin can do this, but it is too early to consider the matter settled.

One study examined the progression of osteoarthritis in 119 people for three years. In this double-blind, placebo-controlled trial, those who took 1,200 mg of chondroitin daily showed lower rates of severe joint damage. Only 8.8 percent of the chondroitin group developed severely damaged joints during the three years of the study, compared with almost 30 percent of the placebo group. This suggests that chondroitin was slowing the progression of osteoarthritis. Protective effects were also seen in three one-year studies enrolling a total of more than 200 people.

Animal studies provide some additional evidence

for a joint-protecting benefit. However, as with studies of chondroitin for treating osteoarthritis, too high a proportion of the research record involving prevention of osteoarthritis has involved industry-funded research.

How chondroitin works for osteoarthritis. Scientists are unsure how chondroitin sulfate works (if indeed it does). At its most basic level, chondroitin may help cartilage by providing it with the building blocks it needs to repair itself. Chondroitin is also believed to block enzymes that break down cartilage in the joints. Another theory holds that chondroitin increases the amount of hyaluronic acid in the joints. Hyaluronic acid is a protective fluid that keeps the joints lubricated. Finally, chondroitin may have a mild anti-inflammatory effect.

SAFETY ISSUES

Chondroitin generally does not cause much in the way of side effects, besides occasional mild digestive distress. However, there is one case report of an exacerbation of asthma caused by use of a glucosamine-chondroitin product. In addition, there are theoretical concerns that chondroitin might have a mild blood-thinning effect, based on its chemical similarity to the anticoagulant drug heparin. Reassuringly, there are no case reports of any problems relating to this, and studies suggest that chondroitin has at most a mild anticoagulant effect. Nonetheless, prudence suggests that, based on these findings, chondroitin should not be combined with blood-thinning drugs, such as warfarin (Coumadin), heparin, and aspirin, except under physician supervision. In addition, individuals with bleeding problems, such as hemophilia, or who are temporarily at risk for bleeding (for example, undergoing surgery or labor and delivery) should avoid chondroitin.

IMPORTANT INTERACTIONS

Persons using drugs that impair blood coagulation, such as warfarin (Coumadin), heparin, aspirin, clopidogrel (Plavix), ticlopidine (Ticlid), or pentoxifylline (Trental), should not use chondroitin except under physician supervision.

EBSCO CAM Review Board

FURTHER READING

Braun, W. A., et al. "The Effects of Chondroitin Sulfate Supplementation on Indices of Muscle Damage In-

duced by Eccentric Arm Exercise." *Journal of Sports Medicine and Physical Fitness* 45 (2006): 553-560.

Cohen, M., et al. "A Randomized, Double Blind, Placebo Controlled Trial of a Topical Cream Containing Glucosamine Sulfate, Chondroitin Sulfate, and Camphor for Osteoarthritis of the Knee." *Journal of Rheumatology* 30 (2003): 523-528.

Nguyen, P., et al. "A Randomized Double-Blind Clinical Trial of the Effect of Chondroitin Sulfate and Glucosamine Hydrochloride on Temporomandibular Joint Disorders: A Pilot Study." *Cranio* 19 (2001): 130-139.

Palylyk-Colwell, E. "Chondroitin Sulfate for Interstitial Cystitis." *Issues in Emerging Health Technologies* 84 (2006): 1-4.

Richy, F., et al. "Structural and Symptomatic Efficacy of Glucosamine and Chondroitin in Knee Osteoarthritis: A Comprehensive Meta-analysis." *Archives of Internal Medicine* 163 (2003): 1514-1522.

Tallia, A. F., and D. A. Cardone. "Asthma Exacerbation Associated with Glucosamine-chondroitin Supplement." *Journal of the American Board of Family Practice* 15 (2002): 481-484.

Uebelhart, D., et al. "Intermittent Treatment of Knee Osteoarthritis with Oral Chondroitin Sulfate: A One-year, Randomized, Double-blind, Multicenter Study Versus Placebo." *Osteoarthritis Cartilage* 12 (2004): 269-276.

See also: Cartilage; Glucosamine; Herbal medicine; Osteoarthritis.

Chopra, Deepak

CATEGORY: Biography
IDENTIFICATION: Indian-born American physician and proponent of mind/body medicine and Ayurveda
BORN: October 22, 1946; New Delhi, India

OVERVIEW

Deepak Chopra, an American physician born in India, is a best-selling writer and popular public speaker whose work centers on mind/body medicine and health, spirituality, quantum mechanics, and Ayurveda, a traditional medicine system native to India. Ayurveda in the West is largely classified as alternative medicine.

As a youth, Chopra yearned to become a journalist

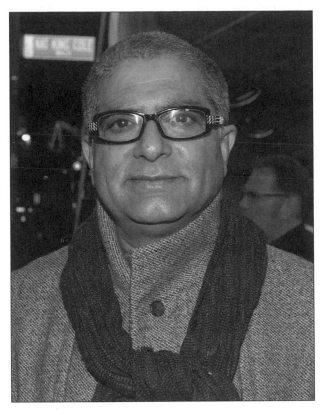

Deepak Chopra. (FilmMagic/Getty Images)

or actor, but he was later inspired to become a physician by a character in the Sinclair Lewis novel *Arrowsmith*. Chopra completed his medical education at the All India Institute of Medical Sciences in New Delhi. He began his medical career as an endocrinologist, obtaining certification in internal medicine with a specialty in endocrinology. However, Chopra later shifted to a career focused in alternative medicine. Before embarking on his own productive medical career, Chopra studied, for several years, with Maharishi Mahesh Yogi, who developed Transcendental Meditation and is regarded as the guru of the movement associated with the technique.

Chopra moved to the United States in 1968 and completed his medical internship and residency in New Jersey, Massachusetts, and Virginia. He obtained his medical license in Massachusetts in 1973 and another in California in 2004. During his early career, Chopra also served as a professor, both at Tufts University and at Boston University. In addition, he was chief of staff at Boston Regional Medical Center. He

later went on to establish a private practice. He has been a longtime member of many respected societies, including the American College of Physicians, the American Medical Association (AMA), and the American Association of Clinical Endocrinologists.

In 1985, Chopra met Maharishi Mahesh Yogi. The well-known alternative practitioner offered to mentor Chopra in the study of Ayurveda. Soon after studying with the Maharishi, Chopra was appointed founding president of the American Association of Ayurvedic Medicine. He later was named the medical director of the Maharishi Ayurveda Health Center for Stress Management and Behavioral Medicine.

Chopra was later appointed executive director of the Sharp Institute for Human Potential and Mind-Body Medicine. Around 1993, he moved with his family to Southern California. The following year, Chopra formally left the Transcendental Meditation movement, reportedly making this decision after his former mentor accused him of trying to compete with his position and to obtain the qualification of "guru."

Chopra resigned from the Sharp Institute in 1996. With David Simon, a medical doctor and an authority in mind/body medicine, he founded the Chopra Center for Well Being in La Jolla, California. The center offers courses in Ayurveda and other alternative medicine techniques. In recent years, some notable institutions (such as the AMA and the University of California) have granted education credits for physicians studying at the center.

Chopra has written more than sixty books that have been translated into dozens of languages. His books are concerned with New Age spirituality, alternative medicine, and peace, among other topics. More than one dozen have been *New York Times* best sellers. He has sold more than twenty million copies worldwide. Chopra also has hosted a weekly radio show, in which he interviewed scientists and others working in alternative medicine. He has been vocal about his opposition to the over-prescribing of drugs and to drug dependency, especially after the death of his friend, singer-songwriter Michael Jackson.

Chopra has received various awards for his work in alternative medicine. *Esquire* magazine named him one of the "top ten motivational speakers" in the United States. He has served as an adviser to the National Ayurveda Medical Association since 2002, and in 2005 he was also appointed senior scientist at the Gallup Organization. In addition, he has served as an adjunct professor at the Kellogg School of Management at Northwestern University. Chopra also contributes significantly to various media, acting as a columnist for the *San Francisco Chronicle* and *The Washington Post*, and he regularly contributes to Intent.com and the HuffingtonPost.com.

Like other alternative and complementary medicine practitioners, Chopra has many critics. Some opponents of his work argue that he misleads and exploits the ill. In particular, critics claim that he creates false hope in the weak, deterring them from seeking traditional, possibly more effective, medical care. Furthermore, some of his critics argue that much of Chopra's popularity comes from his public speaking abilities, not from his teachings. Chopra has said that "perfect health is a matter of choice," and *Business Week* indicated that one of Chopra's main teachings is that health can be improved by ridding oneself of negative emotions and by developing intuitive communication with one's own body. These views trouble a number of traditional clinicians and scientists.

Brandy Weidow, M.S.

FURTHER READING

Chopra, Deepak. "Medicine's Great Divide: The View from the Alternative Side." *American Medical Association Journal of Ethics* 13, no. 6 (2011): 394-398. Also available at http://virtualmentor.ama-assn.org/2011/06/oped2-1106.html. Chopra discusses his perspective on the controversy between modern medicine and complementary and alternative practices.

_____. *Perfect Health: The Complete Mind/Body Guide.* Rev. ed. New York: Harmony, 2001. In this bestselling self-help book, Chopra provides the reader with a step-by-step program of mind/body medicine tailored to individual needs.

_____. *Reinventing the Body, Resurrecting the Soul: How to Create a New You.* New York: Three Rivers Press, 2010. In this *New York Times* best-selling self-help book, Chopra presents the reader with steps toward mind/body healing.

Ninivaggi, Frank John. *Ayurveda: A Comprehensive Guide to Traditional Indian Medicine for the West.* Westport, Conn.: Praeger, 2008.

See also: Ayurveda; Charaka; Diet-based therapies; Mind/body medicine; Spirituality; Traditional healing; Whole medicine; Yoga.

Chromium

CATEGORY: Herbs and supplements
RELATED TERMS: Chromium chloride, chromium picolinate, chromium polynicotinate, high-chromium brewer's yeast
DEFINITION: Essential natural substance used as a dietary supplement for specific health benefits.
PRINCIPAL PROPOSED USES: Diabetes, insulin resistance and abnormal glucose tolerance, heart disease prevention
OTHER PROPOSED USES: Acne, depression, functional hypoglycemia, high cholesterol, metabolic syndrome (syndrome X), migraine headaches, psoriasis, sports performance enhancement, weight loss

OVERVIEW

Chromium is a mineral the body needs in very small amounts, but it plays a significant role in human nutrition. Chromium's most important function in the body is to help regulate the amount of glucose (sugar) in the blood. Insulin plays a starring role in this fundamental biological process by regulating the movement of glucose from the blood and into cells.

Scientists believe that insulin uses chromium as an assistant (technically, a cofactor) to "unlock the door" to the cell membrane, allowing glucose to enter the cell. In the past, it was believed that to accomplish this the body first converted chromium into a large chemical called glucose tolerance factor (GTF). Intact GTF was thought to be present in certain foods, such as brewer's yeast, and for that reason such products were described as superior sources of chromium. However, subsequent investigation indicated that researchers were actually creating GTF inadvertently during the process of chemical analysis. Scientists now believe that there is no such thing as GTF. Rather, chromium appears to act in concert with a very small protein called low molecular weight chromium-binding substance (LMWCr) to assist insulin's action. LMWCr does not permanently bind chromium and is not a likely source of chromium in foods.

Based on chromium's close relationship with insulin, this trace mineral has been studied as a treatment for diabetes. The results have been somewhat positive: It seems fairly likely that chromium supplements can improve blood sugar control in people with diabetes. Chromium also might be helpful for milder abnormalities in blood sugar metabolism. One study suggests that chromium might aid in weight loss too, but other studies failed to find this effect.

REQUIREMENTS AND SOURCES

The official U.S. recommendations for daily intake of chromium (in micrograms) are as follows: infants to six months (0.2) and seven to twelve months of age (5.5); children one to three years (11) and four to eight years (15); girls age nine to thirteen years (21) and fourteen to eighteen years (24); boys age nine to thirteen years (25); males age fourteen to fifty years (35); women age nineteen to fifty years (25), men age fifty-one and older (30), women age fifty-one and older (20), pregnant girls (29), pregnant women (30), nursing girls (44) and nursing women (45).

Some evidence suggests that chromium deficiency may be relatively common. However, this has not been proven, and the matter is greatly complicated because a good test to identify chromium deficiency is not available.

Severe chromium deficiency has been seen only in hospitalized persons receiving nutrition intravenously. Symptoms include problems with blood sugar control that cannot be corrected by insulin alone.

Corticosteroid treatment may cause increased chromium loss in the urine. It is possible that this loss of chromium may contribute to corticosteroid-induced diabetes.

Chromium is found in drinking water, especially hard water, but concentrations vary widely. Many good sources of chromium, such as whole wheat, are depleted of this important mineral during processing. The most concentrated sources of chromium are brewer's yeast (not nutritional or torula yeast) and calf liver. Two ounces of brewer's yeast or four ounces of calf liver supply between 50 and 60 micrograms (mcg) of chromium. Other good sources of chromium are whole grains, beer, and cheese. Also, calcium carbonate interferes with the absorption of chromium.

THERAPEUTIC DOSAGES

The dosage of chromium used in studies ranges from 200 to 1,000 mcg daily, mostly in the form of chromium picolinate. However, there may be potential risks in the higher dosages of chromium. These and all other dosages of chromium cite the amount of the actual chromium ion in the supplement ("elemental chromium"), discounting the weight of the substances, such as picolinate, attached to it.

Selected Food Sources of Chromium, in Micrograms

Food	Chromium
Broccoli, ½ cup	11
Grape juice, 1 cup	8
English muffin, whole wheat, 1	4
Potatoes, mashed, 1 cup	3
Garlic, dried, 1 teaspoon	3
Basil, dried, 1 tablespoon	2
Beef cubes, 3 ounces	2
Orange juice, 1 cup	2
Turkey breast, 3 ounces	2
Whole wheat bread, 2 slices	2
Red wine, 5 ounces	1-13
Apple, unpeeled, 1 medium	1
Banana, 1 medium	1
Green beans, ½ cup	1

Some products state that they contain "GTF chromium." Some of these products are manufactured from brewer's yeast, which was once thought to contain GTF. Others contain chromium as chromium nicotinate, which bears a faint resemblance to the proposed GTF molecule. However, because GTF is no longer believed to exist, this claim should be disregarded.

THERAPEUTIC USES

Chromium has principally been studied for its possible benefits in improving blood sugar control in people with diabetes. Several studies suggest that people with type 2 diabetes may show some improvement when given appropriate dosages of chromium. One study suggests that chromium may also be useful for diabetes that occurs during pregnancy. In addition, nondiabetic persons with mildly impaired blood sugar control might attain better control of blood sugar with chromium supplementation. Because mild impairment of blood sugar control is believed to increase the risk of heart disease, chromium supplementation might help reduce heart disease rates.

Chromium has been sold as a "fat burner" and is

also said to help build muscle tissue. However, most studies evaluating chromium's ability to promote weight loss have not found benefits. One study failed to find benefit with a combination of chromium and conjugated linoleic acid. Studies evaluating chromium as a performance enhancer or aid to body-building have yielded almost entirely negative results.

Studies on whether chromium can improve cholesterol levels have returned mixed results. However, one study suggests that chromium combined with grape seed extract might have a beneficial effect. In addition, among persons taking beta-blockers, chromium may raise levels of HDL (good) cholesterol.

When depression is characterized by rapid mood changes, excessive sleeping and eating, a sense of leaden paralysis, and extreme sensitivity to negative life events, the condition is called atypical depression. A small (fifteen participants) double-blind, placebo-controlled study found that chromium picolinate might be helpful for this form of depression; however, a much larger study failed to find statistically significant benefits.

According to some researchers, impaired blood sugar control, high cholesterol, weight gain, and high blood pressure are all part of a larger condition called metabolic syndrome, or syndrome X. Because chromium may be helpful for the first three of these conditions, chromium deficiency has been proposed as the cause of syndrome X. However, this has not been proven.

One study failed to find that chromium picolinate at 200 mcg per day can improve symptoms of polycystic ovaries, which is a common cause of infertility. Chromium has also been proposed as a treatment for acne, migraine headaches, and psoriasis, but there is no real evidence that it works for these conditions.

SCIENTIFIC EVIDENCE

Diabetes. The evidence regarding use of chromium for type 2 diabetes and other forms of diabetes remains incomplete and inconsistent. In a double-blind, placebo-controlled study, 180 people with type 2 diabetes were given placebo, 200 mcg of chromium picolinate, or 1,000 mcg chromium picolinate daily. The results showed that HbA1c values (a measure of long-term blood sugar control) improved significantly after two months in the group receiving 1,000 mcg and in both chromium groups after four months. Fasting glucose (a measure of short-term blood sugar

control) was also lower in the group taking the higher dose of chromium.

A double-blind trial of seventy-eight people with type 2 diabetes compared two forms of chromium (brewer's yeast and chromium chloride) with placebo. This rather complex crossover study consisted of four eight-week intervals of treatment in random order. The results in the sixty-seven people who completed the study showed that both forms of chromium significantly improved blood sugar control.

Positive results were also seen in three other double-blind, placebo-controlled studies enrolling more than 130 people with type 2 diabetes. However, several other studies have failed to find benefit for people with type 2 diabetes. These contradictory findings suggest that the benefit, if it really exists, is small at best.

A combination of chromium and biotin might be more effective. Following positive results in a small pilot trial, researchers conducted a double-blind study of 447 people with poorly controlled type 2 diabetes. One-half the participants were given placebo, and the rest were given a combination of 600 mcg chromium (as chromium picolinate) with 2 mg of biotin daily. All participants continued to receive standard oral medications for diabetes. In the ninety-day study period, participants given the chromium-biotin combination showed significantly better glucose regulation than those given placebo. The relative benefit was clear in levels of fasting glucose and in HgA1c.

One placebo-controlled study of thirty women with pregnancy-related diabetes found that supplementation with chromium (at a dosage of 4 or 8 mcg chromium picolinate for each kilogram of body weight) significantly improved blood sugar control. Also, chromium has shown some promise for treating diabetes caused by corticosteroid treatment.

Improved blood sugar control in people without diabetes. Many people develop impaired responsiveness to insulin (insulin resistance) and mildly abnormal blood sugar levels. A few small, double-blind trials have found that chromium supplementation may be helpful, although two studies found no benefit. Another small, double-blind trial found that chromium improved the body's response to insulin among overweight people at risk of developing diabetes. There is growing evidence that mildly impaired blood sugar control increases the risk of heart disease, suggesting that chromium supplementation might be useful.

Weight loss. The evidence is mixed on whether chromium is an effective aid for reducing weight or improving body composition (improving the ratio of fatty tissue to lean tissue). In one study, 219 people were given either placebo or 200 or 400 mcg of chromium picolinate daily. Participants were not advised to follow any particular diet. In seventy-two days, people taking chromium experienced significantly greater weight loss than those not taking chromium, more than two-and-one-half pounds versus about one-quarter pound. People taking chromium actually gained lean body mass, so the loss of fatty tissue was even more dramatic: more than four pounds versus less than one-half pound. However, a high dropout rate makes the results of this study somewhat unreliable.

However, in another double-blind study by the same researcher, 130 moderately overweight people attempting to lose weight were given either placebo or 400 mcg of chromium daily. At the end of the trial, no statistically significant differences in weight or body composition were seen between groups. Researchers were able to show benefit only by resorting to fairly complicated statistical maneuvers.

In a third study, forty-four overweight women were given either placebo or 400 mcg of chromium per day. All participants were placed on an exercise program. Through twelve weeks, no differences were seen between the two groups in terms of body weight, waist circumference, or percentage of body fat. A small double-blind trial of older women undergoing resistance training also failed to find evidence of benefit. Generally negative results also have been seen in other small double-blind trials.

When larger studies find positive results and smaller studies do not, it often indicates that the treatment under study is only weakly effective. This may be the case with chromium as a weight-loss treatment. If chromium is effective for weight loss, one small study suggests it may work by influencing the brain and its role in appetite and food cravings.

Heart disease prevention. Insulin resistance and mildly elevated blood sugar levels appear to increase the risk of heart disease. Chromium supplementation might help by improving insulin responsiveness and by normalizing blood sugar. In support of this, an observational trial found associations between higher chromium intake and reduced risk of heart attack.

SAFETY ISSUES

Although the precise upper limit of safe chromium intake is not known, it is believed that chromium is safe when taken at a dosage of 50 to 200 mcg daily. Side effects appear to be rare. However, chromium is a heavy metal and might conceivably build up and cause problems if taken to excess.

There is one report of kidney, liver, and bone marrow damage in a person who took 1,200 to 2,400 mcg of chromium for several months; in another report, as little as 600 mcg for six weeks was enough to cause damage. Such problems appear to be quite rare, and it is possible that these persons already had health problems that predisposed them to such a reaction. The risk of chromium toxicity is believed to be higher in people who already have liver or kidney disease.

Nonetheless, based on these reports, it is possible that the dosage of chromium found most effective for persons with type 2 diabetes (1,000 mcg daily) might present some health risks. For example, there is some evidence that if chromium is taken in high enough amounts, it may be converted from its original safe form (chromium 3) into a known carcinogen, chromium 6. One should consult a doctor before taking more than 200 mcg of chromium daily.

Persons who have diabetes and for whom chromium is effective may need to cut down the dosage of any medication taken for diabetes. Again, one should consult a doctor before continuing chromium use.

There are also several concerns about the picolinate form of chromium in particular. Picolinate can alter levels of neurotransmitters. This has led to concern among some experts that chromium picolinate might be harmful for persons with depression, bipolar disease, or schizophrenia. There also has been one report of a severe skin reaction caused by chromium picolinate.

Finally, there are fairly theoretical and uncertain concerns that chromium picolinate could have adverse effects on deoxyribonucleic acid (DNA). Also, the maximum safe dosage of chromium for women who are pregnant or nursing and for persons with severe liver or kidney disease has not been established.

IMPORTANT INTERACTIONS

One may need extra chromium if also taking calcium carbonate supplements or antacids. The chromium supplement and the doses of these substances should not be taken within two hours of each other, because the two together may interfere with chromium's absorption.

People who are taking corticosteroids may need extra chromium. Also, people who are taking oral diabetes medications or insulin should seek medical supervision before taking chromium, because the dosages of these drugs might need to be reduced. Finally, chromium supplementation may improve levels of HDL (good) cholesterol if the individual is also taking beta-blockers.

EBSCO CAM Review Board

FURTHER READING

Albarracin, C. A., et al. "Chromium Picolinate and Biotin Combination Improves Glucose Metabolism in Treated, Uncontrolled Overweight to Obese Patients with Type 2 Diabetes." *Diabetes/Metabolism Research and Reviews* 24 (2008): 41-51.

Anton, S. D., et al. "Effects of Chromium Picolinate on Food Intake and Satiety." *Diabetes Technology and Therapeutics* 10 (2008): 405-412.

Diaz, M. L., et al. "Chromium Picolinate and Conjugated Linoleic Acid Do Not Synergistically Influence Diet- and Exercise-Induced Changes in Body Composition and Health Indexes in Overweight Women." *Journal of Nutritional Biochemistry* 19 (2008): 61-68.

Docherty, J. P., et al. "A Double-Blind, Placebo-Controlled, Exploratory Trial of Chromium Picolinate in Atypical Depression: Effect on Carbohydrate Craving." *Journal of Psychiatric Practice* 11 (2005): 302-314.

Lucidi, R. S., et al. "Effect of Chromium Supplementation on Insulin Resistance and Ovarian and Menstrual Cyclicity in Women with Polycystic Ovary Syndrome." *Fertility and Sterility* 84 (2005): 1755-1757.

Pei, D., et al. "The Influence of Chromium Chloride-Containing Milk to Glycemic Control of Patients with Type 2 Diabetes Mellitus." *Metabolism* 55 (2006): 923-927.

Yazaki, Y., et al. "A Pilot Study of Chromium Picolinate for Weight Loss." *Journal of Alternative and Complementary Medicine* 16 (2010): 291-299.

See also: Diabetes; Insulin.

Chronic fatigue syndrome

CATEGORY: Condition

RELATED TERMS: Chronic fatigue and immune dysfunction syndrome, myalgic encephalomyelitis, post-viral fatigue syndrome

DEFINITION: Treatment of a chronic disease characterized by debilitating and unexplained low energy, tiredness, and other symptoms.

PRINCIPAL PROPOSED NATURAL TREATMENTS: None

OTHER PROPOSED NATURAL TREATMENTS: Acupuncture, beta-carotene, carnitine, chocolate, dehydroepiandrosterone, echinacea, *Eleutherococcus*, essential fatty acids (gamma-linolenic acid and fish oil), licorice, melatonin, multivitamin-multimineral supplementats, nicotinamide adenine dinucleotide, *Panax ginseng*, traditional Chinese herbal medicine

INTRODUCTION

Chronic fatigue syndrome (CFS) has been a subject of controversy for many years. Medical authorities were once quite skeptical regarding whether it even existed. However, in 1988, the Centers for Disease Control and Prevention (CDC) officially recognized CFS. Today, CFS is defined essentially as follows: unexplained, persistent, or relapsing fatigue with a definite beginning that is not the result of exertion, that is not relieved by rest, and that results in significant reduction of daily activities. Also, a minimum of four of the following symptoms persist or recur for six or more consecutive months of the illness: impairment in short-term memory or concentration; sore throat; tender lymph nodes in the neck or armpits; muscle pain; pain in many joints, without redness or swelling; headache of new pattern or severity; unrefreshing sleep; and malaise following exercise that lasts for more than twenty-four hours. Frequently, symptoms of CFS follow a viral infection; some persons with CFS describe their symptoms as a flu that never goes away.

The cause (or causes) of CFS remains unknown. Because its symptoms somewhat resemble those of mononucleosis (caused by the Epstein-Barr virus), for a time CFS was called chronic Epstein-Barr syndrome. However, further investigation disclosed that evidence of past or current Epstein-Barr infection is no more common in persons with CFS than in the general population. Nonetheless, this erroneous and misleading term still crops up in literature on CFS.

Other syndromes with a pattern of symptoms similar to CFS include fibromyalgia, multiple chemical sensitivities, and food allergies; some consider these conditions to be closely related to each other, but there is no real evidence to support this hypothesis.

There is no dramatically effective treatment for CFS. Antidepressants (such as Prozac and Zoloft) may improve energy and mood; older antidepressants (such as amitriptyline) may improve sleep; antihistamines and decongestants can help allergic symptoms that frequently occur in CFS; and nonsteroidal anti-inflammatory drugs (such as ibuprofen and naproxen) may help pain. Other approaches to CFS that have been tried include magnesium injections, corticosteroid treatment, and a graded exercise program either alone or with the antidepressant fluoxetine.

For a time, researchers expressed some excitement over initial findings that deliberately raising blood pressure might help persons with CFS. However, a double-blind, placebo-controlled study of twenty-five people given a six-week course of fludrocortisone and increased dietary sodium to raise blood pressure found no improvement in CFS symptoms.

PROPOSED NATURAL TREATMENTS

There are some promising natural treatments for CFS, but the scientific evidence for them is not strong.

Essential fatty acids. In a double-blind, placebo-controlled study, sixty-three people were given either a combination of essential fatty acids containing evening primrose oil (a source of gamma-linolenic acid) and fish oil, or liquid paraffin placebo for three months. At one and three months, participants in the treatment group reported significant improvement in CFS symptoms compared with the placebo group. The researchers also found that at the beginning of the study, many participants had abnormal essential fatty acid levels, and these improved with treatment.

However, in 1999, researchers tried to replicate this study with fifty other participants, using more precise means of measuring CFS symptoms. The results showed no difference between persons given essential fatty acids and those given placebo (sunflower oil). These researchers also found no difference in fatty acid levels between persons with CFS and persons without CFS who served as controls.

Nicotinamide adenine dinucleotide. Nicotinamide adenine dinucleotide (NADH) is a naturally occurring chemical that plays a significant role in cellular en-

ergy production. NADH supplements have been tried in hopes that they might improve energy levels in athletes and in persons with chronic fatigue.

A double-blind, placebo-controlled crossover trial that followed twenty-six people given 10 milligrams of NADH for a four-week period showed some improvement in symptoms during NADH treatment compared to the period of placebo treatment (31 versus 8 percent). However, larger studies will have to be performed to actually prove a benefit with this supplement.

Carnitine. Carnitine is a substance the body uses to convert fatty acids to energy. Early studies reported decreased carnitine levels in people with CFS. Based on these studies, an unblinded crossover trial (eight weeks with each treatment, and a two-week "washout" period between) enrolled thirty persons with CFS to evaluate the potential benefits of carnitine supplements. The results suggest potential benefit with this supplement.

This study, however, was severely flawed. Rather than use a placebo group for comparison, researchers chose to investigate the antiviral drug amantadine. This drug has no proven efficacy in CFS, and it caused so many side effects that more than one-half of the participants dropped out during the period when they were taking amantadine. This high dropout rate makes statistical interpretation of the results unreliable. In addition, the lack of blinding in the study reduces the trustworthiness of the results.

Other herbs and supplements. Traditional Chinese herbal medicine is part of a comprehensive and unique approach to healing developed through many centuries in Asia. A double-blind, placebo-controlled study of twenty-nine people suggests that the use of an herbal formula originating in this system may be helpful for CFS. Another double-blind, placebo-controlled study reportedly found dark chocolate helpful for CFS, and another study performed in Hong Kong provides weak evidence that acupuncture might be helpful for chronic fatigue syndrome.

A test-tube study of echinacea and *Panax ginseng* found that both increased cellular immune function in cells taken from people with CFS. However, many herbs and supplements can cause measurable changes in immune function, and such observations do not prove that there will be an actual benefit in people with the disease.

Both beta-carotene and dehydroepiandrosterone

have been suggested as treatments for CFS, but the evidence that they work remains extremely preliminary at best. Based on the theory that CFS might be related to low blood pressure, the herb licorice has been recommended for CFS by some herbalists. Licorice raises blood pressure (and causes other potentially harmful effects) when taken in high doses for a long time. However, there is no evidence that licorice works for CFS, and other treatments to raise blood pressure have proven ineffective for CFS.

Although some authorities have suggested that CFS might be caused by deficiencies of multiple vitamins and minerals, a double-blind, placebo-controlled study of forty-two people found no significant improvement in CFS symptoms when a vitamin-mineral supplement was given four times daily after meals for three months. Another trial failed to find benefit with a multivitamin-multimineral supplement.

A fairly substantial (ninety-six-participant) double-blind, placebo-controlled study failed to find *Eleutherococcus senticosus* (Siberian ginseng) helpful for people with CFS. During the two-month study period, both *Eleutherococcus* and placebo reduced fatigue symptoms, but there was no statistically significant difference. Another study failed to find melatonin helpful for CFS. A special bran extract marketed for enhancing immunity failed to prove more effective than placebo for CFS symptoms (although placebo was quite effective).

People with CFS may at times attribute their symptoms to chemical exposures, thereby relating chronic fatigue syndrome to another loosely defined condition known as multiple chemical sensitivities. One study evaluated people with chronic fatigue syndrome who believed that certain chemical triggers affected their mental function, causing mental sluggishness and confusion. The results showed decreased mental function on testing following exposure to supposed chemical triggers; however, the decrease was the same whether the actual chemical or a substitute placebo was used. In other words, it was the belief that a substance causes harm, rather than actual harm caused by the substance, that produced the symptoms.

HOMEOPATHIC REMEDIES

A six-month double-blind study failed to find constitutional, or classical, homeopathy convincingly more effective than placebo for the treatment of chronic fatigue syndrome. However, homeopathic consultation itself proved to have a dramatically beneficial effect, regardless of whether participants were subsequently given placebo or the actual prescribed homeopathic treatment.

EBSCO CAM Review Board

FURTHER READING

Brouwers, F. M., et al. "The Effect of a Polynutrient Supplement on Fatigue and Physical Activity of Patients with Chronic Fatigue Syndrome." *QJM: Monthly Journal of the Association of Physicians* 95 (2002): 677-683.

CFIDS Association of America. http://www.cfids.org.

Edmonds, M., H. McGuire, and J. Price. "Exercise Therapy for Chronic Fatigue Syndrome." *Cochrane Database of Systematic Reviews* (2004): CD003200. Available through *EBSCO DynaMed Systematic Literature Surveillance* at http://www.ebscohost.com/dynamed.

Smith, S., and K. Sullivan. "Examining the Influence of Biological and Psychological Factors on Cognitive Performance in Chronic Fatigue Syndrome." *International Journal of Behavioral Medicine* 10 (2003): 162-173.

Weatherley-Jones, E., et al. "A Randomised, Controlled, Triple-Blind Trial of the Efficacy of Homeopathic Treatment for Chronic Fatigue Syndrome." *Journal of Psychosomatic Research* 56 (2004): 189-197.

Williams, G., et al. "Therapy of Circadian Rhythm Disorders in Chronic Fatigue Syndrome: No Symptomatic Improvement with Melatonin or Phototherapy." *European Journal of Clinical Investigation* 32 (2002): 831-837.

See also: Fatigue; Fibromyalgia: Homeopathic remedies; Immune support; Insomnia; Lupus; Melatonin; Memory and mental function impairment.

Chronic obstructive pulmonary disease (COPD)

CATEGORY: Condition
RELATED TERMS: Chronic bronchitis, emphysema
DEFINITION: Treatment of lung disease causing chronic coughing and severe shortness of breath.
PRINCIPAL PROPOSED NATURAL TREATMENT: N-acetylcysteine (NAC)

OTHER PROPOSED NATURAL TREATMENTS: Antioxidant-rich diet, Ayurvedic herbal medicine, L-carnitine, coenzyme Q_{10}, creatine, echinacea with wild indigo and white pine, essential oil monoterpenes, fish oil, high-fat and low-carbohydrate diet, ivy leaf, plantain

INTRODUCTION

Chronic obstructive pulmonary disease (COPD) is a permanent lung condition most often caused by cigarette smoking. The disease begins with a wheezing cough and gradually progresses to a shortness of breath that accompanies even the slightest exertion, such as dressing or eating. COPD encompasses both emphysema and chronic bronchitis.

Emphysema consists of the destruction of the tiny air sacs (alveoli) in the lungs and the weakening of the support structure around them. This leads to a collapse of the small airways in the lungs, especially on inhalation, and reduces the body's ability to take in oxygen and expel carbon dioxide.

Chronic bronchitis consists of chronic inflammation of the airways, causing a persistent productive cough. This inflammation also impairs the body's ability to exchange new air for old. COPD also involves spasm of the airways similar to what occurs in asthma. Finally, occasional flare-ups occur when bacteria grow in the lungs, leading to acute exacerbation of symptoms.

Because cigarette smoking contributes to both emphysema and chronic bronchitis, smokers who have COPD should stop smoking. Quitting smoking will not reverse the condition, but it might stop COPD from getting worse. Airborne irritants such as chemical fumes exacerbate symptoms and should also be avoided. Standard treatment for COPD includes using bronchodilators, such as ipratropium and albuterol, to reduce muscle spasms and taking corticosteroids to control inflammation in the airways. Acute flare-ups are treated with antibiotics. Severe COPD may require continuous oxygen therapy.

Malnutrition is common among people with COPD and seems to correspond to the severity of the condition. It has been suggested that the caloric needs of people with COPD increase as the disease progresses. Because malnutrition in turn can worsen lung function and make people more prone to infection, many researchers now recommend that persons with COPD receive supplemental nutrition as part of their treatment.

COPD's Effect on the Lungs

In the United States, the phrase "chronic obstructive pulmonary disease" (COPD) refers to two main conditions: emphysema and chronic bronchitis.

In emphysema, the walls between many of the air sacs of the lung are damaged, causing them to lose their shape and become floppy. This damage also can destroy the walls of the air sacs, leading to fewer and larger air sacs instead of many tiny ones. When this happens, the amount of gas exchange in the lungs is reduced.

In chronic bronchitis, the lining of the airways is constantly irritated and inflamed. This causes the lining to thicken. Thick mucus forms in the airways, making it difficult to breathe.

Most people who have COPD have both emphysema and chronic obstructive bronchitis. Thus, the general condition known as COPD is a more accurate descriptor.

PRINCIPAL PROPOSED NATURAL TREATMENTS

N-acetylcysteine (NAC) may improve breathing in people with COPD. NAC is a specially modified form of the dietary amino acid cysteine. Regular use of NAC may diminish the number of severe bronchitis attacks. A review and meta-analysis of available research focused on eight reasonably well-designed double-blind, placebo-controlled trials of NAC in COPD. The results of these studies, involving about fourteen hundred persons, suggest that NAC taken daily at a dose of 400 to 1,200 milligrams (mg) can reduce the number of acute attacks of severe bronchitis. However, a subsequent three-year, double-blind, placebo-controlled study of 523 people with COPD failed to find benefit with the use of 600 mg of NAC daily.

NAC was once thought to aid lung conditions by helping to break up mucus. However, continuing research casts doubt on this explanation of its action.

OTHER PROPOSED NATURAL TREATMENTS

Evidence from three double-blind, placebo-controlled studies that enrolled forty-nine persons suggests that the supplement L-carnitine can improve exercise tolerance in COPD, presumably by improving muscular efficiency in the lungs and other muscles.

Eucalyptus is a standard ingredient in cough drops and in oils sometimes added to humidifiers. A combination essential oil therapy containing cineole from eucalyptus, d-limonene from citrus fruit, and alpha-pinene from pine has been studied for a variety of respiratory conditions. Because these oils are in a chemical family called monoterpenes, the treatment is called essential oil monoterpenes. A three-month double-blind trial of 246 persons with chronic bronchitis found that oral treatment with essential oil monoterpenes helped prevent acute flare-ups of chronic bronchitis. A previous double-blind study, too small to provide reliable results, hints that oral use of essential oil monoterpenes can enhance the effects of antibiotics for acute flare-ups once they do occur. It is thought that essential oil monoterpenes work by improving the lungs' ability to clear secretions.

A mixture of extracts from echinacea, wild indigo, and white cedar has shown promise for treating a variety of respiratory infections. A well-designed double-blind, placebo-controlled trial of fifty-three people tested its benefits in acute exacerbations of chronic bronchitis. All participants in this trial received standard antibiotic therapy. The results showed that people receiving the herbal medication experienced more rapid improvements in lung function than those given placebo.

In one poorly designed and reported study, the use of an Ayurvedic herbal combination appeared to offer some benefit. It also has been suggested that the sports supplement creatine might improve muscle strength in people with COPD, but results from small double-blind studies have been inconsistent. Slight evidence from a small open trial suggests that coenzyme Q_{10} improves lung function in persons with COPD.

The herbs ivy leaf and plantain have been suggested for chronic bronchitis, but there is no meaningful evidence that they actually help. Another study failed to find pomegranate juice helpful for COPD.

Observational studies suggest a correlation between respiratory problems and diets low in antioxidants from food, such as vitamin A, vitamin E, vitamin C, and beta-carotene. However, such studies do not prove that taking supplements of such nutrients will help. A double-blind study of vitamin E and beta-carotene supplementation found no effect on COPD symptoms. The effects of other antioxidant supplements on COPD have not been studied.

Evidence from several studies suggests that the standard approved diet, low in fat and high in carbohydrates, worsens exercise performance and lung function in people with COPD, whereas a low-carbo-hydrate diet may improve COPD symptoms. Carbohydrates cause the body to produce increased amounts of carbon dioxide, and people with COPD have trouble getting rid of carbon dioxide.

HERBS AND SUPPLEMENTS TO USE ONLY WITH CAUTION

Various herbs and supplements may interact adversely with drugs used to treat chronic obstructive pulmonary disease, so one should be cautious when considering the use of herbs and supplements.

EBSCO CAM Review Board

FURTHER READING

Cerdá, B., et al. "Pomegranate Juice Supplementation in Chronic Obstructive Pulmonary Disease." *European Journal of Clinical Nutrition* 60 (2006): 245-253.

Deacon, S. J., et al. "Randomised Controlled Trial of Dietary Creatine as an Adjunct Therapy to Physical Training in COPD." *American Journal of Respiratory and Critical Care Medicine* 178 (2008): 233-239.

Decramer, M., et al. "Effects of N-acetylcysteine on Outcomes in Chronic Obstructive Pulmonary Disease." *The Lancet* 365 (2005): 1552-1560.

Faager, G., et al. "Creatine Supplementation and Physical Training in Patients with COPD." *International Journal of Chronic Obstructive Pulmonary Disease* 1 (2006): 445-453.

Fuld, J. P., et al. "Creatine Supplementation During Pulmonary Rehabilitation in Chronic Obstructive Pulmonary Disease." *Thorax* 60 (2005): 531-537.

Hauke, W., et al. "Esberitox N as Supportive Therapy When Providing Standard Antibiotic Treatment in Subjects with a Severe Bacterial Infection (Acute Exacerbation of Chronic Bronchitis)." *Chemotherapy* 48 (2002): 259-266.

Kuethe, F., et al. "Creatine Supplementation Improves Muscle Strength in Patients with Congestive Heart Failure." *Pharmazie* 61 (2006): 218-222.

Murali, P. M., et al. "Plant-Based Formulation in the Management of Chronic Obstructive Pulmonary Disease." *Respiratory Medicine* 100 (2005): 39-45.

Sridhar, M. K. "Nutrition and Lung Health: Should People at Risk for Chronic Obstructive Lung Disease Eat More Fruit and Vegetables?" *British Medical Journal* 310 (1995): 75-76.

See also: Allergies; Asthma; Bronchitis; Cough; N-acetylcysteine; Smoking addiction.

Cinnamon

CATEGORY: Herbs and supplements

RELATED TERM: *Cinnamomum zeylanicum, Cinnamon cassia*

DEFINITION: Natural plant product used to treat specific health conditions.

PRINCIPAL PROPOSED USES: Diabetes, high cholesterol

OTHER PROPOSED USES: Antimicrobial, improving appetite, indigestion, polycystic ovary disease, ulcers

OVERVIEW

Most Americans consider cinnamon a simple flavoring, but in traditional Chinese medicine, it is one of the oldest remedies, prescribed for everything from diarrhea and chills to influenza and parasitic worms. Cinnamon comes from the bark of a small Southeast Asian evergreen tree and is available as an oil, extract, or dried powder. It is closely related to cassia (*Cinnamon cassia*) and contains many of the same components, but the bark and oils from *Cinnamomum zeylanicum* are thought to have a better flavor.

THERAPEUTIC DOSAGES

Typical recommended dosages of ground cinnamon bark are 1 to 4 grams (g) daily. Cinnamon oil is generally used at a dose of 0.05 to 0.2 g daily.

THERAPEUTIC USES

Based on the results of one preliminary double-blind, placebo-controlled study, cinnamon has been widely advertised as an effective treatment for type 2 diabetes as well as high cholesterol. However, the evidence for this is mixed.

Germany's Commission E approves cinnamon for improving appetite and relieving indigestion; however, these uses are not backed by reliable scientific evidence. Two animal studies weakly suggest that an extract of cinnamon bark taken orally may help prevent stomach ulcers.

Preliminary results from test-tube and animal studies suggest that cinnamon oil and cinnamon extract have antifungal, antibacterial, and antiparasitic properties. For example, cinnamon has been found to be active against *Candida albicans*, the fungus responsible for vaginal yeast infections and thrush (oral yeast infection), *Helicobacter pylori* (the bacterium that causes stomach ulcers), and even head lice. However, it is a long way from studies of this type to actual proof

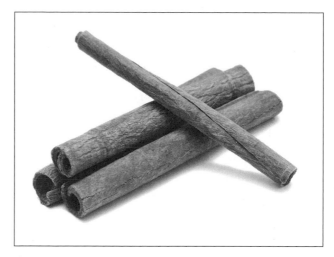

Cinnamon is one of the oldest remedies in traditional Chinese medicine. (©Christian Draghici/Dreamstime.com)

of effectiveness. Until cinnamon is tested in double-blind human trials, it remains unclear if it can successfully treat these or any other infections.

SCIENTIFIC EVIDENCE

Based on previous animal studies that had suggested potential benefits of cinnamon for diabetes, researchers in Pakistan performed a double-blind, placebo-controlled trial. In this forty-day study, sixty people with type 2 diabetes were given cinnamon at a dose of 1, 3, or 6 g daily. The results reportedly indicated that use of cinnamon improved blood sugar levels by 18 to 29 percent, total cholesterol by 12 to 26 percent, low density lipoproteins (LDL, or bad cholesterol) by 7 to 27 percent, and triglycerides by 23 to 30 percent. These results were said to be statistically significant, compared with the beginning of the study and to the placebo group.

However, this study has some odd features. The most important is that it found no significant difference in benefit between the various doses of cinnamon. This is called lack of a dose-related effect, and it generally casts doubt on the results of a study. The researchers counter that perhaps even 1 g of cinnamon is sufficient to produce the maximum cholesterol-lowering effect, and therefore, higher doses simply did not add any further benefit. There is another problem with this study as well: no improvements were seen in the placebo group. This too is unusual, and it also casts doubt on the results.

In an attempt to replicate these results, a group of Dutch researchers performed a carefully designed six-week double-blind, placebo-controlled study of twenty-five people with diabetes. All participants were given 1.5 g of cinnamon daily. The results failed to show any detectable effect on blood sugar, insulin sensitivity, or cholesterol profile. Although this second study was smaller than the first because it had fewer groups, overall, its statistical validity is similar. These unsupportive results were confirmed in a Thai study enrolling sixty people: 1.5 g of cinnamon daily failed to produce any benefit. On the other hand, a double-blind study of seventy-nine people that used 3 g instead of 1.5 g daily did find that cinnamon improved blood sugar levels. A randomized trial involving fifty-eight people with type 2 diabetes also concluded that 2 g of cinnamon daily reduced HbA1c levels (a measurement of blood sugar levels over time), as well as high blood pressure.

In yet another small study involving twenty-two pre-diabetic patients with metabolic syndrome, researchers found that an extract containing 500 mg cinnamon given once daily was effective at modestly reducing fasting blood sugar and systolic blood pressure and increasing lean body weight. However, the low dosage of cinnamon used raises concern about the reliability of the results. A very small study that evaluated cinnamon for improving blood sugar control in women with polycystic ovary disease found evidence of benefit.

At present, it would be premature to consider cinnamon an evidence-based treatment for type 2 diabetes or high cholesterol, but it has definitely shown some promise. Regarding type 1 diabetes, a study of seventy-two adolescents failed to find benefit with cinnamon taken at a dose of 1 g daily. A meta-analysis (formal statistical review) of all published evidence concluded that, thus far, cinnamon has not been shown to have any effect on blood sugar levels in people with diabetes. The evidence regarding cinnamon as a treatment for diabetes is highly inconsistent, suggesting that if cinnamon is indeed effective, its benefits are minimal at most.

SAFETY ISSUES

As a widely used food spice, ground cinnamon bark is believed to be safe. However, cinnamon's essential oil is much more concentrated than the powdered bark commonly used for baking. There is some evidence that high doses of cinnamon oil might depress the central nervous system. Germany's Commission E recommends that pregnant women should avoid taking cinnamon oil or high doses of the bark. Maximum safe doses in young children, nursing women, or individuals with severe liver or kidney disease have not been determined.

When used topically, cinnamon bark oil may cause flushing and a burning sensation. Some people have reported strong burning sensations or mouth ulcers after chewing cinnamon-flavored gum or candy. However, these reactions disappeared within days of discontinuing the gum.

EBSCO CAM Review Board

FURTHER READING

Altschuler, J. A., et al. "The Effect of Cinnamon on A1C Among Adolescents with Type 1 Diabetes." *Diabetes Care* 30 (2007): 813-816.

Khan, A., et al. "Cinnamon Improves Glucose and Lipids of People with Type 2 Diabetes." *Diabetes Care* 26 (2003): 3215-3218.

Mang, B., et al. "Effects of a Cinnamon Extract on Plasma Glucose, HbA, and Serum Lipids in Diabetes Mellitus Type 2." *European Journal of Clinical Investigation* 36 (2006): 340-344.

Suppapitiporn, S., N. Kanpaksi, and S. Suppapitiporn. "The Effect of *Cinnamon cassia* Powder in Type 2 Diabetes Mellitus." *Journal of the Medical Association of Thailand* 89 (2006): S200-S205.

Vanschoonbeek, K., et al. "Cinnamon Supplementation Does Not Improve Glycemic Control in Postmenopausal Type 2 Diabetes Patients." *Journal of Nutrition* 136 (2006): 977-980.

Wang, J. G., et al. "The Effect of Cinnamon Extract on Insulin Resistance Parameters in Polycystic Ovary Syndrome." *Fertility and Sterility* 88, no. 1 (2007): 240-243.

Ziegenfuss, T. N., et al. "Effects of a Water-Soluble Cinnamon Extract on Body Composition and Features of the Metabolic Syndrome in Pre-diabetic Men and Women." *Journal of the International Society of Sports Nutrition* 3 (2006): 45-53.

See also: Cholesterol, high; Diabetes; Herbal medicine.

Cirrhosis

CATEGORY: Condition
RELATED TERMS: Alcoholic liver cirrhosis, biliary cirrhosis, liver cirrhosis
DEFINITION: Treatment of diseases of the liver.
PRINCIPAL PROPOSED NATURAL TREATMENTS: Milk thistle, reduced alcohol consumption
OTHER PROPOSED NATURAL TREATMENTS: Antioxidants, Ayurvedic herbal combinations, branched-chain amino acids, calcium and vitamin D, oligomeric proanthocyanidins, ornithine alpha-ketoglutarate, phosphatidylcholine, S-adenosylmethionine, taurine
HERBS AND SUPPLEMENTS TO USE ONLY WITH CAUTION: Barberry, beta-carotene, blue-green algae, borage, carnitine, chaparral, coltsfoot, comfrey, germander, germanium, greater celandine, kava, kombucha, mistletoe, pennyroyal, pokeroot, sassafras, skullcap, spirulina, traditional Chinese herbal medicine, vitamin A, vitamin B_3, vitamin K

INTRODUCTION

The liver is a sophisticated chemical laboratory, capable of carrying out thousands of chemical transformations on which the body depends. The liver produces vital chemicals from scratch, modifies others to allow the body to use them better, and neutralizes an enormous range of toxins.

A number of influences can severely damage the liver. Alcoholism is the most common. Alcohol is a powerful liver toxin that harms the liver in three stages: alcoholic fatty liver, alcoholic hepatitis, and alcoholic cirrhosis. Although the first two stages of injury are usually reversible, alcoholic cirrhosis is not. Generally, more than ten years of heavy alcohol abuse is required to cause liver cirrhosis. Other causes include hepatitis C infection, primary biliary cirrhosis, and liver damage caused by occupational chemicals and drugs.

A cirrhotic liver is firm and nodular to the touch and, in advanced cases, is shrunken in size. These changes reflect severe damage to its structure. A high percentage of liver cells have died, and fibrous scar-like tissue permeates the organ.

A cirrhotic liver cannot perform its chemical tasks, leading to wide-ranging impairment of bodily functions, such as the development of jaundice (yellowing of the skin from unprocessed toxins), mental confu-

sion, emaciation, and skin changes. In addition, the fibrous tissue impedes blood that is supposed to pass through the liver. This leads to abdominal swelling as fluid backs up (ascites) and to bleeding in the esophagus as veins expand to provide an alternative fluid path. Ultimately, coma develops, often triggered by internal bleeding or infection.

Treatments for liver cirrhosis begin with stopping the use of alcohol and all other liver-toxic substances. A number of treatments such as potassium-sparing diuretics can ameliorate symptoms to some extent, but they do not cure the disease.

The liver is too complex for a machine to duplicate its functions, so there is no equivalent of kidney dialysis for liver cirrhosis. Only a liver transplant can help, but a liver transplant is a difficult operation, with a high failure rate. In addition, the supply of usable livers is inadequate to meet the need.

Persons with cirrhosis of the liver should not take any medications, herbs, or dietary supplements without first consulting a physician. The liver processes many substances taken into the body, and if it is severely damaged, as during liver cirrhosis, ordinarily benign substances may become toxic.

PRINCIPAL PROPOSED NATURAL TREATMENTS

The herb milk thistle might offer various liver-protective benefits. In Europe, it is used to treat viral hepatitis, alcoholic fatty liver, alcoholic hepatitis, liver cirrhosis and drug- or chemical-induced liver toxicity. An intravenous preparation made from milk thistle is used as an antidote for poisoning by the liver-toxic deathcap mushroom, *Amanita phalloides*. However, the supporting evidence for the use of milk thistle in any of these conditions remains far from definitive.

A double-blind, placebo-controlled study of 170 persons with alcoholic or nonalcoholic cirrhosis found that in the group treated with milk thistle, the four-year survival rate was 58 percent, while the placebo group's rate was 38 percent. This difference was statistically significant.

A double-blind, placebo-controlled trial that enrolled 172 persons with cirrhosis for four years also found reductions in mortality, but the researchers just missed the conventional cutoff for statistical significance. A two-year, double-blind, placebo-controlled study of two hundred persons with alcoholic cirrhosis found no reduction in mortality attributable to the use of milk thistle. Other double-blind studies

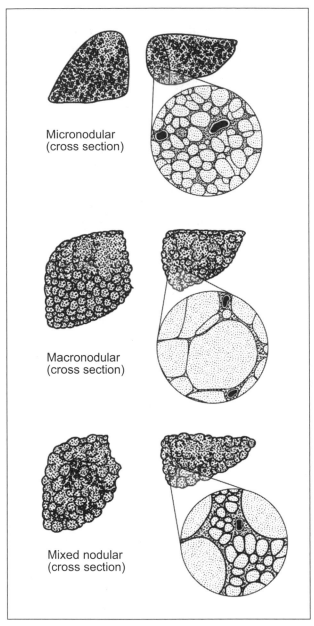

Micronodular
(cross section)

Macronodular
(cross section)

Mixed nodular
(cross section)

Cirrhosis appears in three forms, detectable under the microscope, each depending primarily on the cause of the liver damage. All are characterized by the replacement of normally soft, spongy tissue with hard, fibrous scarring. Alcohol-related cirrhosis usually produces the micronodular form.

of cirrhotic persons have found improvements in tests of liver function, although one did not.

A 2007 review of published and unpublished studies on milk thistle as a treatment for liver disease con-cluded that benefits were seen only in low-quality trials, and even in those, milk thistle did not show more than a slight benefit. However, in a 2008 analysis of nineteen randomized trials, researchers concluded that milk thistle was significantly more effective at reducing mortality from liver cirrhosis (mostly alcohol-related) compared with placebo but no more effective at reducing mortality from any cause.

OTHER PROPOSED NATURAL TREATMENTS

Persons with liver cirrhosis have difficulty synthesizing the substance S-adenosylmethionine (SAMe) from the amino acid methionine. For this reason, supplemental SAMe (best known as a treatment for depression and osteoarthritis) has been tried as a treatment for cirrhosis. However, no strong evidence exists for its effectiveness.

A two-year, double-blind, placebo-controlled trial followed 117 people with alcoholic liver cirrhosis. Overall, those given SAMe did not do significantly better than those given placebo. However, when the results were reevaluated to eliminate persons with severe liver cirrhosis, a significant reduction in mortality and liver transplantation was seen with SAMe. SAMe has also shown some promise for primary biliary cirrhosis, though evidence is not consistent.

Branched-chain amino acids (BCAAs) are naturally occurring molecules (leucine, isoleucine, and valine) that the body uses to build proteins. Because of how they are metabolized, BCAAs might be helpful for persons with liver cirrhosis. However, the evidence that BCAAs actually help is not conclusive. Furthermore, persons with cirrhosis of the liver should not increase amino acid or protein intake except under physician supervision.

Persons with cirrhosis are susceptible to internal bleeding. Preliminary evidence suggests that oligomeric proanthocyanidins (OPCs) might help prevent this problem. OPCs are best documented as a treatment for venous insufficiency (closely related to varicose veins), in which they are thought to work in part by stabilizing blood vessels. Persons with cirrhosis have what amounts to internal varicose veins, caused by the shunting of fluid around the damaged liver.

OTHER NATURAL TREATMENTS

One small study suggests that the supplement carnitine might be helpful for people with hepatic encephalopathy, a life-threatening brain abnormality

Milk Thistle for Cirrhosis

Milk thistle (*Silybum marianum*) is a flowering herb native to the Mediterranean region. It has been used for thousands of years as a remedy for a variety of ailments, particularly liver problems. It is believed to have protective effects on the liver and to improve its function. It is typically used to treat liver cirrhosis, chronic hepatitis (liver inflammation), and gallbladder disorders.

Common names for milk thistle include Mary thistle and holy thistle, and it is sometimes called silymarin, which is actually a mixture of the herb's active components, including silybinin (also called silibinin or silybin). Silymarin, which can be extracted from the seeds (fruit) of the milk thistle plant, is believed to be the biologically active part of the herb. The seeds are used to prepare capsules, extracts, powders, and tinctures.

associated with severe cirrhosis. The amino acid taurine might help reduce muscle cramps in persons with cirrhosis.

One study suggests that protein from vegetable sources might be preferable to protein from animal sources for people with liver cirrhosis, presumably because of differences in amino acid content.

Preliminary evidence from animal studies suggests that the supplement phosphatidylcholine might help prevent alcoholic liver cirrhosis. The supplement ornithine alpha-ketoglutarate and the related substance ornithine-l-aspartate have shown promise for treating hepatic encephalopathy. Vitamin K has shown some promise for helping prevent liver cancer in people with cirrhosis of the liver. An Ayurvedic herbal combination has been studied for the treatment of cirrhosis, but evidence supporting its use remains incomplete and contradictory.

Antioxidants have been proposed for the treatment of primary biliary cirrhosis, based on the theory that free radicals play a role in the disease process. However, despite apparent promise seen in open trials, a double-blind, placebo-controlled study of sixty-one persons failed to find that a combination of vitamins A, C and E, selenium, methionine and CoQ_{10} produced any benefit in terms of fatigue or other liver-related symptoms.

The bones of persons with biliary cirrhosis often become thin. Taking calcium and vitamin D supplements might help. Antioxidants such as vitamin C, vitamin E, and lipoic acid have been tried for biliary cirrhosis, with promising results in preliminary trials.

HERBS AND SUPPLEMENTS TO USE ONLY WITH CAUTION

Many natural products have the capacity to harm the liver. Furthermore, because of the generally inadequate regulation of dietary supplements, there are real risks that herbal products may contain liver-toxic contaminants even if the actual herbs listed on the label are safe. It is recommend that persons with liver disease not use medicinal herbs except under the supervision of a physician. Listed here is specific information to aid in the decision-making process.

Vitamin A and beta-carotene supplements might cause alcoholic liver disease to develop more rapidly. All forms of vitamin B_3 may damage the liver when taken in high doses, including niacin, niacinamide (nicotinamide), and inositol hexaniacinate. Nutritional supplementation at the standard daily requirement level should not cause a problem.

A great many herbs and supplements have known or suspected liver-toxic properties, including barberry, borage, chaparral, coltsfoot, comfrey, germander, germanium (a mineral), greater celandine, certain green tea extracts, kava, kombucha, mistletoe, pennyroyal, pokeroot, sassafras, and various herbs and minerals used in traditional Chinese herbal medicine.

In addition, herbs that are not liver-toxic in themselves are sometimes adulterated with other herbs of similar appearance that are accidentally harvested in a misapprehension of their identity (for example, germander found in skullcap products). Furthermore, blue-green algae species such as spirulina may at times be contaminated with liver-toxic substances called microcystins, for which no highest safe level is known. Some articles claim that the herb echinacea is potentially liver-toxic, but this concern appears to have been based on a misunderstanding of its constituents. Echinacea contains substances in the pyrrolizidine alkaloid family. However, while many pyrrolizidine alkaloids are liver-toxic, those found in echinacea are not believed to have that property.

Whole valerian contains liver-toxic substances

called valepotriates; however, valepotriates are thought to be absent from most commercial valerian products, and case reports suggest that even very high doses of valerian do not harm the liver.

EBSCO CAM Review Board

FURTHER READING

Charlton, M. "Branched-Chain Amino Acid Enriched Supplements as Therapy for Liver Disease." *Journal of Nutrition* 136 (2005): 295S-298S.

Habu, D., et al. "Role of Vitamin K2 in the Development of Hepatocellular Carcinoma in Women with Viral Cirrhosis of the Liver." *Journal of the American Medical Association* 292 (2004): 358-361.

Jiang, Q., et al. "L-Ornithine-L-Aspartate in the Management of Hepatic Encephalopathy." *Journal of Gastroenterology and Hepatology* 24 (2008): 9-14.

Kobayashi, M., et al. "Inhibitory Effect of Branched-Chain Amino Acid Granules on Progression of Compensated Liver Cirrhosis Due to Hepatitis C Virus." *Journal of Gastroenterology* 43 (2008): 63-70.

Malaguarnera, M., Gargante, M. P., et al. "Acetyl-L-Carnitine Treatment in Minimal Hepatic Encephalopathy." *Digestive Diseases and Science* 53 (2008): 3018-3025.

Malaguarnera, M., Pistone, G., et al. "Effects of L-Carnitine in Patients with Hepatic Encephalopathy." *World Journal of Gastroenterology* 11 (2006): 7197-7202.

Marchesini, G., et al. "Nutritional Treatment with Branched-Chain Amino Acids in Advanced Liver Cirrhosis." *Journal of Gastroenterology* 35, suppl. (2000): 7-12.

Rambaldi, A., B. Jacobs, and C. Gluud. "Milk Thistle for Alcoholic and/or Hepatitis B or C Virus Liver Diseases." *Cochrane Database of Systematic Reviews* (2007): CD003620. Available through *EBSCO DynaMed Systematic Literature Surveillance* at http://www.ebscohost.com/dynamed.

Saller, R., et al. "An Updated Systematic Review with Meta-analysis for the Clinical Evidence of Silymarin." *Forschende Komplementärmedizin* 15 (2008): 9-20.

See also: Alcoholism; Branched-chain amino acids; Gastrointestinal health; Hepatitis, alcoholic; Liver disease; Milk thistle; Oligomeric proanthocyanidins; SAMe.

Cisplatin

CATEGORY: Drug interactions

DEFINITION: A chemotherapy drug used to treat cancer of the testicles, bladder, lung, stomach, esophagus, and ovaries, and other forms of cancer.

INTERACTIONS: Acetyl-L-carnitine, antioxidants, black cohosh, ginger, magnesium, melatonin, milk thistle, potassium

TRADE NAME: Platinol

BLACK COHOSH

Effect: Possible Harmful Interaction

The herb black cohosh is often used for menopausal symptoms. Because women receiving cancer chemotherapy may experience menopausal symptoms, black cohosh may appear a promising option. However, one test-tube study found that use of black cohosh may decrease the effectiveness of cisplatin.

MAGNESIUM AND POTASSIUM

Effect: Possibly Helpful Interaction

There is some evidence that use of cisplatin may cause the body to develop potentially dangerous deficiencies of potassium and magnesium. Taking supplements of these nutrients may be advisable.

MELATONIN

Effect: Possible Helpful Interaction

Weak preliminary evidence hints that use of melatonin may reduce side effects and increase efficacy of chemotherapy regimens that include cisplatin.

ANTIOXIDANTS

Effect: Possible Helpful Interaction

It has been suggested that many of the undesired effects of cisplatin are because of the creation of free radicals, dangerous, naturally occurring substances that can damage many cells. For this reason, treatment with antioxidants has been proposed for preventing toxic side effects. However, as yet there is no more than minimal evidence for benefit. One animal study tested a combination of substances with strong antioxidant properties (vitamin E, *Crocus sativus,* and *Nigella sativa*) and found evidence that this mixture reduced the kidney toxicity of cisplatin. A small human trial found evidence that use of vitamin E might help prevent nerve injury (peripheral neuropathy) caused by cisplatin, but because this was an open study, its results are not reliable. Another open study found possible benefits with selenium.

In open studies, the placebo effect and other confounding factors can play a significant role. In a better-designed, double-blind, placebo-controlled study of forty-eight people undergoing cancer treatment with cisplatin, participants were given either placebo or a combination of vitamin E, vitamin C, and selenium in hopes of reducing toxicity to the ears and kidneys. No significant benefits were seen. Note that there are concerns that use of antioxidants could potentially decrease the effectiveness of some forms of chemotherapy. For this reason, experts strongly suggest that people on cancer chemotherapy not use antioxidants, or any herbs or supplements, except in consultation with a physician.

MILK THISTLE
Effect: Possible Helpful Interaction

Animal and test-tube studies hint that the herb milk thistle might decrease the kidney toxicity of cisplatin and also possibly increase cisplatin efficacy.

However, no studies in humans have been reported.

ACETYL-L-CARNITINE
Effect: Possible Helpful Interaction

One study found evidence that the supplement acetyl-L-carnitine might reduce symptoms of peripheral neuropathy caused by cisplatin.

GINGER
Effect: No Benefit

The herb ginger is widely used for treatment of nausea. However, one study failed to find ginger helpful for nausea caused by cisplatin.

EBSCO CAM Review Board

FURTHER READING
Argyriou, A. A., et al. "Vitamin E for Prophylaxis Against Chemotherapy-Induced Neuropathy." *Neurology* 64 (2005): 26-31.

Maestri, A., et al. "A Pilot Study on the Effect of Acetyl-L-Carnitine in Paclitaxel- and Cisplatin-Induced Peripheral Neuropathy." *Tumori* 91 (2005): 135-138.

Manusirivithaya, S., et al. "Antiemetic Effect of Ginger in Gynecologic Oncology Patients Receiving Cisplatin." *International Journal of Gynecological Cancer* 14 (2004): 1063-1069.

Rockwell, S., Y. Liu, and S. Higgins. "Alteration of the Effects of Cancer Therapy Agents on Breast Cancer Cells by the Herbal Medicine Black Cohosh." *Breast Cancer Research and Treatment* 90 (2005): 233-239.

Sieja, K., and M. Talerczyk. "Selenium as an Element in the Treatment of Ovarian Cancer in Women Receiving Chemotherapy." *Gynecologic Oncology* 93 (2004): 320-327.

Van de Loosdrecht, A. A., J. A. Gietema, and W. T. van der Graaf. "Seizures in a Patient with Disseminated Testicular Cancer Due to Cisplatin-Induced Hypomagnesaemia." *Acta Oncologica* 39 (2000): 239-240.

Weijl, N. I., et al. "Supplementation with Antioxidant Micronutrients and Chemotherapy-Induced Toxicity in Cancer Patients Treated with Cisplatin-Based Chemotherapy." *European Journal of Cancer* 40 (2004): 1713-1723.

See also: Acetyl-L-carnitine; Antioxidants; Black cohosh; Food and Drug Administration; Ginger; Magnesium; Melatonin; Milk thistle; Potassium; Supplements: Introduction.

Citrulline

CATEGORY: Herbs and supplements
RELATED TERM: L-citrulline malate
DEFINITION: Natural substance of the human body used as a supplement to treat specific health conditions.
PRINCIPAL PROPOSED USE: Enhancing sports performance
OTHER PROPOSED USES: Alzheimer's disease, fatigue, male sexual dysfunction

OVERVIEW
Citrulline is a nonessential amino acid, meaning that the body can manufacture it from other nutrients. Within the body, citrulline is converted to the amino acid L-arginine. Some of the proposed uses of citrulline supplements are based on raising levels of arginine. Citrulline also plays a role in a physiological process called the urea cycle, in which toxic ammonia is converted to urea.

REQUIREMENTS AND SOURCES
The body manufactures citrulline from the essential

amino acid glutamine. Deficiency of citrulline is unlikely to occur.

THERAPEUTIC DOSAGES

A typical dose of citrulline is 6 to 18 grams daily. It is commonly sold in the form of citrulline malate.

THERAPEUTIC USES

There is little scientific support for any use of citrulline supplements. Citrulline is most commonly marketed today as a supplement for enhancing sports performance. Based on exceedingly speculative reasoning, it is often described as an aerobic complement to the supplement creatine. Supposedly, citrulline enhances aerobic exercise capacity (relatively low-intensity exercise), while creatine enhances anaerobic exercise capacity (high-intensity exercise). However, while there have been numerous double-blind studies on creatine, available evidence on citrulline as a sports supplement is so scant that no conclusions whatsoever can be based on it. The only meaningful study reported thus far found that citrulline reduced rather than enhanced exercise capacity. Current enthusiasm for the supplement is therefore based entirely on testimonials. Since placebos increase sense of energy and well-being and may even enhance performance, enthusiastic testimonials about a new and exciting supplement should be received with considerable caution.

Other proposed uses of citrulline are based on the fact that the body converts citrulline to the amino acid arginine. It is claimed by some that citrulline supplements are actually more effective at raising arginine levels than arginine supplements. However, this has not been established in any scientific sense. Furthermore, arginine itself is not a proven treatment for any condition. For example, citrulline is marketed as a treatment for impotence based on the assumption that arginine is effective for impotence. However, current evidence supporting arginine as an impotence treatment is weak at best, and citrulline itself has not been studied for this use in any meaningful way. Again, numerous testimonials are offered, but they mean little: placebos are very effective for impotence.

Very preliminary studies conducted in France in the late 1970s hint that citrulline may improve mental function in people with Alzheimer's disease and also reduce general fatigue. However, these studies were not conducted at the level of modern scientific standards and have not been followed up.

SAFETY ISSUES

As a naturally occurring amino acid, citrulline is believed to be safe. However, maximum safe doses in young children, pregnant or nursing women, and people with severe liver or kidney disease have not been established.

EBSCO CAM Review Board

FURTHER READING

Bendahan, D., et al. "Citrulline/Malate Promotes Aerobic Energy Production in Human Exercising Muscle." *British Journal of Sports Medicine* 36 (2002): 282-289.

Hickner, R. C., et al. "L-citrulline Reduces Time to Exhaustion and Insulin Response to a Graded Exercise Test." *Medicine and Science in Sports and Exercise* 38 (2006): 660-666.

See also: Creatine; Herbal medicine; Sexual dysfunction in men; Sports and fitness support: Enhancing performance.

Citrus aurantium

CATEGORY: Herbs and supplements

RELATED TERMS: Bitter orange, Seville orange, sour orange

PRINCIPAL PROPOSED USE: Weight loss

OTHER PROPOSED USES: Anxiety, cancer prevention, depression, viral infection

OVERVIEW

Citrus aurantium is the Latin name for a fruit best known as Seville orange, or sour or bitter orange. The juice, peel, and essential oil have all been used medicinally. Traditionally uses include digestive problems, epilepsy, fatigue, insomnia, infections, respiratory problems, and skin problems. As a flavoring, essence of bitter orange is found in the beverages Triple Sec and Cointreau.

THERAPEUTIC DOSAGES

Many *Citrus aurantium* products are made from the juice and concentrated extracts of the peel and are

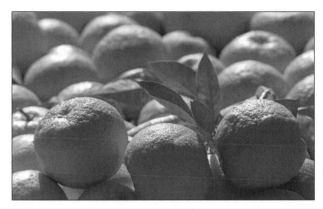

The juice and peel of the Seville orange have been used medicinally. (Adrian Pope/Getty Images)

said to contain a fixed percentage of synephrine or total amines. A typical recommended dosage of such products ranges from 100 to 150 milligrams (mg) two to three times daily. However, these doses may be unsafe.

THERAPEUTIC USES

Citrus aurantium juice and peel contain the stimulant chemical synephrine as well as related stimulants, such as octopamine, tyramine, N-methyltyramine, and hordeline. On this basis, *Citrus aurantium* has been widely marketed as a weight-loss product. However, there is no reliable evidence that *Citrus aurantium* is effective, and considerable reason to worry that it may cause harm. The reassuring statement made by some manufacturers that *Citrus aurantium* offers the "benefits of ephedra without the risks" is not supported by scientific evidence.

The only published double-blind, placebo-controlled trial on *Citrus aurantium* juice did not test the herb alone but, rather, evaluated a combination product that also contained caffeine and St. John's wort. While the results were somewhat positive, overall the study was too preliminary to reach reliable conclusions. An even less reliable study evaluated the synephrine constituent of *Citrus aurantium* and found possible fat-burning actions. In view of the weakness of the evidence in favor of *Citrus aurantium,* and in view of the considerable evidence that it presents health risks, experts recommend against using it for weight loss. Other evidence, far too weak to rely upon, hints that synephrine-rich *Citrus aurantium* extracts might have antidepressant effects.

Besides synephrine and other stimulants, whole *Citrus aurantium* peel contains citral, limonene, and several citrus bioflavonoids, including hesperidin, neohesperidin, naringin, and rutin. Weak evidence hints that these substances might have cancer-preventive and antiviral actions.

The essential oil of *Citrus aurantium* contains linalool and the fragrant substance limonene and might have antianxiety and sedative effects. However, neither of these proposed uses has more than extremely preliminary supporting evidence.

SAFETY ISSUES

Most of the safety concerns regarding *Citrus aurantium* relate to its stimulant constituents. The drug synephrine is known to produce many unpleasant and possibly dangerous side effects, including headache, agitation, rapid heart rate, and heart palpitations. In some people, it can cause angina pectoris, kidney damage, increased pressure in the eye, and reduced blood circulation to the heart and the extremities. The other stimulant amines in *Citrus aurantium* may increase such effects. There is one case report of a heart attack that appears possibly related to use of a *Citrus aurantium* supplement and another that links the herb to stroke. *Citrus aurantium* juice or concentrated extracts can raise blood pressure and increase heart rate and therefore should not be used by individuals with cardiovascular disease or high blood pressure. The herb should also be avoided by people with glaucoma.

Synephrine can also interact with numerous medications and other drugs, including stimulants (including ephedrine, pseudoephedrine [Sudafed], Ritalin, and even caffeine) and anesthetics. The tyramine constituent of *Citrus aurantium* can cause deadly side effects when combined with drugs in the MAO inhibitor family.

The peel and essential oil of *Citrus aurantium* may cause photosensitivity (increased tendency to react to sun exposure). For this reason, combination treatment with drugs that cause the same side effect (such as sulfa antibiotics) is not recommended.

Finally, *Citrus aurantium* juice can alter the way that the liver processes various medications, potentially raising or lowering their levels. In particular, the drugs cyclosporine and felodipine (a calcium channel blocker) are thought to be affected by *Citrus aurantium* juice, but numerous other drugs may interact with it as well. For this reason, experts recommend that persons taking any medications that are critical to their health should not take *Citrus aurantium* juice at the same time. Furthermore, safety in young children, pregnant or nursing women, and people with severe liver or kidney disease has not been established.

IMPORTANT INTERACTIONS

Citrus aurantium should not be taken by persons using medications in the MAO inhibitor family, and it should not be used without consulting a physician if one is taking ephedrine, pseudoephedrine (Sudafed), Ritalin, cyclosporine, calcium channel blockers, drugs that cause photosensitivity (such as sulfa antibiotics), or any medication that is critical to one's health.

EBSCO CAM Review Board

FURTHER READING

Bouchard, N. C., et al. "Ischemic Stroke Associated with Use of an Ephedra-free Dietary Supplement Containing Synephrine." *Mayo Clinic Proceedings* 80 (2005): 541-545.

Bui, L. T., D. T. Nguyen, and P. J. Ambrose. "Blood Pressure and Heart Rate Effects Following a Single Dose of Bitter Orange." *Annals of Pharmacotherapy* 40 (2006): 53-57.

Carvalho-Freitas, M. I., and M. Costa. "Anxiolytic and Sedative Effects of Extracts and Essential Oil from *Citrus aurantium* L." *Biological and Pharmaceutical Bulletin* 25 (2002): 1629-1633.

Hou, Y. C., et al. "Acute Intoxication of Cyclosporin Caused by Coadministration of Decoctions of the Fruits of *Citrus aurantium* and the Pericarps of *Citrus grandis*." *Planta Medica* 66 (2000): 653-655.

Kim, K. W., et al. "Characterization of Antidepressant-like Effects of P-synephrine Stereoisomers." *Naunyn Schmiedeberg's Archives of Pharmacology* 364 (2001): 21-26.

Malhotra, S., et al. "Seville Orange Juice-Felodipine Interaction: Comparison with Dilute Grapefruit Juice and Involvement of Furocoumarins." *Clinical Pharmacology and Therapeutics* 69 (2001): 14-23.

Nykamp, D. L., M. N. Fackih, and A. L. Compton. "Possible Association of Acute Lateral-Wall Myocardial Infarction and Bitter Orange Supplement." *Annals of Pharmacotherapy* 38 (2004): 812-816.

See also: Herbal medicine; Obesity and excess weight.

Citrus bioflavonoids

CATEGORY: Herbs and supplements

RELATED TERMS: Diosmetin, diosmin, hesperidin, naringin, narirutin, neohesperidin, nobiletin, rutin, tangeretin, bioflavonoid

DEFINITION: Natural substance used as a dietary supplement for specific health benefits.

PRINCIPAL PROPOSED USES: Chronic venous insufficiency, hemorrhoids

OTHER PROPOSED USES: Easy bruising, hypertension, leg ulcers, lymphedema following breast cancer surgery, nosebleeds

OVERVIEW

Citrus fruits are well known for providing ample amounts of vitamin C, but they also supply bioflavonoids, substances that are not required for life but that may improve health. The major bioflavonoids found in citrus fruits are diosmin, hesperidin, rutin, naringin, tangeretin, diosmetin, narirutin, neohesperidin, nobiletin, and quercetin. The first five bioflavonoids listed here are discussed in this article.

Citrus bioflavonoids and related substances are widely used in Europe to treat diseases of the blood vessels and lymph system, diseases including hemorrhoids, chronic venous insufficiency, leg ulcers, easy bruising, nosebleeds, and lymphedema following breast cancer surgery. These compounds are thought to work by strengthening the walls of blood vessels. Bioflavonoids are also often said to act as antioxidants; however, while they do have antioxidant activity in the test tube, growing evidence suggests that they do not act as antioxidants in humans.

REQUIREMENTS AND SOURCES

Citrus fruits contain citrus bioflavonoids in varying proportions. Even different brands of citrus juice may vary widely in their bioflavonoid concentrations and composition. For use as a supplement, bioflavonoids are extracted either from citrus fruits or from other plant sources, such as buckwheat.

THERAPEUTIC DOSAGES

A typical dosage of citrus bioflavonoids is 500 milligrams twice daily. The most-studied citrus bioflavonoid treatment is a special micronized (finely ground) combination of diosmin (90 percent) and hesperidin (10 percent).

THERAPEUTIC USES

Double-blind trials suggest (but do not prove conclusively) that a micronized combination preparation of diosmin and hesperidin may be helpful for hemorrhoids. Diosmin and hesperidin, and the bioflavonoid rutin, may also be helpful for chronic venous insufficiency, a condition in which the veins in the legs begin to weaken. One good double-blind trial found diosmin and hesperidin also to be helpful for persons who develop bruises or nosebleeds easily.

Citrus bioflavonoids have also been tried, with some success, for treating lymphedema (arm swelling) following breast cancer surgery. One should not use bioflavonoid combinations containing tangeretin if taking tamoxifen for breast cancer.

In addition, preliminary evidence suggests that citrus bioflavonoids may help reduce cholesterol levels, control inflammation, benefit people with diabetes, reduce allergic reactions, and prevent cancer. "Sweetie fruit," a bioflavonoid-rich hybrid of grapefruit and pummelo, has shown some promise for the treatment of high blood pressure.

SCIENTIFIC EVIDENCE

Hemorrhoids. A two-month, double-blind, placebo-controlled trial of 120 persons with recurrent hemorrhoid flare-ups found that treatment with combined diosmin and hesperidin significantly reduced the frequency and severity of hemorrhoid attacks. Another double-blind, placebo-controlled trial of one hundred persons had positive results with the same bioflavonoids in relieving symptoms once a flare-up of hemorrhoid pain had begun. A ninety-day, double-blind trial of one hundred persons with bleeding hemorrhoids also found significant benefits for both treatment of acute attacks and prevention of new ones. Finally, this bioflavonoid combination was found to compare favorably with surgical treatment of hemorrhoids. However, less impressive results were seen in a double-blind, placebo-controlled study in which all participants were given a fiber laxative with either combined diosmin and hesperidin or placebo.

Two studies claimed to find that diosmin-hesperidin reduces pain after hemorrhoid surgery. These studies, though, show little to nothing, as the researchers failed to use a placebo group and simply compared treated participants to untreated participants. Overall, the evidence remains incomplete, though promising.

Chronic venous insufficiency. A two-month, double-blind, placebo-controlled trial of two hundred people with relatively severe chronic venous insufficiency found that treatment with diosmin-hesperidin significantly improved symptoms compared with placebo. Another double-blind, placebo-controlled trial of diosmin-hesperidin enrolled 101 people with relatively mild chronic venous insufficiency. The results showed little difference between the two groups; the authors theorize that diosmin-hesperidin might be more effective in severe chronic venous insufficiency.

A two-month, double-blind, placebo-controlled trial evaluated the effects of diosmin-hesperidin in 107 people with nonhealing leg ulcers (sores) caused by venous insufficiency or other conditions. The results indicated that treatment significantly improved the rate of healing. Also, a three-month, double-blind, placebo-controlled trial of sixty-seven persons evaluated buckwheat tea (a good source of rutin) for chronic venous insufficiency. The results showed less leg swelling in the treated group. One study reportedly showed that the supplement oxyrutin is more effective than diosmin-hesperidin for chronic venous insufficiency, but the study was too poorly designed to provide meaningful results.

Easy bruising. Some people bruise particularly easily because of fragile capillaries. A six-week, double-blind, placebo-controlled study of ninety-six people with this condition found that combined diosmin and hesperidin decreased symptoms of capillary fragility, such as bruising and nosebleeds. Two rather poorly designed studies from the 1960s found benefits with a combination of vitamin C and citrus bioflavonoids for decreasing bruising in college athletes.

Lymphedema. Breast cancer surgery sometimes causes persistent swelling of the arm (lymphedema) caused by damage to lymph vessels. Citrus bioflavonoids and other natural supplements have shown promise for this condition. In a three-month, double-blind study, fifty-seven women with lymphedema received either placebo or combination therapy consisting of the modified citrus bioflavonoid trimethylhesperidin chalcone plus the bioflavonoid-rich herb butcher's broom. The results indicated that the use of the bioflavonoid combination resulted in significantly less swelling.

Cancer. In a review of twelve studies involving more than five thousand cases, researchers found that people who consumed the highest amounts of flavonoids in their diets had a lower risk of lung cancer than those who consumed less. The significance of these results is weakened because none of the studies were controlled trials, and because the most favorable among them did not account for the quantity of fruits, vegetables, or vitamins in the participants' diets.

SAFETY ISSUES

Extensive investigations of diosmin and hesperidin have found them to be essentially nontoxic and free of drug interactions. The combination has been given to fifty pregnant women in a research study, without apparent harm to women or fetuses.

Some evidence suggests that the bioflavonoid naringen may interact with medications in the calcium channel blocker family, increasing blood levels of the drug. This may necessitate a reduction in drug dosage.

The citrus bioflavonoid tangeretin may reduce the effectiveness of tamoxifen, a drug used to treat breast cancer. One highly preliminary study suggests that some citrus bioflavonoids in the diet of pregnant women might increase the risk of infant leukemia; hesperidin did not produce this effect, and diosmin was not tested.

IMPORTANT INTERACTIONS

The use of the bioflavonoid naringen may necessitate a reduction in medication dose for those who take calcium channel blockers. Persons taking tamoxifen for breast cancer should avoid citrus fruits and juices and the citrus bioflavonoid tangeretin.

EBSCO CAM Review Board

FURTHER READING

Alonso-Coello, P., et al. "Meta-analysis of Flavonoids for the Treatment of Haemorrhoids." *British Journal of Surgery* 93 (2006): 909-920.

Liu, B., et al. "Low-Dose Dietary Phytoestrogen Abrogates Tamoxifen-Associated Mammary Tumor Prevention." *Cancer Research* 65 (2005): 879-886.

Lotito, S. B., and B. Frei. "Consumption of Flavonoid-Rich Foods and Increased Plasma Antioxidant Capacity in Humans: Cause, Consequence, or Epiphenomenon?" *Free Radical Biology and Medicine* 41 (2006): 1727-1746.

Tang, N. P., et al. "Flavonoids Intake and Risk of Lung Cancer." *Japanese Journal of Clinical Oncology* 39 (2009): 352-359.

See also: Calcium channel blockers; Quercetin.

Cleavers

CATEGORY: Herbs and supplements
RELATED TERM: *Galium aparine*
DEFINITION: Natural plant product used to treat specific health conditions.
PRINCIPAL PROPOSED USES: None
OTHER PROPOSED USES: Bladder infection, fluid retention, swollen glands

OVERVIEW

The leaves of the cleavers plant (*Galium aparine*) have small hooked hairs that cause it to cleave to the fingers when touched, hence the name. The whole leaf has been used as a flavoring in soups and stews. Roasted seeds are used as a coffee substitute. The leaves and flowers are used medicinally. Cleavers is primarily used for urinary problems and fluid retention, on the basis of its apparent diuretic (urine-stimulating) effects. It has also been recommended for enlarged lymph nodes, tonsillitis, hepatitis, and snake bites.

THERAPEUTIC DOSAGES

A typical recommended dose of cleavers is one cup of tea three times daily, made by steeping 10 to 15 grams of the herb in a cup of hot water.

THERAPEUTIC USES

Cleavers is often included in herbal mixtures offered for the treatment of kidney and bladder problems, including bladder infections, kidney stones, and prostatitis. It is also said to help cleanse the lymph system. However, there has not been any meaningful scientific evaluation of the herb. Even animal and test-tube studies are essentially lacking.

SAFETY ISSUES

Cleavers has not undergone any meaningful safety testing. Safety in young children, pregnant or nursing women, and people with severe liver or kidney disease has not been established. Just in case cleavers does in fact have the diuretic effects that are claimed for it, people taking the medication lithium should use cleavers only under the supervision of a physician. This is because as dehydration can be dangerous with this medication.

EBSCO CAM Review Board

FURTHER READING
Pyevich, D., and M. P. Bogenschutz. "Herbal Diuretics and Lithium Toxicity." *American Journal of Psychiatry* 158 (2001): 1329.

See also: Diuretics, loop; Diuretics, potassium-sparing; Diuretics, thiazide; Herbal medicines.

Clinical trials

CATEGORY: Issues and overviews
RELATED TERMS: Biomedical research studies, clinical studies, health-related experiments, medical research, research studies
DEFINITION: Observed studies of the effect of medications, supplements, vitamins, treatments, and other interventions on the human body.

OVERVIEW

Clinical trials in complementary and alternative medicine (CAM) are most frequently systematic research studies designed to evaluate the effectiveness and safety of CAM for humans. Clinical trials address the question, What does a particular CAM treatment do to the human body? Other CAM clinical trials may involve a researcher who systematically observes and collects data on the activities and behaviors of specific persons to answer a specific research question.

Clinical trials are developed by a wide range of researchers, including CAM practitioners, traditional doctors, and sponsoring companies. All treatments that must be approved by the U.S. Food and Drug Administration (FDA) must first undergo a clinical trial to prove that the medication or supplement is effective and safe for human use. Even for those treatments that do not require FDA approval, the CAM industry still often uses clinical trials to show health consumers that a product or treatment is effective and safe.

TRIAL DESIGN

To conduct a quality clinical trial, studies must begin with a research question and effective research design. First, the researchers must develop a specific testable question known as a hypothesis. A CAM trial hypothesis might be the following: Massage is as effective as acetaminophen in relieving headaches caused by stress. Next, the researchers select a series of tests and questions that can accurately assess the hypothesis and provide information or data to support the study's conclusion. This is known as a study protocol.

The study protocol explains the trial's purpose, function, and methods (or the way it is to be conducted). Protocols often also include information about the reason for the study, any past research relating to the study, the number of subjects (persons) needed to perform an effective study, eligibility and exclusion criteria, details of the CAM intervention or therapy the participants will receive, what data to gather, what demographic information about the participants to gather, steps for clinical care givers to carry out, and the study endpoints. If a protocol is being run by several different investigators, a single standard protocol must be used without deviation to ensure that the resulting data will be consistent and reliable. All parts of the protocol should answer the hypothesis and should try to eliminate conflicting factors that might lead to false conclusions. In the foregoing hypothesis example, if the investigators do not ask trial participants about their use of ibuprofen or other pain killers for headaches, then false conclusions could be drawn by researchers about the effectiveness of massage therapy for the relief of headaches.

Depending on the design of the study protocol, the clinical trial may be given one of two overall design labels: case-control study or double-blind study. In a case-control study, a group of persons affected by the disease being studied is compared with a group without the disease. In a double-blind study, neither the study personnel nor the study participants know who is assigned to a particular intervention.

Clinical trials are also labeled by the types of questions they are attempting to answer. The first type is a phase I trial, applied to first-ever studies of a particular treatment or product and to early studies in an overall series of clinical trials. After conclusions about the basic safety of the treatment in humans have been drawn from phase I, phase II clinical trials continue to test the safety of the drug and begin to evaluate how effective the drug is in the target population. Phase III studies compare the new treatment to the current standard treatment. This phase is particularly crucial in that it produces the primary data the FDA reviews before approving or rejecting a particular treatment.

Once the clinical trial is properly designed, human volunteers can be asked to participate in the study.

Annotated Sampling of Completed Clinical Trials in Complementary and Alternative Medicine, 2011

- "For Minor Depression, Study Shows No Benefit Over Placebo from St. John's Wort, Citalopram"

  An extract of the herb St. John's wort and a standard antidepressant medication both failed to outdo a placebo in relieving symptoms of minor depression in a clinical trial comparing the three.

- "Omega-3 Fatty Acids May Reduce Inflammation and Anxiety in Healthy Young Adults"

  Study suggests that omega-3 fatty acids from fish oil reduce inflammation and anxiety in healthy young adults.

- "Massage Therapy Holds Promise for Low-Back Pain"

  Comparison of structural and relaxation massage shows that both reduce low-back pain and improve function, compared with usual medical care.

- "Health Behaviors Differ Between Two Groups of CAM Users"

  People who use CAM to promote health differ in health status, behaviors, and health care use from those who use CAM to treat an illness.

- "New Approach for Peanut Allergy in Children Holds Promise"

  Sublingual (under the tongue) immunotherapy may help children with peanut allergy.

- "Mindfulness Meditation Is Associated with Structural Changes in the Brain"

  Mindfulness meditation may increase gray matter in the hippocampus and other brain regions associated with learning, memory, and emotion.

- "Study Shows Cranberry Juice Cocktail Is No Better than Placebo at Preventing Recurrent UTIs"

  Compared with placebo, cranberry juice cocktail is no better at preventing recurrent urinary tract infections in college-aged women.

After all the procedures, tests, and questions are finished, the investigators analyze the data using statistical techniques and then draw a conclusion about their original hypothesis. In many cases, the conclusions establish the overall risks and benefits of any CAM intervention.

To distribute the information learned from clinical trials to the widest audience, most investigators will present their hypotheses, procedures, results, and conclusions in oral presentations, conference posters, and journal articles. Before publication or acceptance for conference presentation, most studies undergo peer review, in which other specialists and investigators in the original author or authors' field examine the clinical trial and support or reject the accuracy and conclu-

sions of the research. The reviewers will determine the validity of a clinical trial based on the researcher's performance in accurately testing the hypothesis. Determination of validity is based on the use of a strong set of tests and evaluations, the repeatability of the study, and the accuracy of data collection and interpretation. Studies that receive positive peer review can be published.

TRIAL IMPORTANCE

Well-designed clinical research trials in CAM are critical to practitioners and users of CAM therapies. CAM clinical trials help prove the validity of CAM treatments. Although CAM treatments have a long history, scientific knowledge about these alternative therapies is often lacking. Without scientific evidence, people already using CAM treatments may be at risk as they many be taking the wrong dose, using the treatment in the wrong way, or using it with other medications that may cause a dangerous interaction. Clinical trial data help consumers and CAM practitioners determine which treatment should be the most safe and effective for a particular issue. Knowing the most effective CAM treatment and using it first can also decrease the amount of time an individual suffers from a particular health issue.

Accurate CAM clinical trials can help validate treatments that are considered nonstandard by mainstream medical practitioners in a way that anecdotal stories about a particular treatment or person cannot. This is helpful when there are multiple CAM treatment options for specific conditions. Clinical research studies can suggest effective ways to combine multiple therapies, such as yoga and dietary supplements.

Manufacturers seeking FDA approval also require clinical trials to prove the safety and efficacy of their products. FDA approval brings an additional level of oversight to a product, and, critical to a manufacturer, also adds validation.

TRIAL OVERSIGHT

A clinical research trial usually has several layers of oversight to ensure that the study is designed well and that the participants will not be harmed. These layers of oversight were created to keep scientists, including medical doctors and other health practitioners, from performing unethical experiments on humans. The history of unethical research includes that conducted by the Nazis during World War II and that conducted by the U.S. government from 1932 to 1972 with poor African American men in Tuskegee, Alabama; the men studied had syphilis but were not treated for the disease.

Institutional Review Boards (IRBs), developed in response to unethical experimentation on humans, review and monitor every clinical trial in the United States. An IRB consists of an independent committee of physicians, medical professionals, statisticians, community advocates, and others that ensure that a clinical trial is ethical and that the rights of study participants are protected. One of the main responsibilities of IRBs is to ensure that research participants are fully informed of a study's purpose, procedures, risks, benefits, and costs through a process called informed consent.

The U.S. government also plays a role in the regulatory oversight of clinical research trials. The Department of Health and Human Service's Office for Human Research Protections (OHRP) oversees and regulates IRBs and human research in general. OHRP helps ensure the rights of persons in clinical trials by providing clarification and guidance, developing educational programs and materials, and providing advice on ethical and regulatory issues in biomedical and behavioral research. The FDA helps investigators create effective, ethical treatment studies on humans.

Many clinical trials (particularly those with more than one study site) also have data-safety-monitoring committees or boards. These independent committees are formed of experts who are familiar with the conditions and treatments under study but who are not involved in the clinical research trials themselves. The committee members review any adverse events, experimental errors, or other issues to make sure the study can continue and to ensure that investigators are performing research appropriately and effectively.

TRIAL PARTICIPATION

Clinical research trials are possible only because volunteers agree to participate in the studies. Participants often volunteer to have a more active role in their own health care, to gain early access to new research treatments, and to help others by contributing to medical research. The decision to join a research trial should be a reasoned one and may involve the help of friends or family members. Before participating in a clinical trial, it is critical to know the key facts about a particular trial. One should understand the trial's procedures, risks, benefits, and personal costs. These answers are provided to volunteers through the informed consent process. The main portion of informed consent occurs before a prospective volunteer agrees to join the study. Only after the conclusion of informed consent can a study subject begin his or her participation in a clinical trial.

Clinical research trials in CAM can be found through the Web, particularly through Clinicaltrials. gov, run by the National Institutes of Health. Investigators around the world submit information to this site about ongoing research. Another option for finding clinical trials is to identify the researchers who have done past work and to contact them about recruitment for future studies.

One can find published research studies through Web-based databases such as Pubmed, provided by the National Library of Medicine. A searchable database of published CAM research studies is available through the Web site of the National Center for Complementary and Alternative Medicine, part of the NIH.

Dawn Laney, M.S., CGC, CCRC

FURTHER READING

Boissel, J. P. "Planning of Clinical Trials." *Journal of Internal Medicine* 255, no. 4 (2004): 427-438. An article focused on the steps in planning clinical trials. Includes information about forming a scientific question for trial design and protocol.

National Center for Complementary and Alternative Medicine. http://nccam.nih.gov. A comprehensive site of a leading U.S. agency for scientific research on complementary and alternative medicine. Provides results and information on CAM obtained from clinical trials.

National Institute of Child Health and Human Development. http://www.nichd.nih.gov/health/clinicalresearch. Provides information about clinical research and the NICHD's role in this research

National Institutes of Health. ClinicalTrials.gov. http://clinicaltrials.gov. A detailed listing of clinical trials in the United States and around the world.

National Library of Medicine. http://www.pubmed.gov. Pubmed contains publication information and (in most cases) brief summaries of articles from scientific and medical journals.

See also: Double-blind, placebo-controlled studies; Education and training of CAM practitioners; Placebo effect; Pseudoscience; Regulation of CAM; Scientific method.

Clomiphene

CATEGORY: Drug interactions
DEFINITION: A drug used to enhance female fertility.
INTERACTIONS: N-acetylcysteine, traditional Chinese herbal medicine
TRADE NAMES: Clomid, Serophene

N-ACETYLCYSTEINE
Effect: Possible Helpful Interaction

The supplement N-acetylcysteine (NAC) has shown promise for enhancing the effectiveness of clomiphene. A double-blind study enrolled 150 women with polycystic ovary syndrome for whom clomiphene had not been effective. One-half of the women were given NAC at a dose of 1.2 grams per day, while the other half received placebo. All participants continued to receive clomiphene. The results showed that the use of NAC significantly improved both ovulation rate and pregnancy rate.

TRADITIONAL CHINESE HERBAL MEDICINE
Effect: Possible Helpful Interaction

Traditional Chinese herbal medicine employs complex combinations of herbs. Several studies conducted in China reported that the use of such combinations can enhance the effectiveness of clomiphene. None of these studies achieved the minimum standards necessary for scientific validity.

EBSCO CAM Review Board

FURTHER READING
Chao, S. L., L. W. Huang, and H. R. Yen. "Pregnancy in Premature Ovarian Failure After Therapy Using Chinese Herbal Medicine." *Chang Gung Medical Journal* 26 (2003): 449-452.
Rizk, A. Y., et al. "N-acetyl-cysteine Is a Novel Adjuvant to Clomiphene Citrate in Clomiphene Citrate-Resistant Patients with Polycystic Ovary Syndrome." *Fertility and Sterility* 83 (2005): 367-370.

See also: Infertility, female; Food and Drug Administration; Herbal medicine; N-acetylcysteine; Polycystic ovary syndrome; Supplements: Introduction; Traditional Chinese herbal medicine; Women's health.

Clonidine

CATEGORY: Drug interactions
DEFINITION: A drug often used to reduce blood pressure and to counter symptoms that occur during withdrawal from alcohol and other addictive substances.
INTERACTIONS: Coenzyme Q_{10}, *Coleus forskohlii*, Yohimbe
TRADE NAME: Catapres

COENZYME Q_{10} (CoQ_{10})
Effect: Supplementation Possibly Helpful

There is some evidence that clonidine might impair the body's ability to manufacture the substance CoQ_{10}. However, it has not yet been shown that CoQ_{10} supplements offer any particular benefit to those taking this medication.

YOHIMBE
Effect: Probable Dangerous Interaction

Persons taking clonidine should not take yohimbe.

Coleus forskohlii
Effect: Theoretical Interaction

The herb *Coleus forskohlii* relaxes blood vessels and might have unpredictable effects if combined with clonidine.

EBSCO CAM Review Board

FURTHER READING
Brinker, F. *Herb Contraindications and Drug Interactions.* 2d ed. Sandy, Oreg.: Eclectic Medical, 1998.
Kishi, H., et al. "Bioenergetics in Clinical Medicine IIII: Inhibition of Coenzyme Q10-Enzymes by Clinically Used Anti-hypertensive Drugs." *Research Communications in Chemical Pathology and Pharmacology* 12, no. 3 (1975): 533-540.

See also: Alcoholism; Coenzyme Q$_{10}$; *Coleus forskohlii*; Food and Drug Administration; Hypertension; Supplements: Introduction; Yohimbe.

Codex Alimentarius Commission

Category: Organizations and legislation
Definition: A commission of the United Nations that creates standards for food nutrition, food safety, and fair trade of food and food products.
Date: Founded in 1963

Establishment and Function

The Codex Alimentarius Commission (CAC) is an agency of the United Nations (U.N.) that creates global standards and guidelines for food nutrition, food safety, and trade practices. These standards and guidelines are known collectively as the Codex Alimentarius (Latin for "food book" or "food code").

The commission was founded in 1963 by two U.N. agencies, the Food and Agriculture Organization (FAO) and the World Health Organization (WHO). The idea for the commission was first formulated in 1961 by the FAO; WHO added its formal support in 1963. The commission comprises 180 member countries, including those of the European Union, and nongovernmental organizations.

The Codex

Codex standards cover a wide range of issues, including maximum allowable levels of pesticides and drugs in plants and food animals, the use of irradiation in food processing, product labeling, and consumer protection. The CAC does not attempt to completely restrict possibly harmful substances; rather, the twenty technical subcommittees that make up the CAC use risk analysis to establish margins of safety for food products. The commission also examines the safety of genetically modified foods, but it has not established official standards in this area of concern. All codex standards are available on the CAC website.

The CAC does not have legal power, so the standards are considered simply guidelines for each nation. Legislation regarding food standards and labeling is the responsibility of each respective member country. Nevertheless, in 1994, the World Trade Organization (WTO) adopted the Codex Alimentarius for world trade, to be used as a reference in settling disputes between countries. This adoption by the WTO effectively turned codex recommendations into international "rules" of trade.

Controversy

The Codex Alimentarius has had a tremendous global affect on the growth, processing, distribution, and consuming of food, yet most consumers have never heard of the commission or its standards. Still, the codex remains a source of controversy. Objections have been raised against the codex's infringement on freedom of trade and personal choice, among other issues. One objection is that the codex institutionalizes practices that are in the interests of global agribusiness instead of in the interests of the consumer.

Of particular controversy is the "Guidelines for Vitamin and Mineral Food Supplements," a standard that was passed in 2005 by the CAC's Committee on Nutrition and Foods for Special Dietary Uses. Consumer groups favoring the use of over-the-counter nutritional supplements, for example, have claimed that codex standards were written to favor the pharmaceutical industry. Such groups believe that under codex standards, unregulated diet supplements, such as vitamins and minerals, will be available only by prescription and that some supplements currently available will be banned.

In response, the CAC stated that it had no intention of banning supplements or of requiring prescriptions for their use. According to the commission, the guidelines concern the composition of the supplements to ensure safety and purity. Herbal medicine is not addressed in codex guidelines.

Despite commission assertions, the adoption of codex standards by the WTO has increased concern, and for some consumer groups the codex remains an intensely emotional issue.

David Hutto, Ph.D.

Further Reading

Codex Alimentarius Commission. "Codex Alimentarius." Available at http://www.codexalimentarius.net.

Food and Agriculture Organization and World Health Organization. "Understanding the Codex Alimentarius." Available at http://www.fao.org/docrep/008/y7867e/y7867e00.htm.

Lee, Kelley. *Historical Dictionary of the World Health*

Organization. Langham, Mass.: Rowman & Little-field, 1998.

U.S. Department of Agriculture, Food Safety and Inspection Service. "Codex Alimentarius." Available at http://www.fsis.usda.gov/codex_alimentarius.

See also: Dietary Supplement Health and Education Act of 1994; Food and Drug Administration; Office of Dietary Supplements.

Coenzyme Q_{10}

CATEGORY: Herbs and supplements

RELATED TERM: Ubiquinone

DEFINITION: Natural substance of the human body used as a supplement to treat specific health conditions.

PRINCIPAL PROPOSED USES: Cardiomyopathy, congestive heart failure, heart attack recovery, hypertension, nutrient depletion/interference caused by various medications

OTHER PROPOSED USES: Amyotrophic lateral sclerosis (Lou Gehrig's disease), asthma, diabetes, kidney failure, migraine headaches, Parkinson's disease, periodontal disease, preeclampsia and pregnancy-induced hypertension, sports performance enhancement, tinnitus

OVERVIEW

Coenzyme Q_{10} (CoQ_{10}), also known as ubiquinone, is a major part of the body's mechanism for producing energy. The name of this supplement comes from the word "ubiquitous," which means "found everywhere." Indeed, CoQ_{10} is found in every cell in the body. It plays a fundamental role in the mitochondria, the parts of the cell that produce energy from glucose and fatty acids.

Japanese scientists first reported therapeutic properties of CoQ_{10} in the 1960s. Some evidence suggests that CoQ_{10} might assist the heart during times of stress on the heart muscle, perhaps by helping it use energy more efficiently.

CoQ_{10}'s best-established use is for congestive heart failure, but the evidence that it works is not entirely consistent. Ongoing research suggests that it may also be useful for other types of heart problems, Parkinson's disease, and several additional illnesses. It is gen-erally used in addition to, rather than instead of, standard therapies. CoQ_{10} supplementation might also be of value for counteracting the side effects of certain prescription medications.

REQUIREMENTS AND SOURCES

Every cell in the human body needs CoQ_{10}, but there is no dietary requirement because the body can manufacture CoQ_{10} itself.

THERAPEUTIC DOSAGES

The typical recommended dosage of CoQ_{10} is 30 to 300 milligrams (mg) daily; higher daily intakes have been used in some studies. CoQ_{10} is fat soluble and may be better absorbed when taken in an oil-based soft gel form rather than in a dry form such as tablets and capsules. Dividing the total daily dosage up into two or more separate doses may produce higher blood levels. A finely ground-up (nanoparticular) form of the supplement appears to be much better absorbed than standard CoQ_{10} products.

THERAPEUTIC USES

Although not all studies have been positive, some evidence supports the use of CoQ_{10} for treating congestive heart failure. CoQ_{10} is taken with conventional medications, not as a replacement for them.

Weaker evidence suggests that this supplement may be useful for heart attack recovery, cardiomyopathy, hypertension, diabetes, strengthening the heart before heart surgery, and migraine headaches. Although CoQ_{10} has been widely advertised as effective for treating Parkinson's disease, in fact, there is only minimal evidence that it works, and some evidence that it does not work.

CoQ_{10} has shown the potential to prevent heart damage and other side effects caused by certain types of cancer chemotherapy. This evidence is weak, however, and as yet it cannot be stated with any certainty that CoQ_{10} is actually helpful.

CoQ_{10} has shown some preliminary promise as an aid to the treatment of kidney failure. People with severe illnesses, such as heart disease, cancer, or kidney failure, should not use CoQ_{10}, or any supplement, except under a physician's supervision.

Highly preliminary studies suggest CoQ_{10} might be helpful for amyotrophic lateral sclerosis. CoQ_{10} has been tried, but not found effective, for the treatment of Huntington's disease.

Coenzyme Q$_{10}$ and Cancer

Coenzyme Q$_{10}$ (CoQ$_{10}$) was first isolated in 1957, and its chemical structure (benzoquinone compound) was determined in 1958. Interest in CoQ$_{10}$ as a therapeutic agent in cancer began in 1961, when a deficiency was noted in the blood of both Swedish and American cancer patients, especially in the blood of patients with breast cancer. A subsequent study showed a statistically significant relationship between the level of plasma CoQ$_{10}$ deficiency and breast cancer prognosis. Low blood levels of this compound have been reported in patients with malignancies other than breast cancer, including myeloma, lymphoma, and cancers of the lung, prostate, pancreas, colon, kidney, and head and neck. Furthermore, decreased levels of CoQ$_{10}$ have been detected in malignant human tissue, but increased levels also have been reported.

Certain medications may interfere with the body's production of CoQ$_{10}$ or partially block its function. The best evidence regards cholesterol-lowering drugs in the statin family, such as lovastatin (Mevacor), simvastatin (Zocor), and pravastatin (Pravachol), along with the supplement red yeast rice (which contains naturally occurring statins). These medications impair CoQ$_{10}$ synthesis as an inevitable side effect of their mechanism of action. Since these drugs are used to protect the heart and since CoQ$_{10}$ deficiency could in theory impair heart function, it has been suggested that this side effect may work against the intended purpose of taking statins. Furthermore, one might naturally guess that some of the side effects of statins could be caused by this induced CoQ$_{10}$ deficiency. However, studies designed to determine whether the use of CoQ$_{10}$ supplements actually offers any benefit to people taking statins have returned inconsistent results at best.

For several other categories of drugs, the evidence that they interfere with CoQ$_{10}$ is provocative but even less reliable. These include oral diabetes drugs (especially glyburide, phenformin, and tolazamide), beta-blockers (specifically propranolol, metoprolol, and alprenolol), antipsychotic drugs in the phenothiazine family, tricyclic antidepressants, methyldopa, hydrochlorothiazide, clonidine, and hydralazine. Again, while in theory CoQ$_{10}$ supplementation might be helpful for people using these medications, there is no direct evidence to support this hypothesis.

CoQ$_{10}$ has also been suggested as a performance enhancer for athletes. However, while one double-blind study of twenty-five highly trained cross-country skiers found some benefit, most studies evaluating potential sports supplement uses of CoQ$_{10}$ have returned negative rather than positive results.

CoQ$_{10}$ is also sometimes claimed to be an effective treatment for periodontal disease. However, the studies on which this idea is based are too flawed to be taken as meaningful. Even weaker evidence, far too weak to rely upon, hints that CoQ$_{10}$ might be useful in some cases of tinnitus (ringing in the ear).

One preliminary study of CoQ$_{10}$ for people undergoing treatment for human immunodeficiency virus (HIV) infection found conflicting results; the supplement appeared to improve general well-being, but it did not protect mitochondria (as the researchers had hoped it would) and actually seemed to worsen symptoms of nerve-related pain (peripheral neuropathy).

Preliminary evidence, far too weak to be relied upon, has been used to suggest that CoQ$_{10}$ might be helpful for asthma, as well as reducing the side effects (specifically, cardiac toxicity) of the cancer chemotherapy drug doxorubicin. CoQ$_{10}$ has additionally been proposed as a treatment for a wide variety of other conditions, including angina, cancer, male infertility, muscular dystrophy, and obesity, but there is, as yet, no evidence that it is effective. There is also some evidence that CoQ$_{10}$ may reduce the risk of pre-eclampsia (high blood pressure during pregnancy) in women who are at risk for this condition.

SCIENTIFIC EVIDENCE

Congestive heart failure. Most but not all studies suggest that CoQ$_{10}$ can be helpful for people with congestive heart failure (CHF). In this serious condition, the heart muscles become weakened, resulting in poor circulation and shortness of breath.

People with CHF have significantly lower levels of CoQ$_{10}$ in heart muscle cells than do healthy people. This fact alone does not prove that the supplements will help CHF; however, it prompted medical researchers to try using CoQ$_{10}$ as a treatment for heart failure.

The largest study was a one-year, double-blind, placebo-controlled trial of 641 people with moderate to severe congestive heart failure. Half were given 2 mg per kilogram body weight of CoQ$_{10}$ daily; the rest were given a placebo. Standard therapy was continued in both groups. The participants treated with CoQ$_{10}$ experienced a significant reduction in the severity of their symptoms. No such improvement was seen in the placebo group. The people who took CoQ$_{10}$ also had significantly fewer hospitalizations for heart failure.

Similarly positive results were also seen in other double-blind studies involving a total of more than 270 participants. One double-blind study found that in people with heart failure so severe they were waiting for a heart transplant, use of CoQ$_{10}$ improved subjective symptoms.

However, two very well-designed double-blind studies published in 1999 and 2000, enrolling a total of about eighty-five people with congestive heart failure, failed to find any evidence of benefit. The reason for this discrepancy is not clear.

Cardiomyopathy. Cardiomyopathy is the general name given to conditions in which the heart muscle gradually becomes diseased. Several small studies suggest that CoQ$_{10}$ supplements are helpful for some forms of cardiomyopathy.

Hypertension. An eight-week double-blind, placebo-controlled study of fifty-nine men already taking medications for high blood pressure found that 120 mg daily of CoQ$_{10}$ reduced blood pressure by about 9 percent, compared with a placebo.

A twelve-week double-blind, placebo-controlled study of eighty-three people with isolated systolic hypertension (a type of high blood pressure in which only the "top" number is high) found that use of CoQ$_{10}$ at a dose of 60 mg daily improved blood pressure measurements to a similar extent.

Similarly, in a twelve-week double-blind, placebo-controlled trial of seventy-four people with diabetes, use of CoQ$_{10}$ at a dose of 100 mg twice daily significantly reduced blood pressure, compared with a placebo. Antihypertensive effects were also seen in previous smaller trials, most of which were not double-blind.

CoQ$_{10}$ may also be beneficial in reducing the risk of high blood pressure during pregnancy (preeclampsia). In one study, 235 pregnant women at risk for preeclampsia were randomized to receive CoQ$_{10}$ (200 mg daily) or a placebo for twenty weeks until they delivered their babies. The women in the treatment group had fewer cases of preeclampsia, compared with those who took the placebo.

Heart attack recovery. In a double-blind trial, 144

people who had recently experienced a heart attack were given either placebo or 120 mg of CoQ$_{10}$ daily for one year, along with conventional treatment. The results showed that participants receiving CoQ$_{10}$ experienced significantly fewer heart-related problems, such as episodes of angina pectoris or arrhythmia, or recurrent heart attacks.

A double-blind study of forty-nine people who had suffered a full cardiac arrest requiring cardiopulmonary resuscitation (CPR) found that use of CoQ$_{10}$ along with mild hypothermia (chilling of the body) was more effective than mild hypothermia plus a placebo. Individuals recovering from a heart attack should not take any herbs or supplements except under the supervision of a physician.

Parkinson's disease. A study published in 2002 raised hopes that CoQ$_{10}$ might help slow the progression of Parkinson's disease. In this sixteen-month double-blind, placebo-controlled trial, eighty people with Parkinson's disease were given either CoQ$_{10}$ (at a dose of 300 mg, 600 mg, or 1,200 mg daily) or a placebo. Participants in this trial had early stages of the disease and did not yet need medication. The results appeared to suggest that CoQ$_{10}$, especially at the highest dose, might have slowed disease progression. However, for a variety of statistical reasons, the results were in fact quite inconclusive.

A subsequent double-blind, placebo-controlled study of 28 people with Parkinson's disease, which was well controlled by medications, indicated that 360 mg of CoQ$_{10}$ daily could produce a mild improvement in some symptoms. Based on these results, a more substantial study was undertaken, enrolling 131 people with Parkinson's disease (again, well controlled by medications). This repeat trial used an especially finely ground form of CoQ$_{10}$ that, though taken at a dose of only 300 mg daily, produced blood levels of the supplement equivalent to those produced by 1,200 mg daily of ordinary CoQ$_{10}$; it did not work. While benefits were seen in both the placebo and the CoQ$_{10}$ group, CoQ$_{10}$ failed to prove more effective than placebo. Further trials will be necessary to confirm (or deny) these results.

Diabetes. In the twelve-week double-blind, placebo-controlled trial of people with diabetes mentioned above, use of CoQ$_{10}$ at a dose of 100 mg twice daily significantly improved blood sugar control, compared with a placebo. Similar benefits were seen in the eight-week double-blind, placebo-controlled study of fifty-nine men also described above. However, a third study failed to find any effect on blood sugar control.

SAFETY ISSUES

In general, CoQ$_{10}$ appears to be extremely safe. No significant side effects have been found, even in studies that lasted a year. However, people with severe heart disease should not take CoQ$_{10}$ (or any other supplement) except under a doctor's supervision.

As noted above, two studies suggest that CoQ$_{10}$ might reduce blood sugar levels in people with diabetes. While this could potentially be helpful for treatment of diabetes, it might present a risk as well; people with diabetes who are using CoQ$_{10}$ might inadvertently push their blood sugar levels dangerously low. However, another trial in people with diabetes found no effect on blood sugar control. Persons with diabetes should track their blood sugar closely if they start taking CoQ$_{10}$ (or, indeed, any herb or supplement).

CoQ$_{10}$ chemically resembles vitamin K. Since vitamin K counters the anticoagulant effects of warfarin (Coumadin), it has been suggested that CoQ$_{10}$ may have the same effect. However, a small, double-blind study found no interaction between CoQ$_{10}$ and warfarin. Nonetheless, in view of warfarin's low margin of safety, prudence indicates physician supervision before combining CoQ$_{10}$ with warfarin.

CoQ$_{10}$ might also interact with reverse transcriptase inhibitors used for treatment of HIV (for example, lamivudine and zidovudine). These medications can cause damage to the mitochondria, the energy-producing subunits of cells, leading in turn to a variety of side effects, including lactic acidosis (a dangerous metabolic derangement), peripheral neuropathy (injury to nerves in the extremities), and lipodystrophy (cosmetically undesirable rearrangement of fat in the body). The supplement CoQ$_{10}$ has been tried for minimizing these side effects, but unexpected results occurred. In a double-blind, placebo-controlled study, use of CoQ$_{10}$ improved general sense of well-being in people with HIV-infection using reverse transcriptase inhibitors; however, for reasons that are unclear, it actually worsened symptoms of peripheral neuropathy. For this reason, people with HIV who have peripheral neuropathy symptoms should use CoQ$_{10}$ only with caution.

The maximum safe dosages of CoQ$_{10}$ for young children, pregnant or nursing women, or those with severe liver or kidney disease have not been determined.

IMPORTANT INTERACTIONS

Persons taking cholesterol-lowering drugs in the statin family, red yeast rice, beta-blockers (specifically propranololmetoprolol and alprenolol), antipsychotic drugs in the phenothiazine family, tricyclic antidepressants, methyldopa, hydrochlorothiazide, clonidine, hydralazine, and oral diabetes drugs (especially glyburide, phenformin, and tolazamide) may need more CoQ$_{10}$. Persons taking Coumadin (warfarin) should not take CoQ$_{10}$ except on a physician's advice. In those taking reverse-transcriptase inhibitors (for HIV infection), CoQ$_{10}$ might improve their general sense of well-being but worsen peripheral neuropathy symptoms.

EBSCO CAM Review Board

FURTHER READING

Christensen, E. R., et al. "Mitochondrial DNA Levels in Fat and Blood Cells from Patients with Lipodystrophy or Peripheral Neuropathy and the Effect of Ninety Days of High-Dose Coenzyme Q Treatment." *Clinical Infectious Diseases* 39 (2004): 1371-1379.

Gvozdjakova, A., et al. "Coenzyme Q$_{10}$ Supplementation Reduces Corticosteroids Dosage in Patients with Bronchial Asthma." *Biofactors* 25 (2006): 235-240.

Khan, M., et al. "A Pilot Clinical Trial of the Effects of Coenzyme Q$_{10}$ on Chronic Tinnitus Aurium." *Otolaryngology and Head and Neck Surgery* 135 (2007): 72-77.

Sandor, P. S., et al. "Efficacy of Coenzyme Q$_{10}$ in Migraine Prophylaxis." *Neurology* 64 (2005): 713-715.

Singh, R. B., et al. "Effect on Absorption and Oxidative Stress of Different Oral Coenzyme Q$_{10}$ Dosages and Intake Strategy in Healthy Men." *Biofactors* 25 (2006): 219-224.

Strey, C. H., et al. "Endothelium-Ameliorating Effects of Statin Therapy and Coenzyme Q$_{10}$ Reductions in Chronic Heart Failure." *Atherosclerosis* 179 (2005): 201-206.

Zhou, S., et al. "Muscle and Plasma Coenzyme Q$_{10}$ Concentration, Aerobic Power and Exercise Economy of Healthy Men in Response to Four Weeks of Supplementation." *Journal of Sports Medicine and Physical Fitness* 45 (2005): 337-346.

See also: Cardiomyopathy; Congestive heart failure; Heart attack; Herbal medicine; Hypertension; Parkinson's disease; Preeclampsia and pregnancy-induced hypertension.

Cola nut

CATEGORY: Herbs and supplements
RELATED TERMS: *Cola acuminata, C. nitida*
DEFINITION: Natural plant product used to treat specific health conditions.
PRINCIPAL PROPOSED USE: Fatigue

OVERVIEW

Indigenous to Western Africa, the cola tree is cultivated in many tropical climates, including Central America and South America, the West Indies, Sri Lanka, and Malaysia. Cola nuts are actually seeds removed from their seed coats. Traditionally, they are chewed raw or taken in pulverized or liquid extract form. Of the various species of cola nuts, the two most commonly edible kinds are *Cola acuminata* and *C. nitida*.

Cola contains caffeine and related chemicals and for this reason is a stimulant. For thousands of years, people in Africa have chewed the seeds to enhance mental alertness and fight fatigue. Centuries ago, Arabs traded gold dust for cola nuts before starting out on long treks across the Sahara.

Cola nut has been used in folk medicine as an aphrodisiac and an appetite suppressant and to treat morning sickness, migraine headache, and indigestion. It has also been applied directly to the skin to treat wounds and inflammation. The tree's bitter twig has been used as well, to clean the teeth and gums.

THERAPEUTIC DOSAGES

Germany's Commission E recommends the following daily dosage of cola: 2 to 6 grams (g) of cola nut, 0.25 to 0.75 g of cola extract, 2.5 to 7.5 g of cola liquid extract, 10 to 30 g of cola tincture, or 60 to 180 g of cola wine.

THERAPEUTIC USES

Based on the cola nut's caffeine content, Germany's Commission E has approved its use for the treatment of fatigue. Cola is ingested daily by millions as one of the main ingredients in cola soft drinks. It is also used in diet and high-energy products such as food bars and as a flavoring in alcoholic beverages, frozen dairy desserts, candy, baked goods, gelatins, and puddings. However, the caffeine-containing cola nut, used in original recipes for Coca-Cola, should

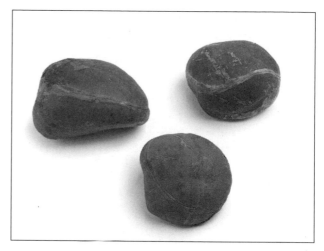

Cola nuts can be chewed raw or taken in pulverized or liquid extract form. (©Pipa100/Dreamstime.com)

not be confused with gotu kola. Because of its caffeine content, cola nut would be expected to increase urination, stimulate the heart and lungs, and help analgesics such as aspirin to function more effectively.

SAFETY ISSUES

Although comprehensive safety studies have not been performed, moderate amounts of cola nut are generally regarded as safe. The Council of Europe and the U.S. Food and Drug Administration have approved it as a food additive. The typical side effects associated with cola nut are those of caffeine, including nervousness, heart irregularities, headaches, and sleeplessness.

Cola is not advised for individuals with stomach ulcers because of both its caffeine and its tannin content. Tannins, found in many plants, are substances that can irritate the stomach.

EBSCO CAM Review Board

FURTHER READING

Ibu, J. O., et al. "The Effect of *Cola acuminata* and *Cola nitida* on Gastric Acid Secretion." *Scandinavian Journal of Gastroenterology* 124 (1986): 39-45.

Newall, C., L. A. Anderson, and J. D. Phillipson. *Herbal Medicines: A Guide for Health-Care Professionals.* London: Pharmaceutical Press, 1996.

See also: Fatigue; Herbal medicine.

Colchicine

Category: Drug interactions
Definition: Drug used to treat attacks of gout and used as a gout preventive.
Interaction: Vitamin B$_{12}$

Vitamin B$_{12}$

Effect: Supplementation Possibly Helpful

Colchicine can impair intestinal absorption of vitamin B$_{12}$, so taking a vitamin B$_{12}$ supplement during extended colchicine therapy may be warranted.

EBSCO CAM Review Board

Further Reading

Webb, D. I., et al. "Mechanism of Vitamin B12 Malabsorption in Patients Receiving Colchicine." *New England Journal of Medicine* 279 (1968): 845-850.

See also: Food and Drug Administration; Gout; Vitamin B$_{12}$; Vitamins and minerals.

Colds and flu

Category: Condition
Definition: Treatment for common respiratory infections caused by viruses.
Principal proposed natural treatments: Andrographis (often combined with *Eleutherococcus*), echinacea (sometimes combined with wild indigo and white pine), essential oil monoterpenes, garlic, *Panax ginseng*, probiotics, vitamin C, zinc
Other proposed natural treatments: Arginine, ashwagandha, astragalus, chlorella, colostrum, combination product containing horseradish and nasturtium, elderberry, ginger, glutamine, green tea extract, hyssop, ivy leaf, kelp, kudzu, linden, maitake, marshmallow, mistletoe, mullein, multivitamin-multimineral supplements, oregano, osha, *Pelargonium sidoides*, peppermint, propolis, reishi, thymus extract, traditional Chinese herbal medicine, sage, suma, yarrow
Probably not effective treatment: *Hippophae rhamnoides* (sea buckthorn)

Introduction

A cold is a respiratory infection caused by one of hundreds of possible viruses. However, because these viruses are so widespread, it is perhaps more accurate to say that colds are caused by a decrease in immunity that allows one of these viruses to take hold.

Colds occur more frequently in winter, but no one knows exactly why. Nearly everyone catches colds occasionally, but some people catch colds quite frequently; others tend to stay sick an unusually long time.

Influenza B, commonly called the flu, occurs in the form of a worldwide epidemic every winter. The predominant symptoms of flu are fever, malaise, and muscle aches. Coldlike respiratory symptoms are usually fairly minor with the flu, but a dangerous type of pneumonia can develop as a complication of influenza, especially in the elderly.

Conventional medicine can neither cure nor prevent the common cold. Furthermore, no over-the-counter treatments have been found to shorten the duration of a cold or even provide significant temporary relief. Cough syrup, in studies, seems to be no better than placebo. Some of the natural treatments described in this section may be able to do better.

People often want to take antibiotics for colds, and many physicians will prescribe them (even though antibiotics have no effect on viruses). Many believe that when associated mucus turns yellow, it means that a bacterial infection has occurred for which antibiotic treatment is indicated. However, viruses can also produce yellow mucus. Even if bacteria have made a home in the excess mucus, they may be only "innocent bystanders" and produce no symptoms. Colds, however, can be complicated by bacterial infections. In such cases, antibiotic treatment may be indicated.

The situation is somewhat better for influenza. The flu shot provides protection against several strains of influenza. There are also prescription antiviral medications that can help prevent flu and also reduce its length and severity.

Principal Proposed Natural Treatments

Various natural treatments have shown promise for treating or preventing colds and flu.

Zinc. One well-known alternative treatment for colds and flu is the use of zinc in nasal gel or lozenges. When zinc is taken this way, it is not being used as a nutrient. Rather, certain forms of zinc release ions that are thought to directly inhibit viruses in the nose and throat.

Taking zinc orally as a nutrient might also be useful

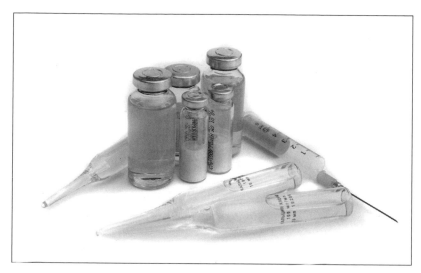

Syringe and bottle of medicine. (©Niderlander/Dreamstime.com)

in some cases. The immune system does not function properly if one does not have enough zinc in his or her body. Because zinc is commonly deficient in the diet, especially among children and the elderly, nutritional zinc supplementation may certainly be useful for those who get sick easily.

A one-year double-blind study of fifty nursing home residents found that zinc supplements compared with placebo reduced rates of infection. In addition, more than ten other studies performed in developing countries have found that zinc supplements at nutritional doses can increase resistance to respiratory and other infection in children, and that they might reduce symptom severity. With zinc, more is not better; once one has enough zinc, getting extra will not help and might even be harmful.

Scientific evidence for zinc nasal gel and lozenges. The use of lozenges containing zinc gluconate or zinc acetate has shown somewhat inconsistent but generally positive results for reducing the severity and duration of the common cold. For example, in a double-blind trial, one hundred people who were experiencing the early symptoms of a cold were given a lozenge that contained either 13.3 milligrams (mg) of zinc from zinc gluconate or a placebo. Participants took the lozenges several times daily until their cold symptoms subsided. The results were impressive. Coughing disappeared within two days in the treated group versus four days in the placebo group. Sore throat disappeared after one day versus three days in the placebo

group, nasal drainage in four days (versus seven days), and headache in two days (versus three days). Positive results have also been seen in double-blind studies of zinc acetate. Not all studies have shown such positive results. However, the overall results appear to be favorable.

It has been suggested that the exact formulation of the zinc lozenge plays a significant role in its effectiveness. According to this view, certain flavoring agents, such as citric acid and tartaric acid, might prevent zinc from inhibiting viruses. In addition, chemical forms of zinc other than zinc gluconate or zinc acetate might be ineffective. Zinc sulfate in particular might not work. Along the same lines, sweeteners such as sorbitol, sucrose, dextrose, and mannitol are said to be fine, while glycine has been discussed in an equivocal manner.

The use of zinc in the nose is somewhat more controversial. In addition to showing inconsistent results in studies, the use of zinc nasal gel can cause pain and possibly loss of sense of smell. In one double-blind, placebo-controlled trial, 213 people with a newly starting cold used one squirt of zinc gluconate gel or placebo gel in each nostril every four hours while awake. The results were significant: Treated participants stayed sick an average of 2.3 days, while those receiving placebo were sick for an average of 9 days, a 75 percent reduction in the duration of symptoms. Somewhat more modest but still significant relative benefits were seen with zinc nasal gel in a double-blind, placebo-controlled study of eighty people with colds. However, a slightly larger study of a similar zinc gluconate nasal gel found no benefit. Another study, this one involving seventy-seven people, failed to find benefit, even with nearly constant saturation of the nasal passages with zinc gluconate nasal spray.

Echinacea. Until the 1930s, echinacea was the number-one cold and flu remedy in the United States. It lost its popularity with the arrival of sulfa antibiotics. Ironically, sulfa antibiotics are as ineffective against colds as any other antibiotic, while echinacea does seem to be at least somewhat helpful. In Germany, echinacea remains the main remedy for minor respiratory infections.

Echinacea is generally thought to work by temporarily stimulating the immune system, although most later evidence has tended to cast doubt on this belief. Contrary to popular belief, however, there is little reason to believe that echinacea strengthens or "nourishes" the immune system when taken over the long term.

There are three main species of echinacea: *E. purpurea*, *E. angustifolia*, and *E. pallida*. A mixture containing all the parts of *E. purpurea* found above ground (flowers, leaves, stems) has the best supporting evidence for effectiveness in treating colds and flu; the root of *E. purpurea* is probably not effective, while the root of *E. pallida* may be the active part of that species.

Echinacea has shown promise for reducing the symptoms and duration of colds and aborting a cold once it has started. However, echinacea does not appear to be helpful for preventing colds. It may also not be effective in children.

Reducing the symptoms and duration of colds. Double-blind, placebo-controlled studies enrolling more than one thousand people have found that various forms and species of echinacea can reduce the symptoms and duration of a common cold. This is true for adults. In one double-blind, placebo-controlled trial, eighty persons with early cold symptoms were given either *E. purpurea* extract or placebo. The results showed that those who were given echinacea recovered significantly more quickly: in just six days among the echinacea group versus nine days among the placebo group.

Another double-blind, placebo-controlled trial looked at the reduction of the severity of cold symptoms. The results in 246 participants showed that treatment with *E. purpurea* significantly improved cold symptoms such as runny nose, sore throat, sneezing, and fatigue. Symptom reduction with *E. purpurea* was also seen in a double-blind, placebo-controlled study of 282 people.

In addition, three double-blind, placebo-controlled studies enrolling about six hundred persons found similar benefits with a combination product containing *E. purpurea* and *E. pallida* root, along with wild indigo and white pine.

While the evidence tends to suggest that the aboveground portion of *E. purpurea* is active against the common cold, two studies have failed to find benefit. One of these was a double-blind, placebo-controlled study enrolling 120 adults, the other an even larger trial (407 participants) involving children. The reason for these negative outcomes is not clear. *E. angustifolia* root has also failed to prove effective in a large study.

Aborting a cold. A double-blind study suggests that echinacea, in addition to making colds shorter and less severe, might also be able to stop a cold that is just starting. In this study, 120 people were given *E. purpurea* or a placebo as soon as they started showing signs of getting a cold.

Participants took either echinacea or placebo at a dosage of twenty drops every two hours for one day, then twenty drops three times a day for a total of up to ten days of treatment. The results were promising. Fewer people in the echinacea group felt that their initial symptoms actually developed into "real" colds (40 percent of those taking echinacea versus 60 percent taking the placebo actually became ill). Also, among those who did come down with "real" colds, improvement in the symptoms started sooner in the echinacea group (four days instead of eight days). Both of these results were statistically significant.

Preventing colds. Several studies have attempted to discover whether the daily use of echinacea can prevent colds from even starting, but the results have not been promising. In one double-blind, placebo-controlled trial, 302 healthy volunteers were given an alcohol tincture containing *E. purpurea* root, *E. angustifolia* root, or placebo for twelve weeks. The results showed that *E. purpurea* was associated with perhaps a 20 percent decrease in the number of people who got sick, and *E. angustifolia* with a 10 percent decrease. However, the difference was not statistically significant. This means that the benefit, if any, was so small that it could have come from chance alone.

Another double-blind, placebo-controlled study enrolled 109 persons with a history of four or more colds during the previous year and gave them either *E. purpurea* juice or placebo for a period of eight weeks. No benefits were seen in the frequency, duration, or severity of colds. Four other studies also failed to find statistically significant preventive effects.

A study often cited as evidence that echinacea can prevent colds actually found no benefit in the 609 participants taken together. Only by looking at subgroups of participants (a statistically questionable procedure) could researchers find any evidence of benefit, and it was still slight.

However, a more recent study using a combination product containing echinacea, propolis, and vitamin C

Common Cold Therapies

- *Pelargonium sidoides.* A typical adult dose of *Pelargonium sidoides* extract is thirty drops three times daily. However, one should follow the instructions on the label for proper dosage.

- *Zinc* (in the form of zinc gluconate or zinc acetate). The official United States dietary recommendations for daily intake of zinc (in milligrams [mg]) are as follows:

  – Infants to age six months (2) and age seven to twelve months (3); children age one to three years (3) and age four to eight years (5); boys age nine to thirteen years (8) and age fourteen years and older (11); girls age nine to thirteen years (8) and age fourteen to eighteen years (9) and women (8); pregnant girls (13) and pregnant women (11); nursing girls (14) and nursing women (12).

  – In studies using zinc to treat the common cold, the doses used were much higher. For example, in one study, participants received 12.8 mg of zinc (42 mg of zinc acetate) every two to three hours while cold symptoms persisted.

- *Echinacea.* Echinacea is usually taken at the first sign of a cold and continued for seven to fourteen days. The three main types of echinacea can be used interchangeably. Depending on the form, dosages are as follows: echinacea powdered extract (300 mg, three times a day), alcohol tincture (1:5) at 3 to 4 milliliters (ml), three times daily; echinacea juice (2 to 3 ml, three times daily); whole dried root (1 to 2 grams, three times daily).

- *Andrographis.* A typical dosage of andrographis is 400 mg three times a day. Doses as high as 2,000 mg three times daily have been used in some studies. Andrographis is usually standardized to its content of andrographolide, typically 4 to 6 percent.

- *Vitamin C.* Vitamin C is available as a single dietary supplement. There is as much controversy about recommended levels as there is about the true health benefits of this vitamin. Many nutritional experts, though, recommend 500 mg of vitamin C daily. This dose is almost undoubtedly safe. The age Upper Limits (ULs) established by the U.S. Food and Nutrition Board are as follows: one to three years (400 mg), four to eight years (650 mg), nine to thirteen years (1,200 mg), fourteen to eighteen years (1,800 mg), age nineteen and older (2,000 mg).

- *Honey.* One should consider taking 1 to 5 tablespoons several times daily. However, infants younger than twelve months of age should not consume honey.

Karen Schroeder, M.S., RD;
reviewed by Brian Randall, M.D.

did find preventive benefits. In this double-blind, placebo-controlled study, 430 children ages one to five years were given either the combination or the placebo for the months during the winter. The results showed a statistically significant reduction in frequency of respiratory infections. It is not clear which of the components of this mixture was responsible for the apparent benefits seen.

Andrographis. Andrographis is a shrub found throughout India and other Asian countries, sometimes called Indian echinacea because it is believed to provide much the same benefits. It has been used historically in epidemics, including the Indian flu epidemic in 1919, during which andrographis was credited with stopping the spread of the disease. It is now popular in Scandinavia as a treatment for colds.

Although it is not known how andrographis might work for colds, some evidence suggests that it might stimulate immunity. The ingredient of andrographis used for standardization purposes, andrographolide, does not appear to affect the immune system as much as the whole plant extract.

According to a few well-designed studies (almost all of which used the proprietary extract produced by a single company), andrographis can reduce the symptoms of colds. It may offer the additional useful benefit of helping to prevent colds.

Reducing cold symptoms. Seven double-blind, placebo-controlled studies enrolling almost one thousand people have found that andrographis (or a combination containing it as the presumed primary ingredient) significantly reduces the duration and severity of cold symptoms.

For example, a four-day, double-blind, placebo-controlled trial of 158 adults with colds found that treatment with a proprietary andrographis extract significantly reduced cold symptoms. Participants were given either placebo or 1,200 mg daily of an andrographis extract standardized to contain 5 percent andrographolide. The results showed that by day two of treatment, and even more by day four, participants given the actual treatment experienced significant improvements in symptoms compared to participants in the placebo group. The greatest response was seen in earache, sleeplessness, nasal drainage, and sore throat, but other cold symptoms improved too.

Three other double-blind, placebo-controlled studies, enrolling about four hundred people, evaluated a proprietary herbal combination treatment containing both andrographis and *Eleutherococcus senticosus* (Russian ginseng) and found benefit. Another study suggests that this combination may be more effective than echinacea. (Somewhat confusingly, this proprietary combination is sold under the same name, Kan Jang, as the pure andrographis product already noted; the manufacturer regards this combination as more effective than andrographis alone, and the combination version of the product has now superseded the previous single-herb version.) The same combination has also shown promise in two double-blind studies for reducing the duration, severity, and rate of complications of influenza.

Andrographis has also been compared to acetaminophen (Tylenol). In a double-blind study of 152 adults with sore throat and fever, participants received andrographis (in doses of 3 or 6 g per day for seven days) or acetaminophen. The higher dose of andrographis (6 g) decreased symptoms of fever and throat pain to about the same extent as acetaminophen, but the lower dose of andrographis (3 g) was not as effective. There were no significant side effects in either group. This study used a different form of andrographis than the proprietary product already noted.

Preventing colds. According to one double-blind, placebo-controlled study, andrographis may increase resistance to colds. A total of 107 students, all eighteen years of age, participated in this three-month trial that used the same proprietary extract of andrographis noted earlier. Fifty-four of the participants took two 100 mg tablets standardized to 5.6 percent andrographolide daily, considerably less than the 1,200 to 6,000 mg per day that has been used in studies on treatment of colds. The other fifty-three students were given placebo tablets with a coating identical to the treatment. Then, once a week throughout the study, a clinician evaluated all the participants for cold symptoms.

By the end of the trial, only sixteen people in the group using andrographis had experienced colds, compared to thirty-three of the placebo-group participants. This difference was statistically significant, indicating that andrographis reduces the risk of catching a cold by a factor of two compared with placebo.

Vitamin C. Vitamin C may mildly reduce symptoms of colds when they occur, but it probably does not help prevent colds.

Treating colds. Numerous studies have found that vitamin C supplements taken at a dose of 1,000 mg or more daily can reduce the severity of cold symptoms and shorten their duration. However, the effect is modest at best. In addition, at least one study suggests that vitamin C can enhance the effect of standard cold treatments, such as acetaminophen. According to most of these studies, using vitamin C throughout the cold season, rather than intermittently, appears to be beneficial. For example, a review of twenty-nine placebo-controlled trials involving almost one thousand episodes of illness concluded that taking a minimum of 2,000 mg per day seems to result in shorter and less severe colds when they occur. However, high doses of vitamin C do not appear to decrease the number of colds experienced during a season.

Many people use vitamin C for colds in a different way: They begin taking it only after cold symptoms first appear. In a review of seven randomized and non-randomized trials, researchers found that this approach–taking high doses of vitamin C (for example, 2,000 to 4,000 mg) at the first sign of illness–does not seem to affect the cold's severity or duration.

Preventing colds. Although some studies suggest that regular use of vitamin C throughout the cold season can help prevent colds, most other studies have found little to no benefit along these lines. Vitamin C has shown a bit more promise for prevention of one type of cold, the so-called postmarathon sniffle. These are colds that develop after endurance exercise; the use of vitamin C before and during competition may help keep a person cold-free afterward. In addition, vitamin C seems to help prevent respiratory infections among persons who are actually deficient in the vitamin.

Essential oils. Eucalyptus is a standard ingredient in cough drops and in oils meant to be added to humidifiers. A standardized combination of three essential oils has been tested for its usefulness in respiratory conditions. The studied combination, called essential oil monoterpenes, includes cineole from eucalyptus, d-limonene from citrus fruit, and alpha-pinene from pine. Numerous double-blind trials have found them effective when taken orally for acute bronchitis, chronic bronchitis, sinus infections, and other respiratory conditions, in both adults and children. Cineole alone at a dose of 200 mg three times daily showed benefit in a double-blind, placebo-controlled study of 152 people with cold symptoms. A second study involving 150 persons also demonstrated favorable results of cineole compared to a combination of five other herbal products.

Ginseng. Although most people in the West think of ginseng as a stimulant, in Eastern Europe ginseng is widely believed to improve overall immunity to illness. As noted, echinacea does not seem to prevent respiratory infections, but it appears that the regular use of ginseng might be able to provide this important benefit.

There are three different herbs commonly called ginseng: Asian or Korean ginseng (*Panax ginseng*), American ginseng (*Panax quinquefolius*), and Siberian ginseng (*Eleutherococcus senticosus*). The latter herb, which is not discussed here, is actually not ginseng.

A double-blind, placebo-controlled study of 323 people found meaningful evidence that an extract of American ginseng taken at 400 mg daily may help prevent the common cold. Participants who used the extract for four months experienced a reduced number of colds compared to those taking placebo. Comparative benefits were also seen regarding the percentage of participants who developed two or more colds and the severity and duration of cold symptoms that did develop. Similar benefits were also seen in a study of forty-three people. Two double-blind, placebo-controlled studies enrolling about one hundred people indicate that American ginseng may also help prevent flulike illness in the elderly.

Garlic. The herb garlic has a long history of use for treating or preventing colds. However, until 2001, there was no scientific evidence that it actually works for this purpose. In one twelve-week, double-blind, placebo-controlled trial, 146 persons received either placebo or a garlic extract between November and February. The results showed that participants receiving garlic were almost two-thirds less likely to catch cold than those receiving placebo. Furthermore, participants who did catch cold recovered about one day faster in the garlic group compared with the placebo group. Note that these studies do not indicate that taking garlic will help once a person already has a cold.

Probiotics. Probiotics are healthful organisms that colonize the digestive tract. Not only can they help prevent intestinal infections, they also appear to help prevent colds.

A seven-month, double-blind, placebo-controlled study of 571 children in day care centers in Finland found that the use of milk fortified with the probiotic bacterium *Lactobacillus* GG modestly reduced the number and severity of respiratory infections. In another controlled trial, probiotics (*L. rhamnosus* GG and *Bifidobacterium lactis* Bb-12) given daily to infants in their formula significantly reduced the risk of acute otitis media and recurrent respiratory infections during the first year of life compared with placebo. Benefits were also seen in three other large studies, in which probiotics, alone or combined with multivitamins-multiminerals, helped prevent colds or reduce their duration and severity in adults.

Another controlled trial involving twenty healthy elite distance runners found that *L. fermentum* given for four months during winter training was significantly more effective at reducing the number and severity of respiratory symptoms than a placebo. In addition, a small double-blind study found evidence that the use of the probiotic bacterium *L. fermentum* improved the effectiveness of the influenza vaccine. The probiotic supplement was taken in two doses: the first two weeks before the vaccine, and the other two weeks after.

OTHER PROPOSED NATURAL TREATMENTS

Various other natural treatments have shown some promise for preventing or treating colds and flu.

Preventing respiratory infections. The use of multivitamin-multimineral supplements, or supplements containing zinc and selenium alone, may help prevent respiratory infections in the elderly, according to some studies. One small double-blind study suggests that the supplement arginine might be helpful for preventing colds in children.

A gargle made from green tea extract has shown promise for preventing influenza. In a double-blind, placebo-controlled study, 124 residents of a Japanese nursing home gargled with green tea catechins or placebo for three months. All participants received standard influenza vaccine. The results showed that those who gargled with the tea extract were less likely to develop influenza than those using placebo. In addition, another double-blind study found preliminary evidence that oral consumption of a green tea extract might help prevent both colds and flu.

There is some evidence that the supplement glutamine may, like vitamin C, help prevent postexercise infections. For example, a double-blind, placebo-controlled study evaluated the benefits of supplemental glutamine (5 g) taken at the end of exercise in 151 endurance athletes. The result showed a significant decrease in infections among those treated. Only 19 percent of the athletes taking glutamine got sick, compared to 51 percent of those on placebo. Echinacea has also shown some promise for this purpose.

In contrast, some evidence suggests that a combination of vitamin E and beta-carotene treatment might increase the risk of exercise-associated colds. The evidence regarding whether vitamin E taken alone can prevent respiratory infections is conflicting.

The thymus gland plays a role in immunity. A one-year, double-blind, placebo-controlled trial of sixteen children with frequent respiratory infections found that treatment with thymus extract could reduce the rate of infection. However, a double-blind, placebo-controlled trial of sixty athletes failed to find any significant evidence of benefit with thymus extract for preventing postexercise infections.

An extract of rice bran has shown some promise for preventing or treating colds in the elderly. Also, a throat spray made from sage has shown considerable promise for reducing sore throat pain. A study widely reported as showing that the supplement colostrum can help prevent colds was actually far too preliminary to prove anything. There is some evidence that elements in kelp might help to prevent infection with several kinds of viruses, including influenza. However, the evidence thus far is more theoretical than practical.

Various herbs, including ashwagandha, astragalus, garlic, maitake, reishi, and suma, are said to enhance immunity over the long term. However, there is no meaningful evidence that they really work. In addition, several herbs, including ginger, kudzu, osha, and yarrow, are said to help avert colds when taken at the first sign of infection; but again, there is no scientific evidence that they are effective.

Products containing colloidal silver are sometimes used in the belief that they will prevent colds and otherwise strengthen the immune system; however, because colloidal silver can cause permanent color changes in the skin, its use is not recommended.

Some older persons do not respond fully to the influenza vaccine. There is some evidence that vitamin E supplements may strengthen the immune response to vaccinations. Similarly, evidence from two double-blind trials, but not a third, suggests that combined multivitamin-multimineral supplements may improve their response. However, in another trial, a multivitamin tablet without minerals actually worsened participants' response to the vaccine.

Two studies suggest that combined multivitamin-multimineral supplements can also improve immune response to the vaccine. However, two others failed to find benefit, and in one study a multivitamin tablet without minerals actually worsened participants' responses to the vaccine. The reason for these discrepancies is unclear. In a double-blind, placebo-controlled study of 124 people, the supplement chlorella at a dose of 200 or 400 mg daily failed to enhance response to influenza vaccine. Another study failed to find benefit with a remedy from the traditional Chinese herbal medicine Hochu-ekki-to.

Treatment of respiratory infections. A standardized product containing elderberry combined with small amounts of echinacea and bee propolis has been widely marketed as a cold and flu remedy. Weak evidence suggests that this mixture may stimulate the immune system and also inhibit viral growth. In a preliminary double-blind study, the combination significantly reduced the recovery time from epidemic influenza B (a relatively mild form of influenza). Another small double-blind study found similar benefits in both influenza A and B.

One small study found that the popular Throat Coat brand of medicinal beverage teas actually does reduce sore throat discomfort, compared with placebo tea. Also, inhaled essential oils have shown some slight promise for the treatment of colds.

The herb *Pelargonium sidoides* is used in Europe for the treatment of colds and other respiratory infections. A double-blind study of 133 adults who had just come down with the common cold found that taking a standardized *Pelargonium* extract at a dose of

30 milliliters three times daily significantly reduced the severity and duration of symptoms compared with placebo.

In double-blind, placebo-controlled studies enrolling more than three hundred people, a combination of four herbs (primrose, gentian root, elderberry, common sorrel, and vervain) has shown promise for treatment of sinusitis. Another study provides weak evidence that a standardized combination of horseradish and nasturtium might be helpful for the treatment of the common cold in children. Other herbs sometimes recommended to reduce cold symptoms, but that lack meaningful supporting scientific evidence, include hyssop, ivy leaf, linden, marshmallow, mistletoe, mullein, oregano, and peppermint.

In a double-blind, placebo-controlled trial, colostrum was not helpful for people with sore throat. (The researchers were sure to exclude people with strep throat, but some participants may have had sore throat caused by bacteria rather than cold viruses.) A substantial (254-participant) double-blind, placebo-controlled study failed to find that the use of the berry of *Hippophae rhamnoides* (sea buckthorn) reduced the number or duration of colds. Finally, a 2009 review of seventeen trials found that there is limited evidence to support the use of traditional Chinese herbal preparations for the common cold.

EBSCO CAM Review Board

FURTHER READING

Cox, A. J., et al. "Oral Administration of the Probiotic *Lactobacillus fermentum* VRI-003 and Mucosal Immunity in Endurance Athletes." *British Journal of Sports Medicine* 44 (2010): 222-226.

Eby, G. A., and W. W. Halcomb. "Ineffectiveness of Zinc Gluconate Nasal Spray and Zinc Orotate Lozenges in Common-Cold Treatment." *Alternative Therapies in Health and Medicine* 12 (2006): 34-38.

Goel, V., et al. "A Proprietary Extract from the Echinacea Plant (*Echinacea purpurea*) Enhances Systemic Immune Response During a Common Cold." *Phytotherapy Research* 19 (2005): 689-694.

Halperin, S. A., et al. "Safety and Immunoenhancing Effect of a Chlorella-Derived Dietary Supplement in Healthy Adults Undergoing Influenza Vaccination." *CMAJ: Canadian Medical Association Journal* 169 (2003): 111-117.

Hemila, H., E. Chalker, and B. Douglas. "Vitamin C for Preventing and Treating the Common Cold." *Cochrane Database of Systematic Reviews* (2010): CD000980. Available through *EBSCO DynaMed Systematic Literature Surveillance* at http://www.ebscohost.com/dynamed.

Hubbert, M., et al. "Efficacy and Tolerability of a Spray with *Salvia officinalis* in the Treatment of Acute Pharyngitis." *European Journal of Medical Research* 11 (2006): 20-26.

Kurugol, Z., N. Bayram, and T. Atik. "Effect of Zinc Sulfate on Common Cold in Children." *Pediatrics International* 49 (2007): 842-847.

Larmo, P., et al. "Effects of Sea Buckthorn Berries on Infections and Inflammation." *European Journal of Clinical Nutrition* 62 (2008): 1123-1130.

Linde, K., et al. "Echinacea for Preventing and Treating the Common Cold." *Cochrane Database of Systematic Reviews* (2006): CD000530. Available through *EBSCO DynaMed Systematic Literature Surveillance* at http://www.ebscohost.com/dynamed.

O'Neil, J., et al. "Effects of Echinacea on the Frequency of Upper Respiratory Tract Symptoms." *Annals of Allergy, Asthma, and Immunology* 100 (2008): 384-388.

Olivares, M., et al. "Oral Intake of *Lactobacillus fermentum* CECT5716 Enhances the Effects of Influenza Vaccination." *Nutrition* 23 (2007): 254-260.

Rautava, S., S. Salminen, and E. Isolauri. "Specific Probiotics in Reducing the Risk of Acute Infections in Infancy." *British Journal of Nutrition* 101 (2009): 1722-1726.

Rowe, C. A., et al. "Specific Formulation of *Camellia sinensis* Prevents Cold and Flu Symptoms and Enhances T Cell Function." *Journal of the American College of Nutrition* 26 (2007): 445-452.

Tesche, S., et al. "The Value of Herbal Medicines in the Treatment of Acute Non-purulent Rhinosinusitis." *European Archives of Oto-Rhino-Laryngology* 265 (2008): 1355-1359.

Zhang, X., et al. "Chinese Medicinal Herbs for the Common Cold." *Cochrane Database of Systematic Reviews* (2007): CD004782. Available through *EBSCO DynaMed Systematic Literature Surveillance* at http://www.ebscohost.com/dynamed.

See also: Andrographis; Bronchitis; Common cold: Homeopathic remedies; Echinacea; Essential oil monoterpenes; Eucalyptus; Garlic; Ginseng; Horseradish; Immune support; Influenza: Homeopathic remedies; Influenza vaccine; Probiotics; Vitamin C; Zinc.

Coleus forskohlii

CATEGORY: Herbs and supplements
DEFINITION: Natural plant product used to treat specific health conditions.
PRINCIPAL PROPOSED USES: Allergies, asthma, bladder infections (for pain relief), eczema, glaucoma, hypertension, irritable bowel syndrome, menstrual cramps, weight loss
OTHER PROPOSED USE: Psoriasis

OVERVIEW

A member of the mint family, *Coleus forskohlii* grows wild on the mountain slopes of Nepal, India, and Thailand. In traditional Asian systems of medicine, it was used for a variety of purposes, including treating skin rashes, asthma, bronchitis, insomnia, epilepsy, and angina. However, modern interest is based almost entirely on the work of a drug company, Hoechst Pharmaceuticals.

Like other drug manufacturers, Hoechst regularly screens medicinal plants in hopes of discovering new medications. In 1974, work performed in collaboration with the Indian Central Drug Research Institute found that the rootstock of *Coleus forskohlii* could lower blood pressure and decrease muscle spasms. Intensive study identified a substance named forskolin that appeared to be responsible for much of this effect.

Like certain drugs used for asthma, forskolin increases the levels of a fundamental natural compound known as cyclic AMP. Cyclic AMP plays a major role in many cellular functions, and some drugs that affect it relax the muscles around the bronchial tubes.

THERAPEUTIC DOSAGES

A common dosage recommendation is 50 milligrams (mg) two or three times a day of an extract standardized to contain 18 percent forskolin. However, because such an extract provides significant levels of forskolin, a drug with wide-ranging properties, experts recommend that *Coleus forskohlii* extracts be taken only with a doctor's supervision.

THERAPEUTIC USES

The scientific evidence for the herb *Coleus forskohlii* as a treatment for any disease is weak. What is known relates to the substance forskolin rather than to the whole herb.

Two preliminary controlled studies have found that oral forskolin may be beneficial for treatment of asthma. Forskolin may work by stabilizing the cells that release histamine and other inflammatory compounds, as well as by relaxing smooth muscle tissue.

Based on these apparent effects, *Coleus forskohlii* has been suggested as a useful treatment for eczema and other allergic conditions, dysmenorrhea (menstrual cramps), angina, irritable bowel syndrome (spastic colon), crampy bladder pain (as in bladder infections), and hypertension (high blood pressure). However, there is no direct evidence that it works.

One small double-blind study indicates that a concentrated forskolin extract might increase the rate of fat burning, thereby potentially enhancing weight loss. In addition, forskolin eyedrops have shown promise in improving glaucoma. *Coleus forskohlii* has also been proposed as a treatment for psoriasis, because that disease appears to be at least partly related to low levels of cyclic AMP in skin cells.

SAFETY ISSUES

The safety of *Coleus forskohlii* and forskolin has not been fully evaluated, although few significant risks have been noted in studies done so far. Caution should be exercised when combining this herb with blood pressure medications and blood thinners.

In 2005, several cases of acute poisoning were reported in Italy, apparently caused by accidental contamination of *Coleus forskohlii* products with similar-appearing plants in the deadly nightshade family. Safety in young children, pregnant or nursing women, and those with severe liver or kidney disease has not been established.

IMPORTANT INTERACTIONS

Those taking blood pressure medications such as beta-blockers, clonidine, or hydralazine or blood-thinning drugs such as warfarin (Coumadin), heparin, clopidogrel (Plavix), ticlopidine (Ticlid), or pentoxifylline (Trental) should use *Coleus forskohlii* only under the supervision of a physician.

EBSCO CAM Review Board

FURTHER READING

Godard, M. P., et al. "Body Composition and Hormonal Adaptations Associated with Forskolin Consumption in Overweight and Obese Men." *Obesity Research* 13 (2005): 1335-1343.
Gonzalez-Sanchez, R., et al. "Forskolin Versus Sodium

Cromoglycate for Prevention of Asthma Attacks." *Journal of Internal Medicine Research* 34 (2006): 200-207.

See also: Allergies; Asthma; Herbal medicine.

Colic

CATEGORY: Condition
RELATED TERM: Infantile colic
DEFINITION: Treatment of excessive and frequently inconsolable crying by an infant.
PRINCIPAL PROPOSED NATURAL TREATMENTS: Behavioral methods, dietary changes, fennel seed oil
OTHER PROPOSED NATURAL TREATMENTS: Acupuncture, chiropractic spinal manipulation, herbal combinations, prebiotics, rooibos (red tea)

INTRODUCTION

The mere thought of a colicky baby is often enough to strike fear in the heart of the parents of a newborn child. A baby with colic may cry for hours despite the parents' attempts at consolation; although the colicky phase will eventually end, it may seem like an eternity while it continues.

Colic is generally defined as excessive (frequently inconsolable) crying that lasts for more than three hours at least three days per week, continuing for at least three weeks; additionally, there must be no medical problem causing the crying. Other symptoms frequently associated with colic include pulling the knees up toward the stomach, a hard or swollen stomach (or both), and excessive gas. Crying occurs most often in the evening. Colic typically ends by the age of four to five months.

Colicky babies may be at an increased risk of abuse at the hands of exhausted and frustrated parents. Additionally, the parent may not properly bond with the child because of feelings of inadequacy and anger, leading to developing behavioral problems as the child grows.

No one knows for sure what causes colic, although there are many theories. One view attributes it to painful digestive cramps or excessive gas (or both) caused by an allergic reaction to foods (such as milk). Another theory suggests that some babies may simply have a sensitive temperament, possibly compounded

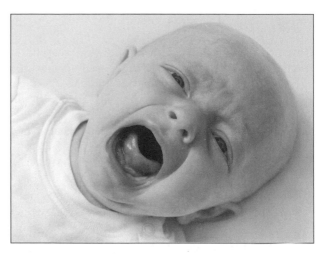

Excessive (usually inconsolable) crying is a symptom of colic. (©Lauriey/Dreamstime.com)

by a parental inability to respond to the infant's needs. Finally, colic may simply be an extreme version of normal infant crying or an increased perception of normal crying by parents with less tolerance for it.

The antispasmodic and sedating drugs dicyclomine and dicycloverine appear to be effective for colic, but they can have dangerous side effects in infants and are not recommended. The gas-relieving drug dimethicone is also sometimes recommended, but evidence suggests that it does not work.

PRINCIPAL PROPOSED NATURAL TREATMENTS

A number of natural approaches to colic have preliminary supporting evidence.

Fennel seed oil. In a double-blind, placebo-controlled study, 125 infants with colic were given either placebo or fennel seed oil at a dose of 12 milligrams (mg) daily per kilogram of body weight. The results were promising. About 40 percent of the infants receiving fennel showed relief of colic symptoms, compared to only 14 percent in the placebo group, a significant difference. Another way to look at the results involves hours of inconsolable crying. In the treated group, infants cried about nine hours per week, compared to twelve hours in the placebo group.

While these are encouraging results, confirmation by an independent research group is necessary before the treatment can be accepted as effective. Furthermore, the safety of fennel seed oil for infants has not been conclusively established.

Dietary changes. Cow's milk can cause allergic reactions. Most infant formula contains cow's milk and can cause reactions in allergic babies. There is also some evidence that breast-fed infants may have allergic responses to cow's milk proteins in the mother's diet.

Numerous small, open, and double-blind studies have evaluated the effects of cow's milk or cow's milk protein in the diet of infants with colic. Most of these studies found an improvement in crying when cow's milk protein was removed from the diet of formula-fed infants or from the diet of the mothers in breast-fed infants.

As an alternative to standard cow's-milk-based formula, researchers primarily used hypoallergenic formula made from hydrolyzed (processed) whey or casein. Formula based on these sources of protein may be superior to those based on soy, because soy itself can cause allergic reactions in sensitive children.

If no improvement is seen through eliminating cow's milk, some experts recommend searching in the breast-feeding mother's diet for other potential food allergens, such as wheat, soy, or eggs. However, it is important to keep nutritional needs in mind: The nursing mother who eliminates certain foods also needs to maintain an adequate intake of calcium, protein, and other nutrients.

It should be noted that most infants with colic are able to tolerate cow's milk protein as they get older. Researchers propose that this early intolerance might be the result of an immature digestive system; according to this theory, the maturation of the digestive tract is the reason that colic usually disappears on its own in time.

Milk also contains lactose, a form of sugar that many adults cannot digest. However, reducing the lactose content of infant formula has not been found helpful in treating colic.

Behavioral methods. Many doctors believe that the cause of colic is not physical but rather results from an infant's oversensitivity to stimuli in the environment. Overanxious parents might contribute to the problem by adding more stimulation in an attempt to calm their child. Other parents might under-react in the belief that paying too much attention to the infant's cries will "spoil" him or her. Either response could set up a cycle leading to long periods of inconsolable crying.

Based on these theories, some authorities recommend counseling the parents of a colicky infant on appropriate coping strategies, including building a personal support system and occasionally leaving the child with a different caregiver to provide a respite. Also, studies evaluating the effects of increased carrying of a colicky child, or of using a motion-simulation device, have not found benefit.

OTHER PROPOSED NATURAL TREATMENTS

A one-week, double-blind, placebo-controlled study of ninety-three breast-fed colicky infants found benefits with a standardized extract of fennel, lemon balm, and chamomile. Another double-blind, placebo-controlled study found benefits with a combination of chamomile, vervain, licorice, fennel, and lemon balm. However, the safety of these herbal combinations in infants has not been established.

A mixture of hydrolyzed whey protein and prebiotics has shown some promise for reducing colic symptoms. Also, a controlled study found that the use of a special type of bottle for bottle feeding reduced colic symptoms.

Chiropractic spinal manipulation has also been tried for colic. One controlled study compared chiropractic treatments with the drug dimethicone. Fifty infants were randomly assigned one of the treatments for two weeks. By the sixth day of treatment, the spinal manipulation group cried significantly less than those on dimethicone. Whether this was a specific effect of the manipulation or a general response to attention and touch is difficult to determine. In one small study, light needling at one acupuncture point on both hands was more effective than no needling among forty infants with colic.

In Great Britain, a preparation called gripe water is widely sold for the treatment of colic. Varying formulations exist, but all include aromatic oils such as dill, spearmint, or caraway combined with alcohol, sucrose (sugar), and sodium bicarbonate. There is no scientific evidence to show whether or not gripe water works. It should be noted that at the recommended dosage, the infant would receive the equivalent of five shots of whiskey. (This would be enough to calm anyone.)

Other herbs sometimes recommended for colic include cardamom, angelica, peppermint, lemon balm, rooibos (red tea) and yarrow. However, no scientific evidence supports their use. The use of salt substitutes containing potassium has also been recommended, but they can be dangerous.

EBSCO CAM Review Board

FURTHER READING

Alexandrovich, I., et al. "The Effect of Fennel (*Foeniculum vulgare*) Seed Oil Emulsion in Infantile Colic." *Alternative Therapies in Health and Medicine* 9 (2003): 58-61.

Cirgin Ellett, M. L., and S. M. Perkins. "Examination of the Effect of Dr. Brown's Natural Flow Baby Bottles on Infant Colic." *Gastroenterology Nursing* 29 (2006): 226-231

Reinthal, M., et al. "Effects of Minimal Acupuncture in Children with Infantile Colic." *Acupuncture in Medicine* 26 (2008): 171-182.

Savino, F., and F. Cresi et al. "A Randomized Double-Blind Placebo-Controlled Trial of a Standardized Extract of *Matricariae recutita, Foeniculum vulgare,* and *Melissa officinalis* (Colimil) in the Treatment of Breast-Fed Colicky Infants." *Phytotherapy Research* 19 (2005): 335-340.

Savino, F., and E. Palumeri et al. "Reduction of Crying Episodes Owing to Infantile Colic: A Randomized Controlled Study on the Efficacy of a New Infant Formula." *European Journal of Clinical Nutrition* 60 (2006): 1304-1310.

Swadling, C., and P. Griffiths. "Is Modified Cow's Milk Formula Effective in Reducing Symptoms of Infant Colic?" *British Journal of Community Nursing* 8 (2003): 24-27.

See also: Acupuncture; Breast-feeding support; Children's health; Fennel; Lactose intolerance; Nondairy milk.

Color therapy

CATEGORY: Therapies and techniques

RELATED TERMS: Chromotherapy, colored light therapy, colorology, gemstone healing

DEFINITION: An energy therapy based on the use of colored light, the choice of colors in one's personal environment, or Ayurvedic chakra theory.

PRINCIPAL PROPOSED USES: Energy balance (physical or spiritual), relief of anxiety or depression, personality analysis

OTHER PROPOSED USES: Treatment of asthma, stress-related disorders, insomnia, and disorders of the immune system

OVERVIEW

The effects of color on human mood have been known for centuries. Prehistoric cave art dated to 90,000 B.C.E. reflects the use of color for this purpose. Colors have symbolic value in many human societies, although the specific associations vary from culture to culture.

Ancient Egyptian and Hindu medical texts mention the use of different colors on the walls of sickrooms to treat various illnesses. In the eleventh century, the Persian physician Avicenna maintained that disease symptoms are associated with different colors. For example, he thought that blue should be used to reduce fever, red to stimulate blood flow, and yellow to relieve muscular pain and inflammation.

In 1671, Sir Isaac Newton demonstrated that white light can be broken into the colors of the visible spectrum when that light is passed through a prism. In 1810, the German writer Johann Wolfgang von Goethe published a book on color theory that dealt with human perception of color, as distinct from its electromagnetic spectrum as analyzed by Newton. Goethe was followed in the twentieth century by researchers interested in the psychological effects of color on humans and the possibility of using color preferences to gain insight into personality structure. The best-known psychological color test is the Lüscher test, invented by the Swiss psychotherapist Max Lüscher. According to Lüscher, a preference for blue indicates contentment; green, self-respect; red, self-confidence; and yellow, an interest in self-development. A newer test, the Manchester Color Wheel, was developed by a group of British psychologists in 2010 as a way to predict responses to various psychotherapies and to detect mood disorders.

MECHANISM OF ACTION

Human perception of color results from the activity of photoreceptor cells known as cones in the retina of the eye. There are three different types of cone cells, which respond to blue (short), green (medium), and red-yellow (long) light waves, respectively. Practitioners of color therapy maintain that the differences in wavelength of the colors in the visible light spectrum (from 390 nanometers for blue-violet to 720 nanometers for red) can be utilized to stimulate or slow down various bodily functions, regulate the secretions of the endocrine glands, affect the brain and central nervous system, and diagnose

Psychological and Physiological Effects of Color

In his book Psychology of Color *(1921), Jesse Charles Fremont Grumbine explains his theory of the impact of color on human psychology.*

Magnetic colors [such] as the reds are thermal and stimulating, the electrical colors, [such] as the blues, are chemical and cooling, and in cases of headache, insanity, fever, the blues and violets should be used, while in cases of tuberculosis, paralysis, melancholia, loneliness, debility, the reds and purples should be employed.

From a purely psychological standpoint, along lines of psychotherapy, red and pinks excite hope, inspire optimism and so neutralize the results or reactions of fear, distrust, despair, while the blues and violets increase a fondness for books, stimulate a love of intellectual, scientific and spiritual pursuits, and so neutralize the results of materialism in all of its forms.

and treat energy imbalances in a person's body, mind, or spirit.

Those who follow the chakra theory of Ayurvedic medicine maintain that each of the seven chakras (energy centers) in the body is associated with a specific color, from red for the chakra at the base of the spine to violet for the crown chakra on the head. Application of light, cloths, crystals, gemstones, or water of the appropriate color to the affected chakra is thought to rebalance the energy centers. This type of color therapy is generally considered pseudoscience.

USES AND APPLICATIONS

It is important to distinguish color therapy, particularly colored-light therapy, from the phototherapy used to treat seasonal affective disorder or such skin diseases as psoriasis or eczema. Mainstream phototherapy makes use of white full-spectrum light or light in the invisible (infrared or ultraviolet) range, whereas color therapy is based on a person's perception of color and may involve cloth, tinted water, or other colored objects as well. As noted, alternative color therapy is used to rebalance energy, treat a range of disorders, and offer insight into one's own personality.

SCIENTIFIC EVIDENCE

No scientific evidence exists that colored light or gemstone therapy is effective in treating physical or mental disorders. Although some studies indicate that persons with mood disorders benefit from wearing or surrounding themselves with bright or cheerful colors, such improvement often reflects a placebo effect.

With regard to color-related personality analysis, a number of double-blind studies of the Lüscher color test have been conducted since the 1980s; most concluded that the test has low test-retest reliability, among other shortcomings. The Manchester Color Wheel is still under investigation as a potentially useful clinical tool for evaluating depressed persons. With regard to the use of chromotherapy in neurology, researchers in Russia and the Balkan countries have investigated the effects of colored light on the secretion of neurotransmitters in the brain; results remain inconclusive.

CHOOSING A PRACTITIONER

The International Association of Colour (IAC), based in London and affiliated with the British Holistic Medicine Association, sets standards for practitioners of color therapy. Most practitioners in the United States, however, are not credentialed by the IAC.

SAFETY ISSUES

There are no known negative effects of chromotherapy, provided it is used alongside conventional medicine rather than as a replacement for it.

Rebecca J. Frey, Ph.D.

FURTHER READING

Ashby, Nina. *Simply Color Therapy*. New York: Sterling, 2006. Part of the publisher's Simply series of books on New Age topics, this is a brief and inexpensive introduction to chromotherapy for general readers.

Carruthers, Helen R., et al. "The Manchester Color Wheel: Development of a Novel Way of Identifying Color Choice and Its Validation in Healthy, Anxious, and Depressed Individuals." *BMC Medical Research Methodology* 10 (2010): 12-25. Includes an image of the color wheel and an account of its development and applications.

Chiazzari, Suzy. *The Complete Book of Color*. Boston: Element, 1999. Also for general readers, this book offers a complete overview of the different forms of color therapy. Lavishly illustrated with diagrams of color theory and with photographs.

"Color Therapy." Available at http://www.therapycolor. com. Basic online introduction to the different types of color therapy, history of color therapy, and the psychological associations of different colors.

Greenfield, Brian. "Color Therapy." Available at http://www.holisticonline.com/color/color_ brian_greenfield.htm. A short article by a color therapist who explains what happens during a color therapy session and explains how color therapy is supposed to work.

See also: Aromatherapy; Art therapy; Ayurveda; Crystal healing; Energy medicine; Magnet therapy; Music therapy; Polarity therapy; Traditional healing.

Colostrum

CATEGORY: Herbs and supplements

DEFINITION: Natural substance from a woman's body used as a supplement to treat specific health conditions.

PRINCIPAL PROPOSED USES: Prevention and treatment of infectious diarrhea

OTHER PROPOSED USES: Lichen planus, Sjögren's syndrome, sore throat and other upper respiratory infections, sports supplement, ulcer prevention

OVERVIEW

Colostrum is the fluid that women's breasts produce during the first day or two after giving birth. It gives newborn infants a rich mixture of antibodies and growth factors that help them get a nutritional good start.

Although colostrum has been available since the first mammals walked the earth, it is relatively new as a nutritional supplement. The resurgence of breast-feeding in the 1970s sparked a revival of interest in colostrum for both infants and adults.

However, most commercial colostrum preparations come from cows, not humans. The antibodies a mother cow gives to her calf are designed to fend off bacteria that are dangerous to cows; these may be very different from those that pose risks to humans. Nonetheless, colostrum also contains substances that

might offer general benefits, such as growth factors (which stimulate the growth and development of cells in the digestive tract and perhaps elsewhere) and transfer factor (which may have general immune-activating properties). In addition, some researchers have used a special form of colostrum called hyperimmune colostrum, created by inoculating cows with bacteria and viruses that affect humans. The cow in turn makes antibodies to them and secretes those antibodies into its colostrum. Hyperimmune colostrum has shown considerable promise as an infection-fighting agent.

Hyperimmune colostrum, however, is not available over the counter as a dietary supplement. Non-hyperimmune colostrum might have some value too, but the evidence is much weaker.

REQUIREMENTS AND SOURCES

Breast-feeding is the healthiest way to nourish a newborn, and a woman's colostrum is undoubtedly good for a baby. However, one should not believe claims (by some manufacturers) that most newborns would die without colostrum. Colostrum is good for health, but it is not essential for life. Colostrum is available in capsules that contain its immune proteins in dry form.

THERAPEUTIC DOSAGES

The usual recommended dosage of colostrum is 10 grams (g) daily. In studies of colostrum as a sports supplement for athletes, the much higher dose of 60 g a day was used.

THERAPEUTIC USES

Many, but not all, studies have found that hyperimmune colostrum might be able to help prevent or treat various forms of infectious diarrhea. Colostrum has also shown some promise as a sports supplement, presumably because it contains growth factors, but study results are inconsistent.

For years, people with ulcers were advised to eat a bland diet and drink lots of milk. Although this treatment was eventually found to be ineffective, according to one study in rats and a small human trial, ordinary colostrum (although not milk) might help protect the stomach from damage caused by anti-inflammatory drugs. It has been hypothesized that colostrum's growth factors help stimulate the stomach to regenerate.

Weak evidence suggests that oral hygiene products containing ordinary colostrum might have beneficial effects in a disease of the mouth called lichen planus, as well as in the condition known as Sjogren's syndrome (which also affects the mouth by reducing salivary flow). One study found that colostrinin, a substance extracted from colostrum, might be helpful for Alzheimer's disease.

Ordinary colostrum has been suggested as a treatment for short bowel syndrome (a condition following digestive tract surgery), chemotherapy-induced mouth ulcers, and inflammatory bowel disease (Crohn's disease and ulcerative colitis), but as yet there is no real evidence that it is effective.

A study cited by some colostrum manufacturers as showing that colostrum can prevent or treat upper respiratory infections (such as colds) was actually far too preliminary to do more than hint at benefits. A proper double-blind, placebo-controlled study of 148 adults failed to find colostrum helpful for shortening the duration of sore throat.

SCIENTIFIC EVIDENCE

Infectious diarrhea. Preliminary evidence suggests that hyperimmune colostrum might help prevent or possibly treat infectious diarrhea. For example, a double-blind, placebo-controlled trial of 80 children with rotavirus diarrhea found that hyperimmune colostrum (prepared by immunizing cows with rotavirus) reduced symptoms and shortened recovery time. Similar results were seen in another double-blind trial of about the same size. However, colostrum prepared by immunizing cows with a monkey form of rotavirus was not found effective for treating rotavirus in a double-blind trial of 135 children. The difference between these results may lie in the level and type of antibodies found in the particular colostrums used. Both hyperimmune and normal colostrum have been tried for prevention or treatment of *Cryptosporidium* infection in people with acquired immunodeficiency syndrome, but the evidence that it works is weak at best.

Other studies suggest that hyperimmune colostrum might help prevent infection with *Shigella* and *E. coli* (a common cause of travelers' diarrhea). However, studies have not found it effective for treating the diarrhea resulting from *Shigella* or *E. coli* infection once it takes hold. A study of Bangladeshi children infected with *Helicobacter pylori* (the organism that

causes digestive ulcers) found no benefits with hyperimmune colostrum.

Sports performance. Colostrum contains the growth factor IGF-1, which may help build muscle, and on this basis colostrum has been proposed as a sports supplement. However, results are conflicting on whether it really works.

In a double-blind, placebo-controlled study, use of colostrum over an eight-week training period did not improve performance on an exercise-to-exhaustion test; however, it did improve performance on a repeat bout twenty minutes later. This suggests potential benefits for enhancing recovery of energy following heavy exercise.

Another eight-week double-blind study found that use of colostrum enhanced sprinting performance, but not endurance exercise, in elite hockey players. Previous double-blind studies found improvements in rowing performance and vertical jump.

A small double-blind study found that colostrum, compared with whey protein, increased lean mass in healthy men and women undergoing aerobic and resistance training. However, no improvements in performance were seen in this trial.

It appears that the IGF-1 in colostrum is not directly absorbed into the body. Nonetheless, consumption of colostrum does appear to increase IGF-1 levels in the blood. The explanation for this is unclear.

SAFETY ISSUES

Colostrum does not seem to cause any significant side effects. However, comprehensive safety studies have not been performed. Safety in young children and in women who are pregnant or nursing has not been established.

EBSCO CAM Review Board

FURTHER READING

Bilikiewicz, A., and W. Gaus. "Colostrinin (A Naturally Occurring, Proline-rich, Polypeptide Mixture) in the Treatment of Alzheimer's Disease." *Journal of Alzheimer's Disease* 6 (2004): 17-26.

Brinkworth, G. D., et al. "Oral Bovine Colostrum Supplementation Enhances Buffer Capacity but Not Rowing Performance in Elite Female Rowers." *International Journal of Sport Nutrition and Exercise Metabolism* 12 (2002): 349-365.

Brinkworth, G. D., and J. D. Buckley. "Concentrated Bovine Colostrum Protein Supplementation Reduces the Incidence of Self-reported Symptoms of Upper Respiratory Tract Infection in Adult Males." *European Journal of Nutrition* 42 (2003): 228-232.

Buckley, J. D. "Bovine Colostrum: Does It Improve Athletic Performance?" *Nutrition* 18 (2002): 776-777.

Hofman, Z., et al. "The Effect of Bovine Colostrum Supplementation on Exercise Performance in Elite Field Hockey Players." *International Journal of Sport Nutrition and Exercise Metabolism* 12 (2002): 461-469.

Mero, A., et al. "IGF-I, IgA, and IgG Responses to Bovine Colostrum Supplementation During Training." *Journal of Applied Physiology* 93 (2002): 732-739.

See also: Diarrhea; Herbal medicine; Sports and fitness support: Enhancing performance.

Coltsfoot

CATEGORY: Herbs and supplements
RELATED TERM: *Tussilago farfara*
DEFINITION: Natural plant product used to treat specific health conditions.
PRINCIPAL PROPOSED USES: Not recommended for any purpose

OVERVIEW

The herb coltsfoot has a long history of use in the herbal medicine of Europe and Asia as a treatment for coughs and sore throats. It does not appear that traditional herbalists recognized that this treatment, which they often recommended for use by children, may cause liver damage.

THERAPEUTIC DOSAGES

Horticulturists have developed a form of coltsfoot that does not carry toxic pyrrolizidine alkaloids. Products of this type, when available, should be safer. Nonetheless, because experts do not know if coltsfoot offers any benefit, it is not possible to state an effective dosage.

THERAPEUTIC USES

Germany's Commission E, the scientific body assigned to approving the use of herbal treatments in Germany, once approved coltsfoot for the treatment of sore throat. However, coltsfoot was subsequently

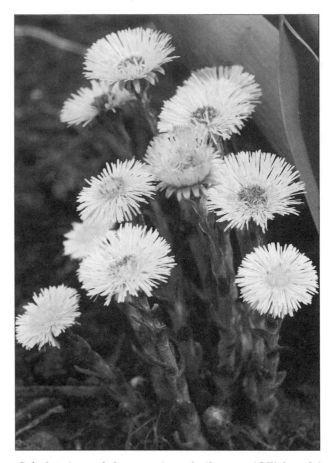

Coltsfoot is used for a variety of ailments. (©Fishrnd/Dreamstime.com)

banned due to its content of potentially liver-toxic substances called pyrrolizidine alkaloids.

Safety aside, there is no meaningful evidence that coltsfoot has any medicinal effects. Only double-blind, placebo-controlled trials can prove a treatment effective, and none have been reported for coltsfoot. Much the same situation prevails for conventional cough syrups, none of which have been proven effective. However, they appear to be safe.

SAFETY ISSUES

The pyrrolizidine alkaloids found in coltsfoot are known to have potential liver-toxic and cancer-promoting effects. One case report indicates that use of a coltsfoot tea in an infant caused severe liver problems that gradually disappeared when the tea was stopped. In another case, an infant developed liver disease and died because the mother drank tea containing coltsfoot during her pregnancy. Similar pyrrolizidine alkaloids are found in the herb comfrey, which has been associated with additional cases of liver injury.

Supporters of herbal therapy have defended the use of coltsfoot on the grounds that it was used for many thousands of years without harm. A flaw exists in this reasoning. Traditional herbalists would be expected to notice immediate, dramatic reactions to herbal formulas, and one can assume with some confidence that treatments used for thousands of years are unlikely to cause such immediate problems in very many people who take them. However, certain types of harm could be expected to elude the detection of traditional herbalists. These include safety problems that are delayed, occur relatively rarely, or are difficult to detect without scientific instruments. How would a traditional herbalist ever know, for example, if a treatment caused liver failure in 1 of 100,000 people who used it, especially if such failure took two or more years to develop? If such a death did occur in the herbalist's patient population, it would probably be attributed to hepatitis or some other common cause. These factors may explain why traditional Chinese herbal medicine uses treatments that are now recognized as dangerous, such as mercury, arsenic, lead, and the kidney toxic herbs in the Aristolochia family.

Coltsfoot appears to fall into the same category. Most people can probably take coltsfoot for a short time and suffer no injury. A few people (especially infants), however, may have greater sensitivity and may suffer harm. Many more people may experience harm if they use coltsfoot for a prolonged period of time. For all these reasons, experts strongly recommend against using coltsfoot.

EBSCO CAM Review Board

Further Reading

Blumenthal M, et al., eds. *The Complete German Commission E Monographs: Therapeutic Guide to Herbal Medicines.* Austin, Tex.: American Botanical Council, 1998.

Schroeder, K., and T. Fahey. "Over-the-Counter Medications for Acute Cough in Children and Adults in Ambulatory Settings." *Cochrane Database of Systematic Reviews* January 23, 2008.

Stickel, F., and H. K. Seitz. "The Efficacy and Safety of Comfrey." *Public Health Nutrition* 3 (2000): 501-508.

Wawrosch, C., B. Kopp, and H. Wiederfield. "Permanent Monitoring of Pyrrolizidine Alkaloid Content in Micropropagated *Tussilago farfara*: A Tool to Fulfill Statutory Demands for the Quality of Coltsfoot in Austria and Germany." *Acta Horticulturae* 530 (2000): 469-472.

See also: Comfrey; Herbal medicine.

Comfrey

Category: Herbs and supplements
Related term: *Symphytum officinale*
Definition: Natural plant product used to treat specific health conditions.
Principal proposed uses: Back pain, sports injures (sprains and strains)
Other proposed uses: Broken bones, bruises, varicose veins, open wounds (not recommended)

Overview

Comfrey is a high-yielding leafy green plant that has been used for centuries as a feed crop for animals and a medicine for humans. However, in 2001, it was removed as an oral dietary supplement from the American market, and soon afterwards, it was removed as a commercial animal food source. These actions were taken because comfrey contains dangerous levels of toxic pyrrolizidine alkaloids, and its use has led to severe liver injury and death.

Traditionally, oral or topical use of comfrey was said to help bones heal more rapidly, and this is the origin of its Latin name *Symphytum* ("drawing together"). It was also used orally for the treatment of digestive and lung problems. Topical comfrey creams have been used to treat minor wounds, bruises, sprains, and varicose veins.

Therapeutic Dosages

The tested form of topical comfrey contains 10 percent of a 2.5:1 juice extract made from fresh pressed plant sap; in other words, every 100 grams (g) of cream contains the equivalent of 25 g of comfrey sap.

Therapeutic Uses

Comfrey is commonly included in salves and creams that also contain such herbs as aloe, goldenseal, calendula, and vitamin E. Such preparations are

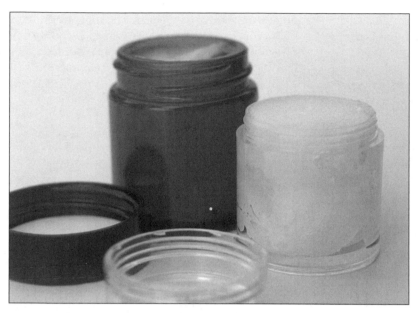

Comfrey ointment. (Tim Winter/Getty Images)

marketed for treatment of minor wounds. However, for safety reasons, comfrey should not be applied to broken skin. Therefore, it should not be used for the treatment of lacerations or abrasions (cuts and scrapes). There is some evidence that topical comfrey might be useful in the treatment of various conditions involving pain in the joints or muscles where skin is unbroken. Safety, however, does remain a concern.

In a double-blind, placebo-controlled study of 142 people with acute ankle sprain, use of comfrey cream for eight days significantly enhanced rate of recovery. Comfrey proved more effective than a placebo in measurements of pain, swelling, and mobility. More modest benefits were seen in another double-blind trial, this one enrolling 203 people with ankle sprain and comparing a high-comfrey product to a low-comfrey product.

Another double-blind, placebo-controlled study, this one enrolling 215 people, found comfrey cream helpful for treatment of back pain. Finally, in a three-week double-blind study of 220 people with osteoarthritis of the knee, comfrey cream reduced symptoms significantly more than a placebo cream.

In a recent, well-designed trial, two concentrations of comfrey creams were evaluated for the treatment of fresh abrasions among 278 patients (almost one-quarter of whom were under age twenty). The higher-concentration cream (10 percent) contained ten times more comfrey than the low-concentration cream (considered the reference or placebo cream). The 10 percent comfrey cream led to significantly faster wound healing than the reference cream after two to three days of application. Although the researchers reported no adverse effects in either group, the use of comfrey has been associated with severe and even life-threatening, toxic effects when used orally, and its use over open wounds should be undertaken with extreme caution.

Additional studies, generally of lower quality, suggest possible benefit for shoulder tendonitis and knee injuries. The active ingredients in comfrey are not known but may include rosmaric acid, choline, and allantoin.

SAFETY ISSUES

As noted above, comfrey contains substances called pyrrolizidine alkaloids that are both toxic to the liver and carcinogenic. The main form of liver disease seen with comfrey is a blockage of small veins that can lead to liver cirrhosis and eventually liver failure (hepato-occlusive disease). Liver transplantation may be required. Oral use of comfrey for as brief a time as five to seven days in a child and nineteen to forty-five days in adults has resulted in severe liver disease and death. Long-term use of very low dosages may also cause harm.

In general, the root of the plant contains more pyrrolizidine alkaloids than the leaves. Related species of comfrey such as *S. uplandicum* and *S. asperum* contain even higher levels of these toxins and may be mistakenly sold as ordinary comfrey.

Pyrrolizidine alkaloids in comfrey can be absorbed through the skin. For this reason, it has been recommended that when using comfrey preparations, the daily amount of pyrrolizidine alkaloids should not exceed 100 micrograms (mcg). Few products are labeled to indicate their pyrrolizidine alkaloid content. Furthermore, the common analytic methods used for testing pyrrolizidine alkaloid content may fail to measure a certain chemical form of these toxins (the

N-oxide form), leading to results that are too low by a factor of ten or more. For all these reasons, it may be prudent to avoid topical comfrey products entirely. If comfrey is used as a topical treatment, experts recommend that it not be applied for more than four to six weeks per year or more than ten days in a row and that it never be applied on broken skin. In addition, comfrey should not be used by children, pregnant or nursing women, or people with liver disease.

EBSCO CAM Review Board

FURTHER READING

Barna, M., et al. "Wound Healing Effects of a *Symphytum* Herb Extract Cream." *Wiener Medenzinische Wochenschrift* 157 (2007): 569-574.

Grube, B., et al. "Efficacy of a Comfrey Root (*Symphyti offic. radix*) Extract Ointment in the Treatment of Patients with Painful Osteoarthritis of the Knee." *Phytomedicine* 14, no. 1 (2007): 2-10.

Koll, R., et al. "Efficacy and Tolerance of a Comfrey Root Extract (*Extr. Rad. Symphyti*) in the Treatment of Ankle Distorsions." *Phytomedicine* 11 (2004): 470-477.

Kucera, M., et al. "Topical Symphytum Herb Concentrate Cream Against Myalgia." *Advances in Therapy* 22 (2005): 681-692.

Oberlies, N. H., et al. "Analysis of Herbal Teas Made from the Leaves of Comfrey (*Symphytum officinale*): Reduction of N-oxides Results in Order of Magnitude Increases in the Measurable Concentration of Pyrrolizidine Alkaloids." *Public Health Nutrition* 7 (2004): 919-924.

Stickel, F., and H. K. Seitz. "The Efficacy and Safety of Comfrey." *Public Health Nutrition* 3 (2000): 501-508.

See also: Aloe; Calendula; Coltsfoot; Goldenseal; Herbal medicine; Vitamin E; Wounds, minor.

Common cold: Homeopathic remedies

CATEGORY: Homeopathy

DEFINITION: The use of highly diluted remedies to treat a common viral infection of the upper respiratory system.

STUDIED HOMEOPATHIC REMEDIES: *Eupatorium perfo-*

liatum; Euphrasia; homeopathic cough syrup (*Drosera, Arnica,* belladonna, *Artemisia cina, Cuprum, Ferrosi phosphas, Uragoga ipecacuanha, Solidago*); homeopathic remedy containing *Aconitum, Bryonia, Lachesis, Eupatorium,* and phosphorus; individualized (classical) homeopathy; *Phytolacca*

INTRODUCTION

The common cold is an infection caused by one of hundreds of related viruses, causing symptoms of sore throat, sneezing, headache, congestion, runny nose, and fatigue. These symptoms are self-limited, meaning that they will go away on their own. The onset of symptoms of a common cold is often sudden, and the cold tends to resolve in four days to two weeks.

A severe sore throat can be caused by the bacterium *Streptococcus.* Strep throat, as it is commonly called, can cause heart damage. Antibiotic treatment is necessary to prevent this complication.

SCIENTIFIC EVALUATIONS OF HOMEOPATHIC REMEDIES

Weak evidence suggests that homeopathic remedies might have a place in the treatment of colds. However, the best-designed studies (including one that evaluated classical homeopathy) failed to find evidence of benefit.

The homeopathic remedy *Phytolacca* was tested in two double-blind, placebo-controlled trials to evaluate its potential benefit for sore throat symptoms caused by colds. In these studies, involving about three hundred people, the remedy appeared to reduce the duration of symptoms. However, these studies had several weaknesses in design, making the results unreliable.

A small double-blind, placebo-controlled trial of sixty adults and children found positive results with a homeopathic cough syrup as a treatment for a dry cough. The syrup contained *Drosera, Arnica,* belladonna, *Artemisia cina, Cossus cacti, Corallium rubrum, Cuprum Ferrosi phosphas, Uragoga ipecacuanha,* and *Solidago.*

A study of fifty-three persons compared the homeopathic remedy *Eupatorium perfoliatum* D2 with aspirin as a treatment for the common cold and found them equally effective. However, this was not a double-blind study; furthermore, aspirin itself has not been shown effective for the common cold.

A double-blind study compared aspirin with a combination homeopathic medicine that included *Aconitum, Bryonia, Lachesis, Eupatorium,* and phosphorus.

Again, the treatment proved to be as effective (or as ineffective) as aspirin, but in the absence of a placebo group, the results are difficult to interpret.

A well-designed, double-blind, placebo-controlled study enrolling 170 children with recurrent colds found no benefit with classical homeopathic treatment. All participants were evaluated by trained homeopathic practitioners and were prescribed remedies, but only about one-half of the participants received the remedy; the others received placebo treatment. The results failed to show any benefit with classical homeopathy versus placebo.

A double-blind, placebo-controlled study involving 994 children (age four to fifteen years) evaluated treatment with *Euphrasia* 30c (centesimal) dilution for the prevention of conjunctivitis (essentially, a cold in the eye). The investigators chose this remedy because it is frequently self-prescribed by people with conjunctivitis and often recommended by practitioners outside traditional medicine. However, no benefits were seen.

In a twelve-week double-blind study, 251 children were given either placebo or one of three homeopathic remedies selected according to a standard Norwegian, simplified, constitutional, homeopathic protocol. The homeopathic remedies failed to prove more effective than placebo.

TRADITIONAL HOMEOPATHIC TREATMENTS

Classical homeopathy offers many possible homeopathic treatments for the common cold, all of which are chosen based on various specific details of the person seeking treatment. For example, persons who are restless and who experience deep aches in addition to other cold symptoms will fit the symptom picture for *Eupatorium*. For this use, the remedy is generally recommended in a potency between 6c and 30c, which is a significantly more dilute dosage than the 2x potency used for some conditions. Persons who have primarily a sore throat and swollen tonsils (relieved by cold drinks but not hot drinks), accompanied by shooting pain in the ears, aching joints, muscle soreness, restlessness, and prostration, more closely fit the homeopathic indication for *Phytolacca*.

EBSCO CAM Review Board

FURTHER READING

Mokkapatti, R. "An Experimental Double-Blind Study to Evaluate the Use of Euphrasia in Preventing Conjunctivitis." *British Homeopathic Journal* 81 (1992): 22-24.

Ramchandani, N. M. "Homoeopathic Treatment of Upper Respiratory Tract Infections in Children." *Complementary Therapies in Clinical Practice* 16 (2010): 101-108.

Schmiedel, V., and P. Klein. "A Complex Homeopathic Preparation for the Symptomatic Treatment of Upper Respiratory Infections Associated with the Common Cold." *Explore* (New York) 2 (2006): 109-114.

Steinsbekk, A., et al. "Self-Treatment with One of Three Self-Selected, Ultramolecular, Homeopathic Medicines for the Prevention of Upper Respiratory Tract Infections in Children." *British Journal of Clinical Pharmacology* 59 (2005): 447-455.

See also: Colds and flu; Ear infections; Homeopathy; Influenza: Homeopathic remedies.

Compulsive overeating

CATEGORY: Condition

RELATED TERMS: Binge-eating disorder, food addiction, food-related impulse disorder

DEFINITION: A pattern of behavior in which a person routinely ingests large quantities of food beyond the feeling of fullness without the ability to stop.

SIGNS

It is estimated that 4 million American adults are compulsive overeaters.

The behavior is nearly twice as common in women as in men, and it typically begins before the age of twenty years. The primary sign of compulsive overeating is regularly eating large quantities of food uncontrollably without physical hunger. Other food-related behaviors include eating rapidly, eating to the point of physical discomfort, eating alone and secretly, hiding food to eat later, hiding the evidence of eating, stealing other people's food, and eating food that has been discarded or is about to be discarded.

Compulsive overeaters have a preoccupation with food, spending inordinate amounts of time on meal planning, food shopping, and cooking and eating.

They make furtive trips to convenience stores, fast-food restaurants, and late-night grocery stores. They recognize that their eating habits are not normal and feel powerless to stop eating voluntarily. They turn to food for comfort and yet use it as a reward. Their rapid weight gain brings them feelings of guilt, shame, disgust, and self-loathing. They cannot separate their identify from their weight; in weighing themselves, for example, how they feel about themselves is dictated by the number on the scale. They believe that they will be better persons once they are thin, so they try various diets with a sense of desperation. Although weight may be lost initially, it is often regained, plus more.

UNDERLYING CAUSES

Researchers have not conclusively determined the underlying causes of compulsive overeating. Studies have investigated genetic predispositions to food addiction, in which a person's metabolism of foods, such as sugar, wheat, and fats, affects the same areas of the brain affected by other addictive substances, such as cocaine. Other brain studies have examined compulsive overeating as a biochemically based impulse disorder somewhat similar to kleptomania, hypersexuality, compulsive shopping, and gambling addiction. A connection to dopamine in the brain has been shown, as well as hypersensitivity to the pleasurable properties of foods.

Some medical professionals consider compulsive overeating to be a means of self-medicating for clinical depression. In some cases, the resulting rapid weight gain may be a protective mechanism to cope with physical or sexual abuse. The behavior also may serve to numb painful emotions of rejection, abandonment, and low self-esteem. One study showed that compulsive overeaters produce more cortisol in response to stress than do normal eaters; cortisol is known to stimulate the drive to eat, leading to obesity. Chronic stress has an apparent connection to the preference for high-energy foods that contain large amounts of sugar and fat.

NEGATIVE EFFECTS

The unbalanced diet of the compulsive overeater, who typically chooses sweets and starches, has adverse health consequences, such as high serum cholesterol level, high blood pressure, and increased risks for heart attack, stroke, kidney failure, and diabetes. This diet also may result in lethargy, moodiness, irritability, and depression.

In some cases, self-harming may be used to dissociate from emotional pain by substituting physical pain that releases endorphins. Compulsive overeaters who self-harm usually hold themselves to unreasonably high standards, have difficulty expressing their emotions, and are repulsed by their own bodies. The extreme and rapid weight gain contributes to varicose veins, blood clots in the legs, sciatica, arthritis, and bone deterioration. It may also cause shortness of breath and sleep apnea.

TREATMENT

Like alcoholism, compulsive overeating is considered to be a disease in that it involves treatment and recovery and cannot be overcome by willpower alone. However, it is also a behavior that may be managed with behavior modification therapy. A typical initial exercise is to keep a food diary, a written record of the kind and quantity of food eaten, the time and place of eating, and the emotional context. This diary is then analyzed to identify habits, underlying emotions, and foods that trigger uncontrollable eating. The next step usually is to consult a nutritionist to devise a healthy food plan with adequate calories for energy, necessary nutrients, and fiber for improved digestion. A third step is to identify and practice healthy activities–emotional coping mechanisms–that substitute for food; these activities may include exercise, meditation, and spending time with friends.

Persons can seek support from professional counseling or from a twelve-step program such as Overeaters Anonymous. In some cases, drug therapy with antidepressants may be appropriate.

Bethany Thivierge, M.P.H.

FURTHER READING

Academy for Eating Disorders. http://www.aedweb.org.

National Eating Disorders Association. http://www.nationaleatingdisorders.org.

Ross, Carolyn Coker. *The Binge Eating and Compulsive Overeating Workbook: An Integrated Approach to Overcoming Disordered Eating.* Oakland, Calif.: New Harbinger, 2009. With distinct sections on healing the body, mind, and spirit, this book offers a whole-body plan for regaining physical and emotional health.

Sheppard, Kay. *Food Addiction: The Body Knows*. Rev. ed. Deerfield Beach, Fla.: Health Communications, 1993. Written by a certified eating-disorder specialist, this book addresses the addictive influences of the metabolism of flour and sugar, as well as the psychological need for support and self-healing.

See also: Depression, mild to moderate; Eating disorders; Gastroesophageal reflux disease; Gastrointestinal health; Obesity and excessive weight; Obsessive-compulsive disorder; Weight loss, undesired.

Congestive heart failure

CATEGORY: Condition
DEFINITION: Treatment of the weakened pumping ability of the heart.
PRINCIPAL PROPOSED NATURAL TREATMENTS: Coenzyme Q_{10}, hawthorn, vitamin B_1
OTHER PROPOSED NATURAL TREATMENTS: Arginine, creatine, L-carnitine, magnesium, ribose, taurine, Transcendental Meditation, yoga

INTRODUCTION

When the heart sustains injury that weakens its pumping ability, a complicated physiological state called congestive heart failure (CHF) can develop. Fluid builds up in the lungs and lower extremities, the heart enlarges, and many symptoms develop, including severe fatigue, difficulty breathing while lying down, and altered brain function. Medical treatment for this condition is quite effective and sophisticated, consisting of several drugs used in combination.

PRINCIPAL PROPOSED NATURAL TREATMENTS

CHF is too serious a condition for self-treatment. The supervision of a qualified health-care professional is essential. However, given medical supervision, some of the following treatments may be quite useful.

The herb hawthorn appears to be effective for mild CHF and also may be helpful for more severe CHF. However, while standard drugs have been shown to help reduce hospitalizations and mortality associated with CHF, there is no similar evidence for hawthorn. Also, adding the supplement coenzyme Q_{10} to standard treatment may improve results. Finally, the supplement vitamin B_1 (thiamin) may be helpful for persons who take loop diuretics (such as furosemide) for CHF.

Hawthorn. Several double-blind, placebo-controlled trials, involving about 750 participants, have found hawthorn helpful for the treatment of mild to moderate CHF. In one of the best of these studies, 209 people with relatively advanced CHF (technically, New York Heart Association class III) were given either 900 milligrams (mg) or 1,800 mg of standardized hawthorn extract or matching placebo. The results after sixteen weeks of therapy showed significant improvements in the hawthorn groups compared with the placebo groups. Benefits in the high-dose hawthorn group included a reduction in subjective symptoms and an increase in exercise capacity. Subjective symptoms improved to about the same extent in the lower-dose hawthorn group, but there was no improvement in exercise capacity.

In an analysis that mathematically combined the results of ten controlled trials involving 855 persons, hawthorn extract was found to be significantly better than placebo for improving exercise tolerance, decreasing shortness of breath and fatigue, and enhancing the physiologic function of an ailing heart in mild to moderate CHF. In another study, however, researchers found that persons with mild to moderate CHF taking a special extract of hawthorn, 900 mg daily, were more likely to experience an initial worsening of their condition compared to those taking placebo. By the end of six months, however, there was no difference in the two groups. In light of numerous other studies supporting the safety and effectiveness of hawthorn in CHF, the results of this special extract study need to be repeated before drawing any firm conclusions.

A comparative study suggests that hawthorn extract (900 mg) is about as effective as a low dose of the conventional drug captopril. However, while captopril and other standard drugs in the same family have been shown to help reduce hospitalizations and mortality associated with CHF, there is no similar evidence for hawthorn.

Like other treatments used for CHF, hawthorn improves the heart's pumping ability. However, it may offer some important advantages over certain conventional drugs used for this condition.

Digoxin, and other medications that increase the power of the heart, also make the heart more susceptible to dangerous irregularities of rhythm. In

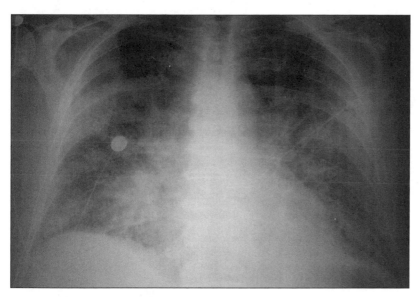

An X ray showing congestive heart failure. (Visuals Unlimited, Inc./Charles McRae, MD/Getty Images)

contrast, preliminary evidence indicates that hawthorn may have the unusual property of both strengthening the heart and stabilizing it against arrhythmias. It is thought to do so by lengthening what is called the refractory period. This term refers to the short period following a heartbeat during which the heart cannot beat again. Many irregularities of heart rhythm begin with an early beat. Digoxin shortens the refractory period, making such a premature beat more likely, while hawthorn seems to protect against such potentially dangerous breaks in the heart's even rhythm.

Another advantage of hawthorn involves toxicity. With digoxin, the difference between the proper dosage and the toxic dosage is dangerously small. Hawthorn has an enormous range of safe dosing.

However, digoxin is itself an outdated drug. There are many newer drugs for CHF (such as angiotensin I-converting enzyme inhibitors) that are much more effective than digoxin. Many of these have been proven to prolong life in people with severe CHF. There is no reliable evidence that hawthorn offers the same benefit (although one large study found hints that it might). Also, it is not clear whether one can safely combine hawthorn with other drugs that affect the heart.

Coenzyme Q_{10}. People with CHF have significantly lower levels of coenzyme Q_{10} (CoQ_{10}) in heart muscle cells than healthy people. This fact alone does not prove that CoQ_{10} supplements will help CHF; however, it prompted medical researchers to try using this supplement as a treatment for heart failure.

In the largest study, 641 people with moderate to severe CHF were monitored for one year. One-half were given 2 mg per kilogram of body weight of CoQ_{10} daily; the rest were given placebo. Standard therapy was continued in both groups. The participants treated with CoQ_{10} experienced a significant reduction in the severity of their symptoms. No such improvement was seen in the placebo group. The people who took CoQ_{10} also had significantly fewer hospitalizations for heart failure. Similarly positive results were also seen in other double-blind studies involving a total of more than 270 participants. However, two later and very well-designed double-blind studies enrolling about eighty-five persons with CHF failed to find any evidence of benefit. The reason for this discrepancy is not clear.

Vitamin B_1. Evidence suggests that the strong diuretics (technically, "loop diuretics," such as furosemide) commonly used to treat CHF may interfere with the body's metabolism of vitamin B_1 (thiamin). Because the heart depends on vitamin B_1 for proper function, this finding suggests that taking a supplement may be advisable; preliminary evidence suggests that thiamin supplementation may indeed improve heart function in persons with CHF.

OTHER PROPOSED NATURAL TREATMENTS

A large Italian trial involving almost seven thousand persons found that fish oil may modestly reduce the risk of death or admission to the hospital for cardiovascular reasons in persons with CHF. Several studies (primarily by one research group) suggest that the amino acid taurine may be useful in CHF and could be more effective than CoQ_{10}.

Another treatment for CHF that has some evidence is the supplement L-carnitine, especially when given in the special form called propionyl-L-carnitine. Carnitine is frequently combined with CoQ_{10}. Three small double-blind studies enrolling about seventy persons with CHF found that the supplement arginine significantly improved symptoms of CHF and improved objective measurements of heart function.

Evidence suggests that the sports supplement creatine may offer some help for the sensation of fatigue that often accompanies CHF. One small double-blind study found preliminary evidence that the supplement ribose may improve CHF symptoms.

Combination therapy with several of the supplements mentioned here may also be helpful. A double-blind trial of forty-one persons found that the use of a supplement containing taurine, CoQ_{10}, creatine, and carnitine, along with other nutrients, improved objective measures of heart function. Also, a study performed in China reported that berberine (a constituent of various herbs, including goldenseal and Oregon grape) can decrease mortality and increase quality of life in CHF.

There is some evidence that supplementing with magnesium may be helpful for persons taking both digoxin and diuretics; diuretics can deplete the body of magnesium, and this, in turn, may increase the risk of digoxin side effects. One study found that the use of magnesium (as magnesium orotate) may improve exercise capacity and reduce heart arrhythmias in people with CHF who have just undergone bypass graft surgery. Additionally, in a well-designed trial involving seventy-nine persons with severe CHF, magnesium orotate significantly improved survival and clinical symptoms after one year compared with placebo.

Weak evidence suggests that relaxation therapy (specifically Transcendental Meditation), Tai Chi, and yoga may improve functional capacity and quality of life in people with CHF. Also, vitamin E has been proposed as a treatment for CHF, but a small double-blind study did not find it effective.

HERBS AND SUPPLEMENTS TO USE ONLY WITH CAUTION

One study found hints that supplementation with vitamin C at a dose of 4 grams daily might worsen muscle function in people with CHF. Various other herbs and supplements may interact adversely with drugs used to treat CHF.

EBSCO CAM Review Board

FURTHER READING

Belardinelli, R., et al. "Coenzyme Q10 and Exercise Training in Chronic Heart Failure." *European Heart Journal* 27 (2006): 2675-2681.

GISSI-HF Investigators et al. "Effect of N-3 Polyunsaturated Fatty Acids in Patients with Chronic Heart Failure (The GISSI-HF Trial)." *The Lancet* 372 (2008): 1223-1230.

Jayadevappa, R., et al. "Effectiveness of Transcendental Meditation on Functional Capacity and Quality of Life of African Americans with Congestive Heart Failure." *Ethnicity and Disease* 17 (2007): 72-77.

Keith, M. E., et al. "A Controlled Clinical Trial of Vitamin E Supplementation in Patients with Congestive Heart Failure." *American Journal of Clinical Nutrition* 73 (2001): 219-224.

Nightingale, A. K., et al. "Chronic Oral Ascorbic Acid Therapy Worsens Skclctal Muscle Metabolism in Patients with Chronic Heart Failure." *European Journal of Heart Failure* 9 (2007): 287-291.

Omran, H., et al. "D-Ribose Improves Diastolic Function and Quality of Life in Congestive Heart Failure Patients." *European Journal of Heart Failure* 5 (2003): 615-619.

Pittler, M., R. Guo, and E. Ernst. "Hawthorn Extract for Treating Chronic Heart Failure." *Cochrane Database of Systematic Reviews* (2008): CD005312. Available through *EBSCO DynaMed Systematic Literature Surveillance* at http://www.ebscohost.com/dynamed.

Pullen, P. R., et al. "Effects of Yoga on Inflammation and Exercise Capacity in Patients with Chronic Heart Failure." *Journal of Cardiac Failure* 14 (2008): 407-413.

Stepura, O. B., and A. I. Martynow. "Magnesium Orotate in Severe Congestive Heart Failure (MACH)." *International Journal of Cardiology* 134 (2008): 145-147.

Yeh, G. Y., P. M. Wayne, R. S. Phillips. "Tai Chi Exercise in Patients with Chronic Heart Failure." *Medicine and Sport Science* 52 (2008): 195-208.

Zick, S. M., B. Gillespie, and K. D. Aaronson. "The Effect of *Crataegus oxycantha* Special Extract WS 1442 on Clinical Progression in Patients with Mild to Moderate Symptoms of Heart Failure." *European Journal of Heart Failure* 10 (2008): 587-593.

See also: Angina; Atherosclerosis and heart disease prevention; Cardiomyopathy; Coenzyme Q_{10}; Fatigue; Hawthorn; Heart attack; Hypertension; Strokes; Vitamin B_1.

Conjugated linoleic acid

CATEGORY: Herbs and supplements

DEFINITION: Natural substance of the human body used as a supplement to treat specific health conditions.

PRINCIPAL PROPOSED USE: Improving body composition

OTHER PROPOSED USES: Allergic rhinitis, cancer prevention, diabetes, high cholesterol, metabolic syndrome

OVERVIEW

Conjugated linoleic acid (CLA) is a mixture of different isomers, or chemical forms, of linoleic acid. Linoleic acid is an essential fatty acid, a type of fat that the body needs for optimum health.

Based on preliminary evidence, CLA has been promoted as a fat-burning supplement and as a treatment for diabetes. However, there is little evidence that it works and growing evidence that CLA might actually worsen blood sugar control in people who are overweight.

REQUIREMENTS AND SOURCES

Although linoleic acid itself is an important nutritional source of essential fatty acids, there is no evidence that people need to get conjugated linoleic acid in their diet. CLA does occur in food, but it would be very difficult to get the recommended dose that way. Supplements are the only practical source.

THERAPEUTIC DOSAGES

The typical dosage of CLA ranges from 3 to 5 g daily. As with all supplements taken at this high a dosage, it is important to purchase a reputable brand, as even very small amounts of a toxic contaminant could quickly add up.

THERAPEUTIC USES

While CLA is often recommended for aiding weight loss or improving body composition (ratio of muscle to fat), evidence from studies is conflicting. One meta-analysis (systematic statistical review) of all the data found minimal benefits at most. Another meta-analysis concluded that, when taken at a dose of 3.2 grams (g) per day, CLA slightly reduces body fat levels. Finally, in one study, a combination of CLA and chromium failed to improve body composition.

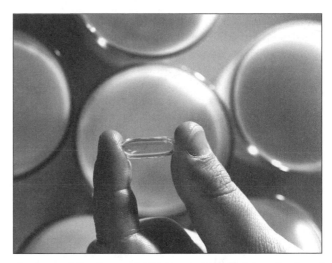

Conjugated linoleic acid (CLA) capsule. CLA is a fat found in milk. (James King-Holmes/Photo Researchers, Inc.)

It should be noted that some, but not all, studies have raised concerns that use of CLA by overweight people could raise insulin resistance and therefore increase the risk of diabetes. In addition, its use might increase a person's cardiovascular risk in other ways, as described in the following Safety Issues section.

One study failed to find that CLA-enriched milk is helpful for metabolic syndrome, a condition associated with increased risk of heart disease. Another study failed to find that CLA can enhance immune function.

A twelve-week double-blind, placebo-controlled study of forty subjects tested CLA as a treatment for people with allergies to birch pollen (a common cause of hay fever) and found some evidence of benefit. A small double-blind trial found weak evidence that CLA might be useful for high cholesterol. Some animal and test-tube studies suggest that CLA might help prevent cancer, but the evidence is preliminary and inconsistent.

SAFETY ISSUES

CLA appears to be a generally safe nutritional substance. However, there are some concerns with its use. During the course of investigations into its effect on fat, CLA was found to act somewhat similarly to some oral medications used for diabetes. This led to research into the possible usefulness of CLA as a treatment for diabetes. In one study, CLA reduced blood sugar levels in diabetic rats as effectively as a standard diabetes treatment. The same researchers also performed a small double-blind, placebo-controlled trial in humans. The results indicated that CLA improved insulin responsiveness in people with type 2 (adult onset) diabetes. However, several subsequent studies found opposite and rather alarming results: Use of CLA by people with diabetes may worsen blood sugar control; in overweight people without diabetes, CLA might decrease insulin sensitivity, creating a prediabetic state. In contrast, a study using the most precise method of measuring insulin sensitivity failed to find any harmful effect. Nonetheless, at present, individuals with diabetes or who are at risk for it should not use CLA except under a physician's supervision.

One study found that CLA impairs endothelial function and another that it increases levels of C-reactive protein; both of these effects suggest a possible increase in cardiovascular risk.

Concerns have also been raised regarding use of CLA by nursing mothers. A double-blind, placebo-controlled study indicates that use of CLA reduces the fat content of human breast milk. Since infants depend on the fat in breast milk to provide adequate calories and on certain fats to aid proper growth and development, it is probably prudent for nursing mothers to avoid CLA supplements. Maximum safe dosages of CLA for young children, pregnant women, and those with severe liver or kidney disease have not been determined.

EBSCO CAM Review Board

FURTHER READING

Close, R. N., et al. "Conjugated Linoleic Acid Supplementation Alters the Six-Month Change in Fat Oxidation During Sleep." *American Journal of Clinical Nutrition* 86 (2007): 797-804.

Gaullier, J. M., et al. "Supplementation with Conjugated Linoleic Acid for Twenty-four Months Is Well Tolerated by and Reduces Body Fat Mass in Healthy, Overweight Humans." *Journal of Nutrition* 135 (2005): 778-784.

Larsen, T. M., et al. "Conjugated Linoleic Acid Supplementation for One Year Does Not Prevent Weight or Body Fat Regain." *American Journal of Clinical Nutrition* 83 (2006): 606-612.

Nugent, A. P., et al. "The Effects of Conjugated Linoleic Acid Supplementation on Immune Function in Healthy Volunteers." *European Journal of Clinical Nutrition* 59, no. 6 (2005): 742-750.

Steck, S. E., et al. "Conjugated Linoleic Acid Supplementation for Twelve Weeks Increases Lean Body Mass in Obese Humans." *Journal of Nutrition* 137 (2007): 1188-1193.

Voevodin, M., et al. "The Effect of CLA on Body Composition in Humans." *Asia Pacific Journal of Clinical Nutrition* 14 (2005): S55.

Whigham, L. D., A. C. Watras, and D. A. Schoeller. Efficacy of Conjugated Linoleic Acid for Reducing Fat Mass." *American Journal of Clinical Nutrition* 85 (2007): 1203-1211.

See also: Diabetes; Herbal medicine; Obesity and excess weight.

Conjunctivitis

CATEGORY: Condition
RELATED TERM: Pink eye
DEFINITION: Treatment of inflammation of the conjunctiva, the clear membrane that covers the eyeball.
PRINCIPAL PROPOSED NATURAL TREATMENTS: None
OTHER PROPOSED NATURAL TREATMENTS: Barberry, bee propolis, calendula, chamomile, eyebright, goldenseal, Oregon grape, vitamin A

INTRODUCTION

Conjunctivitis is an inflammation of the conjunctiva, which is the clear membrane that covers the eyeball. Symptoms in the affected eye include a bloodshot appearance, crusty discharge, and discomfort that may feel like something has gotten in the eye. Conjunctivitis, also called pink eye, is frequently caused by a viral infection, sometimes of the same viruses that cause colds. In such cases, conjunctivitis could be called "a cold in the eye" and is really no more serious than any other cold. Other causes of conjunctivitis include bacterial infections, allergies, environmental irritants such as smoke or pollution, exposure to chemicals such as chlorine or contact-lens solution, and injuries to the eye.

Medical treatment varies depending on the cause of the inflammation. Common viral conjunctivitis does not require treatment; if the conjunctivitis is caused by the herpes virus, urgent treatment

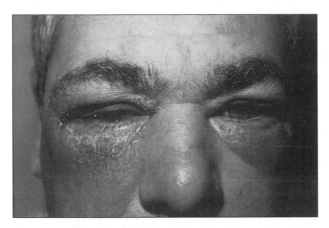

Symptoms of conjunctivitis include a bloodshot appearance, crusty discharge, and discomfort that may feel like something has gotten in the eye. (Biophoto Associates/Photo Researchers, Inc.)

is necessary. For bacterial eye infections, antibiotic ointment or oral antibiotics are usually prescribed; for allergic conjunctivitis, prescription eye drops or antihistamines, or both, may be used.

PROPOSED NATURAL TREATMENTS

Herbal teas. Traditionally, herbal teas have been applied to the eyes directly or in compress or poultice form. This method, however, is not recommended because, if absolute sterility is not ensured, further serious infection may occur. Furthermore, allergic reactions to herbal products are relatively common and may themselves cause eye irritation. Chamomile tea has also traditionally been used to soothe conjunctivitis symptoms.

Vitamin A. There is some evidence that persons with chronic conjunctivitis may have a vitamin A deficiency. However, this does not prove that taking vitamin A supplements would be helpful in treating or preventing conjunctivitis.

Bee propolis. Preliminary studies suggest that bee propolis may be helpful for treating conjunctivitis. However, because it was applied topically to the eye in these trials, this treatment is not recommended out of concerns for sterility.

Other herbs and supplements. As the name indicates, eyebright is a traditional herbal treatment for eye conditions; however, this recommendation may be based more on the bloodshot appearance of its petals than on any actual medicinal effect. The herbs barberry,

Oregon grape, and goldenseal contain berberine, a substance with antimicrobial and antibacterial properties. A special berberine preparation is used as a pharmaceutical treatment for conjunctivitis in Germany, but it is not used widely elsewhere. The herb calendula is thought to possess anti-inflammatory and antiseptic properties and has been used traditionally as an eye compress.

EBSCO CAM Review Board

FURTHER READING

Gaby, A. R. "Nutritional Therapies for Ocular Disorders." *Alternative Medicine Review* 13 (2008): 191-204.

Koby, M. "Conjunctivitis." In *Ferri's Clinical Advisor 2010*, edited by Fred F. Ferri. Philadelphia: Mosby/Elsevier, 2009.

Olitzky, S. E., et al. "Disorders of the Conjunctiva." In *Nelson Textbook of Pediatrics*, edited by Richard E. Behrman, Robert M. Kliegman, and Hal B. Jenson. 18th ed. Philadelphia: Saunders/Elsevier, 2007.

See also: Barberry; Bee propolis; Blepharitis; Calendula; Cataracts; Chamomile; Eyebright; Glaucoma; Goldenseal; Oregon grape; Uveitis; Vitamin A.

Constipation

CATEGORY: Condition

DEFINITION: Treatment of difficult or infrequent bowel movements.

PRINCIPAL PROPOSED NATURAL TREATMENTS: *Cascara sagrada*, dandelion, He Shou Wu, increased dietary fiber (debittered fenugreek seeds, flaxseed, glucomannan, psyllium husks), increased water intake, methyl sulfonyl methane, probiotics (alone or with prebiotics), *Senna*, traditional Chinese herbal medicine

OTHER PROPOSED NATURAL TREATMENTS: Acupuncture, aloe, Ayurvedic herbal combinations, barberry, basil, biofeedback, bladderwrack, buckthorn, cayenne, dandelion, goldenseal, honey, red raspberry, slippery elm

INTRODUCTION

In the nineteenth century, a naturopathic concept came into being whose influence persists today: namely, that regular, frequent, and complete bowel movements are necessary for optimum health. William Harvey Kellogg, of Kellogg's cereal fame, wrote extensively of the dangers of "auto-intoxication" purportedly caused by inadequate elimination. He and others claimed that a concrete-like sludge builds up on the wall of the colon, increasing in thickness over time and destroying the health of the body.

However, in modern times, physicians have performed millions of direct examinations of the colon, using the procedure known as colonoscopy, without finding any evidence of such a coating. Caked colons are a myth.

Furthermore, conventional medicine has never observed any connection between elimination and overall health. Many people eliminate only once a week or so, and their health appears to be no worse than that of the population at large. In addition, one study found that there is no connection between constipation and colon cancer.

Nonetheless, most people find occasional constipation unpleasant. For some, it becomes a severe chronic problem. It can be associated with irritable bowel syndrome (IBS), in which case it is called constipation-predominant IBS. Conventional treatment for constipation involves mainly increasing exercise and intake of dietary fiber and water, while reserving laxatives, suppositories, and enemas for emergencies.

PRINCIPAL PROPOSED NATURAL TREATMENTS

Occasional constipation can be safely self-treated. However, if constipation becomes a chronic problem, it should be evaluated by a physician.

Increasing dietary fiber and water intake is the first treatment to try for chronic constipation. Whole grains and fruits and vegetables add fiber in the diet. In addition, fiber supplements may be taken in the form of psyllium husks, debittered fenugreek seeds, glucomannan, and flaxseed. A typical dosage of fiber is 5 to 10 grams, one to three times daily, with a minimum of sixteen ounces of liquid. One should start with the lower doses and work up gradually, as too much fiber at once can actually worsen constipation.

The herbs *Cascara sagrada* and *Senna* are stimulant laxatives approved as over-the-counter (OTC) treatments for constipation. Another herb, common buckthorn, also contains these substances, but it is not an approved OTC drug in the United States. All of these work by virtue of chemical constituents called anthraquinones that irritate the colon wall. When taken to excess, stimulant laxatives can cause dependence. In addition, if overused, they can cause depletion of potassium. This is especially dangerous for people taking drugs in the digoxin family.

Traditional Chinese herbal medicine offers numerous herbal combinations for the treatment of constipation. One such combination has undergone study: a combination of the herbs rhubarb and licorice called Daio-kanzo-to. In this two-week, double-blind, placebo-controlled trial, 132 people complaining of constipation were randomly assigned to one of three groups: placebo, low-dose Daio-kanzo-to, or high-dose Daio-kanzo-to. The results indicate that the higher-dose group, but not the lower-dose group, experienced statistically significant improvements in constipation compared with placebo.

Some evidence indicates that probiotics (friendly bacteria) alone or taken with prebiotics (nutrients that encourage the growth of probiotics) may improve constipation. For example, 266 women with constipation who consumed yogurt containing the probiotic *Bifidobacterium animalis* and the prebiotic fructoligosaccharide twice daily for two weeks experienced significant improvement compared to women consuming regular yogurt as placebo. In addition, in a six-week, double-blind, placebo-controlled trial of 274 people with constipation-predominant IBS, the use of a probiotic formula containing *B. animalis* significantly reduced discomfort and increased stool frequency. In another double-blind, placebo-controlled study of forty-five children with chronic constipation, researchers found that the use of *Lactobacillus rhamnosus* was more effective than placebo and just as effective as magnesium oxide. Furthermore, a small trial found benefits in children, this time with a mixture of bifidobacteria and lactobacilli, and a study not limited to children found benefit with *L. casei Shirota*. Finally, another study found that a combination of *B. lactis* and *B. longus* improved bowel regularity in the elderly.

The psychological aspect of constipation also should be considered. Like sleep, elimination is inhibited by thinking too much about it. Part of the key to solving chronic constipation problems is to decrease the sense of worry and anxiety about it. Although constipation is certainly unpleasant, its evils have been greatly exaggerated. Thinking less about it will often go a long way toward solving the problem.

OTHER PROPOSED NATURAL TREATMENTS

Numerous herbs are used alone or in combination formulas for the treatment of constipation. These include aloe, Ayurvedic herbal combinations, barberry, bladderwrack, basil, buckthorn, cayenne, dandelion, goldenseal, He shou wu, red raspberry, and slippery elm. Honey has also shown some potential. The effectiveness of these therapies has not been scientifically evaluated to any meaningful extent.

Besides herbs, other alternative medicine therapies have been proposed for use in the treatment of constipation. Biofeedback may be effective for some forms of constipation (particularly those associated with uncoordinated functioning of pelvic muscles), but the evidence is mixed for short-term benefits and is lacking for long-term benefits. One small study failed to find acupuncture helpful.

EBSCO CAM Review Board

FURTHER READING

Bekkali, N. L., et al. "The Role of a Probiotics Mixture in the Treatment of Childhood Constipation." *Nutrition Journal* 6 (2007): 17.

Chiarioni, G., et al. "Bio-feedback Treatment of Fecal Incontinence: Where Are We and Where Are We Going?" *World Journal of Gastroenterology* 11 (2005): 4771-4775.

De Paula, J. A., E. Carmuega, and R. Weill. "Effect of the Ingestion of a Symbiotic Yogurt on the Bowel Habits of Women with Functional Constipation." *Acta Gastroenterologica Latinoamericana* 38 (2008): 16-25.

Guyonnet, D., et al. "Effect of a Fermented Milk Containing *Bifidobacterium animalis* DN-173 010 on the Health-Related Quality of Life and Symptoms in Irritable Bowel Syndrome in Adults in Primary Care." *Alimentary Pharmacology and Therapeutics* 26 (2007): 475-486.

Koh, C. E., et al. "Systematic Review of Randomized Controlled Trials of the Effectiveness of Biofeedback for Pelvic Floor Dysfunction." *British Journal of Surgery* 95 (2008): 1079-1087.

Pitkala, K. H., et al. "Fermented Cereal with Specific Bifidobacteria Normalizes Bowel Movements in Elderly Nursing Home Residents." *Journal of Nutrition, Health, and Aging* 11 (2007): 305-311.

Rao, S. S., et al. "Long-Term Efficacy of Biofeedback Therapy for Dyssynergic Defecation." *American Journal of Gastroenterology* 105 (2010): 890-896.

See also: Aging; Diarrhea; Gastritis; Gastrointestinal health; Herbal medicine; Irritable bowel syndrome (IBS); Lactose intolerance; Probiotics.

Copper

CATEGORY: Herbs and supplements

RELATED TERMS: Copper complexes of various amino acids, copper gluconate, copper picolinate, copper sulfate

DEFINITION: Natural substance of the human body used as a supplement to treat specific health conditions.

PRINCIPAL PROPOSED USE: Balancing high zinc intake

OTHER PROPOSED USES: Heart disease, high cholesterol, osteoarthritis, osteoporosis, rheumatoid arthritis

OVERVIEW

The human body contains only 70 to 80 milligrams (mg) of copper in total, but it is an essential part of many important enzymes. Copper's possible role in treating disease is based on the fact that these enzymes cannot do their jobs without it. However, there is little direct evidence that taking extra copper can treat any disease.

REQUIREMENTS AND SOURCES

The official U.S. recommendations for daily intake of copper are as follows: 200 micrograms (mcg) for infants up to six months of age, 220 mcg for infants seven to twelve months of age, 340 mcg for children one to three years old, 440 mcg for children four to eight years old, 700 mcg for persons nine to thirteen years old, 890 mcg for persons fourteen to eighteen, and 900 mcg for those nineteen and older. Recommended intake is 1,000 mcg for pregnant women and 1,300 mcg for nursing women.

High zinc intake reduces copper stores in the body; therefore, those persons taking zinc in doses above nutritional levels (as, for example, in the treatment of macular degeneration) will need extra copper. In addition, persons taking iron or large doses of vitamin C may need extra copper. Ideally, copper should be taken at least two hours apart from these two nutrients, so that they do not interfere with each other's absorption.

Copper Levels and Too Much Zinc

Copper is a trace mineral that is part of several enzymes and proteins that are essential for adequate use of iron by the body. In some studies, low copper intake has been implicated with other variables, such as heightened cholesterol, as a possible risk factor for cardiovascular disease. Zinc can cause reduced levels of copper in the body.

Zinc is an essential mineral that is naturally present in some foods, added to others, and available as a dietary supplement. Zinc is also found in many cold lozenges and some over-the-counter drugs sold as cold remedies. Intakes of 150 to 450 milligrams (mg) of zinc per day have been associated with such chronic effects as low copper status, altered iron function, reduced immune function, and reduced levels of high-density lipoproteins. Reductions in a copper-containing enzyme, a marker of copper status, have been reported with even moderately high zinc intakes of approximately 60 mg per day for up to ten weeks.

Oysters, nuts, legumes, whole grains, sweet potatoes, and dark greens are good sources of copper. Drinking water that passes through copper plumbing is a good source of this mineral, and sometimes it may even provide too much.

THERAPEUTIC DOSAGES

Copper is often recommended at a high (but still safe) dose of 1 to 3 mg (1,000 to 3,000 mcg) daily.

THERAPEUTIC USES

Copper has been proposed as a treatment for osteoporosis, based primarily on studies that found benefit using combinations of various trace minerals including copper. However, one study found that copper supplements taken alone may not be helpful.

One researcher, L. M. Klevay, has claimed in more than a dozen papers that copper deficiencies increase the risk of high cholesterol and heart disease, but he has failed to supply any real evidence that this idea is true. A small double-blind, placebo-controlled study of copper supplements for reducing heart disease risk factors such as cholesterol profile found no benefit.

Copper has long been mentioned as a possible treatment for osteoarthritis and rheumatoid arthritis, but there is as yet no real evidence that it works.

SAFETY ISSUES

The following daily doses of copper should not be exceeded: 1,000 mcg for children ages one to three years, 3,000 mcg for children ages four to eight, 5,000 mcg for children ages nine to thirteen, 8,000 mcg for persons ages fourteen to eighteen, and 10,000 mcg for persons nineteen and older. Doses for pregnant or nursing women should not exceed 10,000 mcg or 8,000 mcg if the women are eighteen years old or younger. Maximum safe dosages of copper for individuals with severe liver or kidney disease have not been determined.

IMPORTANT INTERACTIONS

Individuals who are taking zinc should be sure to get enough copper. Those persons taking iron supplements or high doses of vitamin C may need extra copper. They should take the copper either two hours before or two hours after taking these other substances.

EBSCO CAM Review Board

FURTHER READING

Cashman, K. D., et al. "No Effect of Copper Supplementation on Biochemical Markers of Bone Metabolism in Healthy Young Adult Females Despite Apparently Improved Copper Status." *European Journal of Clinical Nutrition* 55 (2001): 525-531.

Finley, E. B., and F. L. Cerklewski. "Influence of Ascorbic Acid Supplementation on Copper Status in Young Adult Men." *American Journal of Clinical Nutrition* 37 (1983): 553-556.

See also: Herbal medicine; Zinc.

Cordyceps

CATEGORY: Herbs and supplements
RELATED TERM: *Cordyceps sinensis*
DEFINITION: Fungus and larvae combination used to treat specific health conditions.
PRINCIPAL PROPOSED USES: None
OTHER PROPOSED USES: Cancer prevention, diabetes, fatigue, high blood pressure, high cholesterol, immune support, kidney protection, liver support, lupus, male sexual dysfunction, sports performance, viral hepatitis

OVERVIEW

Although *Cordyceps sinensis* is often described as an herb, it is actually a combination of a parasitic fungus and the larvae of a moth (a caterpillar). The fungus attacks the caterpillar and destroys it from within. The remaining structures of the caterpillar, along with the fungus, are dried and sold as cordyceps.

Cordyceps has a long history of use in China as a tonic, a substance said to generally strengthen the body, particularly following illness. It was also used to treat bronchitis, kidney failure, and tuberculosis.

THERAPEUTIC DOSAGES

Typical traditional recommended doses of cordyceps range from 5 to 10 grams per day. Concentrated extracts are also available, taken at a lower dosage.

THERAPEUTIC USES

Cordyceps is widely marketed today as treatment for many conditions. However, there is no reliable scientific evidence that it actually provides any medical benefits. Most research on cordyceps was done in China and is not up to modern scientific standards. In general, double-blind, placebo-controlled studies are the most reliable form of evidence. However, such studies have to be performed and reported according to certain standards. Although several double-blind studies have been reported on cordyceps, they all fall considerably short of the level necessary for scientific validity. These somewhat dubious double-blind trials hint that cordyceps might be helpful for reducing high cholesterol and improving male sexual function.

Evidence is more negative than positive regarding whether cordyceps is helpful for enhancing sports performance. Weak evidence hints that cordyceps may modulate the immune system, which means that it stimulates some aspects of the immune system while suppressing others. On this basis, it has been tried in China as an aid in organ transplant surgery and for the treatment of viral hepatitis and lupus.

Highly preliminary test-tube and animal studies hint that cordyceps may help fight stress, control blood sugar levels (potentially making it useful in diabetes), reduce cancer risk, lower high blood pressure, and help protect the kidney against damage caused by the drugs cyclosporin and gentamycin.

Other test-tube studies hint that cordyceps may stimulate production of hormones, such as cortisone and testosterone. However, contrary to what some Web sites say, these studies are far too preliminary to indicate any therapeutic hormonal effect.

SAFETY ISSUES

Use of cordyceps does not generally cause apparent side effects. However, comprehensive safety studies have not been reported. In addition, there are two case reports in which cordyceps products contained enough lead to cause lead poisoning. Safety in young children, pregnant or nursing women, or people with severe liver or kidney disease has not been established.

EBSCO CAM Review Board

FURTHER READING

Chiou, W. F., et al. "Protein Constituent Contributes to the Hypotensive and Vasorelaxant Activities of *Cordyceps sinensis*." *Life Sciences* 66 (2000): 1369-1376.

Colson, S. N., et al. "*Cordyceps sinensis* and *Rhodiola rosea*-based Supplementation in Male Cyclists and Its Effect on Muscle Tissue Oxygen Saturation." *Journal of Strength and Conditioning Research* 19 (2005): 358-363.

Koh, J. H., et al. "Activation of Macrophages and the Intestinal Immune System by an Orally Administered Decoction from Cultured Mycelia of *Cordyceps sinensis*." *Bioscience, Biotechnology, and Biochemistry* 66 (2002): 407-411.

_____. "Antifatigue and Antistress Effect of the Hot-Water Fraction from Mycelia of *Cordyceps sinensis*." *Biological and Pharmaceutical Bulletin* 26 (2003): 691-694.

Parcell, A. C., et al. "*Cordyceps sinensis* (CordyMax Cs-4) Supplementation Does Not Improve Endurance Exercise Performance." *International Journal of Sport Nutrition and Exercise Metabolism* 14 (2004): 236-242.

Weng, S. C., et al. "Immunomodulatory Functions of Extracts from the Chinese Medicinal Fungus *Cordyceps cicadae*." *Journal of Ethnopharmacology* 83 (2002): 79-85.

See also: Chinese medicine; Herbal medicine.

Coriolus versicolor

CATEGORY: Herbs and supplements

RELATED TERMS: Kawaratake, *Trametes versicolor*, turkey tail, Yun Zhi

DEFINITION: Fungus used to treat specific health conditions.
PRINCIPAL PROPOSED USE: Cancer treatment support
OTHER PROPOSED USE: Cancer prevention

OVERVIEW

Coriolus versicolor is a common tree fungus often seen by hikers as a stiff, rounded, horizontal protuberance from tree trunks, with concentric lines of varying color. In traditional Chinese herbal medicine, this fungus is used to strengthen overall vitality and treat lung and liver problems, as well as other conditions.

THERAPEUTIC DOSAGES

A typical dosage of PSK or PSP as an adjunct to standard cancer treatment is 2 to 6 grams daily. For prevention of cancer, some experts recommend 500 milligrams daily, but there is no real scientific basis for this recommendation.

THERAPEUTIC USES

Extracts of *Coriolus versicolor* called polysaccharide-K (PSK) and polysaccharopeptide (PSP) are under study as immune stimulants for use alongside chemotherapy in the treatment of cancer. These two related substances, made from slightly different strains of the fungus, are thought to act as biological response modifiers, meaning that they affect the body's response to cancer.

According to most but not all reported trials, most of which were performed in Asia, both PSK and PSP can enhance the effects of various forms of standard cancer treatment. For example, in a twenty-eight-day double-blind, placebo-controlled study of thirty-four people with advanced non-small-cell lung cancer, use of *Coriolus* extracts along with conventional treatment significantly slowed the progression of the disease.

It is thought that *Coriolus* extracts work by stimulating the body's own cancer-fighting cells. PSK and PSP may also have cancer-preventive effects. In addition, very weak evidence hints that extracts of *Coriolus versicolor* might be helpful for human immunodeficiency virus infection.

SAFETY ISSUES

According to Chinese studies, PSP and PSK appear to be relatively nontoxic, in both the short and long term. Few side effects have been reported in clinical trials. However, safety in young children, pregnant or

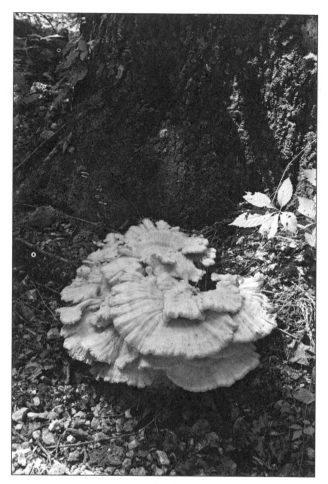

Coriolus versicolor is a tree fungus used in traditional Chinese herbal medicine. (Susan Leavines/Photo Researchers, Inc.)

nursing women, and people with severe liver or kidney disease has not been established.

EBSCO CAM Review Board

FURTHER READING

Chu, K. K., S. S. Ho, and A. H. Chow. "*Coriolus versicolor*: A Medicinal Mushroom with Promising Immunotherapeutic Values." *Journal of Clinical Pharmacology* 42 (2002): 976-984.

Fisher, M., and L. X. Yang. "Anticancer Effects and Mechanisms of Polysaccharide-K (PSK): Implications of Cancer Immunotherapy." *Anticancer Research* 22 (2002): 1737-1754.

Jian, X., et al. "Subchronic Toxicity Test of Polysaccharopeptide of Yun Zhi (PSP)." In *International Sympo-*

sium on Traditional Chinese Medicine and Cancer: Development and Clinical Validation–Advances Research in PSP, edited by Q. Y. Yang. Hong Kong: Hong Kong Association for Health Care, 1999.

Jin, T. Y. "Toxicological Research on Yun Zhi Polysaccharopeptide (PSP)." In *International Symposium on Traditional Chinese Medicine and Cancer: Development and Clinical Validation–Advances Research in PSP*, edited by Q. Y. Yang. Hong Kong: Hong Kong Association for Health Care, 1999.

Tsang, K. W., et al. "*Coriolus versicolor* Polysaccharide Peptide Slows Progression of Advanced Non-Small-Cell Lung Cancer." *Respiratory Medicine* 97 (2003): 618-624.

See also: Cancer treatment support; Chinese medicine; Herbal medicine.

Corticosteroids

CATEGORY: Drug interactions

RELATED TERM: Glucocorticoids

DEFINITION: Anti-inflammatory and immune-suppressant medications.

INTERACTIONS: Aloe (topical), calcium, chromium, creatine, dehydroepiandrosterone, ipriflavone, licorice, vitamin D

DRUGS IN THIS FAMILY: Betamethasone (Celestone), cortisone acetate (Cortone Acetate), dexamethasone (Decadron, Dexameth, Dexone, Hexadrol), hydrocortisone (Cortef, Hydrocortone), methylprednisolone (Medrol), prednisolone (Delta-Cortef, Pediapred, Prelone), prednisone (Deltasone, Liquid Pred, Meticorten, Orasone, Panasol-S, Prednicen-M, Sterapred DS), triamcinolone (Aristocort, Atolone, Kenacort)

CALCIUM, VITAMIN D

Effect: Helpful Interactions

One of the most serious side effects of long-term corticosteroid use is accelerated osteoporosis. Although it is not fully clear how this works, corticosteroid interference with calcium and vitamin D is known to play a major role.

Calcium and vitamin D supplements are definitely beneficial for fighting ordinary osteoporosis; in addition, there is good evidence that they also protect against osteoporosis brought on by corticosteroids. A review of five trials enrolling a total of 274 participants found that calcium and vitamin D supplementation significantly prevented bone loss at the lumbar spine and forearm in corticosteroid-treated persons. For example, in a two-year, double-blind, placebo-controlled study of 130 persons, supplementation with 1,000 mg of calcium and 500 IU of vitamin D daily actually reversed steroid-induced bone loss, causing a net bone gain.

ALOE AND LICORICE (TOPICAL)

Effect: Possible Supportive Interactions with Topical Corticosteroids

Aloe and licorice are two herbs sometimes used topically for skin problems. Preliminary evidence suggests that each one might help topical corticosteroids, such as hydrocortisone, work better.

DEHYDROEPIANDROSTERONE (DHEA)

Effect: Possible Helpful Interaction

There are theoretical reasons (but little direct evidence) to believe that persons taking corticosteroids, such as prednisone, might be protected from some side effects by taking DHEA at the same time.

CHROMIUM

Effect: Supplementation Possibly Helpful

Long-term, high-dose corticosteroid treatment can cause diabetes. This may be at least partly caused by chromium deficiency. A very preliminary study found treatment with corticosteroids caused increased loss of chromium in the urine. Another preliminary study found that persons with corticosteroid-induced diabetes could improve blood sugar control by taking chromium supplements.

CREATINE

Effect: Possible Helpful Interaction

Long-term use of corticosteroids, whether orally or possibly by inhalation can slow a child's growth. One animal study suggests that use of the supplement creatine may help prevent this side effect.

IPRIFLAVONE

Effect: Possible Harmful Interaction

The supplement ipriflavone is used to treat osteoporosis. A three-year, double-blind trial of almost five hundred women, as well as a small study, found worrisome evidence that ipriflavone can reduce white blood cell count in some people. For this reason, anyone taking medications that suppress the immune system should avoid using ipriflavone except under physician supervision.

LICORICE (INTERNAL)

Effect: Possible Harmful Interaction

When taken by mouth, the herb licorice appears to enhance some actions of oral corticosteroids but to interfere with others. Because of the unpredictable nature of this interaction, persons using oral corticosteroids should avoid licorice.

EBSCO CAM Review Board

FURTHER READING

Alexandersen, P., et al. "Ipriflavone in the Treatment of Postmenopausal Osteoporosis." *Journal of the American Medical Association* 285 (2001): 1482-1488.

Ravina, A., et al. "Reversal of Corticosteroid-Induced Diabetes Mellitis with Supplemental Chromium." *Diabetic Medicine* 16 (1999): 164-167.

Robinzon, B., and M. Cutulo. "Should Dehydroepiandrosterone Replacement Therapy Be Provided with Glucocorticoids?" *Rheumatology* 38 (1999): 488-495.

Van Vollenhoven, R. F., et al. "A Double-Blind, Placebo-Controlled, Clinical Trial of Dehydroepianodrosterone in Severe Systemic Lupus Erythematosus." *Lupus* 8 (1999): 181-187.

See also: Food and Drug Administration; Supplements: Introduction.

Corydalis

CATEGORY: Herbs and supplements
RELATED TERMS: *Corydalis turtschaninovii, C. yanhusuo,* Yan Hu So
DEFINITION: Natural plant product used to treat specific health conditions.
PRINCIPAL PROPOSED USE: Pain relief (including peripheral neuropathy, painful menstruation, and pain caused by soft tissue injuries)
OTHER PROPOSED USES: Cataracts, heart arrhythmia, preventing blood clots

OVERVIEW

Widely used in Chinese herbal medicine, the herb corydalis is said to alleviate pain by moving qi (energy) and stimulating the blood. These expressions refer to traditional concepts included within the complex theories of traditional Chinese herbal medicine. In terms of Western diagnostic categories, corydalis may be recommended for soft tissue injuries, menstrual discomfort, and abdominal pain. The part of the plant used medicinally is the rhizome (underground stalk).

THERAPEUTIC DOSAGES

Corydalis is usually taken at a dose of 5 to 10 grams daily, or equivalent quantities of an extract.

THERAPEUTIC USES

There is no reliable evidence that corydalis or its constituents offer any medicinal benefits. Corydalis contains a number of active and potentially dangerous chemicals in the alkaloid family, including tetrahydropalmatine (THP), corydaline, protopine, tetrahydrocoptisine, tetrahydrocolumbamine, and corybulbine. Of these, THP may be the most active, as well as the most toxic.

Only double-blind, placebo-controlled studies can actually show that a treatment works, and there is only one such study that is relevant to corydalis. This trial tested THP as a treatment for a type of heart rhythm abnormality called supraventricular arrhythmia. Reportedly, the use of THP produced significant benefits, compared with a placebo. However, this study was conducted in China, and there is considerable skepticism about the validity of Chinese medical trials.

Much weaker evidence from animal and test-tube studies hints that TNP or corydalis extracts might have pain-relieving, sedative, and anti-inflammatory effects. Corydalis constituents may also affect neurotransmitters in the brain, including dopamine and gamma-aminobutyric acid (GABA). Equally weak evidence hints at benefits for preventing or treating cataracts, reducing blood coagulation, and lowering blood pressure. However, none of this research remotely approaches the level of evidence that can prove a treatment effective.

SAFETY ISSUES

Corydalis has not undergone any meaningful safety testing. The herb is known to produce immediate side effects, including nausea and fatigue, in some people. In addition, there are serious safety concerns related to its alkaloid constituent THP. Use of products containing THP has repeatedly been associated with severe and potentially fatal liver injury. In addition, there are three reports that use of THP by young children has led to life-threatening suppression of the central nervous system. For these reasons, experts strongly recommend against the use of corydalis, especially by young children, pregnant or nursing women, and people with liver disease.

EBSCO CAM Review Board

FURTHER READING

McRae, C. A., et al. "Hepatitis Associated with Chinese Herbs." *European Journal of Gastroenterology and Hepatology* 14 (2002): 559-562.

Picciotto, A., et al. "Chronic Hepatitis Induced by Jin Bu Huan." *Journal of Hepatology* 28 (1998): 165-167.

Stickel, F., G. Egerer, and H. K. Seitz. "Hepatotoxicity of Botanicals." *Public Health Nutrition* 3 (2000): 113-124.

See also: Chinese medicine; Herbal medicine.

Cough

CATEGORY: Condition
DEFINITION: Treatment of the cough reflex.
PRINCIPAL PROPOSED NATURAL TREATMENTS: None
OTHER PROPOSED NATURAL TREATMENTS: Cocoa, elecampane, essential oils of anise, eucalyptus, fennel, peppermint, and thyme, garlic, horehound, hyssop, ivy leaf, lobelia, licorice, marshmallow, mullein, plantain, primula root, sesame oil, slippery elm, soap bark

INTRODUCTION

The cough reflex is intended to expel mucus and other unwanted material from the breathing passages. However, sometimes it causes an unproductive cough that seems to serve no purpose. The most common cause of coughing is a viral infection. Sometimes a chronic cough may indicate asthma, either allergic or created temporarily by a respiratory infection. Other causes of cough include sinus drainage tickling the throat and chronic bronchitis.

First and foremost, medical treatment for cough involves treating the underlying condition, if possible. When appropriate, cough suppressants may be prescribed to hold coughing to manageable levels. Most cough remedies contain codeine or the codeine-like drug dextromethorphan, to suppress the cough reflex, and guaifenesin, which is thought to loosen mucus. Other common ingredients such as decongestants and antihistamines do not directly affect coughs. There is no reliable evidence that any over-the-counter cough suppressant actually works. Furthermore, while it is often said that prescription codeine cough syrups are more effective than dextromethorphan, one study found that neither codeine nor dextromethorphan reduced nighttime coughing in children to any greater extent than placebo. In another study, prescription codeine cough syrup failed to prove more effective than dextromethorphan.

PROPOSED NATURAL TREATMENTS

Although many herbs have been used to treat coughs, none has been shown effective in a double-blind, placebo-controlled trial. Without such trials, it is impossible to know whether a treatment really works, regardless of its reputation. A few studies that lack a placebo group are sometimes cited in support of traditional cough remedies, but these are almost as unreliable as completely unscientific anecdotes.

Weak evidence indicates that the herb marshmallow may help soothe coughs. The herb coltsfoot has been

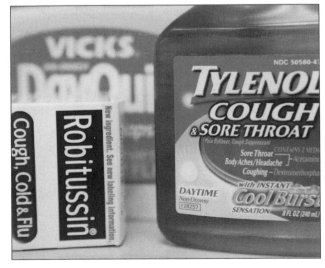

Over-the-counter cough suppressants containing the drug dextromethorphan. (Getty Images)

used since ancient times to relieve cough; its scientific name, *Tusillago farfara,* means "cough dispeller" in Latin. However, there is no scientific evidence to indicate that coltsfoot works. Furthermore, the root of the plant contains high levels of liver-toxic pyrrolizidine alkaloids. The leaves and flowers are safer, but they also may contain these toxins.

Many herbs are categorized as mucilaginous (gluey) and are said to coat the throat. These herbs include marshmallow, mullein, plantain, and slippery elm. The herbs ivy leaf, primula root, and soap bark contain chemicals called saponins, which are said to loosen mucus. Other herbs used for coughs include elecampane, garlic, horehound, hyssop, lobelia, and licorice. Essential oils such as anise, eucalyptus, fennel, peppermint, and thyme are often included in cough preparations or added to a vaporizer. There is no meaningful scientific evidence that any of these treatments are effective. However, because much the same situation exists for standard cough suppressants, these alternative treatments may be worth trying.

Chocolate contains the stimulant substance theobromine. One study hints that theobromine might have a cough-suppressant effect. Another study found that a sesame oil cough preparation was no more effective than placebo.

The most common cause of a cough is a respiratory infection; for this reason, herbs and supplements used to treat colds may be worth considering too.

EBSCO CAM Review Board

FURTHER READING

Saab, B. R., et al. "Sesame Oil Use in Ameliorating Cough in Children." *Complementary Therapies in Medicine* 14 (2006): 92-99.

Schroeder, K., and T. Fahey. "Over-the-Counter Medications for Acute Cough in Children and Adults in Ambulatory Settings." *Cochrane Database of Systematic Reviews* (2001): CD001831. Available through *EBSCO DynaMed Systematic Literature Surveillance* at http://www.ebscohost.com/dynamed.

Usmani, O. S., et al. "Theobromine Inhibits Sensory Nerve Activation and Cough." *FASEB Journal* 19 (2005): 231-233

See also: Bronchitis; Chronic obstructive pulmonary disease (COPD); Colds and flu.

Cranberry

CATEGORY: Functional foods
RELATED TERMS: Cranberry juice, *Vaccinium macrocarpon*
DEFINITION: Natural food promoted as a dietary supplement for specific health benefits.
PRINCIPAL PROPOSED USE: Bladder infection
OTHER PROPOSED USES: Cancer prevention, heart disease prevention, periodontal disease prevention and treatment, ulcer prevention and treatment

OVERVIEW

The cranberry plant is a close relative of the common blueberry. Native Americans used it both as food and for the treatment of bladder and kidney diseases. The pilgrims learned about cranberry from local tribes and quickly adopted it for their own use. Physicians later used it for bladder infections, for "bladder gravel" (small bladder stones), and to remove "blood toxins."

In the 1920s, researchers observed that drinking cranberry juice makes the urine more acidic. Because bacteria that commonly affect the urinary tract, such as *Escherichia coli,* dislike acidic environments, physicians concluded that they had discovered a scientific explanation for the traditional uses of cranberry. This discovery led to widespread medical use of cranberry juice for treating bladder infections. Cranberry fell out of favor with physicians after World War II, but it became popular again during the 1960s, as a self-treatment.

USES AND APPLICATIONS

Cranberry is widely used today to prevent bladder infections, although the evidence to support this use remains limited. Contrary to the research from the 1920s, it now appears that cranberry's acidification of the urine is not likely to play an important role in the treatment of bladder infections; current study has focused instead on cranberry's apparent ability to block bacteria from adhering to the bladder wall. If the bacteria cannot "hold on" to the wall, they will be washed out with the stream of urine. Studies have found that in women who frequently develop bladder infections, bacteria seem to have a particularly easy time holding on to the bladder wall. This suggests that cranberry juice can actually get to the root of the problem.

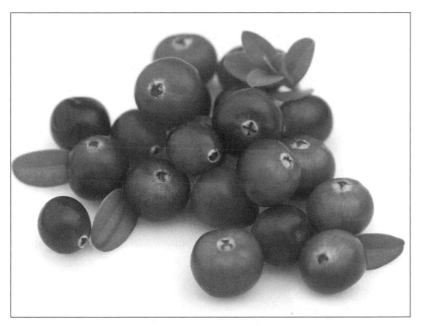

Drinking cranberry juice is thought to help prevent bladder infections.
(©Margo555/Dreamstime.com)

Just as cranberry seems to prevent adhesion of bacteria to the bladder, preliminary evidence suggests that it might also help prevent adhesion of the ulcer-causing bacterium *Helicobacter pylori* to the stomach wall. On this basis, it has been proposed for preventing or treating ulcers, with mixed results.

Other preliminary evidence suggests that the same actions of cranberry juice might make it useful for treating or preventing cavities or gum disease. However, there is one problem to work out before cranberry could be practical for this purpose: The sweeteners added to cranberry juice harm teeth, but without sweeteners, cranberry juice is very bitter.

Cranberry has also been investigated as a possible aid in reducing the risk of heart disease and cancer and as a treatment for diabetes, but there is no meaningful evidence that it is actually helpful for these conditions. Another study failed to find cranberry significantly effective for enhancing mental function.

SCIENTIFIC EVIDENCE

Bladder infection. Probably the best evidence for the use of cranberry juice for preventing bladder infections comes from a one-year, double-blind, placebo-controlled study of 150 sexually active women that compared placebo with both cranberry juice (8 ounces three times daily) and cranberry tablets. The results showed that both forms of cranberry significantly reduced the number of episodes of bladder infections; cranberry tablets were more cost-effective.

A double-blind study of 376 hospitalized elderly people attempted to determine whether a low dose of cranberry juice (as cranberry juice cocktail, 10 ounces daily–a very low dose in comparison to the previous study) would help prevent acute infections. It failed to find benefit, perhaps in part because of the dosage of cranberry and because of the low number of infections that developed overall.

Another double-blind study evaluated cranberry juice cocktail for the treatment of chronic bladder infections. This trial followed 153 women with an average age of 78.5 years for six months. Many women of this age group have chronic asymptomatic bladder infections: signs of bacteria in the urine without any symptoms. One-half of the participants were given 10 ounces a day of a standard commercial cranberry cocktail drink, the other a placebo drink prepared to look and taste the same. Both treatments contained the same amount of vitamin C to eliminate the possible antibacterial influence of that supplement. Despite the weak preparation of cranberry used, the results showed a 58 percent decrease in the incidence of bacteria and white blood cells in the urine.

A one-year-long open trial of 150 women found that the regular use of a cranberry juice and lingonberry combination reduced the rate of urinary tract infection compared with a probiotic drink or no treatment. However, because this study was not double-blind, the results are unreliable.

A review of ten studies investigated the benefits of cranberry juice or tablets, compared with a placebo control, in persons susceptible to urinary tract infections. Among 1,049 participants, researchers found that the cranberry products reduced the incidence of urinary tract infections by 35 percent, a statistically significant amount, in a twelve-month period. The effect was most notable in those with recurrent infections. However, many participants dropped out of the studies early, suggesting that continuous consumption of cranberries is not well tolerated.

On the negative side, three other double-blind, placebo-controlled studies evaluated the effectiveness of cranberry extract for eliminating bacteria in the urine of people with bladder paralysis (neurogenic bladder). The results showed no benefit. However, a subsequent study of forty-seven persons with neurogenic bladder from spinal cord injuries found that the use of cranberry extract tablets for six months significantly reduced the risk of urinary tract infections.

Ulcers. The bacterium *H. pylori* plays a major role in the initiation and maintenance of peptic ulcers, those ulcers in the stomach and duodenum. A ninety-day, double-blind, placebo-controlled study performed in China tested the effects of daily consumption of cranberry juice in persons who were chronically infected with *H. pylori* (but who did not necessarily have ulcers). The results indicated that the use of cranberry significantly decreased levels of *H. pylori* in the stomach, presumably by causing some of the detached bacteria to be "washed away." Another study involving 295 children with *H. pylori* but without ulcer symptoms also demonstrated the ability of cranberry to reduce the levels of the stomach bacteria.

While this was a promising finding on a theoretical level, it did not directly address the treatment or prevention of ulcers.

A more practical study evaluated the use of cranberry as a support to standard therapy. This double-blind trial enrolled 177 people with ulcers who were undergoing treatment with a common triple-drug therapy (omeprazole, amoxicillin, and clarithromycin, known as OAC) used to eradicate *H. pylori*. All participants received this drug treatment for one week. During this week and for two weeks after, they were additionally given either placebo or cranberry juice. Researchers also looked at a third group attending the same clinic, who received only OAC.

The results were somewhat promising. In the study group at large, OAC plus cranberry was no more effective than OAC plus placebo or OAC alone. However, among female participants in the study, the use of cranberry was associated with a significantly increased rate of *H. pylori* eradication compared with placebo or no treatment.

Does this mean that women undergoing ulcer treatment may benefit from cranberry? Perhaps, but not necessarily. When a treatment fails to produce benefit in the entire group studied, researchers may, after the fact, look for a subgroup who did benefit. The laws of chance alone ensure that they can almost always find one. Therefore, it is not clear whether cranberry actually did provide benefit or whether this finding was merely a statistical fluke.

DOSAGE

The usual dosage of dry cranberry juice extract is 300 to 400 milligrams twice daily, and the usual dosage of pure cranberry juice (not cranberry juice cocktail) is 8 to 16 ounces daily.

SAFETY ISSUES

As a widely consumed food, cranberry is thought to have a generally good safety profile. However, several case reports suggest that cranberry could interact with the drug warfarin (Coumadin), potentially leading to internal bleeding. Two formal studies have failed to find evidence of such an interaction, while a third study did find that cranberry can increase the blood thinning effect of warfarin in healthy male participants. One should take caution, especially when consuming more than 8 ounces of cranberry juice daily.

In addition, cranberry juice might allow the kidneys to excrete weakly alkaline drugs more rapidly, thereby reducing their effectiveness. This would include many antidepressants and prescription painkillers. Finally, indirect evidence suggests that the regular use of cranberry concentrate tablets might increase the risk of kidney stones.

IMPORTANT INTERACTIONS

For persons taking warfarin, the use of cranberry might lead to excessive bleeding. Cranberry could decrease the effectiveness of drugs that are weakly alkaline, including many antidepressants and prescription painkillers.

EBSCO CAM Review Board

FURTHER READING

Chambers, B. K., and M. E. Camire. "Can Cranberry Supplementation Benefit Adults with Type 2 Diabetes?" *Diabetes Care* 26 (2003): 2695-2696.

Gotteland, M., et al. "Modulation of *Helicobacter pylori*

Colonization with Cranberry Juice and *Lactobacillus johnsonii* La1 in Children." *Nutrition* 24 (2008): 421-426.

Jepson, R., and J. Craig. "Cranberries for Preventing Urinary Tract Infections." *Cochrane Database of Systematic Reviews* (2008): CD001321. Available through *EBSCO DynaMed Systematic Literature Surveillance* at http://www.ebscohost.com/dynamed.

Pham, D. Q., and A. Q. Pham. "Interaction Potential Between Cranberry Juice and Warfarin." *American Journal of Health-System Pharmacy* 64 (2007): 490-494.

Shmuely, H., et al. "Effect of Cranberry Juice on Eradication of *Helicobacter pylori* in Patients Treated with Antibiotics and a Proton Pump Inhibitor." *Molecular Nutrition and Food Research* 51 (2007): 746-751.

See also: Bladder infections.

Creatine

CATEGORY: Herbs and supplements

RELATED TERM: Creatine monohydrate

DEFINITION: Natural substance of the human body used as a supplement to treat specific health conditions.

PRINCIPAL PROPOSED USE: Sports performance enhancement

OTHER PROPOSED USES: Amyotrophic lateral sclerosis, cancer treatment support, chronic obstructive pulmonary disease, congestive heart failure, dermatomyositis, disuse atrophy following injury, mental function (following sleep deprivation), high triglycerides, Huntington's disease, improved ratio of body fat to muscle, McArdle's disease, mitochondrial illnesses, muscular dystrophy, myotonic dystrophy, Parkinson's, polymyositis, schizophrenia, weight loss

OVERVIEW

Creatine is a naturally occurring substance that plays an important role in the production of energy in the body. The body converts it to phosphocreatine, a form of stored energy used by muscles.

Although the evidence for creatine is not definitive, it has the most evidence behind it among all the sports supplements. Numerous small double-blind studies suggest that it can increase athletic perfor-

mance in sports that involve intense but short bursts of activity. The theory behind its use is that supplemental creatine can build up a reserve of phosphocreatine in the muscles to help them perform on demand. Supplemental creatine may also help the body make new phosphocreatine faster when it has been used up by intense activity.

REQUIREMENTS AND SOURCES

Although some creatine exists in the daily diet, it is not an essential nutrient because the human body can make it from the amino acids L-arginine, glycine, and L-methionine. Provided enough animal protein (the principal source of these amino acids) is consumed, the body will make all the creatine needed for good health.

Meat (including chicken and fish) is the most important dietary source of creatine and its amino acid building blocks. For this reason, vegetarian athletes may potentially benefit most from creatine supplementation.

THERAPEUTIC DOSAGES

For bodybuilding and exercise enhancement, a typical dosage schedule starts with a loading dose of 15 to 30 g daily (divided into 2 or 3 separate doses) for three to four days, followed by 2 to 5 g daily. Some authorities recommend skipping the loading dose. (By comparison, humans typically get only about 1 g of creatine in their daily diet.)

Creatine's ability to enter muscle cells can be increased by combining it with glucose, fructose, or other simple carbohydrates; in addition, prior use of creatine might enhance the sports benefits of carbohydrate-loading. Caffeine may block the effects of creatine.

THERAPEUTIC USES

Creatine is one of the best-selling and best-documented supplements for enhancing athletic performance, but the scientific evidence that it works is far from complete. The best evidence points to potential benefits in forms of exercise that require repeated short-term bursts of high-intensity exercise; this has been seen more in artificial laboratory studies, though, than in studies involving athletes during normal sports performance. It might also be helpful for resistance exercise (weight training), although not all studies have found benefit.

Creatine has also been proposed as an aid to

promote weight loss and to reduce the proportion of fat to muscle in the body, but there is little evidence that it is effective for this purpose. Preliminary evidence suggests that creatine supplements may be able to reduce levels of triglycerides in the blood. (Triglycerides are fats related to cholesterol that also increase risk of heart disease when elevated in the body.) Creatine supplements might also help counter the loss of muscle strength that occurs when a limb is immobilized, such as following injury or surgery; however, not all results have been positive.

Studies, including small double-blind trials, inconsistently suggest that creatine might be helpful for reducing fatigue and increasing strength in various illnesses where muscle weakness occurs, including chronic obstructive pulmonary disease (COPD), congestive heart failure, dermatomyositis, Huntington's disease, McArdle's disease, mitochondrial illnesses, muscular dystrophy, and myotonic dystrophy.

One study claimed to find evidence that creatine supplements can reduce levels of blood sugar. However, because dextrose (a form of sugar) was used as the placebo in this trial, the results are somewhat questionable.

Evidence from animal and open human trials suggested that creatine improved strength and slowed the progression of amyotrophic lateral sclerosis (ALS), and for this reason, many people with ALS tried it. However, these hopes were dashed in 2003 when the results of a ten-month double-blind, placebo-controlled trial of 175 people with ALS were announced. Use of creatine at a dose of 10 grams (g) daily failed to provide any benefit in terms of symptoms or disease progression. Negative results were also seen in subsequent, slightly smaller studies. Creatine also does not appear to strengthen muscles in people with wrist weakness due to nerve injury.

Long-term use of corticosteroid drugs can slow a child's growth. One animal study suggests that use of supplemental creatine may help prevent this side effect. Creatine has also shown some promise for improving mental function, particularly after sleep deprivation. However, in one small study, it showed no similar benefit in young adult subjects who were not sleep-deprived.

One study failed to find creatine helpful for maintaining muscle mass during treatment for colon cancer. Another study found little to no benefits in

Parkinson's disease, and another failed to find any benefit in schizophrenia.

Scientific Evidence

Exercise performance. Several small double-blind studies suggest that creatine can improve performance in exercises that involve repeated short bursts of high-intensity activity. For example, a double-blind study investigated creatine and swimming performance in eighteen men and fourteen women. Men taking the supplement had significant increases in speed when doing six bouts of 50-meter swims starting at three-minute intervals, compared with men taking a placebo. However, their speed did not improve when swimming ten sets of 25-yard lengths started at one-minute intervals. It may be that the shorter rest time between laps was not enough for the swimmers' bodies to resynthesize phosphocreatine.

None of the women enrolled in the study showed any improvement with the creatine supplement. The authors of this study noted that women normally have more creatine in their muscle tissue than men do, so perhaps creatine supplementation (at least at this level) is not of benefit to women, as it appears to be for men. Further research is needed to fully understand this gender difference in response to creatine.

In another double-blind study, sixteen physical education students exercised ten times for six seconds on a stationary cycle, alternating with a thirty-second rest period. The results showed that individuals who took 20 g of creatine for six days were better able to maintain cycle speed. Similar results were seen in many other studies of repeated high-intensity exercise, although benefits are generally minimal in studies involving athletes engaged in normal sports rather than contrived laboratory tests. Isometric exercise capacity (pushing against a fixed resistance) also may improve with creatine, according to some studies.

In addition, two double-blind, placebo-controlled studies, each lasting twenty-eight days, provide some evidence that creatine and creatine plus HMB (beta hydroxymethyl butyrate) can increase lean muscle and bone mass. The first study enrolled fifty-two college football players during off-season training, and the other followed forty athletes engaged in weight training.

However, studies of endurance or nonrepeated exercise have not shown benefits. Therefore, creatine probably will not help those running marathons or single sprints.

High triglycerides. A fifty-six-day double-blind, placebo-controlled study of thirty-four men and women found that creatine supplementation can reduce levels of triglycerides in the blood by about 25 percent. Effects on other blood lipids such as total cholesterol were insignificant.

Congestive heart failure. Easy fatigability is one unpleasant symptom of congestive heart failure. Creatine supplementation has been tried as a treatment for this symptom, with some positive results. A double-blind study examined seventeen men with congestive heart failure who were given 20 g of creatine daily for ten days. Exercise capacity and muscle strength increased in the creatine-treated group. Similarly, muscle endurance improved in a double-blind, placebo-controlled crossover study of twenty men with chronic heart failure. Treatment with 20 g of creatine for five days increased the amount of exercise they could complete before they reached exhaustion. These results are promising, but further study is needed.

SAFETY ISSUES

Creatine appears to be relatively safe. No significant side effects have been found with the regimen of several days of a high dosage (15 to 30 g daily) followed by six weeks of a lower dosage (2 to 3 g daily). A study of one hundred football players found no adverse consequences during ten months to five years of creatine supplementation. Contrary to early reports, creatine does not appear to adversely affect the body's ability to exercise under hot conditions and might even be beneficial.

Dividing the dose may help avoid gastrointestinal side effects (diarrhea, stomach upset, and belching). In one study of fifty-nine male soccer players, administering two separate 5 g doses was associated with less diarrhea than a single 10 g dose.

However, there are some potential concerns with creatine. Because it is metabolized by the kidneys, fears have been expressed that creatine supplements could cause kidney injury, and there are two worrisome case reports. However, evidence suggests that creatine is safe for people whose kidneys are healthy to begin with and who do not take excessive doses. Furthermore, a one-year double-blind study of 175 people with amyotrophic lateral sclerosis found that

use of 10 g of creatine daily did not adversely affect kidney function. Nonetheless, prudence suggests that individuals with kidney disease, especially those on dialysis, should avoid creatine supplements.

Another concern is that creatine is metabolized in the body to the toxic substance formaldehyde. However, it is not clear whether the amount of formaldehyde produced in this way will cause any harm. Three deaths have been reported in individuals taking creatine, but other causes were most likely responsible.

It has also been suggested that use of oral creatine would increase urine levels of the carcinogen N-nitrososarcosine, but this does not seem to be the case. A few reports suggest that creatine could, at times, cause heart arrhythmias. As with all supplements taken in very high doses, it is important to purchase a high-quality form of creatine, because contaminants present even in very low concentrations could conceivably build up and cause problems.

EBSCO CAM Review Board

FURTHER READING

Astorino, T. A., et al. "Is Running Performance Enhanced with Creatine Serum Ingestion?" *Journal of Strength Conditioning Research* 19 (2005): 730-734.

Bemben, M. G., et al. "Creatine Supplementation During Resistance Training in College Football Athletes." *Medicine and Science in Sports and Exercise* 33 (2001): 1667-1673.

Chilibeck, P. D., et al. "Effect of Creatine Ingestion After Exercise on Muscle Thickness in Males and Females." *Medicine and Science in Sports and Exercise* 36 (2004): 1781-1788.

Cramer, J. T., et al. "Effects of Creatine Supplementation and Three Days of Resistance Training on Muscle Strength, Power Output, and Neuromuscular Function." *Journal of Strength Conditioning Research* 21 (2007): 668-677.

Deacon, S. J., et al. "Randomized Controlled Trial of Dietary Creatine as an Adjunct Therapy to Physical Training in COPD." *American Journal of Respiratory and Critical Care Medicine* 178 (2008): 133-139.

Eckerson, J. M., et al. "Effect of Creatine Phosphate Supplementation on Anaerobic Working Capacity and Body Weight After Two and Six Days of Loading in Men and Women." *Journal of Strength Conditioning Research* 19 (2005): 756-763.

Kambis, K. W., and S. K. Pizzedaz. "Short-term Creatine

Supplementation Improves Maximum Quadriceps Contraction in Women." *International Journal of Sport Nutrition and Exercise Metabolism* 13 (2003): 97-111.

Pluim, B. M., et al. "The Effects of Creatine Supplementation on Selected Factors of Tennis Specific Training." *British Journal of Sports Medicine* 40 (2006): 507-511.

See also: Citrulline; Herbal medicine; Sports and fitness support: Enhancing performance.

Crohn's disease

CATEGORY: Condition

RELATED TERMS: Granulomatous ileitis, ileocolitis, inflammatory bowel disease, regional enteritis

DEFINITION: Treatment of a bowel disorder.

PRINCIPAL PROPOSED NATURAL TREATMENT: Nutritional support

OTHER PROPOSED NATURAL TREATMENTS: Acupuncture, avoidance of allergenic foods, boswellia, fish oil, glutamine, probiotics, wormwood

INTRODUCTION

Crohn's disease is a disease of the bowel that is closely related to ulcerative colitis. The two are grouped in a category called inflammatory bowel disease (IBD) because they both involve inflammation of the digestive tract.

The major symptoms of Crohn's disease include fever, nonbloody or bloody diarrhea, abdominal pain, and fatigue. The rectum may be severely affected, leading to fissures, abscesses, and fistulas (hollow passages). Intestinal obstruction can occur, and over time fistulas may develop in the small bowel. Other complications include gallstones, increased risk of cancer in the small bowel and colon, and pain in or just below the stomach that mimics the pain of an ulcer. Arthritis, skin sores, and liver problems also may develop.

Crohn's disease tends to wax and wane, with periods of remission punctuated by severe flare-ups. Medical treatment aims at reducing symptoms and inducing and maintaining remission.

Sulfasalazine is one of the most commonly used medications for Crohn's disease. Given either orally

---

Nutritional Deficiencies and Crohn's Disease

Nutritional complications are common in Crohn's disease. Deficiencies of proteins, calories, and vitamins are well documented. These deficiencies may be caused by inadequate dietary intake, intestinal loss of protein, or poor absorption, also referred to as malabsorption.

Treatment for Crohn's disease may include drugs, nutritional supplements, surgery, or a combination of these options. The goals of treatment are to control inflammation, correct nutritional deficiencies, and relieve such symptoms as abdominal pain, diarrhea, and rectal bleeding.

A doctor may recommend nutritional supplements, especially for children whose growth has been slowed. Special high-calorie liquid formulas are sometimes used for this purpose. A small number of patients may need to be fed intravenously for a brief time through a small tube inserted into the vein of the arm. This procedure, an elemental diet, can help patients who need extra nutrition temporarily, those whose intestines need rest, or those whose intestines cannot absorb enough nutrition from food.

---

or as an enema, it can both decrease symptoms and prevent recurrences. Corticosteroids such as prednisone are used similarly, sometimes combined with immunosuppressive drugs such as azathioprine. In severe cases, partial removal of the bowel may be necessary.

Another approach involves putting people with Crohn's disease on an elemental diet. This involves special formulas consisting of required nutrients but no whole foods. After some time on such a diet, whole foods often can be restarted, but only one item at a time.

PRINCIPAL PROPOSED NATURAL TREATMENTS

People with Crohn's disease can easily develop deficiencies in numerous nutrients. Malabsorption, decreased appetite, drug side effects, and increased nutrient loss through the stool may lead to mild or profound deficiencies of protein; vitamins A, B_{12}, C, D, E, and K; folate; calcium; copper; magnesium; selenium; and zinc. Supplementation to restore adequate body supplies of these nutrients is highly advisable and may improve specific symptoms and overall health. It is recommended that one work closely with a physician to identify any nutrient deficiencies and

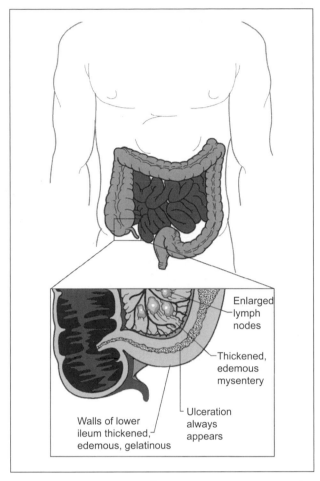

Crohn's disease can cause inflammation and ulceration within any region of the digestive tract, but most often in the ileum.

to evaluate the success of supplementation to correct them.

OTHER PROPOSED NATURAL TREATMENTS

Several natural treatments have shown promise for Crohn's disease, but none have been proven effective. In a ten-week, double-blind, placebo-controlled study, the use of the herb wormwood appeared to successfully enable a reduction of drug dosage in people with Crohn's disease. This German trial enrolled forty people who had achieved good control of their symptoms through the use of steroids and other medications. One-half were given an herbal blend containing wormwood (500 milligrams [mg] three time daily), while the other one-half were given placebo. Beginning at week two, researchers began a gradual tapering

down of the steroid dosage used by participants. Over subsequent weeks, most of those given placebo showed the expected worsening of symptoms that the reduction of drug dosage would be expected to cause. In contrast, most of those receiving wormwood showed a gradual improvement of symptoms. No serious side effects were attributed to wormwood in this study.

Although these findings are promising, many treatments that show promise in a single study fail to hold up in subsequent independent testing. Additional research will be needed to establish wormwood as a helpful treatment for Crohn's disease. In addition, there are concerns that wormwood might have toxic effects in some people.

The herb boswellia is thought to have some anti-inflammatory effects. An eight-week, double-blind, placebo-controlled trial of 102 people with Crohn's disease compared a standardized extract of boswellia with the drug mesalazine. Participants taking boswellia fared at least as well as those taking mesalazine, according to a standard method of scoring Crohn's disease severity.

Fish oil also has anti-inflammatory effects. However, the evidence suggests that it is not helpful for Crohn's disease. A one-year double-blind trial involving seventy-eight participants with Crohn's disease in remission who were at high risk for relapse found that fish oil supplements helped keep the disease from flaring up. A smaller study also found benefit. In contrast, a one-year, double-blind, placebo-controlled trial that followed 120 people with Crohn's disease did not find any reduction of relapse rates. Moreover, two well-designed trials, enrolling 738 persons, convincingly failed to find any benefit for omega-3 fatty acid supplementation in the prevention of Crohn's disease relapse.

One preliminary double-blind study found indications that the probiotic yeast *Saccharomyces boulardii* may be helpful for reducing diarrhea in people with Crohn's disease. However, two studies failed to find diarrhea-reducing benefit with *Lactobacillus* probiotics, and in an analysis of eight randomized, placebo-controlled studies, probiotics were ineffective at maintaining remission in persons with Crohn's disease. Lactobacilli have also failed to prove effective for helping to prevent Crohn's disease recurrences in people who have had surgery for the condition.

Some evidence hints that probiotics might reduce the joint pain that commonly occurs in people with inflammatory bowel disease. Also, glutamine has been suggested as a treatment for Crohn's disease, but the most meaningful of the reported studies on its potential benefits failed to find it helpful. Some evidence hints that acupuncture might be helpful for Crohn's disease. Preliminary investigations hint that food allergies might play a role in Crohn's disease. However, there is no meaningful evidence that avoiding allergenic foods can improve Crohn's symptoms.

HERBS AND SUPPLEMENTS TO USE ONLY WITH CAUTION

Various herbs and supplements may interact adversely with drugs used to treat Crohn's disease.

EBSCO CAM Review Board

FURTHER READING

Bousvaros, A., et al. "A Randomized, Double-Blind Trial of *Lactobacillus* GG Versus Placebo in Addition to Standard Maintenance Therapy for Children with Crohn's Disease." *Inflammatory Bowel Disease* 11 (2005): 833-839.

Feagan, B. G., et al. "Omega-3 Free Fatty Acids for the Maintenance of Remission in Crohn Disease." *Journal of the American Medical Association* 299 (2008): 1690-1697.

Marteau, P., et al. "Ineffectiveness of *Lactobacillus johnsonii* La1 for Prophylaxis of Postoperative Recurrence in Crohn's Disease." *Gut* 55 (2006): 842-847.

Omer, B., et al. "Steroid-Sparing Effect of Wormwood (*Artemisia absinthium*) in Crohn's Disease." *Phytomedicine* 14 (2007): 87-95.

Rahimi, R., et al. "A Meta-analysis on the Efficacy of Probiotics for Maintenance of Remission and Prevention of Clinical and Endoscopic Relapse in Crohn's Disease." *Digestive Diseases and Sciences* 53 (2008): 2524-2531.

Romano, C., et al. "Usefulness of Omega-3 Fatty Acid Supplementation in Addition to Mesalazine in Maintaining Remission in Pediatric Crohn's Disease." *World Journal of Gastroenterology* 11 (2006): 7118-7121.

Van Den Bogaerde, J., et al. "Gut Mucosal Response to Food Antigens in Crohn's Disease." *Alimentary Pharmacology and Therapeutics* 16 (2002): 1903-1915.

See also: Constipation; Diarrhea; Fatigue; Gas, intestinal; Gastritis; Gastrointestinal health; Inflammatory bowel syndrome (IBS); Lactose intolerance; Probiotics; Ulcerative colitis; Wormwood.

Cryotherapy

CATEGORY: Therapies and techniques

RELATED TERMS: Cold therapy, cryoablation, cryosurgery

DEFINITION: The use of extreme cold in medical treatment and surgery.

PRINCIPAL PROPOSED USES: Cancer of the breast, colon, kidney, liver, lung, pancreas, prostate, retina, and skin; cervical dysplasia; inflammation; sprains; warts

OTHER PROPOSED USES: Acne, eye surgery, heart disease, hemorrhoids, Parkinson's disease, spinal cord injuries, tattoo removal

OVERVIEW

Cryotherapy has been used since the time of ancient Egypt to treat external pain and inflammation. In the nineteenth century, freezing was first used to remove external tissue by using ice and salt. With the advent of liquid nitrogen in the early twentieth century, freezing cells became commonplace. Later in the century, with the development of nitrogen and argon gas, scientists were able to develop the medical technology used in what is now known as cryosurgery.

MECHANISM OF ACTION

Applying extreme cold extraneously to inflammation or injuries constricts blood flow and numbs the nerves, reducing pain and swelling. Freezing external skin lesions or cancers kills the tissue and leads to the "shedding" of the skin. Applying extreme cold internally, by using nitrogen or argon gas cryosurgically, kills cells and extracts cancerous tissue from organs.

USES AND APPLICATIONS

Externally, ice packs are commonly used in the treatment of sprains, sports injuries, and general pain and inflammation. In cryosurgery, at −40°Fahrenheit (−40°Celsius) ice crystallizes inside cells, causing them to burst and die. Surgeons use a needle to insert argon or nitrogen gas inside tissue containing precancerous or cancerous cells, freezing the cells and killing them. Dermatologists use freezing to remove warts, skin lesions, and tattoos. Eye surgeons use cryotherapy during cataract and retina surgery to freeze tissue and seal retinal holes. Brain surgeons use cryotherapy to freeze the thalamus and reduce the effects of Parkinson's disease and other brain disorders. Cardiologists use cryotherapy to reduce heart muscle damage in persons who have had a heart attack.

SCIENTIFIC EVIDENCE

In 2009, at the Fifteenth World Congress of the International Society of Cryosurgery, scientific results showed that for persons who were unable to undergo traditional surgery for their cancers because of metastasizing, particularly persons with lung, liver, kidney, prostate, breast, or pancreatic cancer, cryosurgery was highly effective. Cryosurgery, compared with traditional chemotherapy treatments, had an increase of 30 to 50 percent in the partial or complete reduction of tumors.

In a double-blind study in 2005, fourteen youth received dental surgery, in which each had his or her impacted third molar tooth extracted. Some participants were treated with cryotherapy and others not. Those who received cryotherapy treatments reported significantly less pain and swelling in the jaws.

CHOOSING A PRACTITIONER

The American Medical Association recommends that persons choose a qualified, experienced, and licensed physician for all cryosurgery procedures. This doctor should be knowledgeable and accomplished in using state-of-the-art cryotherapy technology.

SAFETY ISSUES

Extreme cold applied to extraneous skin tissue for more than twenty minutes can lead to frostbite. Cryotherapy that is used to treat internal organs rarely results in bleeding, nerve damage, or infection.

Mary E. Markland, M.A.

FURTHER READING

Freiman, Anatoli, and Nathaniel Bouganim. "The History of Cryotherapy." *Dermatology Online Journal* 11, no. 2 (2005). Available at http://dermatology.cdlib.org/112/reviews/hxcryo/freiman.html.

Jackson, Arthur, Graham Colver, and Rodney Dawber. *Cutaneous Cryosurgery: Principles and Clinical Practice.* 3d ed. New York: Taylor & Francis, 2006.

Katz, Aaron, and Philippa Cheetham. *Living a Better Life After Prostate Cancer: A Survivor's Guide to Cryotherapy.* San Diego, Calif.: University Readers, 2009.

Korpin, Nikolai N., ed. *Basics of Cryosurgery.* New York: Springer, 2001.

Sulik, Sandra M., and Cathryn B. Heath. *Primary Care Procedures in Women's Health.* New York: Springer, 2010.

See also: Balneotherapy; Cancer treatment support; Hydrotherapy; Pain management.

Crystal healing

CATEGORY: Therapies and techniques
RELATED TERM: Vibrational medicine
DEFINITION: A therapy that employs crystals to effect or facilitate physical, emotional, and psychospiritual healing.
PRINCIPAL PROPOSED USES: Anxiety, arthritis, back problems, blood pressure, common cold
OTHER PROPOSED USES: Alcoholism, depression, emotional balance, fungal infections, gastritis, kidney function, neuralgia, skin diseases, throat infections, vision problems.

OVERVIEW

Crystals fall into seven structural types, but individual examples range in the thousands, each with its own alleged traditional uses in healing. For example, agate is used for gastritis and skin diseases, chrysoprase is used in the treatment of depression and alcoholism, and jade is used for improving kidney function and emotional balance. These forms are subdivided into more descriptive varieties. In some crystal directories, for instance, agate is divided into blue lace, dendritic, fire, and moss, which may be used, respectively, for throat infections, neuralgia, vision problems, and fungal infections.

The use of crystals to promote healing and wellbeing is attested in many ancient cultures, including Egyptian, Indian, and Native American. Traditional and mythological lore about crystals has continued from the Middle Ages to the present day.

One modern discovery added a scientific veneer to the notion that crystals emit forces. In 1880, brothers Pierre and Jacques Curie found that crystals subjected to mechanical pressure yielded a measurable electrical discharge. This process is called the piezoelectric effect.

MECHANISM OF ACTION

The mechanism of action in crystals varies according

to culture. In Ayurvedic medicine, crystals are said to interact with the energy system of the body, the aura and seven chakras, which are the energy vortices located at different points in the body.

USES AND APPLICATIONS

Crystal healing is said to help alleviate physical, mental, emotional, and spiritual problems.

SCIENTIFIC EVIDENCE

Unsubstantiated scientific explanations often cite the piezoelectric effect as evidence of the positive effects of crystal healing and construct models such as lasers or capacitors (as in the use of quartz to amplify and focus a healer's bioenergy). The absence of a standard transcultural crystal directory that would be recognized by theoreticians and practitioners of crystal healing renders biomedical testing difficult. Remedies vary from directory to directory and depend on cultural context, tradition, and mythology; remedies also depend on the practitioner's own usage or even the intuition of the person seeking help. The notion that agate, because of its layered appearance, is useful in treating organs with different layers of tissue is a type of magical thinking of which the ancient Egyptian physicians would have approved. Also, biomedical explanations would include a placebo effect. Crystal healing may be better accepted by basing itself not on a Western biomechanical paradigm but on an Eastern paradigm of vitalism or energetics.

SAFETY ISSUES

With some exceptions, there exists no obvious risk in wearing or carrying crystals, in temporarily applying a crystal to a person seeking care, in placing crystals around a person in a circular pattern, or in simply placing crystals in view for contemplation. Certain imported gemstones (such as blue topaz, which is sometimes used to treat digestive problems or to stimulate the metabolism) are irradiated to enhance or intensify color. In this case, the blue topaz's radioactivity could be harmful if exposure were repeated or prolonged.

David J. Ladouceur, Ph.D.

FURTHER READING

Gerber, Richard. *Vibrational Medicine: The Number One Handbook of Subtle-Energy Therapies.* 3d ed. Rochester, Vt.: Bear, 2001.
Gienger, Michael. *Crystal Power, Crystal Healing: The Complete Handbook.* Translated by Astrid Mick. London: Cassell, 2009.
Jerome, Lawrence E. *Crystal Power: The Ultimate Placebo Effect.* Buffalo, N.Y.: Prometheus Books, 1989.

See also: Ayurveda; Energy medicine; Folk medicine; Traditional healing.

Cupping

CATEGORY: Therapies and techniques
RELATED TERMS: *Baguanfa*, body vacuuming, *dijiufa*, fire cupping, *hijama*, horn technique, *jiaofa*
DEFINITION: A skin-surface therapy involving cupped vessels under vacuum to suction the skin and relieve local congestion.
PRINCIPAL PROPOSED USES: Abdominal pain, arthritis, asthma, back pain, chronic pain, cough, headache, indigestion, menstrual disturbances, other forms of muscle pain
OTHER PROPOSED USES: Acne, breast enhancement, cellulite, common cold, hypertension, insomnia, paralysis

OVERVIEW

Cupping, typically associated with traditional Chinese medicine, is one of the oldest known therapeutic practices in the world. Cupping involves attaching a hollow cupped vessel to the surface of the skin by heat or air suction. Once a vacuum is created, the underlying tissue is lifted and blood is drawn to the area. The degree of skin discoloration indicates the nature of the congestion. The number, size, type, and movement of the cup and the degree and duration of suction can be varied according to the ailment being treated.

MECHANISM OF ACTION

The exact healing mechanism of cupping is unknown. Cupping is thought to stimulate the body's natural energy to promote healing by reducing stagnant blood, activating the immune system, improving circulation, and helping the body detoxify. Another possible explanation is the placebo effect.

USES AND APPLICATIONS

Cupping therapy is primarily used to relieve pain, gastrointestinal disorders such as abdominal pain and

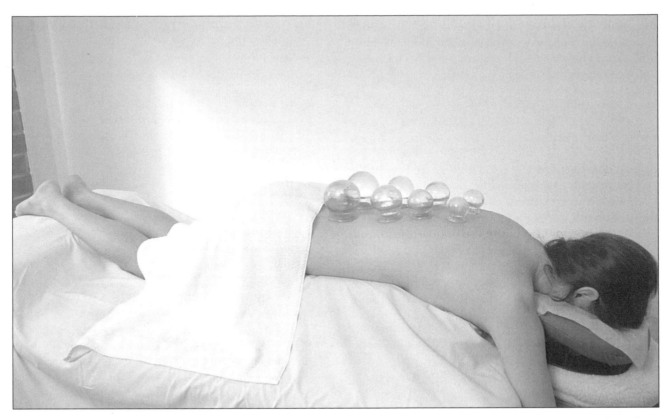

Chinese medicine may employ a technique called cupping, the application to the back of cups that create a vacuum, in order to restore proper circulation. (PhotoDisc)

indigestion, respiratory problems such as chronic cough and asthma, menstrual disturbances, and skin conditions. Cupping is most commonly used in conjunction with acupuncture, acupressure, bleeding treatments, and moxibustion.

SCIENTIFIC EVIDENCE

Cupping has existed for hundreds of years and many researchers have investigated its benefits, but it is a new area of study in Western medicine. Most evidence supporting the use of cupping as a cure for illness is anecdotal.

Various studies have suggested that cupping treatments are effective in temporarily alleviating chronic pain. None, however, were double-blind, placebo-controlled trials, and most proved to be inconclusive because of low enrollment, poor study design, inadequate blinding procedures, and a lack of appropriate scientific control groups. Several studies indicate that cupping treatments combined with other therapies,

such as acupuncture, may improve clinical outcomes, but scientific evidence is limited.

Cupping is an appealing natural treatment option for various illnesses because it is convenient and relatively safe. Some evidence suggests that cupping may be beneficial for various conditions because of its relaxation effect. More rigorous research studies are needed, however, to properly assess the clinical value of cupping in Western medicine.

CHOOSING A PRACTITIONER

Cupping therapy is a relatively unregulated field. Treatments should be performed by skilled practitioners to avoid injury.

SAFETY ISSUES

Cupping therapy, which is considered safe with minimal side effects, may cause marks or bruising. The appearance of blisters, blood spots, or burns indicates an abnormally harsh treatment.

Cupping should be performed only on areas of soft muscle tissue. It should not be performed on persons with skin ulcers, high fever, convulsions, cramps, bleeding disorders, or cardiovascular disease, or on women who are pregnant.

Rose Ciulla-Bohling, Ph.D.

FURTHER READING

Chirali, Ilkay Z. *Traditional Chinese Medicine: Cupping Therapy.* 2d ed. New York: Churchill Livingstone/Elsevier, 2007.

Dharmananda, Subhuti. "Cupping." Institute for Traditional Medicine. Available at http://www.itmonline.org/arts/cupping.htm.

Pringle, Michael. "Some Thoughts on Fire Cupping." *Journal of Chinese Medicine* 83 (2007): 46-51.

Shixi, Huang, and Cao Yu. "Cupping Therapy." *Journal of Chinese Medicine* 82 (2006): 52-57.

See also: Chinese medicine; Folk medicine; Pain management; Soft tissue pain; Traditional Chinese herbal medicine; Traditional healing.

Cyclosporine

TRADE NAMES: Neoral, Sandimmune
CATEGORY: Drug interactions
DEFINITION: Helps prevent rejection of a transplanted organ by suppressing the immune system.
INTERACTIONS: Berberine (found in goldenseal, Oregon grape, and barberry), citrus aurantium, grapefruit juice, ipriflavone, peppermint oil, St. John's wort, *Scutellaria baicalensis*

GRAPEFRUIT JUICE

Effect: Possible Harmful Interaction

Grapefruit juice slows the body's normal breakdown of several drugs, including cyclosporine, allowing it to build up to potentially excessive levels in the blood. A study indicates this effect can last for three days or more following the last glass of juice. If one takes cyclosporine, the safest approach is to avoid grapefruit juice altogether.

CITRUS AURANTIUM

Effect: Possible Harmful Interaction

Like grapefruit juice, bitter orange (citrus auran-

tium) may raise levels of cyclosporine. If one takes cyclosporine, the safest approach is to avoid citrus aurantium altogether.

BERBERINE

Effect: Possible Harmful Interaction

The substance berberine, found in goldenseal, Oregon grape, and barberry, may increase levels of cyclosporine.

ST. JOHN'S WORT

Effect: Possible Harmful Interaction

The herb St. John's wort (*Hypericum perforatum*) is primarily used to treat mild to moderate depression. St. John's wort has the potential to accelerate the body's normal breakdown of certain drugs, including cyclosporine, resulting in lower blood levels of these drugs.

This interaction appears to have occurred in two heart transplant patients taking cyclosporine, leading to heart transplant rejection. These persons had been doing well after transplantation while taking standard immunosuppressive therapy that included cyclosporine. After starting St. John's wort for depression, however, they began experiencing problems and their blood levels of cyclosporine were found to have dipped below the therapeutic range. After St. John's wort was discontinued, cyclosporine levels returned to normal and no further episodes of rejection occurred.

Numerous cases of transplant rejection episodes involving the heart, kidney, and liver have also been reported in people using the herb. Based on this evidence, if one is taking cyclosporine, one should not take St. John's wort.

IPRIFLAVONE

Effect: Possible Harmful Interaction

The supplement ipriflavone is used to treat osteoporosis. A three-year, double-blind trial of almost five hundred women, as well as a small study, found worrisome evidence that ipriflavone can reduce white blood cell count in some people. For this reason, anyone taking medications that suppress the immune system should avoid taking ipriflavone.

PEPPERMINT

Effect: Possible Harmful Interaction

An animal study indicates that use of peppermint oil may increase cyclosporine levels in the body. If one is taking cyclosporine and wishes to use peppermint oil as well, notify a physician in advance, so that blood levels of cyclosporine can be monitored and the dose adjusted if necessary. If one is already taking both peppermint oil and cyclosporine and stops taking the peppermint, the body's cyclosporine levels may fall. Again, consult a physician to make the necessary dosage adjustment.

SCUTELLARIA BAICALENSIS

Effect: Possible Harmful Interaction

The herb *Scutellaria baicalensis* (Chinese skullcap) may impair absorption of cyclosporine, according to a study in animals.

EBSCO CAM Review Board

FURTHER READING

Alexandersen, P., et al. "Ipriflavone in the Treatment of Postmenopausal Osteoporosis." *Journal of the American Medical Association* 285 (2001): 1482-1488.

Barone, G. W., et al. "Drug Interaction Between St. John's Wort and Cyclosporine." *Annals of Pharmacotherapy* 34 (2000): 1013-1016.

Breidenbach, T., et al. "Drug Interaction of St. John's Wort with Cyclosporin." *The Lancet* 355 (2000): 1912.

Ernst, E. "Second Thoughts About Safety of St. John's Wort." *The Lancet* 354 (1999): 2014-2016.

Malhotra, S., et al. "Seville Orange Juice-Felodipine Interaction: Comparison with Dilute Grapefruit Juice and Involvement of Furocoumarins." *Clinical Pharmacology and Therapeutics* 69 (2001): 14-23.

Ruschitzka, F., et al. "Acute Heart Transplant Rejection Due to Saint John's Wort." *The Lancet* 355 (2000): 548-549.

Takanaga, H., et al. "Relationship Between Time After Intake of Grapefruit Juice and the Effect on Pharmacokinetics and Pharmacodynamics of Nisoldipine in Healthy Subjects." *Clinical Pharmacology and Therapeutics* 67 (2000): 201-214.

Wu, X., et al. "Effects of Berberine on the Blood Concentration of Cyclosporin in Renal Transplanted Recipients: Clinical and Pharmacokinetic Study." *European Journal of Clinical Pharmacology* 8 (2005): 567-572.

See also: Barberry; Citrus aurantium; Food and Drug Administration; Goldenseal; Oregon grape; Ipriflavone; Peppermint; St. John's wort; Supplements: Introduction.

Cystoseira canariensis

CATEGORY: Herbs and supplements
RELATED TERM: Brown seaweed
DEFINITION: Natural plant product used to treat specific health conditions.
PRINCIPAL PROPOSED USE: Sports and fitness performance enhancement

OVERVIEW

Because of the high emotional stakes involved in both amateur and professional sports, pharmaceutical and supplement manufacturers continually seek to find products that might add a competitive edge. Findings from test-tube studies suggested that an extract of the brown seaweed *Cystoseira canariensis* might inhibit a substance in the body called myostatin.

THERAPEUTIC DOSAGES

A typical dose of cystoseira is 1,200 milligrams (mg) per day, often divided into three doses.

THERAPEUTIC USES

Myostatin inhibits the growth of muscle cells. It is believed that some animals, and some people, produce relatively less myostatin and therefore develop stronger muscles even without much exercise. Consider chimpanzees that live in a cage but are nonetheless much stronger than similarly sized humans. If a substance could be discovered that effectively blocks the action of myostatin, that substance might logically be hypothesized to aid muscle growth. Therefore, based on findings that can only be characterized as far too preliminary to rely upon, cystoseira became a widely marketed sports supplement.

SCIENTIFIC EVIDENCE

Despite the foregoing test-tube findings, it is a very long way from test tube evidence to real benefits. The vast majority of effects seen in the test tube do not ultimately translate into an effective treatment. To truly determine whether a treatment works, it must undergo human trials, specifically, one type of trial: the double-blind, placebo-controlled study. Only one such study has been performed on cystoseira, and it failed to find any benefits.

In this twelve-week double-blind study, twenty-two males were randomly assigned to receive either a placebo or 1,200 mg per day of cystoseira. Both groups underwent intensive resistance training (weight lifting) for the duration of the trial. The results showed no difference in outcome between the treatment and the placebo groups. Although a single study cannot prove lack of efficacy, this outcome does clearly demonstrate that cystoseira has been brought to market prematurely.

SAFETY ISSUES

Cystoseira is thought to be a safe, foodlike substance. No serious adverse effects were seen in the human study described above. However, comprehensive safety testing has not been performed. Maximum safe doses in pregnant or nursing women, young children, and people with liver or kidney disease have not been determined.

EBSCO CAM Review Board

FURTHER READING

Ramazanov, Z., M. Jimenez del Rio, and T. Ziegenfuss. "Sulfated Polysaccharides of Brown Seaweed *Cystoseira canariensis* Bind to Serum Myostatin Protein." *Acta Physiologica et Pharmacologica Bulgarica* 27 (2003): 101-106.

Willoughby, D. S. "Effects of an Alleged Myostatin-Binding Supplement and Heavy Resistance Training on Serum Myostatin, Muscle Strength and Mass, and Body Composition." *International Journal of Sport Nutrition and Exercise Metabolism* 14 (2004): 461-472.

See also: Herbal medicine; Sports and fitness support: Enhancing performance.